Atlas of Clinical Positron Emission Tomography

Michael N. Maisey MD FRCP FRCR

Department of Radiological Sciences, Guy's, King's and St Thomas' School of Medicine, London

Richard L. Wahl MD FACNP

Division of Nuclear Medicine, University of Michigan Medical Center, Ann Arbor, Michigan

Sally F. Barrington MSc(Dist) MRCP

Clinical PET Centre, Guy's and St Thomas' Hospitals, London

ARNOLD

A member of the Hodder Headline Group
LONDON • SYDNEY • AUCKLAND
Co-published in the USA by Oxford University Press, Inc., New York

First published in Great Britain in 1999 by
Arnold, a member of the Hodder Headline Group,
338 Euston Road, London NW1 3BH

http://www.arnoldpublishers.com

Co-published in the USA by
Oxford University Press Inc.,
198 Madison Avenue, New York, NY10016
Oxford is a registered trademark of Oxford University Press

Whilst the advice and information in this book are believed to be true and accurate at the date of going to press, neither the authors nor the publisher can accept any legal responsibility or liability for any errors or omissions that may be made. In particular (but without limiting the generality of the preceding disclaimer) every effort has been made to check drug dosages; however, it is still possible that errors have been missed. Furthermore, dosage schedules are constantly being revised and new side-effects recognized. For these reasons the reader is strongly urged to consult the drug companies' printed instructions before administering any of the drugs recommended in this book.

British Library Cataloguing in Publication Data
A catalogue record for this book is available from the British Library

Library of Congress Cataloging-in-Publication Data
A catalog record for this book is available from the Library of Congress

ISBN 0 340 74098 1

1 2 3 4 5 6 7 8 9 10

Commissioning Editor: Nick Dunton
Production Editor: Julie Delf
Production Controller: Sarah Kett

Typeset in Hong Kong by Best-set Typesetter Ltd
Printed and bound in China

What do you think about this book? Or any other Arnold title?
Please send your comments to feedback.arnold@hodder.co.uk

Atlas of Clinical Positron Emission Tomography

Contents

Contributors

Sally F. Barrington MSc(Dist) MRCP   Lecturer/Senior Clinical Fellow and Honorary Consultant in Nuclear Medicine, Guy's and St Thomas' Hospitals, London, UK

Gary J.R. Cook MSc MRCP FRCR   Lecturer/Senior Clinical Fellow and Honorary Consultant in Nuclear Medicine, Guy's and St Thomas' Hospitals, London, UK

Michael N. Maisey MD FRCP FRCR   Professor, Department of Radiological Sciences, Guy's, King's and St Thomas' School of Medicine, London, UK

P.K. Marsden PhD   Senior Lecturer in Radiological Sciences, Clinical PET Centre, Guy's, King's and St Thomas' School of Medicine, London, UK

Julie L. Sutcliffe BSc MSc   Lecturer in Radiological Sciences, Clinical PET Centre, Guy's and St Thomas' School of Medicine, London, UK

Richard L. Wahl MD   Professor of Internal Medicine and Radiology, Division of Nuclear Medicine, University of Michigan Medical Center, Ann Arbor, Michigan, USA

Preface

Clinical positron emission tomography (PET) is a rapidly emerging clinical imaging technique. The reasons for the emergence of PET as a clinical tool include improvements in computers and scanners; in particular the ability to perform whole-body scans for cancer staging. Other significant developments include the simplification of hospital based cyclotrons which can be run cost-effectively and reliably in a hospital to support a routine clinical service. Over the last 5 years or so, clinical PET studies have demonstrated significant benefits in patient management, particularly in oncology but also in cardiology, neurology and psychiatry. As with any other new diagnostic modality, there has been a considerable learning period before it could be used with confidence for patient management. This is equally true for PET as for any other imaging technique, even for physicians and radiologists experienced in reporting nuclear medicine procedures.

This atlas attempts to distil more than 5 years' experience of clinical PET imaging in an effort to assist departments setting up clinical PET, shorten the inevitable learning curve and indicate to clinicians the role of PET in improving patient care. Technical aspects of imaging and the scientific bases have been limited to a single introductory chapter, as the intention is to concentrate on the clinical issues.

We have chosen cases to illustrate how clinical PET imaging is being used to improve patient care by influencing management and outcome. Each case presented illustrates an important application, and each example is a real patient seen in one of our departments over the last 5–7 years. Where appropriate we have included the results of other imaging methods, but we have limited this in order to include as many PET images as possible. Generally we have used black and white illustrations because we believe that this is usually the most appropriate way to view and report PET scans.

In each chapter we have provided some clinical background in the introduction, including a section on epidemiology, pathology and, in the case of cancer, the staging methods. A brief review of the important papers in the literature which will provide the basis for further reading has been included. We have then identified the key management issues where PET can play a significant role. For each of these key management issues we have selected cases in which PET scans have been useful. Where appropriate, specific 'teaching points' likely to be of particular importance to students are highlighted (on a green background).

We have attempted to summarize the present situation by tabulating what we consider to be the current clinical indications for a PET scan in each area of application, and where appropriate we have included a suggested algorithm incorporating PET scanning. We have also listed the indications which, although not yet always based on extensive evidence, we believe are likely to become important in the future.

Most of this atlas is devoted to oncology. This is because in most centres practising clinical PET, oncology forms over half of the workload. The cancers discussed in most detail are those with the most published data on clinical accuracy and benefit. We have, however, included a chapter briefly describing other cancers where there are emerging applications which we believe will be important as more experience is obtained.

MNM
RLW
SFB   London and Ann Arbor, January 1999

Acknowledgements

Of all the clinical imaging methods, PET is the most multidisciplinary. Without a good team working closely together it is almost impossible to provide a successful service to patients. We would therefore like to acknowledge that without the contribution of everyone working in the Guy's and St Thomas' Clinical PET Centre and the University of Michigan PET Center this atlas would not have been possible. We would also like to acknowledge the help of Marion Blagg for typing the text and Kathleen Curran for assistance in preparation of the images. Our thanks must also go to the following colleagues:

Paul Marsden PhD, for writing the first chapter of the book on Principles and Methods.

Paul Shreve MD, for contributions of clinical case material to this text and to the development of clinical PET at the University of Michigan. His contributions included, but were not limited to, the sections on prostate cancer imaging, pancreatic cancer imaging, and the images using dual head coincidence detection.

Kirk Frey MD PhD, for his contributions of case material to the section on brain PET and for his efforts in attempting to teach RLW something of neuroscience.

Markus Schwaiger and his former fellows at the University of Michigan, for several key cardiac PET images used in the text and for his efforts to teach RLW something of cardiac PET imaging.

Betty Recker MS, for her major contributions in recruiting patients to be part of the PET imaging studies performed at the University of Michigan.

Susan J. Fisher BS, for contributions to the preclinical development of PET in cancer.

Kenneth R. Zasadny PhD, for his contributions to quantitation of PET.

Chuck Meyer PhD and colleagues in the University of Michigan Radiology Digital Image Processing Laboratory, for fusing PET images with CT and MRI.

Raya S. Brown PhD and Anaira Clavo PhD, for their major contributions to understanding, on a biological basis, the images we see on PET.

Dr David Hawkes and the Computational Imaging Science Division, for developing the co-registration methods; particularly Colin Studholme, for allowing us to use his automatic registration algorithms.

Michael Marber MD, for contributing explanatory diagrams in the cardiac section and helping us to understand cardiac physiology in hibernation.

Adam Steinmetz MD, for his work in providing the brain registered anatomy material and for developing FDG cardiac gating.

Barry Shulkin MD, Associate Professor of Internal Medicine and Director of Pediatric Nuclear Medicine, is thanked for providing images of neuroendocrine tumours and pheochromocytoma.

Thanks also to the many clinicians who have supported our efforts to establish clinical PET in our institutions, in particular Adrian Timothy, Jules Dussek, Mark McGurk, Elfy Chevretton, Michael Webb Peploe and Mike Smith who were particularly encouraging in the early stages.

Guy's and St Thomas' Clinical PET Centre

- Physicians: Professor M.N. Maisey, Dr M.J. O'Doherty, Professor I. Fogelman, Dr T.O. Nunan, Dr S.E.M. Clarke, Dr S.F. Barrington, Dr G.J.R. Cook, Dr J.B. Bingham
- Physicists and computer scientists: Dr P.K. Marsden, Mr R. Badawi, Dr M. Lodge, Mr E.J.R. Somer
- Radiochemistry: J. Sutcliffe, M. Jacobson, G. Brockman
- Cyclotron: P. Halstead, R. Snow, M. Kelly, I. Miller
- Clinical manager: M. Dakin
- Radiographers: B. Cronin, D. Ellwood, A. Dynes, D. Pritchard, N. Benetar
- Secretary: M. Finneran

University of Michigan PET Center

- Physicians: Professor R.L. Wahl, Dr K. Frey, Dr P. Shreve, Dr Barry Shulkin, Professor M. Schwaiger, Dr S. Minoshima, Professor D.E. Kuhl
- Physics and computer: Dr R. Koeppe, Dr K. Zasadny, Dr C. Meyer
- Radiochemistry: Dr M. Kilbourn, L. Tluczek, Dr D. Jewitt
- Technicians: J. Rothley, A. Weeden, P. Kison, T. Hauser
- Cyclotron: J. Moskwa, J. Viola
- Secretary: D. Murphy

The Guy's and St Thomas' Clinical PET Centre owes a great deal to Professor Sir Cyril Chantler, Principal of UMDS for unwavering support, to Lord Whitelaw for chairing the fundraising appeal, to the Trustees of St Thomas' and Guy's Hospitals for their support and Dr Desmond Croft for early efforts to make it happen. Thanks are also given to Professor Emeritus William H. Beierwaltes, Professor Bernard Agranoff and Professor Sid Gilman, who were instrumental in the establishment of the PET Center at the University of Michigan. Professor David Kuhl is thanked for his original efforts in developing tomographic imaging, and for bringing whole body PET to the University of Michigan. We hope that this atlas goes some way to justifying their confidence in PET and us.

Abbreviations

AIB	aminoisobutyric acid
ACC	American College of Cardiology
ACPC	aminocyclopentanecarboxylic acid
AIF	arterial input function
BGO	bismuth germanate
CAD	coronary artery disease
CEA	carcinoembryonic antigen
CNS	central nervous system
CT	computed tomography
DICOM	digital imaging and communications in medicine
DMSA	Dimercaptosuccinic acid
EBV	Epstein–Barr virus
EDE	effective dose equivalent
EDTA	ethylene diamine tetraacetic acid
EEG	electroencephalography
ELND	elective lymph node dissection
FAP	familial adenomatous polyposis
FDG	$[^{18}F]$2-fluoro-2-deoxy-D-glucose
FES	$[^{18}F]$17-β-oestradiol
FU	$[^{18}F]$uracil
FWHM	full width half maximum
HD	Hodgkin's disease
HED	hydroxyephedrine
HMPAO	hexamethylpropyleneamine-oxime
HNPCC	hereditary non-polyposis colorectal cancer
HPLC	high performance liquid chromatography
LAD	left anterior descending artery
LAL	limulus amebocyte lysate
LSO	lutetium oxyorthosilicate
MAO-B	monoamineoxidase-B
MIBG	*meta*-iodobenzylguanidine
MRI	magnetic resonance imaging
MRS	magnetic resonance spectroscopy
NHL	non-Hodgkin's lymphoma
NIH	National Institute of Health
NSCLC	non-small cell lung cancer
OPCA	olivopontocerebellar atrophy
OSEM	ordered subsets estimation maximization
PACS	picture archiving and communications system
PET	positron emission tomography
PM	photomultiplier tubes
PSA	Prostate specific antigen
PTH	parathyroid hormone
PTSM	pyruvaldehyde bis(*N*-4-methylthiosemicarbazone)
PUO	pyrexia of unknown origin

ROI	region of interest
SCC	squamous cell carcinoma
SCLC	small cell lung cancer
sestamibi	^{99m}Tc-labelled methoxymethylpropyl isonitrile
SOL	space-occupying lesion
SPECT	single photon emission computed tomography
SPM	statistical parametric map
SPN	solitary pulmonary nodule
SUV	standardized uptake value
TSH	thyroid stimulating hormone

Part I
Introduction

Chapter 1

Principles and Methods

P.K. Marsden

Positron emission tomography

Until recently, PET has developed largely independently of mainstream nuclear medicine. This distinction is becoming less clear with the advent of clinical PET, but there are still two fundamental features that distinguish PET from conventional radionuclide imaging techniques:
- the radiotracers that are utilized in PET
- the process whereby data is acquired and reconstructed into an image.

PET tracers

The majority of PET tracers are labelled with the biogenic radionuclides ^{15}O, ^{13}N, ^{11}C and ^{18}F. These all have half-lives ($T_{1/2}$) of less than 2 h, and can be incorporated into a large number of biological compounds to create tracer molecules for studying normal and pathophysiological processes. The most important of these tracers is the ^{18}F labelled glucose analogue [^{18}F]2-fluoro-2-deoxy-D-glucose (FDG), which is used to estimate the rate of glucose utilization. The four standard positron emitting radionuclides all require a cyclotron for their production, and their short half-lives dictate that patient scanning must be carried out fairly close to the cyclotron.

The positron emission tomography process

The radionuclides used in PET decay by the emission of a **positron** which behaves in a similar way to an electron but has a positive charge. At the end of its range, which is about 1 mm in tissue, the positron undergoes mutual annihilation with an electron, resulting in the production of two 511 keV γ rays which are emitted at 180° to each other. These γ rays are detected almost simultaneously (or 'in coincidence') by a PET scanner, and an image of the original radionuclide distribution can be reconstructed without the need for a collimator. The combination of high sensitivity, resulting from the absence of collimators, and the ability to perform an accurate correction for photon attenuation, results in the production of images of higher quality and quantitative accuracy than those that can be obtained using single photon emitters.

Components of a PET facility

The scanner itself is only one of several components that are required in order to perform PET scanning, as shown in Figure 1.1.

Cyclotron

^{15}O, ^{13}N, ^{11}C and ^{18}F are all produced by nuclear bombardment in a **cyclotron** (although there are some generator-produced PET radionuclides, notably ^{82}Rb). Cyclotrons are manufactured specifically for PET applications, and may be either self-shielded or situated in a shielded room.

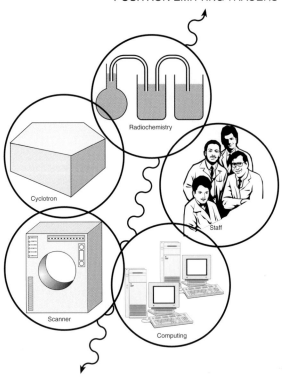

POSITRON EMITTING TRACERS

Radiochemistry

Cyclotron

Staff

Scanner

Computing

POSITRON EMISSION TOMOGRAPHY

Figure 1.1 *The components of PET.*

Radiochemistry laboratory

A radiochemistry laboratory is required for synthesis of the radiotracer, and to perform the appropriate quality control and quality assurance procedures. Automated systems are available for synthesis of the most common tracers, such as FDG and [^{13}N]ammonia, but procedures for synthesizing less common compounds, such as [^{11}C]L-methionine, must often be developed in house.

PET scanner

Current dedicated PET scanners are high performance multi-slice devices usually employing discrete **bismuth germanate (BGO)** scintillation crystals. There is, however, a wide range of scanner configurations including modified single photon emission computed tomography (SPECT) systems capable of performing both PET and SPECT.

Data processing

The data processing requirements for PET are very high. Although initial image reconstruction is performed by a processor incorporated into the scanner itself, a comprehensive network of computer workstations is required for offline processing, reporting and data archiving.

Staff

A fairly large number of staff, including cyclotron technicians, radiochemists, radiographers and medical physics and computing staff, as well as nuclear medicine physicians, are associated with most PET installations. However, as protocols become standardized and PET technology becomes more user-friendly, it is becoming feasible to perform clinical PET studies with a staff contingent similar to that of a conventional nuclear medicine department.

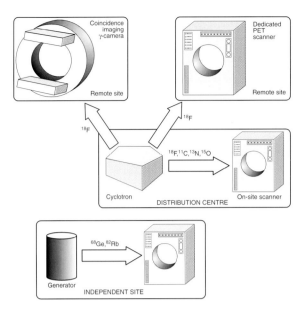

Figure 1.2 *PET tracer distribution options. Very short-lived tracers can only be used near to the cyclotron, but ^{18}F labelled tracers can be transported to remote sites.*

Distribution of PET tracers

For the short lived radionuclides ^{15}O ($T_{1/2} = 2.07\,min$), ^{13}N ($T_{1/2} = 9.96\,min$), and ^{11}C ($T_{1/2} = 20.4\,min$), the scanner must be sited close to the cyclotron. In practice, this distance may be up to several hundred metres if, for example, a pneumatic transport system is used. The most widely used clinical PET tracer, FDG, has a half-life of 109.8 min and transportation over much longer distances (up to several hours' travelling time) is feasible. This gives rise to the concept of a radiotracer distribution facility (Figure 1.2) which supplies FDG once or twice daily to regional centres, each equipped only with a PET scanner or other PET imaging device. The distribution facility may be attached to an active PET centre or may be set up solely for the purpose of exporting tracers to other centres.

Production of PET radiopharmaceuticals

Positron emitting radionuclides

The positron emitting radionuclides relevant to clinical imaging are all proton rich nuclei with relatively short half-lives. Positrons from a given radionuclide are emitted over a continuous range of energies, but can be characterized by a maximum energy (E_{max}). Table 1.1 lists the properties and means of production for the radionuclides most commonly used in clinical PET studies.

The cyclotron

Commercial cyclotrons specifically designed for the production of PET radionuclides are available. A schematic diagram of a negative ion PET cyclotron is shown in Figure 1.3(a). The cyclotron consists of two **dee electrodes**, which are about 1 m in diameter. Negative ions (usually H^-, i.e. a proton and two electrons) are produced from an ion source at the centre of the dees, and an alternating voltage is applied so that the ions move back and forth from one dee to the other. A strong magnetic field (1–2 T) applied at right angles to the plane of the dees constrains the path of the ions to a circular orbit, which increases in diameter as the ions pick up energy from the electric field. On passing through a thin carbon stripping foil inserted into the beam at the edge of the dees, two electrons are stripped from each H^- ion. The resulting H^+ ions move out of the beam under the influence of the

Table 1.1 Positron emitting radionuclides and their means of production

Radio-nuclide	Half-life	E_{max} (MeV)	Production reaction	Target	Product
^{11}C	20.4 min	0.96	$^{14}_{7}N(p,\alpha)^{11}_{6}C$	$^{nat}N_2$ gas	$^{11}CO_2$ gas
^{13}N	9.96 min	1.19	$^{16}_{8}O(p,\alpha)^{13}_{7}N$	^{nat}O water	$^{13}NH_4^+$ ion
^{15}O	2.07 min	1.72	$^{15}_{7}N(p,n)^{15}_{8}O$	$^{15}N_2$ gas	$^{15}O_2$ gas
			$^{14}_{7}N(d,n)^{15}_{8}O$	$^{nat}N_2$ gas	$^{15}O_2$ gas
^{18}F	109.8 min	0.635	$^{18}_{8}O(p,n)^{18}_{9}F$	^{18}O water	$^{18}F^-$ ion
			$^{20}_{10}Ne(d,\alpha)^{18}_{9}F$	^{nat}Ne gas	$^{18}F–F_2$ gas
^{68}Ga	68 min	1.9	$^{68}Ge \rightarrow {}^{68}Ga$	(generator)	Ga metal
^{82}Rb	75 s	3.36	$^{82}Sr \rightarrow {}^{82}Rb$	(generator)	RbCl

a

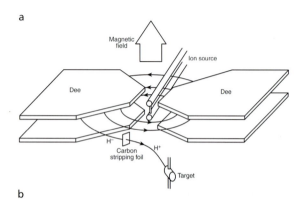

b

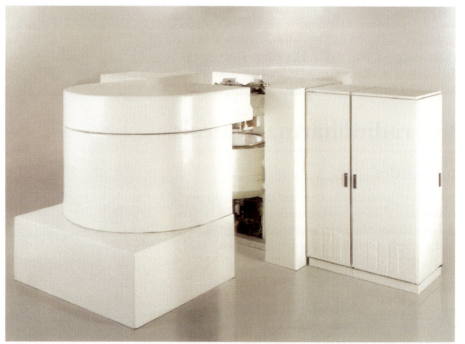

Figure 1.3 *(a) Schematic diagram of a negative ion cyclotron. (b) A modern dedicated PET cyclotron (photograph courtesy of CTI, Inc.).*

magnetic field and are directed on to the target where they undergo a nuclear reaction with the target material. Older cyclotrons accelerate positive ions directly, and the beam has to be extracted electrostatically, which results in dispersion of the beam and the creation of relatively long lived radioactive activation of the components of the cyclotron. Modern negative ion cyclotrons can be opened for maintenance within several hours of bombardment. Another advantage of the negative ion design is that several targets can be bombarded to produce two radionuclides simultaneously. Cyclotrons can either be self shielded, or housed in a concrete vault, which allows easier access for maintenance.

Cyclotrons designed for PET are usually limited to relatively low energies, and hence also limited in the range of nuclear reactions they can induce. A maximum energy of 11 MeV is sufficient to obtain adequate yields of ^{11}C, ^{13}N, ^{15}O and ^{18}F by proton bombardment. Lower energy (3–4 MeV) cyclotrons, presently aimed primarily at the production of ^{15}O, are available, and the range of radionuclides that can be produced by these, and also by small dedicated linear accelerators, is likely to increase.

Target chemistry and tracer synthesis

The yield of the required radionuclide from the cyclotron target depends on many factors relating both to the bombardment process and to the target chemistry, both of which also determine the initial chemical form of the radionuclide. Target materials and the chemical form of the products are given in Table 1.1. The chemical form of the radionuclide will determine what radiopharmaceuticals can be labelled with it. For example, $^{18}F^-$ produced from the $^{18}_{8}O(p,n)^{18}_{9}F$ reaction on an ^{18}O water target can be used to produce FDG via nucleophilic substitution; however, it is very difficult to label fluorodopa with ^{18}F in this form. Fluorodopa is more readily labelled with $^{18}F_2$ obtained from the $^{20}_{10}Ne(d,\alpha)^{18}_{9}F$ reaction. In many cases the target product is converted into a reactive intermediate, which is subsequently reacted with a stable precursor to obtain the final radiopharmaceutical. For example, [^{11}C]methyl iodide can be used to incorporate ^{11}C labelled methyl groups into many complex organic molecules, and this route is used routinely for the production of [^{11}C]L-methionine. The final stage of production usually involves the separation of the radioactive product from non-radioactive by-products using **high performance liquid chromatography (HPLC)** or other standard separation techniques.

All processes must be performed under the constraints imposed by the short half-life of the radionuclide, the large amounts of radioactivity and the very small (picomolar) quantities of material involved. Consequently a great deal of effort has gone into automating the syntheses, and commercial systems are available for the synthesis of the common PET radiopharmaceuticals (see Figure 1.4). More complex systems permit semi-automated production of ^{11}C labelled compounds.

Generator produced radionuclides

^{82}Rb and ^{68}Ga can both be produced from generator systems. ^{82}Rb has a very short half-life (75 s) and results from the decay of ^{82}Sr ($T_{1/2} = 25$ days). ^{82}Sr is loaded on to a stannic oxide column and ^{82}Rb is eluted with saline. ^{82}Rb is used directly to measure myocardial perfusion using a continuous infusion system that allows elution of the generator directly into an intravenous catheter. ^{68}Ga, resulting from the decay of ^{68}Ge ($T_{1/2} = 280$ days), is obtained either in the form of ^{68}Ga-EDTA or more recently in ionic form by eluting a tin dioxide column with 1 M HCl.

Quality control and quality assurance

Quality control is critical in the routine production of PET radiopharmaceuticals as, unlike conventional nuclear medicine tracers, products are synthesized daily and procedures are often specific to the centre using them.

Chemical purity is defined as the fraction of tracer in the formulated radiopharmaceutical that is in the desired molecular form. A test is performed, using HPLC with ultraviolet or conductivity detection, to ensure that no compounds are present in sufficient

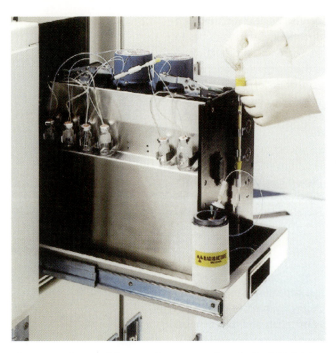

Figure 1.4 *Commercial system for automated synthesis of FDG (photograph courtesy of CTI, Inc.).*

quantities to cause toxicity or to be pharmacologically active. Such compounds will normally all be removed during tracer preparation with preparative HPLC or another separation procedure.

- **Radiochemical purity** is defined as the fraction of the specified radionuclide present in the desired chemical form and in the specified molecular position. It is usually determined using HPLC with radiation detection. Radiochemical impurities can originate from radionuclide production, side reactions or incomplete removal of protecting groups, for example.

- **Radionuclidic purity** is defined as the fraction of total radioactivity present as the specified radionuclide, and is determined either by measurements of energy spectra and physical half-life, or indirectly using HPLC and gas chromatography techniques. In cases where the half-life of radionuclidic impurities is much shorter than that of the desired radionuclide, the purity can be improved by simply letting the impurities decay, e.g. in the case of ^{13}N and ^{15}O impurities which are often present when ^{18}F is produced via the $^{18}_{8}O(p,n)^{18}_{9}F$ reaction.

Microbiological testing

It must also be verified that radiopharmaceuticals are sterile and free from pyrogens. Tests for sterility and pyrogens are too time consuming to be performed before patient administration, but the **limulus amebocyte lysate (LAL)** test is a less general test for pyrogenicity which can be performed in about an hour and is used to test multidose vial preparations of FDG.

Physical principles of PET imaging

Annihilation coincidence detection

The average range of a positron (β^+) in soft tissue is only a few millimetres (e.g. ~0.6 mm for ^{18}F). At the end of its range, a positron combines with an electron (β^-) and undergoes an annihilation reaction in which the mass of the electron and the positron is converted

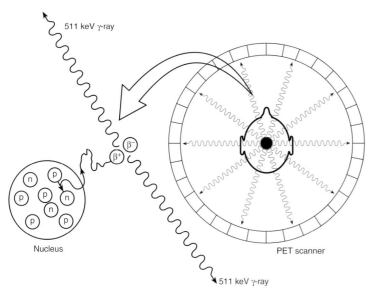

Figure 1.5 *The principle of annihilation coincidence detection. β-decay of a proton rich nucleus results in the conversion of a proton (p) into a neutron (n), and the emission of a positron (β⁺) from the nucleus. The positron follows a convoluted path, with a range of ~1 mm, before interacting with an electron (β⁻) to produce two 511 keV annihilation γ-rays. Detectors on opposite sides of the scanner register the annihilation γ-rays simultaneously or 'in coincidence'.*

into energy in the form of two 511 keV γ rays, which are emitted at (almost) 180° to each other (Figure 1.5). If both γ rays are detected within a certain time of one another (i.e. within a **coincidence time window**), then it is assumed that they both originated from the same annihilation event, and that the original disintegration occurred along a line joining the two detection positions. This is known as **annihilation coincidence detection**. A PET scanner consists of a ring of scintillation detectors, arranged so that pairs of detectors on opposite sides of the ring operate in coincidence with one another, and data acquired in this manner, without a collimator, can be reconstructed into an image using standard algorithms. The lack of a collimator, and the uniform response that is a feature of PET imaging, result in images of higher quality than can be obtained with single photon techniques (i.e. SPECT). The finite range of positrons in tissue and the non-collinearity of the annihilation γ rays (~0.25°) impose a limit on the spatial resolution obtainable with PET. This limit has not been reached by the PET scanners in operation today, but may become an issue in the future. In practice, it is usually the scanner sensitivity and the need to smooth data to reduce noise that limit the spatial resolution obtained in patient images.

Correction for photon attenuation

The fraction of the photon flux attenuated by tissue for any given pair of detectors in a PET scanner is independent of where along the line joining the detectors the radionuclide lies. This means that an accurate attenuation correction of the emission data can be made. Correction factors are obtained by calculating the ratio between two additional scans, a blank scan and a transmission scan, which are performed with external positron emitting sources (for example, rotating rod sources as shown in Figure 1.6). The blank scan is performed when the scanner is empty, and the transmission scan is performed with the patient in position. The transmission scan can also be reconstructed to provide a crude transmission CT image of the patient, which is aligned with subsequent emission images. If the outline of the patient is known, for example, from the outline of an emission scan of the brain, and the linear attenuation coefficient is known to be uniform, then a fairly accurate correction for attenuation can be calculated without actually performing a transmission scan.

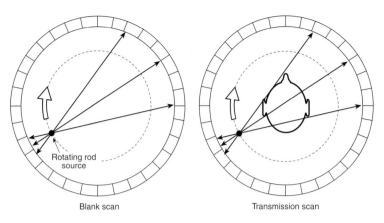

Blank scan   Transmission scan

Figure 1.6 *Attenuation correction using rotating rod transmission sources. Attenuation correction factors are obtained from the ratio of the counts in the blank scan to the counts in the transmission scan for all coincidence pairs of detectors.*

PET scanner

A state-of-the-art commercial PET scanner, as shown in Figure 1.7, consists of several rings of BGO block detectors. Many contiguous planes are imaged simultaneously, so the whole brain or heart can be imaged without moving the patient. A variation on this basic design is a system in which a partial ring of block detectors rotates rapidly around the patient to obtain full angular coverage. There are several transmission source configurations; for example, rotating rod sources which rotate within the field of view and retract into a shielded housing when not in use. Thin lead or tungsten septa are inserted between each imaging plane in order to reject photons, particularly those originating outside of the field of view, that will otherwise degrade the signal to noise ratio. Note that the septa are not collimators – collimation occurs automatically as a result of annihilation coincidence detection. The septa can be retracted out of the field of view so that the scanner can be operated in 3D mode (see below) if desired.

Block detector

Detectors for use in PET scanners must stop high energy 511 keV γ rays with high efficiency and at high rates. The most common design is the **block detector** (Figure 1.8) based on a BGO scintillation crystal. BGO has a higher attenuation coefficient than sodium iodide. The detector consists of a BGO block (typically 5 cm $\times$ 5 cm $\times$ 3 cm) which is divided up into, for example, 64 individual segments. Four photomultiplier tubes detect the scintillation light emitted from the crystal block, and the segment in which a γ ray interacts is identified by comparing the amount of scintillation light detected in each photomultiplier tube in a similar way to a γ-camera. The block detector is a cost-effective solution for the construction of high resolution scanners with large numbers of contiguous rings. In the next generation of scanners, BGO is likely to be superseded by lutetium oxyorthosilicate (LSO), which has a higher light output and a shorter scintillation decay time. LSO will lead to improved spatial resolution, by facilitating new detector designs, and improved signal to noise levels, particularly for 3D acquisition.

Three-dimensional (3D) acquisition

The sensitivity of PET scanners can be increased by a factor of 3–10 by retracting the interslice septa from the field of view and acquiring coincidence events between detectors in different planes of the scanner. This is done at the cost of a large increase in the amount of scatter and other background events detected, particularly from activity outside the field of view. 3D PET is advantageous for studies of the brain, for children, and when the activity in the field of view is small. The computing resources necessary to process 3D data are very large. 2D and 3D acquisition modes are shown schematically in Figure 1.9.

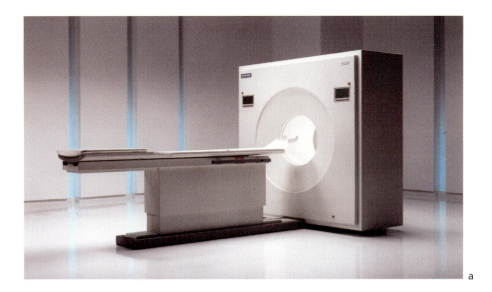

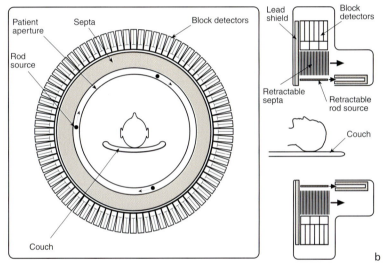

Figure 1.7 *(a) A state of the art BGO dedicated PET scanner. (b) Schematic diagram showing front view and cutaway side view of scanner. The septa are retracted into a housing at the back of the scanner in order to perform acquisitions in 3D mode – some recent systems are built without septa. The transmission rod sources retract into a shielded container when not in use. Some scanners use point sources rather than rods (photograph courtesy of CTI, Inc.).*

511 keV SPECT and coincidence imaging

Several alternatives to dedicated PET scanners are available, primarily for performing clinical PET studies with FDG, and are attractive in that they allow both positron and single photon emitting tracers to be imaged on the same scanner. Most are based on γ-camera technology, usually with each head a single large sodium iodide crystal, as opposed to discrete BGO block detectors. Both 511 keV SPECT and dual head **coincidence imaging** are available as add-ons to standard γ-camera systems, although thicker crystals are usually employed. The simplest approach is to image 511 keV photons with a specially constructed high energy collimator, but there is significant septal penetration by the high energy photons, and this approach results in poor spatial resolution and poor sensitivity. A more promising approach is the use of two opposed γ-cameras operating in coincidence (in 3D mode). Typical images from such a system are shown in Figure 1.10. Manufacturers are also currently developing combined PET/SPECT systems with purpose designed detectors. Although the intrinsic spatial resolution of coincidence imaging γ-cameras is impressive,

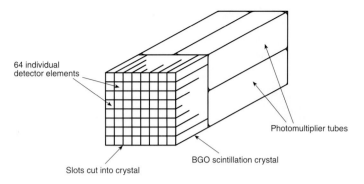

64 individual detector elements

Photomultiplier tubes

BGO scintillation crystal

Slots cut into crystal

Figure 1.8 *A BGO block detector. An individual detector element is identified by comparing the amount of scintillation light detected by the four photomultiplier tubes.*

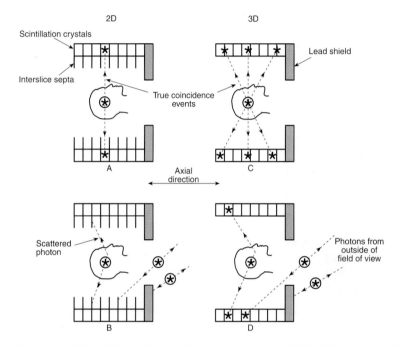

2D

3D

Scintillation crystals

Interslice septa

Lead shield

True coincidence events

Axial direction

A

C

Scattered photon

Photons from outside of field of view

B

D

Figure 1.9 *2D and 3D acquisition. A section through a multislice PET scanner is shown. In 2D, true coincidence pairs are only accepted between detectors in the same ring as shown in (A). The interslice septa serve to shield the detectors from both scattered photons, and, in combination with the lead side shields, from photons originating outside the field of view (B). In 3D, the septa are removed from the field of view, which allows the detection of cross plane coincidences, thus significantly increasing the sensitivity of the scanner (C). Removal of the septa also increases the sensitivity to scattered photons and to photons originating outside the field of view, both of which can degrade image quality (D).*

there are major limitations to sensitivity and count rate, and the problems associated with activity outside the field of view when imaging in 3D mode apply particularly to these systems. Nevertheless, many initial reports are encouraging, and it remains to be seen whether the performance of coincidence imaging γ-camera systems is adequate for routine clinical PET applications.

Comparison of scanners

Figure 1.11 illustrates the various scanner configurations for imaging of PET tracers. Table 1.2 lists some performance parameters for the different configurations – these are typical values and are not representative of any particular scanner.

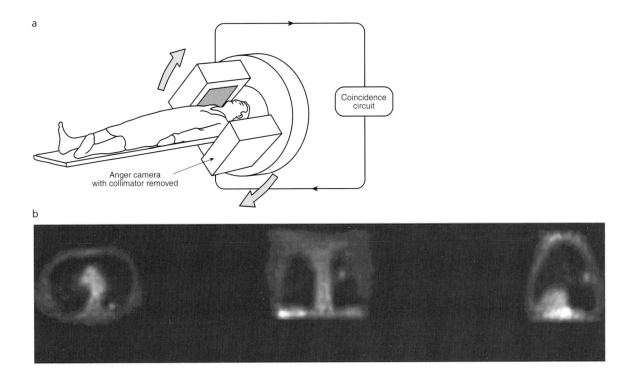

a

Coincidence circuit

Anger camera with collimator removed

b

Transaxial   Coronal   Sagittal

Figure 1.10 *(a) A coincidence imaging γ-camera system. The two Anger camera heads operate without collimators, and data is acquired in 3D mode. (b) An attenuation corrected FDG scan performed with a coincidence imaging γ-camera system (image courtesy of ADAC Laboratories).*

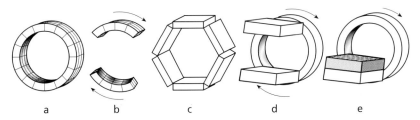

a   b   c   d   e

Figure 1.11 *Different PET scanner configurations: (a) Conventional BGO dedicated PET scanner; (b) partial ring BGO dedicated PET scanner; (c) dedicated PET scanner with six position-sensitive sodium iodide detectors; (d) dual headed γ-camera for coincidence imaging (no collimators); (e) γ-camera with 511 keV collimator.*

Commonly used radiopharmaceuticals

FDG

FDG (Figure 1.12) is by far the most widely used PET tracer. Much of clinical PET is based on the fact that diseased tissue has a different rate of glucose utilization to normal tissue, and in particular, tumours often exhibit high metabolic rates. FDG is used as a metabolic tracer in preference to glucose itself (labelled with ^{11}C, for example) because FDG is trapped in tissue whereas glucose is not, which makes [^{11}C]glucose scans difficult to interpret. The 2 h half-life of ^{18}F is well suited to the rate of uptake for FDG and permits acquisition of images over a period of 30 min or so at reasonable data rates. The kinetics of FDG can be described by a simple three-compartment model, as shown in Figures 1.13 and 1.14.

Table 1.2 Performance parameters for different scanner configurations. These figures are typical values only

	Dedicated PET scanner	Partial ring PET scanner	NaI PET scanner	Dual-head γ-camera
Tomographic spatial resolution (FWHM mm)	4.5	4.5	3.5	3.5
Relative sensitivity	35 (2D) 250 (3D)	65	100	10
Maximum count rate (kcps)	~150	~100	~75	~15
Attenuation correction	Rotating rod sources/point source	Rotating rod sources/point source	Rotating point source	Under development
Scanner configuration	Ring of block detectors	Rotating partial ring of block detectors	Six position sensitive NaI detectors	Dual-head γ-camera with no collimators
Axial field of view (cm)	15	15	25	35
Acquisition mode	2D or 3D	3D only	3D only	3D only
Scintillation crystal	20–30 mm BGO	20 mm BGO	25 mm NaI	9–15 mm NaI

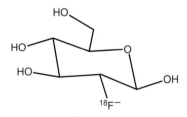

Figure 1.12 *The structure of [^{18}F]2-fluoro-2-deoxy-D-glucose (FDG). ^{18}F is substituted for the hydroxyl (OH) group in the 2-position.*

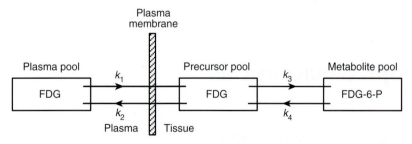

Figure 1.13 *Three-compartment model of FDG kinetics. The compartments represent respectively free FDG in plasma, free FDG in tissue and FDG 6-phosphate. Free FDG is phosphorylated by the action of hexokinase to FDG 6-phosphate but is not metabolized further – it may be dephosphorylated over a timescale of several hours. The rate constants k_1, k_2, k_3, k_4 (in units of min^{-1}) represent the extraction of tracer from plasma into tissue, the return of free FDG to plasma, the rate of phosphorylation, and the rate of dephosphorylation respectively. In many tissues k_4 is very low, in which case the metabolic rate for glucose is given by the expression ([glc]/LC) × ($k_1 k_3$)/($k_1 + k_3$) where [glc] is the plasma glucose concentration and LC is the lumped constant.*

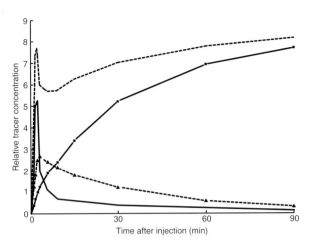

Figure 1.14 *Time activity curves for FDG in cortical grey matter and in plasma (corrected for radio-active decay). Extraction into tissue is rapid over the first 10 min, and then continues less rapidly over the next hour or so. Free FDG in tissue reaches a peak within a few minutes of the injection time and then falls. At 30 min the ratio between bound and free FDG is about 4 to 1. The total labelled FDG, as registered by a PET scanner, includes contributions from FDG and FDG-6-P and from FDG in plasma, although after 30 min the plasma FDG contributes only a few percent of the total activity. Most clinical protocols consist of a 30–60 min uptake period after tracer administration followed by a static scan over a period of ~30–60 min, which results in an image where the greyscale level is roughly proportional to the rate of glucose utilization. - - -, total FDG + FDG-6-P (tissue plus plasma); —■—, FDG-6-P in tissue; - -▲- -, free FDG in tissue; —, FDG in plasma.*

Because the kinetics of FDG and glucose are not identical, the so-called **lumped constant** is invoked to account for the difference between the rate of glucose utilization as measured with FDG and the true rate. The lumped constant is believed to have a constant value over a wide range of situations for a given tissue type – for normal grey matter it has a value of 0.52. Figure 1.15 shows the normal whole body distribution of FDG.

$^{18}F^-$

Uptake of $^{18}F^-$ provides an index of bone metabolism, and has a long history of use in skeletal imaging to investigate focal bone disease such as tumours or infection. $^{18}F^-$ is rapidly cleared from the blood by renal excretion, and by incorporation into bone by exchanging with the hydroxyl ion in hydroxyapatite crystal in bone to form fluoroapatite. Imaging is performed ~60 min after tracer injection (Figure 1.16).

[^{15}O]Water

[^{15}O]Water is a freely diffusible tracer with an extraction fraction of nearly 100%, and is used to measure perfusion using the principles established by Kety and Schmidt (1948). Clinical studies usually employ a bolus injection followed by a static scan of 1–2 min duration which results in an image with values directly proportional to blood flow. [^{15}O]Water is primarily used to image cerebral perfusion, in particular for PET brain activation studies, where its short half-life permits many scans to be performed in rapid succession; however, it can also be used to examine tumour and myocardial perfusion. Because of the very short half-life, large activities of tracer must be handled before administration and high finger doses to technical staff may result unless an automated tracer delivery system is used. The image quality obtained is usually inferior to that obtained with longer lived tracers.

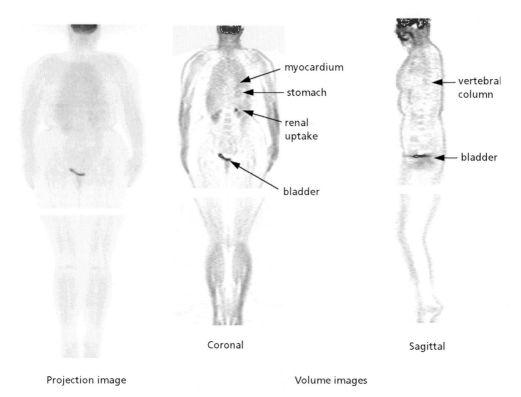

myocardium

stomach

renal uptake

bladder

vertebral column

bladder

Coronal

Sagittal

Projection image

Volume images

Figure 1.15 *Normal FDG whole body distribution. This FDG-PET scan of a normal subject shows that FDG is taken up into all normal tissue except fat. A large fraction of the administered activity is taken up by the brain (~6%) and the myocardium (~4%). FDG is excreted via the kidneys and accumulates rapidly in the bladder (~20% in the first 2 h). Multibed whole body scans such as this can be displayed as a projection image (left), or as individual orthogonal planes (right). The projection image may be used for a preliminary examination of the data before proceeding to the more detailed volume images.*

[^{11}C]L-Methionine

Accumulation of [^{11}C]L-methionine into tumour tissue is believed to be due to increased transport of amino acids and incorporation of amino acids into protein fractions, although it is not clear which of these mechanisms is predominant in PET tumour imaging. Further metabolism also results in the label being incorporated into lipids and nucleic acids. [^{11}C]L-Methionine can be used to delineate tumour extent, and to some extent tumour proliferation rate. The normal whole body distribution of [^{11}C]L-methionine is shown in Figure 1.17.

[^{13}N]Ammonia

[^{13}N]Ammonia is rapidly extracted into the myocardium with a 70% extraction fraction (falling to ~35% at high coronary flows), and is trapped by the glutamic acid–glutamate reaction. It has been suggested that the degree to which ammonia is trapped depends to some extent on the metabolic state of the myocardium; however, due to its ease of use, and the high quality images that can be obtained, [^{13}N]ammonia is the standard tracer for PET myocardial perfusion studies. Clinical protocols consist of a static scan beginning a few

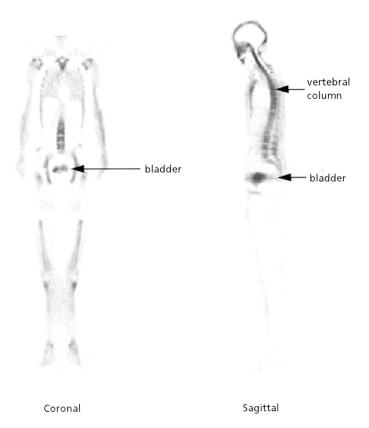

Coronal   Sagittal

Figure 1.16 *Normal ^{18}F whole body distribution.*

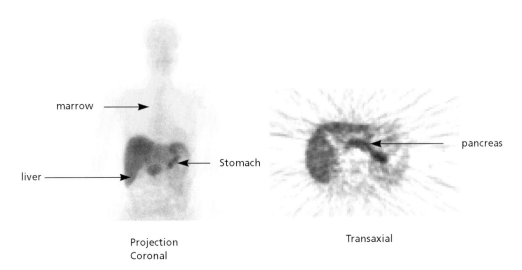

Projection   Transaxial
Coronal

Figure 1.17 *Projection and transaxial (emission) views are shown of a normal [^{11}C]L-methionine body scan. Uptake is seen in the liver, stomach, pancreas and marrow containing areas of the skeleton. Physiological uptake of methionine may also be seen in the gut, lacrimal and salivary glands and the urinary tract (not shown).*

minutes after tracer injection to allow for clearance of the blood pool activity. Several methods have been described for obtaining parametric images of myocardial perfusion, but these are complicated by the appearance of labelled metabolites in the blood which become significant a few minutes after injection. Due to the dependence of trapping on metabolism, [^{13}N]ammonia is seldom used to image cerebral perfusion.

Table 1.3 Potential radiopharmaceuticals for clinical PET

Radiopharmaceutical	Application
[^{11}C]Flumazenil	Localization of epileptic foci
[^{18}F]Fluoromisonidazole	Hypoxic tumour cells, ischaemically compromised myocardium
[^{11}C]Acetate	Cardiac oxidative metabolism
[^{11}C]Palmitate	Cardiac fatty acid metabolism
[^{13}N]Glutamate	Tumour metabolism
[^{18}F]Fluorodopa	Dopamine synthesis
[^{11}C]Aminoisobutyric acid (AIB)	Tumour amino acid uptake
[^{11}C]Aminocyclopentanecarboxylic acid (ACPC)	Tumour amino acid uptake
[^{18}F]Uracil (FU)	Evaluation of response to chemotherapy
[^{11}C]Thymidine	Tumour cellular proliferation rate
[^{68}Ga]EDTA	Blood–brain barrier permeability
[^{62}Cu]PTSM	Blood flow
[^{11}C]Tyrosine	Tumour metabolism

^{82}Rb

The isotope ^{82}Rb is used to measure myocardial perfusion. Rubidium is an analogue of potassium, and its kinetics are similar to those of the single photon emitter ^{201}Tl. Rubidium is extracted rapidly into the myocardium with a 50–60% extraction fraction which falls to 25–30% at high flows. The short half-life of ^{82}Rb (75 s) mean that repeat studies can be performed in rapid succession, however. ^{82}Rb cannot be produced from a cyclotron but is generated by the decay of ^{82}Sr in a generator. An automated system for rapid elution of the generator and rapid infusion of the eluate are therefore required, and this also serves to eliminate the potential high radiation doses to technical personnel.

Other radiopharmaceuticals for clinical PET

Table 1.3 lists other promising PET radiopharmaceuticals that may find a clinical role.

Clinical PET protocols

Some standard protocols are shown diagrammatically in Figure 1.18. The details of each protocol will vary from centre to centre, but these examples illustrate some general points. Protocols for clinical PET studies are the result of a trade-off between the high quality images that can be obtained with long scanning times, and the need to minimize time spent on the patient couch. The emphasis is on obtaining images for visual and semi-quantitative analysis rather than performing the complex procedures required for absolute quantification. Nevertheless, clinical PET protocols are still often very long and the number of studies that can be performed in a working day is limited.

FDG brain scan

A simple static emission scan is shown in Figure 1.19. A calculated attenuation correction is performed, based on the scalp outline as seen in the emission scan. Alternatively, a transmission scan can be performed before the tracer injection; however, this requires that the patient must remain (stationary) on the couch throughout the transmission, uptake and emission periods. With some scanners, the transmission scan can be acquired after injection of the tracer, thus reducing the time spent on the couch.

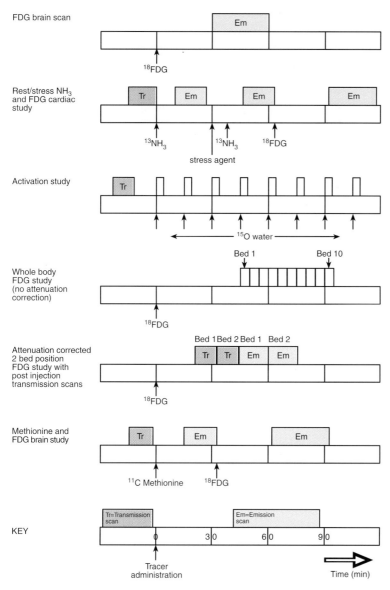

Figure 1.18 *Scanning protocols for common clinical PET studies.*

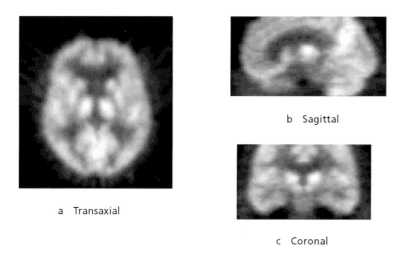

b Sagittal

a Transaxial

c Coronal

Figure 1.19 *FDG brain scan with calculated attenuation correction. Transaxial, sagittal and coronal slices through a selected point in the dataset are shown.*

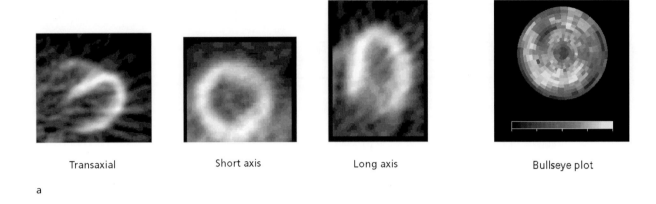

Transaxial   Short axis   Long axis   Bullseye plot

a

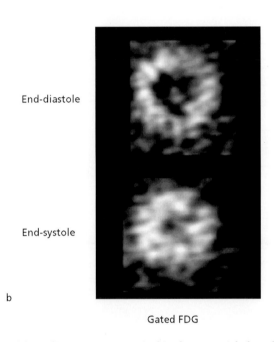

End-diastole

End-systole

b

Gated FDG

Figure 1.20 *(a) Cardiac images are acquired in the transaxial plane, but are often resliced into short axis and long axis slices. In a bullseye plot, the most active part of the myocardium is considered to have normal uptake and other regions are expressed as a percentage of this reference region. In this way, comparisons between studies can be made. For example, the difference between normalized FDG and ammonia bullseyes can be displayed to identify regions of perfusion/metabolism mismatch. (b) Gated FDG cardiac scan. Representative short axis slice shown at end diastole and end systole with uniform contraction and wall thickening.*

Rest/stress ammonia and FDG cardiac study

The times at which the three successive tracer injections are given must be arranged such that an emission scan does not begin until the count rate from the previously administered tracer has fallen to a sufficiently low level. A pharmacological cardiac stressing agent (e.g. adenosine) is administered before the second ammonia injection. Cardiac studies can be performed as simple static emission scans (Figure 1.20a), but higher resolution and more accurate quantitative values can be obtained by performing gated emission scans (Figure 1.20b). The cardiac cycle is divided into 4–8 separate images, each of which can be processed

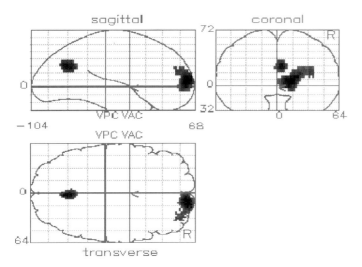

Figure 1.21 *A statistical parametric map derived from a [^{15}O]water activation study. Regions that show statistically significant changes from a series of rest images are displayed as dark areas. This example shows a subject engaged in a task of retrieval from episodic memory. Activation is evident in the precuneus and the right superior frontal gyrus (courtesy of MD Kopelman, P Grasby, T Stevens and S Foli).*

in the same way as a static cardiac scan. Estimates of wall motion and wall thickening can be made from gated cardiac studies if the acquisition time is extended to account for the smaller number of counts in each image.

Brain activation study

Brain activation studies with [^{15}O]water require the tracer to be administered many times in succession at 10–15 min intervals. The patient is subjected to different stimuli (or performs a specific task) during each scan. A simple protocol might consist of eight sequential scans, which alternate between a task (or stimulus) and a control state. A statistical analysis is performed on the image sequence in order to identify regions where there is a statistically significant change between the task and control images, and thus identify the regions of cortex associated with the specified task. Activation studies are usually performed in 3D mode, and results can be visualized as a **statistical parametric map (SPM)** as shown in Figure 1.21.

Whole body scan

Because the axial field of view of most PET scanners is limited to ~15 cm, larger areas of the body can only be imaged by moving the patient couch through the gantry. This is usually performed in a series of steps, the length of each step being slightly smaller than the axial field of view as the end planes have a relatively low sensitivity. As scanning time (and the time the patient can remain on the couch without discomfort) is limited, there is a trade-off between the image quality (related to the time at each position) and the axial coverage. With ^{18}F labelled tracers it is possible to obtain high quality tomographic images of the whole body in about 45 min (Figure 1.15). Complete head to toe coverage can usually be obtained by moving the patient through the scanner in a single pass, although on some scanners the data must be acquired in two passes, the first from head to pelvis and the second from feet to pelvis. Whole body studies are usually performed without attenuation correction as the total scan time for transmission scan, tracer uptake period and emission scan would be prohibitive; however, non-attenuation corrected studies must be interpreted with care as distortions are introduced into the images (Figure 1.22). Conversely, a transmission scan will contribute noise to the emission image, and there is evidence that this may reduce sensitivity for the detection of small lesions. Correction for attenuation is essential if it is

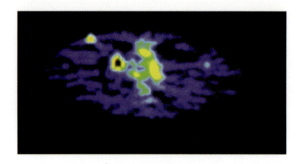
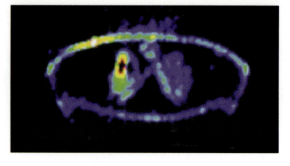

With attenuation correction   No attenuation correction

Figure 1.22 *Image distortions due to the absence of attenuation correction. The uncorrected whole body section demonstrates the high apparent activity that is seen at the body surface, and also the distortion that occurs to tumours of circular cross-section, which are artificially elongated in the direction of least attenuation. From KR Zasadny, PV Kison, LE Quint, RL Wahl. Radiology 1996; 201(3), p. 874, Figs 2b,c. Reproduced with permission.*

Table 1.4 Effective dose equivalent (EDE) values for common PET radiopharmaceuticals				
Tracer	Typical activity		EDE	
	(MBq)	(mCi)	(mSv)	(mR)
FDG	250	7	6.8	705
$^{18}F^-$	250	7	6.7	693
[^{11}C]L-Methionine	370	10	4.6	460
[^{15}O]Water	2000	55	2.3	234
[^{13}N]Ammonia	550	15	1.5	150
^{82}Rb	2000	55	2.4	244

desired to calculate **standardized uptake values (SUVs)** from the image, and to this end several new techniques for performing and processing transmission scans are under development. It is likely that attenuation corrected whole body studies will become routine in the near future.

Static scan with measured attenuation correction

If it is necessary to calculate SUVs, then a static scan of a limited region (1–2 bed positions) with a pre- or postinjection transmission scan must be performed (Figure 1.23) as it is difficult to perform a calculated attenuation correction for regions other than the brain. The static scan can be performed in the same session as a whole body scan (at a set time after injection). The ability to perform a postinjection transmission scan, which is possible if rod transmission sources are used, significantly reduces the time spent on the couch and also reduces the possibility of artefacts due to patient movement between the emission and transmission scans. Figure 1.23 shows static attenuation corrected and non-attenuation corrected scans of the chest.

Methionine and FDG study

In the methionine and FDG protocol, the first tracer ($T_{1/2}$ = 20 min) must be allowed to decay before the second tracer is scanned. The second tracer can be injected immediately after the first has been scanned, provided the uptake period of the second tracer is greater than the time it takes for the first to decay to an acceptable level.

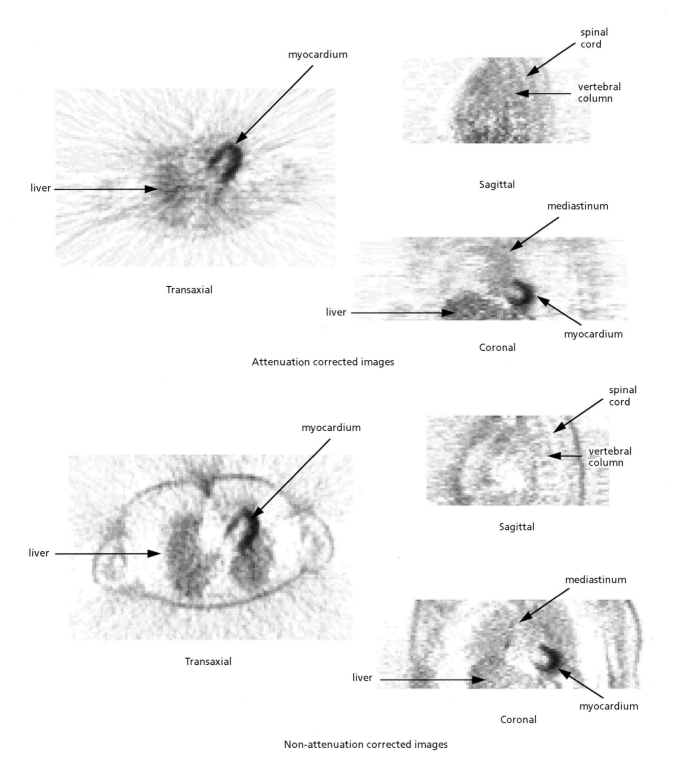

Figure 1.23 *Static attenuation corrected and non-attenuation corrected scans of the chest. The transmission scan (overleaf) is also reconstructed and provides some basic anatomical information.*

Radiation dosimetry

Table 1.4 shows the whole body **effective dose equivalent (EDE)** values for common PET radiopharmaceuticals. Values are on the whole less than for single photon emitters,

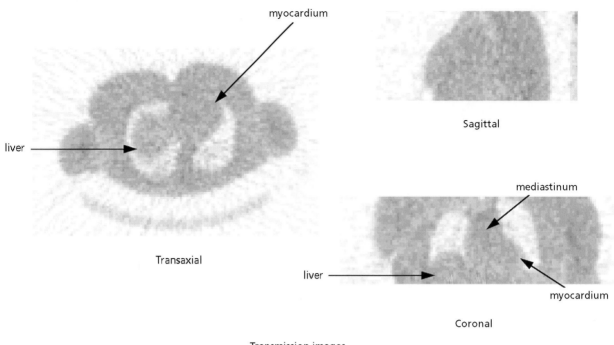

myocardium

liver

Transaxial

Sagittal

mediastinum

liver

myocardium

Coronal

Transmission images

Figure 1.23 *Continued.*

primarily due to the short half-lives of the PET radionuclides. For children, administration of activities reduced in proportion to body weight results in images which are of at least as good quality as those obtained in adults.

Quality control

Clinical scanning must be accompanied by a rigorous quality control program. This is relatively straightforward and involves ensuring that there is a proper correction for the variations in efficiency between the large number of crystals that comprise the scanner. This normalization procedure takes several hours and can be performed infrequently (i.e. monthly), provided there are no detector failures. More infrequently, a setup scan that changes the detector gains to counteract any drift that has occurred, and ensures that all detectors are operating optimally, must be performed. The setup scan also takes a couple of hours. On a daily basis, quality control can consist of a short (30 min) blank scan to check that the detectors have not drifted significantly since the last time the scanner was normalized. This quality control scan also serves as the blank scan for attenuation correction.

Quantification methods

One of the main strengths of PET is the ability to perform quantitative studies. In its most simple form, quantification means simply that average values of tracer uptake in different regions can be directly compared. Absolute quantification, on the other hand, is the determination of physiological parameters in absolute units. All forms of quantification are subject to the limitations imposed by the partial volume effect (see below).

Semi-quantitative methods

Semi-quantitative methods involve simple comparisons of absolute or relative regions of interest (ROI). For example, hypometabolic areas associated with epileptic foci might be characterized by comparison with contralateral regions, or with a brain region, such as the cerebellum, that is believed to be unaffected by the disease. Similarly, lung tumour uptake can be characterized as a ratio to the uptake in normal lung tissue. Cardiac PET images are frequently displayed and manipulated in the form of a bullseye plot, which is usually calibrated so that the region in the image with the highest radiotracer concentration is assumed to be normal.

Normalized semi-quantification

Normalized semi-quantification methods are also referred to as semi-quantitative; however, by correcting for the administered activity it is possible to compare ROI values between patients without having to make any assumptions about normal or reference tissue regions. An example of such an index is the SUV described below.

Absolute quantification

If a curve of the arterial tracer concentration against time, the **arterial input function (AIF),** can be determined, then it is possible to take quantification a stage further and obtain values for physiological parameters in absolute units. For example, using FDG, glucose metabolic rate can be determined in $mol\,min^{-1}g^{-1}$ and with ^{15}O labelled water, blood flow can be determined in units of $ml\,min^{-1}g^{-1}$. Determining the AIF by direct sampling is complex and invasive and not suitable for routine clinical applications. There are various non-invasive alternatives for obtaining the AIF, for example, by rapid dynamic scanning of the heart or the aorta, but in general absolute quantification is not performed for clinical studies.

Partial volume effect

All quantification performed in PET is subject to the limitations imposed by poor spatial resolution, which manifests itself as the **partial volume effect**. For objects of dimensions less than twice the spatial resolution (FWHM) in the image, the apparent activity in the object is decreased (Figure 1.24). For objects of diameter equal to the spatial resolution the maximum apparent activity concentration will be less than 50% of the true value. A simple correction for partial volume, based on phantom measurements, can be made, but this can lead to large errors for objects of dimensions less than the spatial resolution. The situation is complicated further for small objects in a 'warm' background, so quantification of radiotracer uptake for small objects must be treated with great caution.

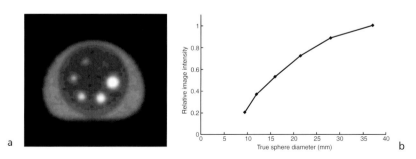

Figure 1.24 *Partial volume effect. The torso phantom (a) contains six spheres filled with the same uniform concentration of tracer. The reduction in apparent activity for the smaller spheres is clearly seen, and is plotted in (b). The spatial resolution of the image is 10 mm FWHM.*

Standardized uptake values

The standardized uptake value (SUV) is widely used in PET oncology studies. It is an index of tracer (usually FDG) uptake in a tumour which may permit differentiation between benign and malignant tumours, and possibly identify tumour stage. The SUV is defined as follows:

$$SUV = \frac{\text{Tracer uptake (MBq ml}^{-1})}{\text{Administered activity (MBq)}/(\text{Patient weight (kg)} \times 1000)}$$

Tracer uptake is determined from a small ROI placed over the tumour in an attenuation corrected image. A scanner calibration factor is required to convert the value measured from the image into $MBq\,ml^{-1}$. SUVs are based on the approximation that the tracer is distributed uniformly throughout the body, so in normal tissue SUVs are very roughly equal to 1. However, since little FDG accumulates in normal fat in fasting patients, many vascular tissues have an SUV of about 2. For tumours, where the metabolic rate is higher, SUVs may range from 2 to 15 or so. Since tumours often have very heterogeneous distributions of tracer uptake, SUVs are generally evaluated for the hottest part of the tumour, which is assumed to be the most malignant. It has been shown that, because FDG is not taken up in adipose tissue, SUVs are more reproducible when the lean body mass (derived from measurements of both height and weight) is substituted for patient weight in the expression above to give SUV_{lean}. A correction depending on blood glucose concentration can also be made which accounts for competition between FDG and glucose, as SUVs are commonly depressed if there are elevated blood glucose levels. When SUVs are quoted, or compared with threshold values taken from the literature, care must be taken to see which of the various corrections have been applied.

Limitations of SUVs

Despite their widespread use, SUVs are subject to several fundamental problems and should be interpreted with care:

- SUVs provide a crude index of the tumour metabolic rate provided that the tracer uptake has saturated at the time of measurement. Various studies have shown that tracer uptake may continue to increase for several hours after administration, and that the shape of the uptake curve is very variable. To minimize errors due to these effects, SUVs should always be acquired at the same time after injection.
- SUVs for small tumours (<1 cm diameter) are particularly vulnerable to partial volume errors. It may be possible in some cases to obtain an accurate estimate of the tumour dimensions, on which to base a partial volume correction, from CT or MRI. However, the anatomical extent of the tumour may well not match the extent of tracer uptake.
- FDG is taken up rapidly in inflamed tissue, which may lead to erroneous SUVs in some situations (e.g. after radiotherapy).
- SUVs are significantly reduced for small lesions in the lower lobes of the lung due to the blurring effect of respiratory motion.

Parametric images

A **parametric image** shows some derived quantity, e.g. blood flow, as opposed to straightforward tracer uptake, and is a powerful way of presenting functional information. One example, which is useful in a clinical environment, is the calculation of parametric images of myocardial perfusion, calibrated in units of $ml\,min^{-1}g^{-1}$ and derived from dynamic $[^{13}N]$ammonia scan data (Figure 1.25). A parametric blood flow image will be able to identify globally reduced perfusion, possibly due to disease of all three coronary arteries – it would not be possible to identify this situation from a simple uptake image. The acquisition protocol involves rapid dynamic scanning for the first few minutes following tracer administration, and the AIF (required to calculate perfusion) is derived from the

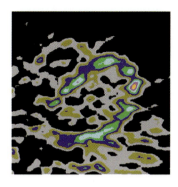 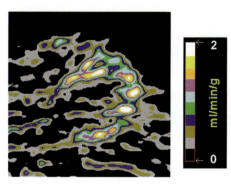

Rest ammonia   Stress ammonia with dipyridamole

Figure 1.25 *Parametric images of myocardial blood flow image derived from a dynamic [^{13}N]ammonia scan. The image is calibrated in ml min^{-1} g^{-1}.*

images of the left ventricle. Images are calculated using the 'Patlak' graphical method (Choi and Huang 1993). Parametric images can be produced for most of the standard clinical PET tracers.

Statistical parametric maps

There is a great deal of interest in using statistical techniques to analyse PET images on a voxel by voxel basis. Many of these techniques were originally developed for analysing data from brain activation studies with ^{15}O labelled water. A statistical test is applied to every pixel in a set of images, in order to identify voxels that differ significantly from either a set of 'rest' images or from a 'normal' population average image. The resulting *p*-value or *z*-score, which represents the degree of statistical significance, can be displayed as a parametric image (an SPM, as shown in Figure 1.21) and used to identify areas of statistically significant change. Although techniques such as SPM are not currently routinely utilized for clinical applications, they are very powerful and their use is likely to increase.

Image display and data processing

Image display programs

In addition to standard features, such as colour scale manipulation and image zoom, display tools must be capable of handling the multidimensional nature of the PET datasets, i.e. time frames, multiple planes, multiple bed positions and cardiac gated studies. Programs must also be capable of displaying several scans simultaneously to allow assessment of follow up studies and to compare scans in multiple tracer protocols. Figure 1.26 shows a general purpose PET display tool.

Image co-registration

Anatomical information in PET images

Many structures within the brain can be clearly delineated in an FDG brain scan. However, there is insufficient anatomical detail to be of use in, for example, the planning of surgery, where the location of a tumour in relation to critical structures must be determined. PET transmission images can provide coarse anatomical information that is sometimes useful, for example, in localizing tumours in the lung, but accurate localization of regions of tracer uptake can only be obtained by co-registering PET data with anatomical images from either CT or MRI.

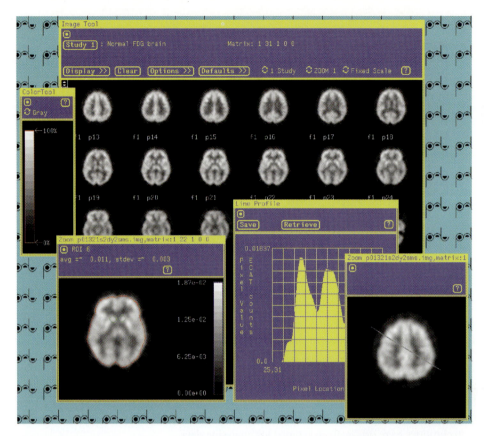

Figure 1.26 *A general purpose image display tool. The facility to normalize data in different ways is useful; for example, consecutive slices can be normalized relative to one another, or it may be desirable to scale each slice to its own maximum value in order to visualize features with low tracer uptake. Images are usually displayed so that the values displayed on the screen are proportional to the radiotracer concentration, and so are not dependent on scan time. Images may also be corrected for radioactive decay relative to the start of the scan. This tool incorporates sophisticated facilities for placing ROIs on an image, which is particularly important when analysing dynamic datasets.*

File transfer and file formats

The problems involved in transferring images from different modalities on to a single workstation and converting them into a common data format before registration cannot be overestimated. Despite the advent of the **picture archiving and communications system (PACS)**, there is still a bewildering variety of different image formats and communications protocols. Many CT, MRI, PET and SPECT scanners are now based around standard UNIX workstations. Open software permits direct access to image data, and most consoles allow this to be exported. However, until universal standards such as DICOM (digital imaging and communications in medicine) achieve wider currency, data transfer and format conversion remains a problem that is mainly addressed by in-house solutions.

Registration algorithms

There are many different algorithms for intermodality image registration. Some utilize external fiducial markers or stereotactic frames, which can be visualized in the two relevant modalities. These are attached to the patient and are subsequently registered using an interactive or automatic program. In practice, markers can be difficult to use as they need to be accurately located on the patient for at least two separate scans, which may be performed on different days. Also, markers require modifications to be made to the standard imaging protocol and so they can only be used prospectively. A more flexible solution is the use of

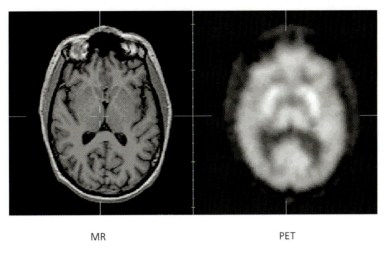

MR   PET

a   Transaxial

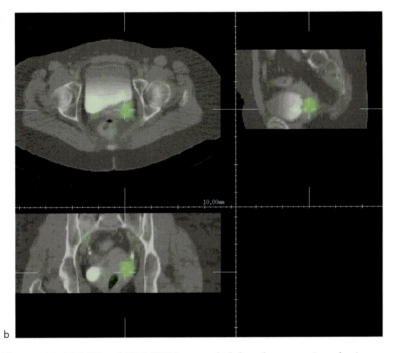

b

Figure 1.27 *(a) MRI and FDG-PET images which have been co-registered using an automatic algorithm. The images are displayed side by side and the cursors on each image move in parallel to identify equivalent points. (b) The image shows an MRI scan and an FDG-PET scan of the pelvis. The registration was performed using anatomical landmarks. The two images have been merged so that the location of the tumour can be visualized.*

anatomical landmarks. In this method a trained user locates a series of points which can be unambiguously located in both images (e.g. the tip of the caudate nuclei on both FDG-PET and MRI). These are then automatically aligned. Many algorithms are now available that use complex image processing techniques to automatically register multimodality brain data with minimal user interaction. A major advantage of these algorithms is that they can be applied retrospectively. Techniques that utilize measures such as image information content result in very robust algorithms. The accuracy for co-registration in the brain, which involves rigid body transformations only, is widely quoted as being ~2 mm. Accurate co-registration in other parts of the body is at present more difficult as non-rigid-body transformations and image warping algorithms are often required. Examples of PET images co-registered with images from other modalities are shown in Figure 1.27.

Data processing and archiving

Volume of data

Current PET scanners acquire 30–50 contiguous slices of image data, and each plane consists of a 128 × 128 or 256 × 256 matrix. Although these image datasets are not particularly large (1–5 Mbyte per static acquisition), the sizes rapidly multiply for dynamic scans, whole body scans and multitracer studies. A centre with a full schedule of clinical PET studies can easily generate upwards of 1 Gbyte of raw scan data and images per week. The amount of data that has to be acquired, processed and archived is very large, and the processing steps are computationally intensive. The computing requirements for clinical PET are therefore considerable.

Image reconstruction

The production of images from raw PET data requires the combination of several auxiliary files (e.g. attenuation correction, normalization, etc.) before the reconstruction step. Reconstruction is usually performed by one or more dedicated processors, which are integrated with the scanner, and commences immediately after data acquisition is complete. A single scan typically takes under a minute to reconstruct, although reconstruction of 3D data may take longer. For whole body and dynamic studies, where a large number of separate acquisitions are acquired sequentially, image reconstruction can proceed in parallel with the acquisition of the next time frame, or bed position, and the reconstructed image is available soon after the end of data acquisition. There is usually a significant amount of processing, much of it interactive, to be performed after image reconstruction. Straightforward reorganization of data, such as the creation of condensed projection and volumetric whole body images or reslicing of cardiac images, and more complex procedures such as the creation of parametric images, image registration and calculation of SUVs, are all time consuming. Final images will therefore often not be available to the clinician for some time after the scan has been completed. Images are usually reconstructed using the standard filtered backprojection algorithm, and 3D extensions of this. In addition, practical and robust iterative reconstruction algorithms are now available which promise better signal to noise properties without loss of spatial resolution, as shown in Figure 1.28. If further post-processing, such as absolute quantification, is required, then additional offline computing power is necessary.

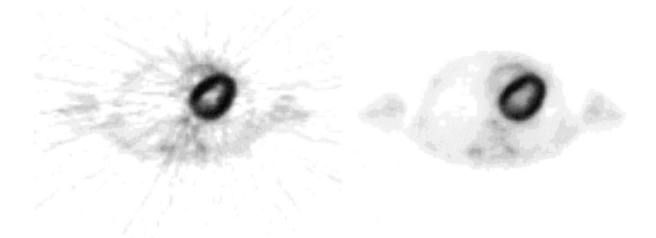

Figure 1.28 *A standard filtered backprojection reconstruction compared with the same data reconstructed using ordered subsets estimation maximization (OSEM) which is a fast, practical iterative reconstruction algorithm. The algorithm is very effective in reducing streak artefacts.*

Data archiving

If raw data is to be archived (permitting data to be processed differently, or reconstructed again in the event of errors) then the 1 Gbyte or so of data produced per week must all be copied and logged onto storage media, i.e. tape or optical disc, in an organized, and preferably automated, fashion. Although the requirement for fast retrieval of raw scan data is small, it is necessary to have fast access to image data for the purposes of comparing repeat scans, performing retrospective studies and audit. This means that although tape or slow optical discs may be adequate for archive, a faster medium, such as hard disc, is required for image data. Technology both for back-up of data (for recovery in the event of disaster) and for long term archiving of data is evolving rapidly, and care must be taken to ensure that a chosen solution will not be rapidly outgrown or become obsolete.

Computer hardware and software

Data processing and display is usually performed using a local area network of UNIX workstations, one of which is the scanner console, with additional PCs for administrative and less computationally intensive tasks. The distinction between a workstation and a PC is rapidly becoming blurred, and many tasks can be performed on either. Software standardization permits users to learn standard software interfaces for all the tasks they wish to perform, independently of the particular machine they are using. The network also requires additional facilities such as a high quality colour printer for production of hard copy, Internet access, printers, archiving devices and so on. The role of the computer network extends to cover a large number of administrative roles, e.g. patient booking systems, databases, information retrieval, patient reports and email, and it is advantageous if these can all be administered centrally. As the network will be used by a wide variety of users with varying degrees of computer literacy, it is essential that it is carefully administered in terms of upgrades, security and documentation.

Further reading

Anon (1991) Clinical PET: its time has come. *J Nucl Med* **32**(4).

Badawi RD (1997) 3D-mode acquisition in clinical PET. *Nucl Med Comms* **18**(9), 801–4.

Badawi RD, Marsden PK (1999) Developments in component based normalisation for 3D-PET. *Phys Med Biol* **44**(2), 571–94.

Badawi RD, Marsden PK, Cronin BF, Sutcliffe JL, Maisey MN (1996) Optimization of noise-equivalent count rates in 3D PET. *Phys Med Biol* **41**, 1755–6.

Bailey DL (1992) 3D acquisition and reconstruction in positron emission tomography. *Ann Nucl Med* **6**(3), 123–30.

Brix G, Zaers J, Adam LE *et al.* (1997) Performance evaluation of a whole-body PET scanner using the NEMA protocol. *Journal Of Nuclear Medicine* **38**, 1614–23.

Budinger TF (1998) PET instrumentation: what are the limits? *Seminars in Nuclear Medicine* **28**, 247–67.

Burns HD, Gibson RE, Dannals RE, Siegl PKS (eds) (1993) *Nuclear Imaging in Drug Discovery, Development, and Approval.* Birkhauser, Boston, MA.

Choi Y, Huang SC (1993) A simplified method for quantification of myocardial blood flow using nitrogen-13-ammonia and dynamic PET. *J Nucl Med* **34**(3), 488–97.

Dahlbom M, Hoffman EJ, Hoh CK *et al.* (1992) Whole-body positron emission tomography: Part 1. Methods and performance characteristics. *J Nucl Med* **33**, 1191–9.

Freifelder R, Karp JS (1997) Dedicated PET scanners for breast imaging. *Physics In Medicine And Biology* **42**, 2463–80.

Freifelder R, Karp JS, Geagan M, Muehllehner G (1994) Design and performance of the HEAD PENN-PET scanner. *IEEE Trans Nucl Sci* **41**(4), 1436–40.

Hamberg LM, Hunter GF, Alpert NM, Choi NC, Babich JW (1994) The dose uptake ratio as an index of glucose metabolism: useful parameter or oversimplification? *J Nucl Med* **35**(8), 1308–12.

Henkin RE, Boles MA, Dillehay GL *et al.* (eds) (1996) *Nuclear Medicine.* Mosby-Year Book, St. Louis, MO.

Hoffman EJ, Huang SC, Phelps ME (1979) Quantitation in positron emission computed tomography: 1. Effect of object size. *Journal Of Computer Assisted Tomography* **3**, 299–308 (Abstract).

Hoh CK, Dahlbom M, Hawkins RA *et al.* (1994) Basic principles of positron emission tomography in oncology: quantitation and whole body techniques. *Wiener Klin Wochenschr* **106**(15), 496–504.

Hoh CK, Hawkins RA, Glaspy JA *et al.* (1993) Cancer detection with whole-body PET using 2-[18F]fluoro-2-deoxy-D-glucose. *J Comput Assist Tomogr* **17**(4), 582–9.

Jarritt PH, Acton PD (1996) PET imaging using gamma-camera systems – a review. *Nucl Med Comms* **17**(9), 758–68.

Kety SS, Schmidt CF (1948) The nitrous oxide method for the quantitative determination of cerebral blood flow in man: theory, procedure and normal values. *J Clin Invest* **27**, 476–83.

Lewellen TK (1998) Time-of-flight PET. *Seminars in Nuclear Medicine* **28**, 268–75.

Links JM (1998) Advances in nuclear medicine instrumentation: considerations in the design and selection of an imaging system. *European Journal Of Nuclear Medicine* **25**, 1453–66.

Lodge MA, Badawi RD, Marsden PK (1998) Quantitative accuracy of simultaneous emission/transmission scanning in whole body PET. *Eur J Nuc Med* **25**(4), 417–23.

Lodge MA, Lucas JD, Marsden PK, Cronin BF, O'Doherty MJ, Smith MA (1999) A PET study of ^{18}FDG uptake in soft tissue masses. *Eur J Nucl Med* **26**(1), 22–30.

McCarthy TJ, Wetch MJ (1998) The state of positron emitting radionuclide production in 1997. *Seminars in Nuclear Medicine*, **28**, 235–46.

Phelps ME, Huang SC, Hoffman EJ, Selin C, Sokoloff L, Kuhl DE (1979) Tomographic measurement of local cerebral glucose metabolic rate in humans with (F-18)2-fluoro-2-deoxy-D-glucose: validation of method. *Ann Neurol* **6**, 371–88.

Phelps ME, Mazziotta JC, Schelbert HR (eds) (1986) *Positron Emission Tomography and Autoradiography: Principles and Applications for the Brain and Heart.* Raven Press, New York.

Stocklin G, Pike VW (eds) (1993) *Radiopharmaceuticals for Positron Emission Tomography.* Kluwer Academic Publishers, Dordrecht, The Netherlands.

Studholme C, Hill DLG, Hawkes DJ (1997) Automated three-dimensional registration of magnetic resonance and positron emission tomography brain images by multiresolution optimization of voxel similarity measures. *Medical Physics* **24**, 25–35.

TerPogossian MM (1992) The rigins of positron emission tomography. *Seminars in Nuclear Medicine* **22**, 140–49.

Tewson TJ, Krohn KA (1998) PET radiopharmaceuticals: state-of-the-art and future prospects. *Seminars in Nuclear Medicine* **28**, 221–34.

Townsend DW, Wensveen M, Byars LG *et al.* (1993) A rotating PET scanner using BGO block detectors: design, performance and applications. *J Nucl Med* **34**, 1367–76.

Wagner HN (1998) A brief history of positron emission tomography (PET). *Seminars in Nuclear Medicine* **28**, 213–20.

Wienhard K, Dahlbom M, Eriksson L *et al.* (1994) The ECAT EXACT HR: performance of a new high resolution positron scanner. *J Comput Assist Tomogr* **18**, 110–18.

Xu M, Cutler PD, Luk WK (1996) Adaptive, segmented attenuation correction for whole-body pet imaging. *IEEE Transactions On Nuclear Science*, **43**, 331–6.

Zasadny KR, Kison PV, Quint LE, Wahl RL (1996) Untreated lung cancer. Quantification of systematic distortion of tumour size and shape on non-attenuation-corrected 2-[fluorine-18]-fluoro-2-deoxy-D-glucose PET scans. *Radiology* **201**(3), 873–6.

Zasadny KR, Wahl RL (1993) Standardized uptake values of normal tissues at PET with 2-[fluorine-18]-fluoro-2-deoxy-D-glucose: variation with body weight and a method for correction. *Radiology* **189**(3), 847–50.

Chapter 2

Clinical applications of PET

It is not possible to be dogmatic about the role of PET imaging, partly because of the limited resources for this imaging modality and partly because the applications are changing and emerging rapidly. Where PET is available it might be the preferred imaging method for a particular clinical problem. However, a patient with a clinical problem would not necessarily be referred over a long distance if PET is not available locally and cheaper alternatives can provide many of the answers. Further, there will always be situations when more than one diagnostic strategy can be used appropriately to give the same results, and choice will depend on factors such as availability, costs and skills. In this summary the American College of Cardiology guidelines have been adopted to classify the evolving role of PET tracers in clinical practice. Using these guidelines, applications fall into four groups: 1, 2a, 2b and 3.

AMERICAN COLLEGE OF CARDIOLOGY CATEGORIES
1 Usually appropriate and considered useful with clinical evidence supporting diagnostic efficacy
2a Generally acceptable and less well established
2b Can be helpful but not well established by evidence
3 Generally not appropriate

Oncology (Chapters 4–11)

Applications in oncology can be considered under a number of headings which have different importance in different tumours:
- differentiating benign from malignant masses (e.g. lung nodules)
- establishing the grade of malignancy (e.g. brain tumours)
- localization of biopsy sites (e.g. tumours of the head and neck)
- treatment planning (e.g. brain tumours)
- establishing the local extent of tumour (e.g. squamous cell cancer of head and neck)
- detecting loco-regional spread (e.g. lung cancer)
- identifying distant metastases (e.g. melanoma)
- treatment monitoring (e.g. remission/response) radiotherapy or chemotherapy (e.g. lymphoma)
- suspected recurrence (e.g. breast cancer)
- staging a relapse to plan treatment (e.g. colorectal tumour)
- identifying primary disease (carcinoma of unknown origin, raised circulating markers, local nodes).

Category 1: Usually appropriate and considered useful

- most cases of suspected tumour recurrence but especially when anatomical imaging is difficult or equivocal and management will be affected (particularly primary brain tumours, colorectal cancers, pelvic cancers, head and neck cancers, lung cancers, some

breast cancers, lymphomas, malignant melanomas and sarcomas; but most malignancies are included)
- residual masses after therapy and where anatomical imaging is equivocal; particular examples are lymphoma in the mediastinum and malignant teratoma in the abdomen
- benign vs. malignant pulmonary nodules, where there is uncertainty on anatomical imaging and a relative contraindication to biopsy or an equivocal biopsy
- presurgical staging of lung cancer (especially when CT is equivocal)
- differentiating malignant from benign pancreatic masses
- recurrence of colorectal cancer for restaging if surgery considered
- restaging of malignant melanoma before further surgery.

Category 2a: Generally acceptable but less well established
- malignant melanoma primary staging for Clark levels 4 and 5, Breslow >1.5 mm
- brachial plexus lesion in breast cancer (radiation effects vs. malignant infiltration)
- local spread of head and neck cancers where clinical or anatomical imaging is equivocal
- localizing differentiated thyroid cancer where circulating markers are raised but the site is not identified
- primary staging for Hodgkin's disease and non-Hodgkin's lymphoma
- monitoring the response to chemotherapy and/or hormone therapy including neoadjuvant treatment before resection of large primary tumours
- site of primary disease in cases of carcinoma of unknown origin if management will be affected by determining the primary
- primary staging of oesophageal cancers
- axillary node status (breast cancer) especially where there is a relative contraindication to axillary dissection.

Category 2b: Can be helpful but not well established by evidence (emerging)
- suspected sarcoma developing in underlying Paget's disease of bone
- determining cancer response to chemotherapy/radiotherapy when anatomical imaging is equivocal
- establishing remission in chemotherapy/radiotherapy treated Hodgkin's disease and non-Hodgkin's lymphomas
- the primary staging and grading of soft tissue sarcomas
- determining local extension of pelvic cancers in difficult cases
- bone lesions (metastases vs. benign lesions) where anatomical imaging and/or biopsy is insufficient and management will be affected.

Neuropsychiatry (Chapter 12)
Category 1: Usually appropriate and considered useful
- presurgical evaluation of partial epilepsy
- suspected recurrence or failed primary treatment of primary malignant brain tumours
- early diagnosis of dementia, when MR or CT is either normal, marginally or equivocally abnormal
- the grading and prognosis of primary brain tumour.

Category 2: Generally acceptable but less well established
- diagnosis of partial epilepsy when MR imaging and/or SPECT imaging is normal or equivocal
- locating the optimal site for biopsy (either primary or recurrent brain tumour)
- differentiating malignancy from infection in HIV subjects where MRI is equivocal
- diagnosis of arteritis in systemic lupus erythematosus when MRI is normal
- assessment of cerebral blood flow/metabolism before neuro-interventional procedures.

- demonstration of dementia where MRI is clearly abnormal
- most instances of stroke
- most psychiatric disorders other than early dementia.

Cardiac applications (Chapter 13)

Category 1: Usually appropriate and considered useful

- diagnosis of hibernating myocardium in patients with poor left ventricular function before revascularization (or cardiac transplantation)
- patients with a fixed SPECT perfusion deficit with poor evidence of prior myocardial infarction who might benefit from revascularization
- diagnosis of coronary artery disease.
- diagnosis of coronary artery disease where other investigations (thallium, ECG, etc.) remain equivocal

Category 2a: Generally acceptable but less well established

- differential diagnosis of cardiomyopathy (ischaemic vs. other types of dilated cardiomyopathy).

Category 2b: Can be helpful but not well established by evidence (emerging)

- medical treatment of ischaemic heart disease in hyperlipidaemic patients.

Category 3: Generally not appropriate

- patients with confirmed coronary artery disease in whom revascularization is not contemplated or indicated.

Miscellaneous

Category 1: Usually appropriate and considered useful

- hyperparathyroidism where other imaging methods have failed to identify a parathyroid adenoma especially where the patient has been previously operated on using ($[^{11}C]$L-methionine).

Category 2a: Generally acceptable but less well established

- identifying the presence of focal bone disease where routine bone scan and/or anatomical imaging has failed to identify the site or presence of bone disease when there is a high clinical suspicion (F⁻scan)
- identifying recurrent functional pituitary tumours when anatomical imaging has not been successful
- sarcoid disease activity extent assessment.

Chapter 3

Oncology: a brief overview

Cancer is the second most common cause of death in western industrialized countries, causing 25% of all deaths. Its incidence is now increasing in most age groups. Reasons for this include increasing levels of environmental carcinogens and the increasing age of the population. There is now approximately a one in three chance of an individual contracting cancer at some time during his or her lifetime. Many of these cancers are now curable, but many others remain without satisfactory therapeutic options. Complete surgical excision remains the best way of treating and curing many cancers, but many patients are either found to be inoperable at surgery, or relapse soon after, because undetected spread has already occurred. The problem of operations being performed on inoperable cancers has a significant cost to the patient as well as being an enormous waste of healthcare resources. For example, the survival of patients with mediastinal spread from lung cancer is approximately 5% whereas those patients without mediastinal spread have a 5 year survival of approximately 50%. It is in the area of reducing unnecessary surgery that PET scanning is making one of its significant contributions. Radiation therapy and chemotherapy are both alternative and additional methods of treatment. Chemotherapy in particular is increasingly used both as primary treatment, adjuvant or neoadjuvant therapy in an effort to render inoperable cancer operable. PET scanning is increasingly being applied to the problem of assessing the metabolic response to treatment, and efforts are also being made to use the methodology to provide early prediction of the effectiveness of a chemotherapy regime which if successful could significantly improve patient management and outcome. In some instances PET scanning is providing more accurate information than more conventional anatomical imaging methods: in other cases it provides unique additional information. One of the most important challenges is to define the most accurate and cost-effective diagnostic pathway for any individual clinical situation.

At initial diagnosis an important question is whether the tumour is localized or disseminated. This often determines whether the tumour is resectable for cure by surgical techniques, or whether it has disseminated to such an extent that it cannot be successfully removed by surgery, and needs additional treatment with radiation therapy or chemotherapy. Basic approaches to tumour staging are quite similar from disease to disease. They generally consider:
- the size of the primary lesion (**T stage**)
- whether the primary tumour has spread to regional lymph nodes (**N stage**)
- whether the tumour has spread beyond the nodes to the rest of the body (**M stage**).

Clearly, resecting a primary tumour alone when disease is disseminated systemically will not be curative. Indeed, such an endeavour can be counterproductive in that there are major risks of morbidity, mortality and cost, associated with surgical procedures which are not curative. As an example, for elderly patients with impaired pulmonary function, thoracotomy can result in a mortality of 5–10%. Such a risk, along with a cost of over $25 000 in the US, can scarcely be justified if the disease has spread beyond the surgical field and satisfactory local tumour control can be achieved by non-surgical methods. This scenario occurs in several common cancers, and accurate diagnostic tests are needed to ensure that aggressive or radical surgical procedures are not undertaken in patients who are unlikely to benefit from them, and are indeed more likely to be harmed. By possessing accurate staging information, a rational choice can be made in therapy. One of the first rules in medicine is to 'do no harm'. An accurate understanding of the location(s) of tumours is needed for this to be achieved.

Once cancer is diagnosed, determining how to treat it or whether the treatment is effective can be challenging. Most tumours will eventually shrink in size with effective treatments, but the shrinkage can be slow and sometimes incomplete even though the tumour is 'dead' and has been replaced with scar. In other situations, the area of the tumour may be very hard to assess after surgery or radiation therapy because of clips which distort anatomy, or because of severe anatomic distortions in the region of the lesion. One of the more empirical aspects of cancer management is the choice of what chemotherapeutic agent to use, how to determine if the treatment is working, and to determine how much treatment is enough . . . or too much. Since chemotherapy causes major toxicity and has substantial costs, excessive treatment is undesirable. Treating a scar with chemotherapy is not particularly useful. However, it is very important to treat residual living cancer aggressively. These determinations are not made optimally with current imaging methods.

LIMITATIONS OF ANATOMICAL IMAGING METHODS

1   Inability to determine if a mass is benign or malignant
2   Inability to determine if enlarged lymph nodes contain cancer
3   Inability to detect small tumour foci in lymph nodes or elsewhere
4   Inability to predict or to rapidly assess the response of a cancer to treatment
5   Inability to determine whether a residual abnormality present after treatment represents scar or tumour
6   Difficulty in assessing the entire body for cancer
7   Extreme difficulty in separating benign postoperative or postradiation changes from viable tumour

CT and MRI, while cornerstones of cancer imaging, have major limitations. For example, a recent lung cancer staging trial showed CT to have an accuracy of only about 52% in staging for the presence or absence of lung cancer in the mediastinum. CT and MRI have difficulty in assessing the entire body for cancer and extreme difficulty in separating benign postoperative/postradiation changes from viable tumour.

ADVANTAGES OF METABOLIC IMAGING

1   Ability to distinguish viable metabolically active tissue from scar
2   Potential to use a variety of metabolic tracers to assess different tissue functions
3   Ability to provide quantitative measurements of metabolic activity of cancer cells
4   Potential to detect change before there is any change in size of a mass
5   Detection is dependent on the intensity of the signal rather than the lesion size
6   Postsurgical or postradiotherapy distortion of anatomy is less important for accurate interpretation than MRI or CT

PET offers the proven ability and potential to improve on CT and MRI in these difficult clinical settings. Metabolic imaging complements anatomical imaging and addresses the shortfalls.

PET and the cancer cell

Until quite recently, the use of PET for imaging cancer was considered a research endeavour, requiring a team of researchers. PET technology remains expensive, but if FDG (the most commonly used PET cancer imaging radiopharmaceutical) can be purchased from a regional cyclotron, PET imaging can be initiated for the cost of purchasing and installing a PET imaging system, which can be less than $1 million, or perhaps even less for a specialized hybrid SPECT/PET γ-camera (if performance characteristics are adequate). In addition, clinical results with FDG-PET and the positron-emitter labelled glucose analogue FDG have been very promising in most common cancers, including many situations where CT and MRI have limitations. Thus, in the past decade PET has moved from being a research tool to a clinical tool. Subsequent chapters of this book will present many examples of the clinical utility of PET.

KEY DEVELOPMENTS

1930	Raised aerobic glycolysis in tumour cells	(Warburg 1930)
1979	FDG for cerebral glucose metabolism	(Phelps *et al.* 1979)
1980	FDG for tumours in animals	(Som *et al.* 1980)
1982	FDG in brain tumour	(Patronas *et al.* 1982)
1982	FDG in colon cancer	(Yonekura *et al.* 1982)
1991	FDG for primary and metastatic breast cancer	(Wahl *et al.* 1991)

METABOLIC DIFFERENCES BETWEEN NORMAL TISSUE AND CANCER

Cancer tissue generally has:

- increased glycolysis
- increased protein synthesis
- more anoxic and hypoxic cells
- increased or decreased receptors
- increased DNA synthesis
- increased blood flow
- increased amino acid transport

Although many metabolic alterations are present in cancers but not normal tissues, and have and potentially can be targeted with PET, this clinical atlas focuses mainly on the excessive glucose metabolism seen in many cancers. The observation that tumours have increased rates of aerobic glycolysis compared with normal tissues was first made by Warburg over 50 years ago, but has been shown to be true in most human cancers as well. ^{18}F has a 109 min half-life and is generally cyclotron produced. FDG was first used in humans for brain imaging in the mid 1970s. In 1980, Som and colleagues demonstrated that FDG accumulated into rodent tumours following iv administration, apparently due to metabolic trapping. In 1982, the first imaging of human tumours was reported, both in brain tumours and colorectal cancer metastatic to the liver (Patronas et al. 1982, Yonekura et al. 1982).

PET imaging often 'works' in cancer imaging because cancers differ from normal tissues in several ways. There are multiple alterations in cancer physiology which can be detected using positron emitting tracers. Tumours commonly grow more rapidly than normal tissues, and thus have higher rates of glucose metabolism, DNA synthesis, and amino acid transport than do normal tissues. Tumours often express qualitatively or quantitatively different antigenic phenotypes from many normal tissues, as well as increased numbers of receptors, such as the oestrogen receptor on some breast cancers.

The use of FDG

Although a rather wide range of biochemical alterations can be observed in cancer cells, the one most clinically applied in PET tumour imaging, to date, has been the relative overconsumption of glucose by tumour cells. FDG, the ^{18}F labelled analogue of 2-deoxy-D-glucose, is transported into the cancer cells like glucose by facilitative glucose transporter molecules (often GLUT1), and is phosphorylated to FDG-6-phosphate by hexokinase (often hexokinase type II). FDG-6-phosphate is polar and does not cross cell membranes well, i.e. it is trapped in cancer cells. FDG-6-phosphate can be dephosphorylated to FDG by glucose-6-phosphatase, but this reaction occurs relatively slowly, particularly in cancer cells, which commonly lack glucose-6-phosphatase, or have relatively low levels of it.

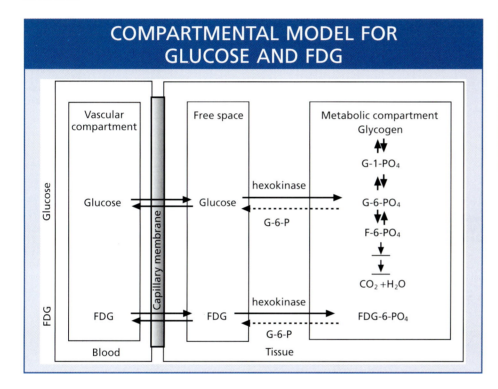

COMPARTMENTAL MODEL FOR GLUCOSE AND FDG

The major tracer used to trace glucose metabolism is FDG, which is transported into cancer cells like glucose and phosphorylated like glucose, but is not substantially moved beyond this point in the intracellular glucose metabolic pathway.

In the past several years, there has been rapid growth in the use of FDG for cancer imaging. This is because, in a wide variety of human cancers, a high tumour/background uptake ratio develops just 0.5–2 h after intravenous injection (Larson *et al.* 1981, Wahl *et al.* 1991) (see Case 3.5 below). The mechanisms for this increased FDG-6-phosphate accumulation in many cancer cells has been shown to be due to:

- increased expression of glucose transporter molecules at the tumour cell surface
- increased levels/activity of hexokinase (and other glycolytic enzymes)
- reduced levels of glucose-6-phosphatase versus most normal tissues (Wahl 1996) and in some instances increased blood flow.

Autoradiographic studies have shown that there is much more FDG uptake into areas of viable tumour than into areas of frank necrosis, but studies in some rodent tumour models and in humans, have shown that the uptake of FDG can be into areas where inflammatory cells are present or into areas of infection (Kubota *et al.* 1992; Brown *et al.* 1993).

BASIS OF FDG USE IN ONCOLOGY

Increased aerobic and anaerobic glycolysis

   increased glucose transport

   increased hexokinase

   decreased glucose-6-phosphatase

Cell surface glucose transporter molecules (GLUT1–5)

Activation of gene coding for synthesis of GLUT1 in tumours

Overexpression of GLUT1 and 3 demonstrated

WHY IS FDG SO USEFUL?

Long half-life for a PET tracer

Availability; regional distribution possible

Relatively high uptake (T/NT) in most human cancers

'Reflects' glycolysis

Cancers often overexpress glucose transporter molecules such as GLUT1, and thus transport in excess glucose; cancers often have elevated levels of hexokinase activity (especially hexokinase type II) and phosphorylate glucose faster than normal tissues; finally some cancers also have slower rates of loss of glucose-6-phosphate from tumours than normal tissues, accentuating the accumulation of phosphorylated glucose analogues in tumours. The quantitative level of alterations in these metabolic pathways will often be greater in the more aggressive than the less aggressive tumours, leading to the potential for characterizing the aggressiveness of human tumours non-invasively.

The normal human *in vivo* distribution of FDG includes the brain, heart, kidneys and urinary tract, at 1 h after tracer injection (Figure 3.1). Myocardial uptake is variable, and highly dependent on the dietary status of the patient. The heart expresses insulin sensitive glucose transporters (GLUT4) and myocardial uptake is thus enhanced in the presence of insulin though in the fasting state there is little uptake of FDG in cardiac or other muscle. Similarly, skeletal muscle has increased uptake of FDG in the presence of insulin. In general, several hours of fasting are recommended before FDG-PET studies in cancer, as fasting lowers insulin levels and also generally reduces blood sugar levels compared to the postprandial state (Wahl *et al.* 1991). Uptake within the myocardium can be variable. Both patients shown in Figure 3.1 were scanned after a 6 h fast, yet uptake within the myocardium is very different.

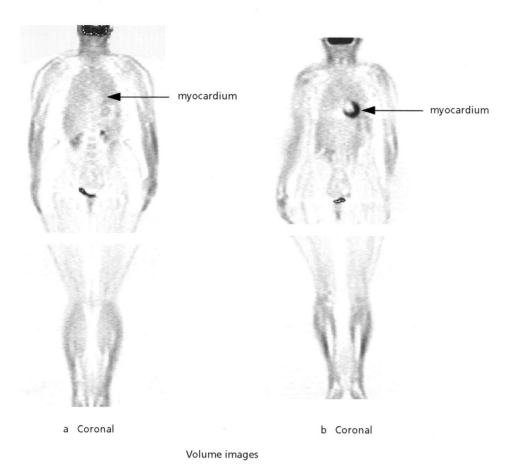

a Coronal   b Coronal

Volume images

Figure 3.1 *Normal human FDG uptake.*

High blood glucose levels can interfere with tumour targeting owing to competitive inhibition of FDG uptake by D-glucose. The latter phenomenon has been shown in preclinical and clinical series, although diabetes does not preclude the possibility of PET imaging of cancer in many patients. At present, the optimal method for handling diabetic patients for PET imaging is uncertain, but many centres have the patients fast and do not administer additional insulin, despite serum glucose level elevations, and obtain useful diagnostic information. Tumour SUVs can be lower than expected in diabetic patients, however.

The exact meaning of the 'signal' seen during PET imaging of cancers remains a matter of intense investigation. FDG does not trace glucose metabolism exactly: FDG has somewhat more uptake into tumours than would be expected for a tracer of glucose metabolism alone. This may be due to differences in transport of FDG and D-glucose, or possibly due to altered affinity of hexokinase for FDG rather than D-glucose, as their metabolism is clearly not identical. Although initial studies in brain tumours suggested that FDG uptake was strongly related to the proliferative activity of tumour cells, this has been questioned. *In vitro* a strong correlation has been seen between the number of viable cancer cells and the extent of FDG uptake, though this area has only had limited careful evaluation. This relationship between FDG uptake and the number of viable cancer cells also been shown *in vivo* in several animal models, in breast cancer, for example (Brown *et al.* 1996). This area remains under intense study, but there seems little question that high levels of FDG uptake are most consistent with a substantial number of viable cancer cells being present. In the absence of overt infectious/inflammatory process, several studies in patients have shown higher uptake in tumour with the highest proliferative rate. It should be noted that preliminary clinical data from several centres suggests that some tumours are less well seen with FDG-PET than others, e.g. prostate cancer and some renal cancers and hepatomas, and the reasons for these disparities are under evaluation. In general, it seems that high FDG uptake is associated with a fairly high number of viable tumour cells, that tumour cell growth may be rapid, and that inflammatory cells may also be present, contributing to a high tumour signal. It should also be noted that FDG is by no means a specific tracer of tumour metabolism; rather it traces glucose utilization, and non-neoplastic conditions such as sarcoidosis and some infections can have intense FDG uptake *in vivo*. It is apparent that several factors govern FDG uptake into tumours, but clinical studies generally show that high FDG uptake is generally associated with tumours which are aggressive.

Future clinical tracers for cancer

While many amino acids and DNA precursors are overtransported or overutilized by cancers, the only such agent extensively applied clinically to date in cancer imaging has been [^{11}C]L-methionine, a tracer with a 20 min half-life. This agent is more restricted in availability than FDG, because of its much shorter half-life (20 min for ^{11}C vs. 109 min for ^{18}F), but can be very helpful in imaging brain and other tumours. Increased transport and metabolism of several amino acids are commonly seen in cancers and represent useful physiological alterations for imaging with PET. Many amino acids have been evaluated, but [^{11}C]L-methionine is the one with which there is the greatest clinical experience in PET imaging. Use of [^{11}C]L-methionine in cancer imaging is based on this experience and the increased activity of the transmethylation pathways in some cancers. There is normally substantial uptake of this tracer in the pancreas, salivary glands, liver, bone marrow and kidneys. [^{11}C]L-Methionine is a natural amino acid, so there is some metabolism of it in the bloodstream and some limited uptake of ^{11}C into the normal brain, though the uptake is much lower there than with FDG. This tracer has been used in brain tumour imaging (including pituitary adenomas), in head and neck cancer imaging, in lymphomas and in lung cancers (Bergstrom *et al.* 1983, Kubota *et al.* 1985). The study of amino acid transport may be all that is possible if ^{11}C with its 20 min half-life is chosen as the tracer, as even with [^{11}C]L-methionine much of the early imaging is of the transport process, with relatively less of the protein synthetic process.

Other alterations in tumour physiology may be more tumour specific than general, allowing for the development of very specific PET radiopharmaceuticals. As an example, radioligands with specificity for the oestrogen receptor expressed on many well-differentiated breast cancers are quite specific for their uptake into tissues rich in oestrogen receptor (Mintun *et al.* 1988). Similarly, PET tracers specific for monoamine uptake pathways are quite specific for adrenergic tissues such as pheochromocytomas (Shulkin *et al.* 1993).

Other PET tracers of interest, but currently much more commonly used in research than in clinical applications include:
- [^{11}C] thymidine and other radiolabelled DNA precursors
- labelled chemotherapeutic agents
- labelled receptor or antigen binding ligands
- agents which trace tumour blood flow and tumour hypoxia.

Perhaps the best studied of such ligands to date is [^{18}F]**17-β-oestradiol (FES)**, which has been used in breast cancer imaging studies in humans. While beyond the scope of this clinical book, such agents have considerable potential for expanding the role of PET into clinical practice as well as being valuable research tools.

How PET can be used clinically

HOW PET CAN BE USED CLINICALLY

		Examples
1	Diagnosis and grading	Benign vs malignant single lung nodule
		Prognostic grading of primary brain tumour
2	Extent of disease (staging/restaging), local and distant	Non-small cell lung cancer or Hodgkin's disease or melanoma
3	Localization of disease	Unknown primary or rising serum tumour markers
4	Treatment response, monitoring treatment	Lymphoma with or without residual mass
5	Suspected relapse of disease localization of raised serum markers, clinical features or radiological changes	Treated squamous cell carcinoma of the head and neck
6	Guiding biopsy	Brain or lung cancer or PUO in immunocompromised patient
7	Planning and guiding therapy	Brain tumour – siting of radioactive implants

Diagnostic

Case 3.1: Benign vs. malignant

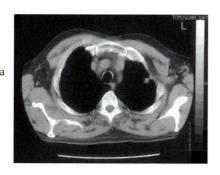

a

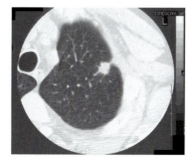

c

CT-bone and lung windows

b   Transaxial FDG

This 71 year old man had long standing pleural calcification secondary to asbestos exposure. Routine chest radiography showed possible new changes at the left apex. CT showed a 1cm pulmonary nodule in the left upper lobe. CT biopsy was unsuccessful with an acellular aspirate. In view of the patient's age and extensive pleural calcification, he was referred for a PET scan to assess the likelihood of malignancy before an open biopsy was attempted. The PET scan showed intense uptake of FDG within the nodule, SUV = 6.8, indicating the lesion was highly likely to be malignant. Open resection was performed and the diagnosis of carcinoma confirmed.

> PET-FDG can distinguish malignant from benign solitary pulmonary nodules. This may be particularly important if there is a contraindication to invasive biopsy or with a failed biopsy.

Extent of disease

Case 3.2: Staging/restaging

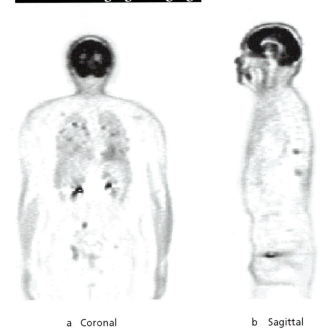

a Coronal   b Sagittal

This 32 year old patient who had malignant melanoma excised from the sternum in December 1993 subsequently developed axillary lymphadenopathy. PET scanning was performed to determine whether there was disease present elsewhere. The scan shows multiple metastases within right infraclavicular fossa, lung, iliac lymph nodes (coronal image) and bone (sagittal).

Localization of disease

Case 3.3

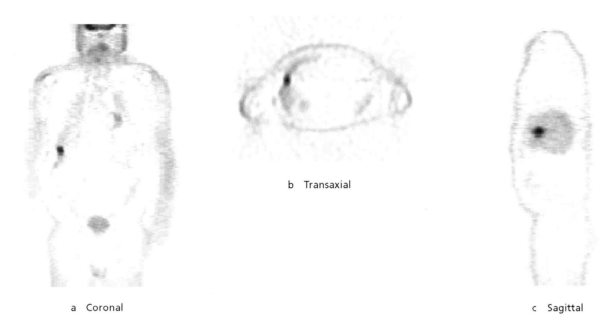

a Coronal

b Transaxial

c Sagittal

Male with rising CEA following hemicolectomy and adjuvant chemotherapy for carcinoma of the colon. Colonoscopy and CT did not reveal active disease. The PET scan revealed a solitary metastasis in the liver with high FDG uptake within the lesion. A wedge resection of the liver was performed. No other disease was identified within the abdomen at laparotomy.

Treatment response

Case 3.4: Hodgkin's disease

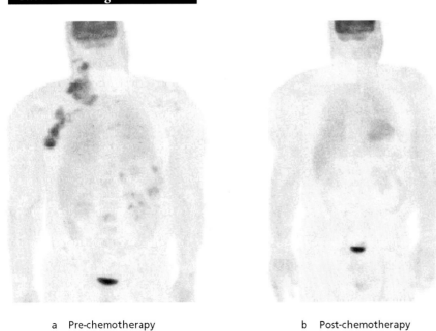

a Pre-chemotherapy

b Post-chemotherapy

This 56 year old man with Hodgkin's disease was scanned prior to treatment, with evidence of lymph node involvement in the right neck, axilla and spleen. After six cycles of chemotherapy, there is complete resolution of FDG uptake.

Suspected relapse

Case 3.5

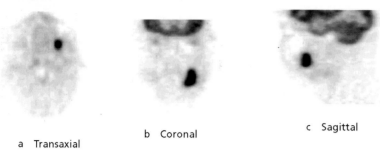

a Transaxial   b Coronal   c Sagittal

This 56 year old woman presented with a recurrent ulcerating lesion in the left retro-molar region clinically invading the mandible. Biopsy revealed recurrent squamous cell carcinoma. CT suggested recurrent disease in the left retromolar region with possible infiltration of mandibular marrow and ipsilateral nodal involvement. The PET scan confirmed recurrent left retromolar cancer with localized involvement of the mandible but no lymphatic spread.

Guiding biopsy

Case 3.6

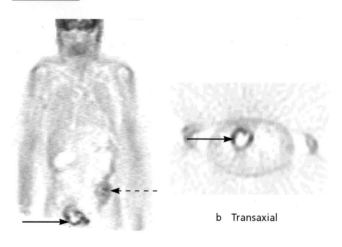

a Coronal   b Transaxial

This 60 year old man with a functioning renal transplant 12 years previously on immunosuppression presented with a pyrexia of unknown origin with no obvious clinical clues as to a possible source. CT scan of the abdomen was reported as showing a renal transplant in the left iliac fossa and a calcified mass in the right iliac fossa due either to a previous transplant or a calcified haematoma. PET scanning revealed a rim of intense uptake of FDG around a photon deficient area (solid arrow), reported as either a tumour with central necrosis or possibly infection or inflammation surrounding a previous transplant. No abnormal uptake was seen elsewhere on the scan to suggest another source for the fever. Physiological uptake was seen in the functioning left renal transplant (broken arrow). Biopsy of the mass revealed lymphoma, which had arisen *de novo* rather than at the site of a previous transplant.

Planning therapy

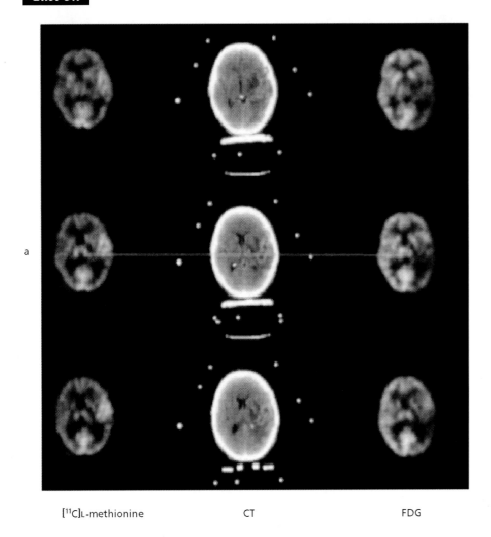

a

[¹¹C]L-methionine   CT   FDG

This patient with a recurrent left parietal lobe glioma underwent registered CT and PET scanning using [¹¹C] L-methionine and FDG. The linked cursor display enables the same reference point to be viewed in the three scans simultaneously, combining the functional and anatomical information required for optimal siting of radioactive implants. Note the external radioactive markers used on the CT to register to the PET images.

References and further reading

Bergstrom M, Collins VP, Ehras E *et al.* (1983) Discrepancies in brain tumor extent as shown by CT and PET using ^{68}Ga-EDTA, ^{11}C-glucose and ^{11}C-methionine. *J Comput Assist Tomogr* **6**, 1062–6.

Brown RS, Fisher SJ, Wahl RL (1993) Autoradiographic evaluation of the intra-tumoral distribution of 2-deoxy-D-glucose and monoclonal antibodies in xenografts of human ovarian adenocarcinoma. *J Nucl Med* **34**(1), 75–82.

Brown RS, Leung JY, Fisher S *et al.* (1996) Intratumoral distribution of tritiated-FDG in breast carcinoma: correlation between glut-1 expression and FDG uptake. *J Nucl Med,* **37**(6), 1042–7.

Erasmus JJ, McAdams HP, Patz EF Jr *et al.* (1998) Thoracic FDG PET: state of the art. *Radiographics* **18**(1), 5–20.

Hoh CK, Schiepers C, Seltzer MA *et al.* (1997) PET in oncology: will it replace the other modalities? *Sem in Nucl Med* **27**(2), 94–106.

Kubota K, Matsuzawa T, Ito M *et al.* (1985) Lung tumor imaging by positron emission tomography using ^{11}C-L-methionine. *J Nucl Med* **26**, 37–42.

Kubota R, Yamada S, Kubota K *et al.* (1992) Intratumoral distribution of fluorine-18 fluorodeoxyglucose in vivo: High accumulation in macrophages and granulation tissues studied. *J Nucl Med* **33**(11), 1972–80.

Larson SM, Weiden PL, Grunbaum Z *et al.* (1981) Positron imaging feasibility studies. II: Characteristics of 2-deoxyglucose uptake in rodent and canine neoplasms. Concise communication. J *Nucl Med* **22**(10), 875–9.

McGuirt WF, Greven K, Williams D 3rd *et al.* (1998) PET scanning in head and neck oncology: a review. *Head & Neck* **20**(3), 208–15.

Mintun MA, Welch MJ, Siegel BA *et al.* (1988) Breast cancer: PET imaging of estrogen receptors. *Radiology* **169**(1), 45–8.

Patronas NJ, DiChiro G, Brooks RA *et al.* (1982) Work in progress: 18F fluorodeoxyglucose and PET in the evaluation of radiation necrosis of the brain. *Radiology* **144**, 885–9.

Paulus P, Hustinx R, Daenen F *et al.* (1997) Usefulness of 18FDG positron emission tomography detection and follow-up of digestive cancers. *Acta Gastroent Belgica* **60**(4), 278–80.

Phelps ME, Huang SC, Hoffman EJ *et al.* (1979) Tomographic measurement of local cerebral glucose metabolic rate in humans with 18F2-fluoro-2-deoxy-D-glucose: validation of method. *Ann Neurol* **5**, 371–88.

Shulkin BL, Koeppe RA, Francis IR *et al.* (1993) Pheochromocytomas that do not accumulate metaiodobenzylguanidine: Localization with PET and administration of FDG. *Radiology* **186**(3), 711–15.

Smith TA (1998) FDG uptake, tumour characteristics and response to therapy: a review. *Nucl Med Commun* **19**(2), 97–105.

Som P, Atkins HL, Bandoypadhyay D *et al.* (1980) A fluorinated glucose analogue 2-fluoro-2-deoxy-D-glucose. Non toxic tracer for rapid tumour detection. *J Nucl Med* **21**, 670–5.

Wahl RL (1996) Targeting glucose transporters for tumor imaging: 'sweet' idea, 'sour' result. *J Nucl Med* **37**(6), 1038–41.

Wahl RL (1997) Clinical oncology update: the emerging role of positron emission tomography: Part I. *PPO Updates: Principles and Practice of Oncology* **11**(1), 1–24.

Wahl RL (1997) Clinical oncology update: the emerging role of positron emission tomography: Part II. *PPO Updates: Principles and Practice of Oncology* **11**(2), 1–23.

Wahl RL, Cody R, Hutchins GD, Mudgett E (1991) Primary and metastatic breast carcinoma: Initial clinical evaluation with PET with the radiolabelled glucose analog 2-[^{18}F]-fluoro-deoxy-2-D-glucose (FDG). *Radiology* **179**, 765–70.

Wahl RL, Hutchins GD, Buchsbaum DJ *et al.* (1991) ^{18}F-2-deoxy-2-fluoro-D-glucose uptake into human tumor xenografts. Feasibility studies for cancer imaging with positron-emission tomography. *Cancer* **67**, 1544–50.

Warburg O (1930) *The Metabolism of Tumors,* trans. F Dickens. Constable, London, pp. 129–69.

Yonekura Y, Benau RS, Brill AB *et al.* (1982) Increased accumulation of 2-deoxy-2-^{18}F fluoro-D-glucose in liver metastases from colon cancer. *J Nucl Med* **12**, 1133–7.

Part II

Applications of PET in oncology

Chapter 4

Lymphoma

Introduction and background

Hodgkin's disease (HD) and non-Hodgkin's lymphoma (NHL) are common and important malignancies which are increasing in frequency (especially NHL). Although they have many features in common and share common treatments, there are significant differences between the two conditions which must be appreciated for both diagnosis and treatment.

- **Hodgkin's disease** starts as a unifocal disease involving a single group of malignant lymph nodes and spreads via adjacent associated lymph node groups. Limited stage disease is treated appropriately with radiation therapy which results in a complete cure in a high proportion of patients. Even after recurrence, treatment can result in a permanent cure. Patients with bulky disease and stage III–IV disease have a poorer prognosis and usually require treatment with chemotherapy in addition to radiotherapy.

- **Non-Hodgkin's lymphoma** is a multifocal disseminated disease usually requiring combined chemotherapy, sometimes radiotherapy and in some instances high dose chemotherapy with bone marrow transplantation. The disease is ultimately fatal in most patients but long remissions and cure can be effectively induced, particularly in high grade tumours which if untreated would be rapidly fatal. Low grade non-Hodgkin's lymphoma, although carrying a better prognosis untreated, fails to respond as well to chemotherapy and consequently may, paradoxically, have a worse prognosis.

Many patients with lymphomas (up to 25%) have systemic symptoms including fever, weight loss and night sweats, which often indicates a poorer prognosis. Disease outside the lymph nodes occurs in 10–20% and is more common in patients with non-Hodgkin's lymphoma. Conventional staging includes clinical examination and CT of the chest, abdomen and pelvis, and is more critical in management of patients with Hodgkin's disease than with non-Hodgkin's lymphoma.

EPIDEMIOLOGY

	Hodgkin's disease	Non-Hodgkin's lymphoma
Incidence	30 per million	100–200 per million
Peak age	<40 years	>40 years
M/F	F = M	M > F

The incidence of lymphoma is increasing in industrialized countries, with significant differences in incidence, age peaks and sex ratios between Hodgkin's disease and non-Hodgkin's lymphoma.

PATHOLOGY

Tumour types	
HD	NHL
Nodular sclerosing (70%)	Low grade
Lymphocyte predominant (15%)	Intermediate grade
Mixed cellularity (10%)	High grade
Lymphocyte depleted (5%)	

There are several systems of classifying lymphoma in current use for pathological classification. This is the most widely used at present.

PROGNOSIS

HD	NHL
75% 5 year survival	Low grade: 70% 5 year survival
	High–intermediate: 40% 5 year survival rate
Overall 40% have disease free survival	

Hodgkin's disease, if localized and effectively treated, can be expected to be cured. Non-Hodgkin's lymphoma is more likely to be fatal, but there is a great deal of variation.

STAGING OF HD AND NHL

Stage I	Single lymph node region or localized (unifocal) extralymphocytic site
Stage II	Two or more lymph node regions on same side of diaphragm or localized extralymphatic site and its regional nodes (± other lymph node regions on same side of diaphragm)
Stage III	Lymph node regions on both sides of the diaphragm ± involvement of an associated extralymphatic site or spleen or both
Stage IV	Multifocal involvement of one or more extralymphatic sites ± associated lymph node or isolated extralymphatic site with distant (non-regional) nodal involvement

Generally staging is more important in Hodgkin's disease than non-Hodgkin's lymphoma as it is more likely to determine the therapeutic regime. Staging should indicate whether it is clinical only or based on pathology (P). The stages are divided into A (no systemic symptoms) or B (systemic symptoms): weight loss, fever, night sweats. Gallium has been used for staging but is poor below the diaphragm and in low grade lymphoma. CT is generally used but suffers from a low sensitivity.

OTHER NON-NODAL METASTATIC SITES (FREQUENCY)

	HD	NHL
Marrow	−	++
Spleen	+	+
Liver	−	+
CNS	−	+
Skin	−	+
GI tract	−	++
Testes	−	+
Bone	+	+

−, uncommon; +, common; ++, very frequent.

Non-Hodgkin's lymphoma is a multifocal disease rather than a spreading nodal disease. Non-Hodgkin's lymphoma patients are much more likely to develop non-nodal metastatic sites than patients with Hodgkin's disease.

Key management issues

PET in lymphoma

Both Hodgkin's disease and non-Hodgkin's lymphoma can be imaged well with PET using either FDG or [^{11}C]L-methionine. The earliest positron imaging of lymphoma was with planar γ cameras and FDG. In this early work, FDG was shown to detect more non-Hodgkin's lymphoma than ^{67}Ga. Most clinical series have shown that PET will detect nearly all untreated lesions of these lymphomas (unlike CT), and that tracer uptake declines promptly with effective therapy, e.g. all (>50) known lesions of a variety of grades and types of lymphoma were detected using attenuation corrected FDG-PET and several additional lesions in normal sized lymph nodes were identified only by PET. Data suggest that FDG uptake is likely to be higher in untreated high grade lymphomas than in low grade lymphomas, but there is considerable overlap in SUVs. In 22 patients with untreated non-Hodgkin's lymphoma studied by PET and flow cytometry, there was a significant correlation between SUV for FDG and the S-phase fraction (proliferative rate). Infrequently PET scans with FDG in low grade lymphomas may have low tracer uptake, sometimes making tumour detection difficult. It has been suggested that [^{11}C]L-methionine may be better in such situations, but this area is not fully studied. It has also been suggested that [^{11}C]L-methionine uptake is not well related to the proliferative state of lymphomas, but these data are very limited. Although PET is widely being applied to lymphoma imaging in many clinical centres, the published literature on PET in lymphomas is still evolving rapidly. At present, many investigators use PET for lymphoma staging, and (at least in the authors' experience) to determine if a residual abnormality present on CT after treatment is metabolically active or inactive, and thus whether additional treatment is required. The quality of FDG-PET images in low grade lymphomas is much better (again in the authors' experience) than with ^{67}Ga (even if high dose and SPECT are used), consistent with the first published report on imaging lymphoma with FDG. We expect Hodgkin's disease and non-Hodgkin's lymphoma to be among the most common clinical indications for PET in the future.

Examples to illustrate key issues

Key issue 1 Staging prior to treatment

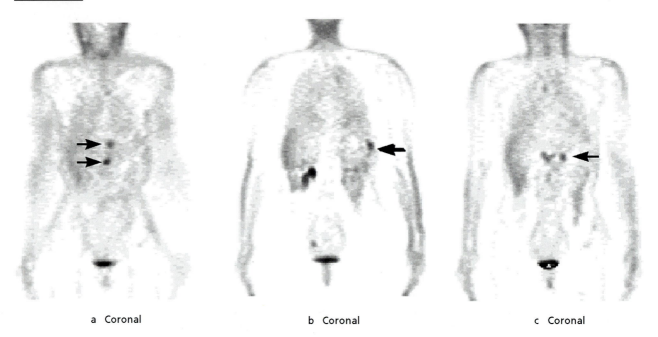

| a Coronal | b Coronal | c Coronal |

A 42 year old woman presented with palpable lymph nodes in the left neck and left supraclavicular fossa; biopsy revealed Hodgkin's disease. CT scan of chest, abdomen and pelvis were normal. The PET scan shows increased uptake of FDG in mesenteric nodes (left coronal image), spleen (middle image) and para-aortic nodes (right image). Hold-up of urine in the right ureter is noted. This PET scan upstaged the patient from stage I to stage III and her treatment was changed from local radiotherapy to systemic chemotherapy.

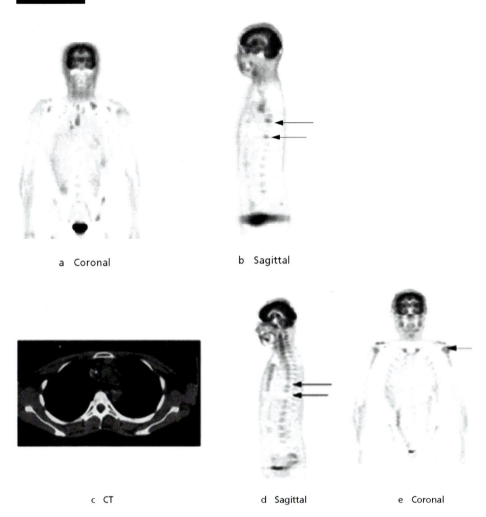

a Coronal

b Sagittal

c CT

d Sagittal

e Coronal

Image (e) from R Carr, SF Barrington, B Madan, CAB Saunders, J van der Walt, AR Timothy. Blood May 1998 91(9), 3340 Fig. 2B. Reproduced with permission.

This 31 year old woman with Hodgkin's disease had evidence of nodal disease (a) and bone infiltration with focal increased uptake in the thoracic spine at T8 and T10 (b). She received local radiotherapy to the thoracic spine together with chemotherapy. There was resolution of nodal disease on the CT, except for a residual mediastinal mass (c). The patient continued to complain of generalized aches and pains. On a repeat PET there was absence of uptake at previously irradiated sites within bone (d); diffusely increased marrow uptake and intense focal uptake within the humeri, more marked on the left. No FDG uptake was seen within the mediastinum and biopsy of the mediastinal mass confirmed absence of viable tumour. Biopsy of the left humerus confirmed infiltration by Hodgkin's disease, whilst iliac crest trephine biopsy showed no evidence of marrow infiltration. The focal changes in bone on the PET scan subsequent to therapy indicated the presence of active disease; the diffuse uptake in bone was likely to be a response to chemotherapy.

> Diffusely increased uptake of FDG within bone marrow may be seen following chemotherapy or treatment with colony stimulating factor, or due to tumour infiltration or marrow hyperplasia of other causes.

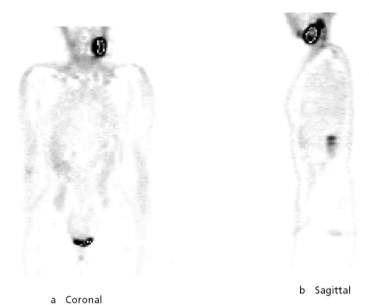

a Coronal

b Sagittal

This 26 year old woman with Hodgkin's disease presented with palpable disease in the left neck. CT indicated bilateral cervical lymphadenopathy and enlarged left supra-clavicular fossa nodes. The PET scan showed disease in the left cervical region only. PET downstaged the patient from stage II to stage I. Note also the uptake within the injection site in the right antecubital fossa (coronal) and the physiological renal activity (sagittal).

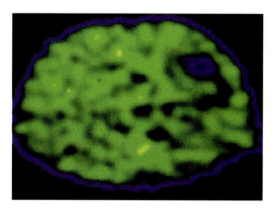

b Transmission

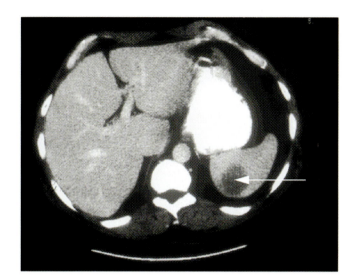

a CT

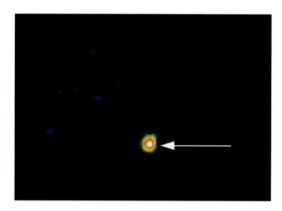

c Emission

From JS Newman, IR Francis, MS Kaminski and RL Wahl. Radiology *190, 111–16, Figs 1a, d. Reproduced with permission.*

This patient with low grade non-Hodgkin's lymphoma had a large hypoattenuating mass within the spleen seen on CT. There was intense uptake of FDG within the splenic mass (arrowed on emission scan), which was subsequently confirmed to contain tumour. The transmission scan is included for anatomical reference.

Non-Hodgkin's lymphoma spreads via the lymphatic system and the pattern of disease is one of multifocal disease within separate lymph node groups. By contrast, Hodgkin's disease spreads locally and disease is most commonly seen in adjacent lymph node groups.

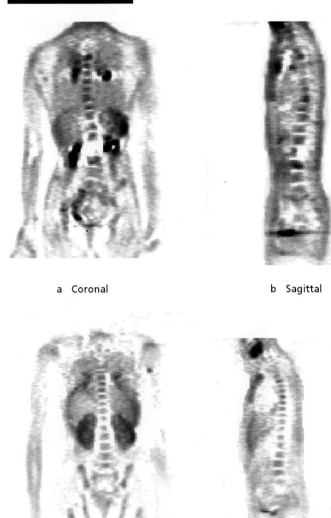

a Coronal   b Sagittal

c Coronal   d Sagittal

Image 4.6c from R Carr, SF Barrington, B Madan, CAB Saunders, J van der Walt, AR Timothy. Blood May 1998 91(9), 3340–46, Fig. 4B. Reproduced with permission.

Coronal and sagittal views are shown of whole body studies using FDG in two patients with Hodgkin's disease; both had increased bone marrow uptake of FDG. The first patient (a,b) had nodal disease (cervical, mediastinal, hilar and splenic uptake is shown) and marrow infiltration by Hodgkin's on iliac crest trephine biopsy. The second patient (c,d) had nodal disease (cervical, supraclavicular and left axillary uptake is shown) with marrow hyperplasia rather than infiltration on trephine biopsy.

Increased uptake of FDG into marrow in patients with lymphoma may be due to tumour infiltration or secondary to marrow hyperplasia. In our experience of scanning 50 patients at initial presentation with lymphoma and correlating marrow uptake of FDG with unilateral iliac crest trephine, provided the primary disease site accumulates FDG, absence of increased marrow uptake indicates that the marrow is not involved. Where increased uptake of FDG is present, marrow biopsy is indicated to distinguish from other causes.

'Cold' artefacts may be produced where they are adjacent to areas of intense uptake of tracer as seen in Case 4.5 where a cold area in L2 is seen adjacent to the high uptake within the renal pelvis. This is particularly true when filtered back projection algorithms are used.

Sagittal views are particularly useful for assessing spinal disease.

Case 4.7

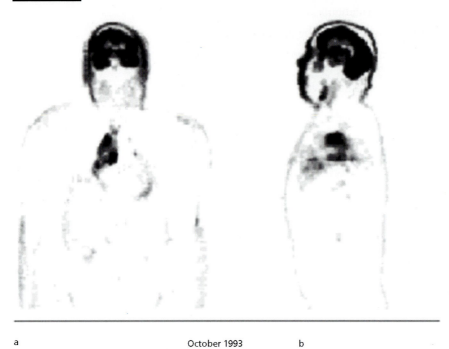

a   October 1993   b

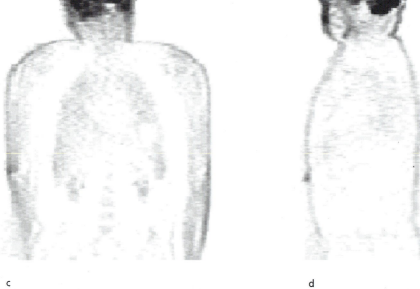

c   d

                    March 1994

At presentation this 36 year old man with Hodgkin's disease had evidence of disease within the right paratracheal region and both lung hila, indicating stage II disease (a,b). Rescanning after radiotherapy (c,d) showed complete resolution of disease.

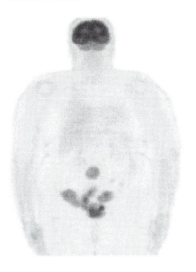
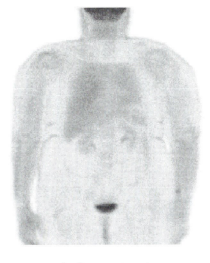

a Pre-treatment   b Post-treatment

This 68 year old woman with high grade non-Hodgkin's lymphoma presented with an abdominal mass. The PET scan showed intense uptake of FDG into small bowel, disease in mesenteric nodes (a) and the right lung (not shown). Following chemotherapy there was complete resolution of disease including bowel (b).

> FDG-PET is particularly valuable in assessing abdominal lymphoma, where other imaging methods are poor.

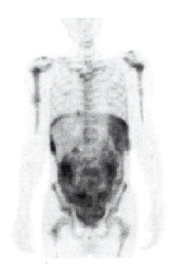
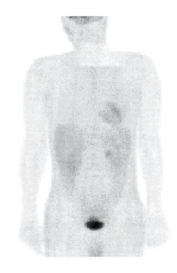

a Pre-treatment   b Post-treatment

From SF Barrington, R Carr. Clin Oncol 7, 334–5. Reproduced with permission.

A 32 year old man presented with a right iliac fossa mass. At surgery the bowel and peritoneum was seen to be heavily infiltrated by tumour. Histology revealed Burkitt's lymphoma and there was marrow involvement by trephine biopsy. CT scan performed at diagnosis was entirely normal. The PET scan showed diffusely increased uptake within marrow, bowel and peritoneum (a). There was clinical response to chemotherapy confirmed by the FDG-PET scan, showing complete resolution of disease, only 9 days after starting chemotherapy (b).

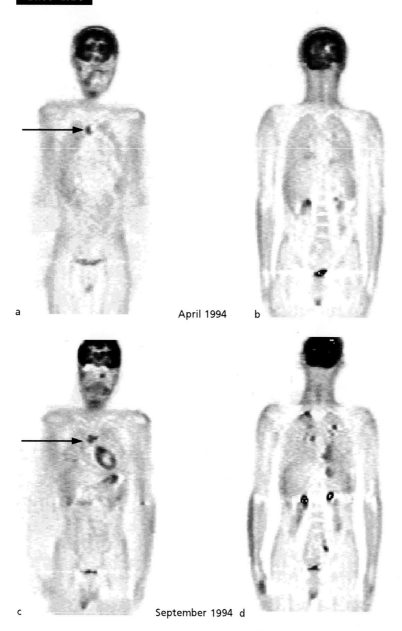

a   April 1994   b

c   September 1994   d

This 19 year old man was diagnosed with Hodgkin's disease in 1993. PET scan performed in April 1994 after treatment with radiotherapy and chemotherapy showed residual disease within the mediastinum (arrowed in a). The patient was treated with further chemotherapy and a bone marrow autograft. Despite this, PET scan performed in September 1994 showed enlargement of mediastinal uptake (c), new lesions in both lung fields and the right hilum (d). The case illustrates progressive disease despite treatment as monitored by PET.

Normal gastric and myocardial uptake often varies within the same patient at different scanning sessions despite the same instructions for patient preparation being given on both occasions. Care must be taken with image displays when comparisons are made. This variability also seems to be true for colonic tracer uptake.

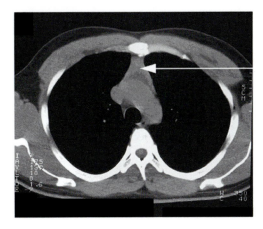

a CT

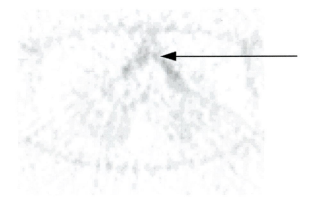

b PET

This 35 year old man was treated with chemotherapy for non-Hodgkin's lymphoma. An increase in thymic size was noted on CT (a) following treatment. PET was performed to assess whether the increase in size represented thymic rebound hyperplasia in response to treatment or residual disease. Low grade FDG uptake was seen in the thymus (b), suggestive of thymic hyperplasia.

Normal thymic (FDG) uptake may be seen in children and young adults, and uptake of FDG in the thymus should not be confused with residual or progressive disease.

Key issue 3 Detection of recurrence

Case 4.12

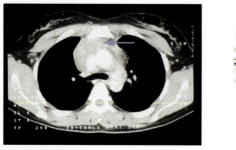 

a CT   b Transaxial

After treatment, the only evidence of residual disease on CT scanning of this 37 year old woman was an anterior mediastinal mass (a). The PET showed no uptake of FDG within the anterior mediastinum, suggesting the residual mass represented fibrotic tissue only (b). At 9 months follow up the patient remained well clinically without evidence of further enlargement of the mass on CT.

> Residual mediastinal masses after treatment for lymphoma may remain for months or years without regressing. Conventional anatomical imaging cannot distinguish tumour from fibrosis. A negative PET may give the clinician the confidence to adopt a conservative observational approach without resort to biopsy.

Case 4.13

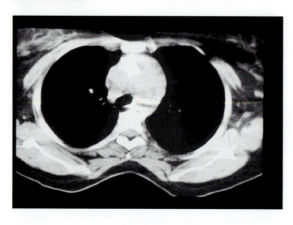 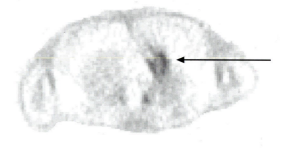

a CT   b Transaxial

This 25 year old patient had FDG uptake within a bulky mediastinal mass following treatment, indicating the presence of active tumour. Biopsy confirmed the presence of residual lymphoma.

Case 4.14

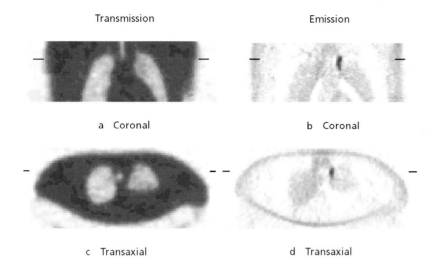

Transmission

a Coronal

c Transaxial

Emission

b Coronal

d Transaxial

This patient with non-Hodgkin's lymphoma and a residual mediastinal mass shown here on the transmission scan (a,c) had evidence of FDG uptake within the mass. Biopsy confirmed the presence of active disease. The Ga^{67} scan was negative.

Case 4.15

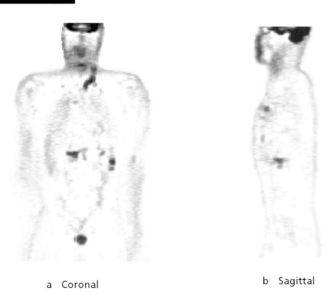

a Coronal

b Sagittal

This 35 year old man with non-Hodgkin's lymphoma responded well to treatment with radiotherapy followed by a stem cell transplant in 1995. At a routine follow up visit in July 1996, thoracic and abdominal CT were performed which indicated the presence of new enlarged lymph nodes at the porta hepatis. There was no evidence of disease elsewhere. FDG-PET scanning showed additional sites in the supraclavicular fossae, spleen (a), mediastinum and abdominal para-aortic nodes (a,b).

> The focal uptake seen within the coronal image in the region of the spleen is distinct from the diffuse uptake seen within the gut which is physiological.

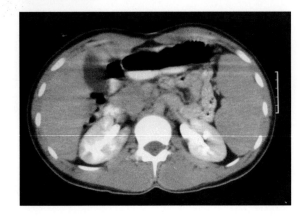

a   CT

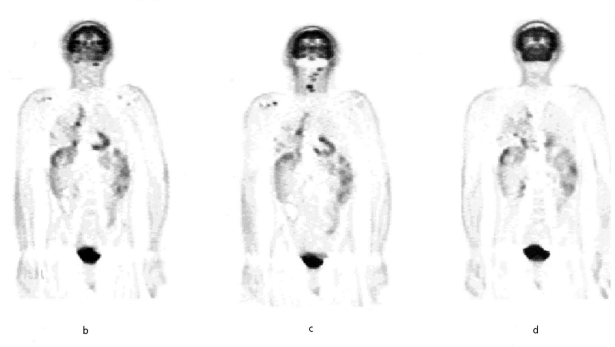

b   c   d

Coronal images

This 25 year old man was diagnosed with Hodgkin's disease in 1992. He was successfully treated and remained in complete remission until 1994, when a routine follow
up CT suggested enlargement of spleen size (a). PET scanning (b–d) indicated multiple
sites of disease with FDG uptake in the neck, supraclavicular fossae, chest, liver and
spleen. Splenectomy confirmed involvement of the spleen with mixed histology of
Hodgkin's disease and non-Hodgkin's lymphoma. The histology was reviewed retrospectively with the original histology, the change in tumour type confirmed, and the
patient's chemotherapy regime altered.

Case 4.17

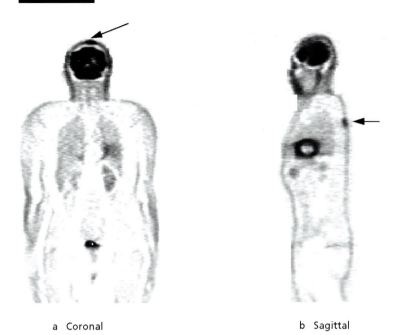

a Coronal   b Sagittal

This 71 year old woman with non-Hodgkin's lymphoma presented to clinic after 2 years in complete remission with a palpable scalp nodule. Uptake of FDG within the scalp nodule was seen (arrowed on a). In addition focal FDG uptake was noted within the skin overlying the region of the left scapula (arrowed on b). The patient was re-examined and a 2 cm skin nodule noted, fine needle aspiration of which revealed the active non-Hodgkin's lymphoma.

> FDG-PET is particularly useful for identifying cutaneous involvement with lymphoma and uptake will appear enhanced without attenuation correction.

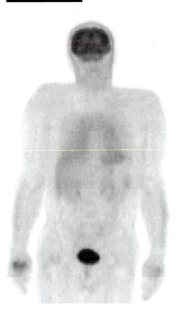
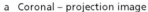
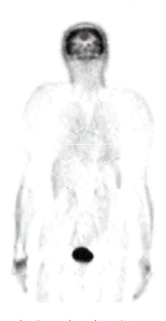

a Coronal – projection image   b Coronal – volume image

This 53 year old patient with Hodgkin's disease developed avascular necrosis of the hips resulting in bilateral hip replacements following treatment in 1988. He remained in complete remission until he re-presented with back pain and right hip pain. ^{99m}Tc bone scan showed increased uptake in L3 and in the right femur distal to the hip replacement. Radiography showed sclerosis in the distal femur. Bilateral hip replacements are more clearly seen in the projection image on PET. There was no evidence of abnormal FDG uptake within the spine or femur. Subsequent biopsy of the right femur showed avascular necrosis only.

> False negative FDG-PET scans in patients with active lymphoma are rare.
>
> Bilateral increased uptake within the hands in this case was due to increased uptake within muscle where the patient had been gripping the couch during the uptake period.

Key issue 4 Differential diagnosis

Case 4.19

Transaxial

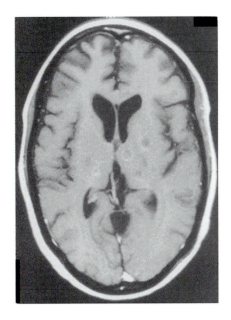

a MRI

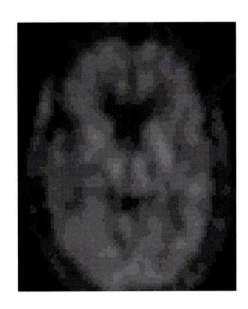

b FDG-PET

From MJ O'Doherty, SF Barrington, M Campbell, J Lowe, CS Bradbeer. Journal of Nuclear Medicine 1997; 38(10), 1575–83, Fig. 2A,B. Reproduced with permission.

This young African woman with known HIV disease had small white matter lesions on MRI, the differential diagnosis of which included toxoplasmosis or lymphoma. Absence of FDG uptake within these lesions was suggestive of toxoplasmosis, which was supported on the basis of a successful response to toxoplasma treatment.

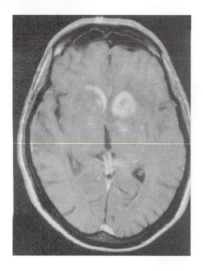

a MRI

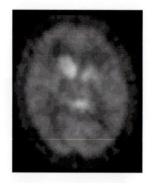

b Transaxial

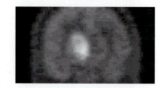

c Coronal

FDG-PET

*From MJ O'Doherty, SF Barrington, M Campbell, J Lowe, CS Bradbeer. Journal of Nuclear Medicine 1997; **38**(10), 1575–83, Fig. 3A,B. Reproduced with permission.*

This man with known HIV disease presented with confusion. Intense uptake of FDG (b,c) within the mass lesions identified on MRI (a) suggested the presence of lymphoma, which was proven on biopsy.

> Differentiating intracerebral lymphoma from toxoplasmosis in HIV positive patients is frequently impossible with MRI/CT: PET scans can usually make the distinction. In a study of 23 patients with HIV and space-occupying lesion, SUVs for toxoplasma ranged from 0.14 to 3.7, for lymphoma from 3.9 to 8.7.

This young man with HIV was initially treated for lymphoma within the right sacroiliac joint. The PET scan done at diagnosis is shown with intense uptake of FDG within the right sacroiliac bone (a,b). There was complete resolution of FDG uptake after treatment (c,d).

Pre-treatment

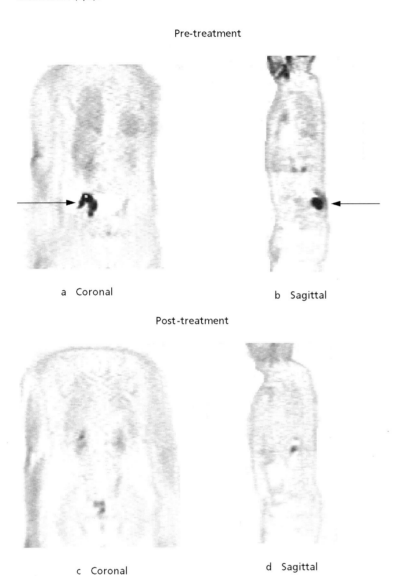

a Coronal

b Sagittal

Post-treatment

c Coronal

d Sagittal

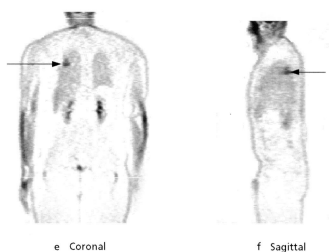

e Coronal   f Sagittal

Case 4.21 Continued

From MJ O'Doherty, SF Barrington, M Campbell, J Lowe, CS Bradbeer. Journal of Nuclear Medicine *1997; 38(10), 1575–83, Fig. 8A,B. Reproduced with permission.*

The patient re-presented with chest pains some months later and was scanned to exclude the presence of infiltration with lymphoma in the chest wall. The PET scan showed focal uptake in the lung, indicative of either pulmonary lymphoma or infection (e,f). Chest radiography was normal but bronchoscopic biopsy revealed the presence of pseudomonas.

Case 4.22

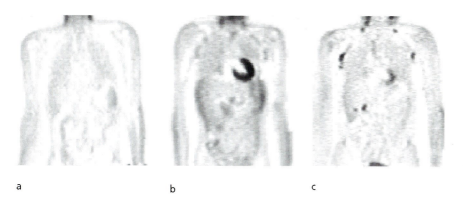

a   b   c

Coronal images

From MJ O'Doherty, SF Barrington, M Campbell, J Lowe, CS Bradbeer. Journal of Nuclear Medicine 1997; 38(10), 1575–83, Fig. 10A,B. Reproduced with permission.

The uptake of FDG within enlarged 'reactive' lymph nodes can be of variable intensity as illustrated by the three patients pictured here. Biopsies of lymph nodes within these patients indicated reactive change or normal lymph nodes, without evidence of tumour.

> Persistent generalized lymphadenopathy cannot be differentiated from lymphoma in patients with HIV using FDG-PET scans. Other conditions which may mimic lymphoma with generalized lymphadenopathy include sarcoidosis, tuberculosis, glandular fever and Epstein–Barr virus (EBV) infection.

Case 4.23

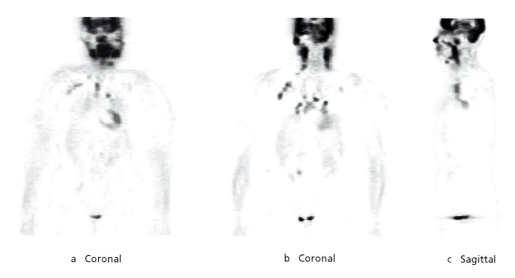

a Coronal   b Coronal   c Sagittal

This 51 year old woman with a history of Hodgkin's disease treated in 1990 presented with lymphadenopathy in both sides of the neck in 1993. Biopsy of the lesions revealed sarcoidosis. She received treatment with a good response clinically. In August 1994 there was no palpable lymphadenopathy but routine follow up CT revealed the presence of a right axillary lymph node. The PET scan showed FDG uptake in the nasal region, salivary glands, lung hilae, mediastinum and right axilla. The pattern of uptake was reported as more suggestive of sarcoid than lymphoma, but the intensity of uptake is indistinguishable in the two disease processes by SUV.

Conclusion

CURRENT CLINICAL INDICATIONS

1 Activity of residual masses

2 Staging (for HD: less important for NHL)

3 Gastrointestinal lymphomas

4 Remission assessment/suspected recurrence

5 CNS: infection vs. lymphoma

POSSIBLE INDICATIONS

1 Replace all anatomical imaging procedures

2 Prediction of response to chemotherapy soon after it is initiated

3 Prognosis assessment

Further reading

Carr R, Barrington SF, Madan B, Saunders CAB *et al.* (1998) Detection of lymphoma in bone marrow by whole body positron emission tomography. *Blood* **91**(9), 3340–46.

De Wit M, Bumann D, Beyer W *et al.* (1997) Whole-body positron emission tomography (PET) for diagnosis of residual mass in patients with lymphoma. *Ann Oncol* **8**(suppl 1), 57–60.

Hoh CK, Glaspy J, Rosen P, Dahlbom M *et al.* (1997) Whole body FDG-PET imaging for staging of Hodgkin's disease and lymphoma. *J Nucl Med* **38**, 343–8.

Lapela M, Leskinen S, Minn HRI *et al.* (1995) Increased glucose metabolism in untreated non-Hodgkin's lymphoma: A study with positron emission tomography and fluorine-18–fluorodeoxyglucose. *Blood* **86**, 3522–7.

Moog F, Bangerter M, Diederichs CG *et al.* (1997) Lymphoma: role of whole-body 2-deoxy-2-[F-18]fluoro-D-glucose (FDG) PET in nodal staging. *Radiology* **203**(3), 795–800.

Moog F, Bangerter M, Diederichs CG *et al.* (1998) Extranodal malignant lymphoma: detection with FDG PET versus CT. *Radiology* **206**(2), 475–81.

Moog F, Bangerter M, Kotzerke J *et al.* (1998) 18-F-fluorodeoxyglucose-positron emission tomography as a new approach to detect lymphomatous bone marrow. *J Clin Onc* **16**(2), 603–9.

Newman JS, Francis IR, Kaminski MS, Wahl RL (1994) FDG-PET imaging in lymphoma: Correlation with CT. *Radiology* **190**, 111–16.

O'Doherty MJ, Barrington SF, Campbell M *et al.* (1997) PET scanning and the HIV positive patient. *J Nucl Med* **38**(10), 1575–83.

Okada J, Yoshikawa K, Imazeki K *et al.* (1991) The use of FDG-PET in the detection and management of malignant lymphoma: Correlation of uptake with prognosis. *J Nucl Med* **32**(4), 686–91.

Paul R (1987) Comparison of fluorine-18–2-fluorodeoxyglucose and gallium-67 citrate imaging for detection of lymphoma. *J Nucl Med* **28**(3), 288–92.

Rodriguez M, Rehn S, Ahlstrom H *et al.* (1995) Predicting malignancy grade with PET in non-Hodgkin's lymphoma. *J Nucl Med* **36**, 1790–6.

Romer W, Hanauske AR, Ziegler S, Thodtmann R, Weber W, Fuchs C *et al.* (1998) Positron emission tomography in non-Hodgkin's lymphoma: assessment of chemotherapy with fluorodeoxyglucose. *Blood* **91**, 4464–71.

Stumpe KD, Urbinelli M, Steinert HC, Glanzmann C, Buck A, von *et al.* (1998) Whole-body positron emission tomography using fluorodeoxyglucose for staging of lymphoma: effectiveness and comparison with computed tomography. *European Journal of Nuclear Medicine* **25**, 721–8.

Chapter 5

Lung cancer

Introduction and background

Lung cancer is among the most frequent and most lethal of cancers in both men and women. It is the most rapidly increasing tumour in the industrialized countries. Most lung cancers are caused by smoking, but smoking appears to be a somewhat less important factor in adenocarcinoma which is the cancer most rapidly increasing in frequency in the US. Lung cancer makes up 22% of all cancers in men and 8% of all cancers in women. Although early lung cancers (non-small cell T1 N0 cancers) are curable by surgery with a greater than 50% 5 year survival, only 13% of all patients with lung cancer survive for 5 years. The basic treatment for non-small cell lung cancer remains surgical, although only approximately one in five patients are operable at the time of presentation. The remainder of the patients receive palliative chemotherapy or radiation therapy. Patients with small cell lung cancer respond well initially to chemotherapy and radiation therapy and are generally not treated surgically.

EPIDEMIOLOGY	
Incidence	
Men	800–1000 cases per million
Women	400–500 cases per million
Male/female ratio	2:1

Lung cancer is increasing in frequency, especially in women.

PATHOLOGY		
Tumour types	UK	USA
Small cell (SCLC)	25%	20%
Non-small cell (NSCLC)		
Adenocarcinoma	15%	40%
Large cell	10%	10%
Squamous	50%	30%

There are significant differences in frequency in different countries, the most noteworthy being the high and increasing incidence of adenocarcinoma in women in the US.

PROGNOSIS

5 year survival	8–10% overall	
Mortality	849 per million males	431 per million females
Stage I	50–70% 5 year survival	
Stage II	25–50% 5 year survival	
Stage III + IV	<20% 5 year survival	
Perioperative mortality	<5% under 60 years of age	>5% over 60 years of age

Generally lung cancer carries a poor prognosis, less than 10% survival overall. However, a young person with a small peripheral NSCLC and no spread has a very good outlook if treated properly.

STAGING

T1	Tumour 3 cm or less	Stage I
T2	Tumour more than 3 cm	T_1 or T_2, N_0
	or involves main bronchus	
	or involves pleura	
	or associated with atelectasis extending to hilum	
T3	Any size of tumour invading	Stage II
	chest wall	T_1 or T_2, N_1, M_0
	diaphragm	
	pericardium	
	main bronchus <2 cm from carina	
	entire lung atelectasis or pneumonitis	
T4	Any size tumour invading	Stage III
	mediastinum	T_1 or T_2, N_2
	heart	T_3 or T_4
	great vessels	N_3
	trachea	
	oesophagus	
	vertebral body	
	carina	
	malignant pleural effusion	
N0	No local nodal metastases	
N1	Ipsilateral peribronchial or hilar nodal metastases	
N2	Ipsilateral mediastinal or subcarinal nodal metastases	
N3	Contralateral mediastinal, hilar or scalene or supraclavicular nodal metastases	
M1	Distant metastases	Stage IV
		M_1

The key issue is the spread to mediastinum which usually renders the patient inoperable. CT is the cornerstone, backed up by mediastinoscopy and biopsy. Unfortunately CT has a poor sensitivity, and consequently many patients are operated on when the disease has spread. The important goal is to decrease the number of patients undergoing surgical treatment unnecessarily.

PREFERENTIAL LOCAL SPREAD

Tumour site

Lower lobe   → Posterior mediastinal nodes, subcarinal nodes

Right upper lobe   → Superior mediastinal nodes

Left upper lobe   → Anterior mediastinal nodes, superior mediastinal nodes

Peripheral lesions   → Pleura, chest wall or diaphragm

Knowledge of the likeliest early site of spread is helpful in getting the best results from staging procedures.

COMMON METASTATIC SITES

Bone

Liver

Adrenal

Brain

At presentation, some patients will have distant metastatic disease: at the time of death, most will have distant disease.

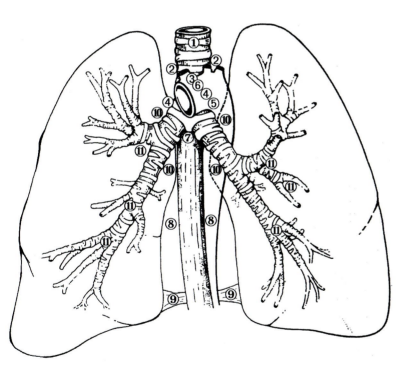

Figure 5.1 *Lymph node drainage from the lung. 1, superior (highest) mediastinal; 2, paratracheal; 3, pretracheal, retrotracheal, or posterior mediastinal (3p) and anterior mediastinal (3a); 4, tracheo-bronchial; 5, subaortic (Botallo's); 6, para-aortic (ascending aorta); 7, subcarinal; 8, paraoesophageal (below carina); 9, pulmonary ligament; 10, hilar; 11, bronchopulmonary.*

Key management issues

PET imaging for a lung mass is particularly helpful in high surgical risk patients, where there has been failure of biopsy or difficult biopsy sites and patients have bleeding disorders.

The role of PET in lung cancer

PET has an important role in the differential diagnosis of focal pulmonary abnormalities, in the locoregional and systemic staging of proven lung cancers and in the follow up of lung cancer therapies. So far it has mainly been applied in NSCLC, the authors' experience is that SCLC cancer can also be imaged well with FDG-PET. Both FDG and [^{11}C]L-methionine have been used in imaging, but there are more data for FDG. Several groups have used FDG-PET to evaluate solitary pulmonary nodules (SPN). The largest series has come from Duke University, and has shown that FDG-PET is very accurate as a non-invasive means of characterizing SPN in a series with 51 patients. In most series, FDG uptake in benign lesions is 10–25% of the uptake seen in malignant ones. Some inflammatory lesions which are benign will accumulate FDG, such as tuberculomas and aspergillomas, so FDG is not specific for cancer. Similarly, on infrequent occasions, false negative PET imaging can be seen in small SPN especially in the lower lung zones, so follow up of some negative lesions may be indicated. Recently some false negative PET scans have been reported in bronchioalveolar carcinomas. In most series, FDG-PET is in excess of 90% sensitive for lung cancers in SPN, making it the most accurate non-invasive method available, often avoiding the morbidity of fine needle biopsy or surgery.

For staging of the mediastinum, FDG-PET has been shown in several series to be more accurate than CT, as PET can detect cancer in normal sized lymph nodes as well as excluding cancer from enlarged nodes. An early series in 23 patients showed PET to be 82% accurate, while CT was only 52% accurate in mediastinal staging. Follow up series have shown even better accuracy for PET. In the authors' experience, false positive uptake of FDG in the mediastinum can occur, particularly in areas of the US where granulomatous disease such as histoplasmosis are endemic, meaning that biopsy confirmation of such nodal involvement is essential. In Europe, it seems that false positive FDG-PET scans in the mediastinum are much less common. Similar excellent staging results have been seen in multiple series and are also seen with [^{11}C]L-methionine.

PET also has an important role in staging the whole body. A paper by one of our group (Lewis *et al.* 1994) showed that additional malignant lesions were found in 41% of 34 patients, with management altered in 29%. Of greatest importance was a change to non-surgical management, found in 18% of cases. The economic consequences of eliminating a thoracotomy are considerable. Finally, PET appears very helpful in following up the response of lung cancers to therapy. At present, the authors believe known or suspected lung cancer is the most common indication for clinical PET scanning.

Normal appearances

Static attenuation corrected and non-attenuation corrected scans of the chest are shown. The transmission scan is also reconstructed and provides some basic anatomical information (shown overleaf).

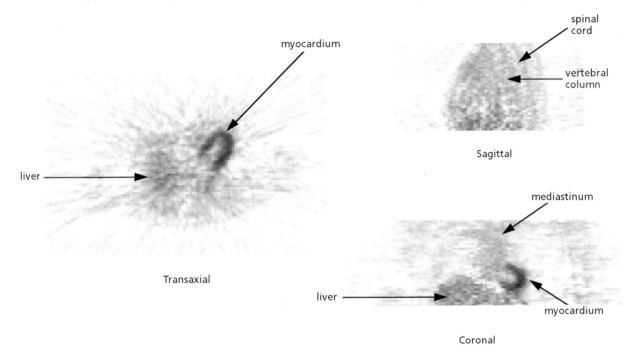

Attenuation corrected emission images of the thorax.

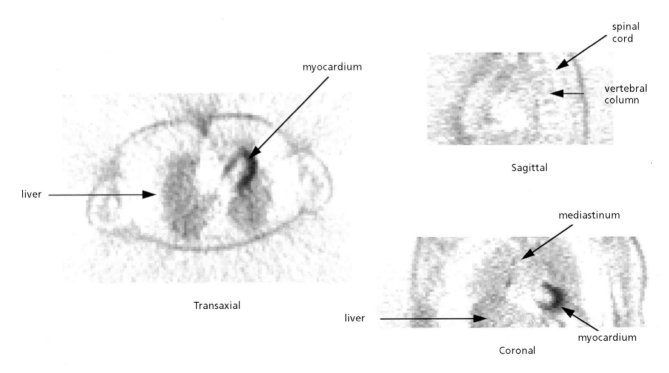

Non-attenuation corrected emission images of the thorax.

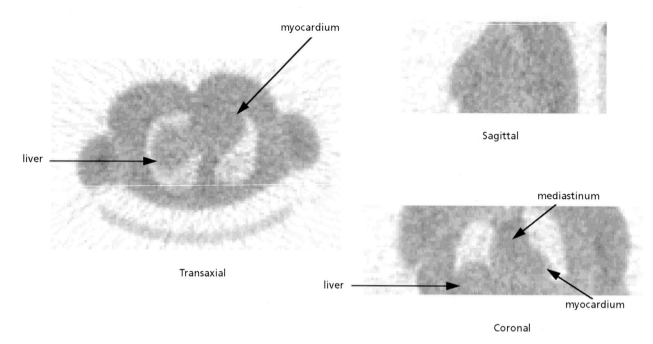

Transmission views of the thorax.

Examples to illustrate key issues

Key issue 1 Diagnosis of a lung mass

Case 5.1

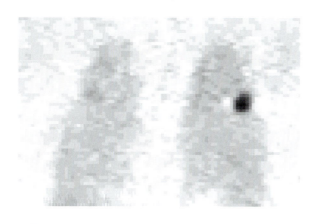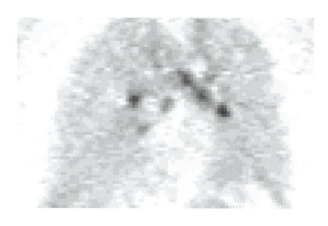

a

b

Coronal images

This female patient with multiple sclerosis was found to have an opacity within the left midzone of the lung on routine chest radiography. The lesion was not visualized at bronchoscopy and washings taken showed no suspicious cells. In view of the patient's medical problems, a PET scan was requested prior to attempting biopsy. The PET scan showed high uptake within the lesion, SUV = 6.2 (a) and in addition intense uptake of FDG within hilar and mediastinal nodes bilaterally (b). The patient did not proceed to surgery, in view of the PET diagnosis of a left lung primary with mediastinal involvement.

> Teaching point: In the US, because of the high incidence of histoplasmosis and other granulomatous disease in which the intensity of uptake of FDG can be similar, biopsy would have been required. In the UK, where histoplasmosis is uncommon, the decision to avoid surgery could be taken with greater certainty without the need for biopsy.

Case 5.2

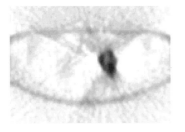

a Transaxial

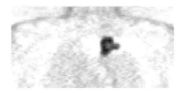

b Coronal

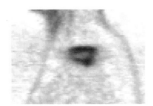

c Sagittal

This 52 year old man presented with a suspected left Pancoast tumour. Biopsy revealed no evidence of tumour but clinical suspicion of malignancy remained high. PET scanning demonstrated intense FDG uptake within the left apical mass, SUV = 6.9, without evidence of local or distant spread. The patient proceeded to resection.

Case 5.3

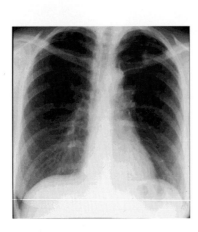

a Chest X-ray

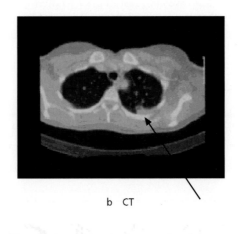

b CT

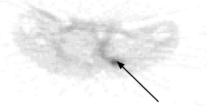

c Transaxial FDG

This 30 year old woman attended a routine medical examination for the purposes of emigration. A chest radiograph (a) showed an opacity within the left apex and CT (b) showed a nodule within the left upper lobe. Needle aspirate from the nodule was reported as containing cells suspicious for malignancy. PET scanning (c) showed intense uptake of FDG within the nodule, SUV = 4.3, also seeming to suggest the presence of malignancy. A wedge resection was performed which revealed the presence of active tuberculosis rather than malignancy.

Case 5.4

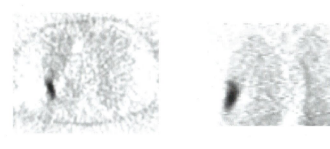

a Transaxial   b Coronal

This 76 year old man was first noted to have a peripheral nodule in the right lung in 1990, with benign radiographic appearances. Serial chest radiographs demonstrated a doubling in size between 1994 and 1996, raising concern that the lesion might have become malignant. The PET scan showed intense uptake of FDG within the lesion, SUV = 7.3. The presumptive diagnosis was of a right lung primary, but exploration of the right lung revealed nodular parenchymal amyloidosis.

Case 5.5

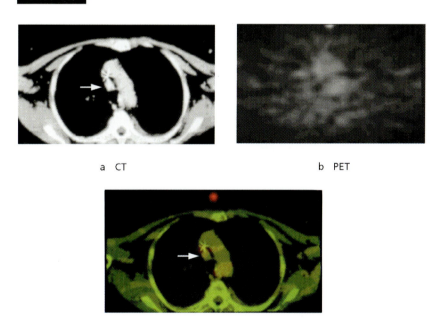

a CT   b PET

c Registered CT/PET

From RL Wahl, LE Quint, RL Greenough, CR Meyer, RI White, MO Orringer. Radiology 1994; **191**, *371–7, Fig 2a,c,d. Reproduced with permission.*

Enlarged (14 mm) right mediastinal lymph node (arrowed) in a patient with a left lung primary lesion is seen on the diagnostic contrast-enhanced CT scan (a). The PET scan (b) shows no FDG uptake into the region of the enlarged node. The areas of residual FDG in the mediastinal blood pool are displayed as grey. The registered CT/PET image (c) shows no increased uptake of FDG by the enlarged node (arrow) or other non-blood pool structures. At surgery this patient was proved to have a benign pulmonary lesion due to anthracosis and no cancer.

Transaxial

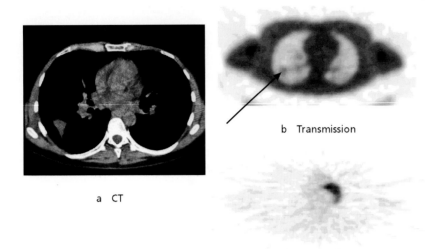

a   CT

b   Transmission

c   Emission

A chest radiograph performed as one of a series of tests to investigate the cause of palpitations in this 32 year old woman demonstrated a lesion in the apical segment of the right lower lobe. Follow up CT (a) confirmed the presence of the lesion, which was reported as suspicious for an adenocarcinoma. No direct biopsy was possible at bronchoscopy but endobronchial biopsies taken from the carina and bronchial washings were normal. The CT lesion is seen also on the PET transmission scan (b) with no evidence of uptake within the site on the emission FDG-PET scan (c), indicating a benign aetiology. Three years after the PET scan the patient remains well, without evidence of a change in the mass on CT or chest radiography.

> Causes of non-malignant increased FDG uptake include TB, sarcoid, amyloid and infection. These false positive cases are rare and do not significantly affect the beneficial impact of FDG-PET for this clinical problem.

Key issue 2 Staging of NSCLC

Case 5.7

a Transmission

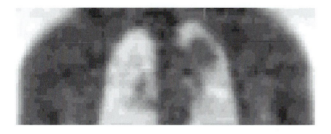

Coronal

b Emission

Coronal

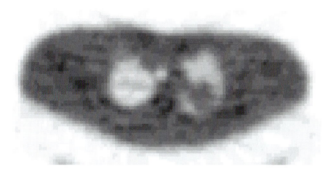

c Transaxial

d Transaxial

The PET scan in this patient referred for staging showed uptake of FDG within the known left upper lobe squamous cell carcinoma. There was no evidence of local or distant spread and the patient was operable and potentially curable.

> The shape and size of the lesion differs between the transmission and emission images. This is commonly due to a central tumour (metabolically active) with distal pulmonary collapse (metabolically inactive).

Transaxial

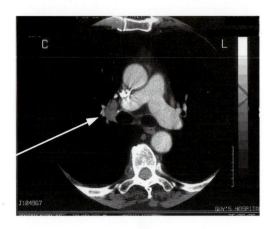

a   CT

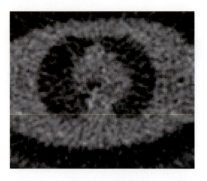

b   Transmission

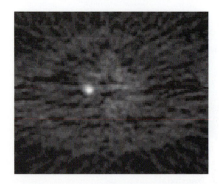

c   Emission

CT and PET were performed for staging in this patient prior to surgery. The tumour is seen on CT (a) abutting the right main bronchus at the level of the carina. The PET (b,c) shows uptake of FDG within this lesion. Adequate resection margins are unlikely to be achieved with a tumour so close to the carina.

> With central lesions, both PET and CT are required for optimal staging.

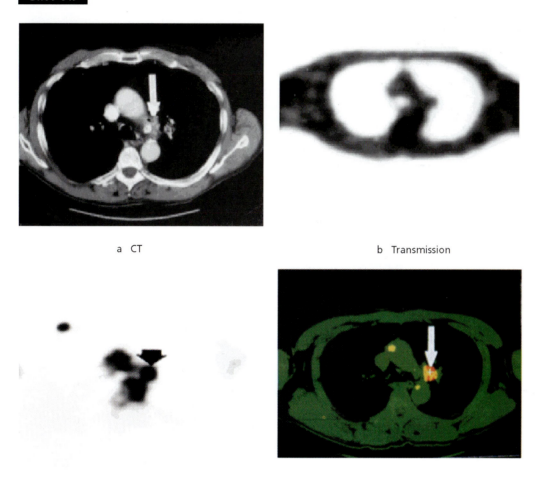

a CT

b Transmission

c Emission

d Registered CT/PET

From RL Wahl, LE Quint, RL Greenough, CR Meyer, RI White, MO Orringer. Radiology *1994;* **191**, *371–7, Fig. 3a–d. Reproduced with permission.*

The mediastinum appeared normal on this CT scan (a). Note that there were normal sized lymph nodes seen (arrowed). The transmission PET scan demonstrates the anatomy around the mediastinum at low resolution (b). The emission PET (c) shows focal uptake in the left mediastinum (arrowed). The registered image (d) shows that the focal increased uptake of FDG is within the 9 mm lymph node (arrowed). Adeno-carcinoma was proved to be present within this normal sized node.

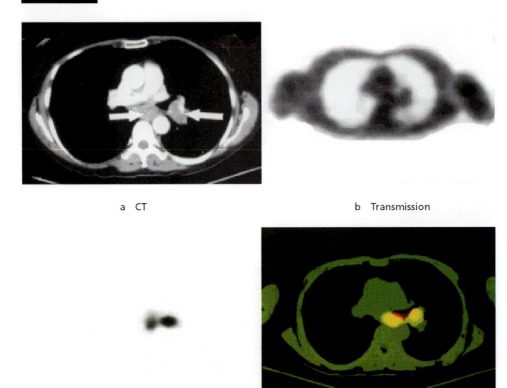

a CT

b Transmission

c Emission

d Registered CT/PET

Reproduced with permission from RL Wahl, LE Quint, RL Greenough, CR Meyer, RI White, MO Orringer. Radiology 1994; **191**, 371–7, Fig. 1a–d.

Enlarged mediastinal lymph nodes (arrowed) are seen on diagnostic contrast enhanced CT scan (a) and in the PET transmission scan (b). The emission scan (c) shows intense uptake of FDG in the mediastinum 50–60 min after tracer injection. The registered CT/PET image (d) shows intense FDG uptake by enlarged nodes. Metastastic (poorly differentiated) cancer was present in mediastinal nodes in this patient.

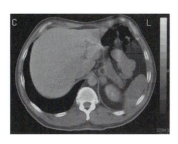

a   CT

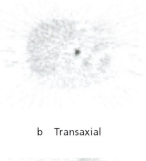

b   Transaxial

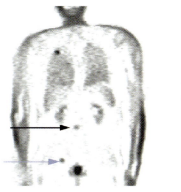

c   Coronal

This 45 year old patient with squamous cell carcinoma of the left main bronchus was referred for PET scanning following a CT which showed mild enlargement of the left adrenal gland (a). The PET scan showed uptake within the primary tumour, SUV = 12(c). A further focus of increased FDG uptake was identified within the left adrenal, SUV = 7.4, indicating an adrenal metastasis (b, c).

> Incidental benign adrenal tumours are frequently found on CT. Adrenal metastases from lung cancer are common. PET is excellent at differentiating these and avoiding unnecessary biopsy as benign adrenal adenomas generally have low FDG uptake while metastases have high FDG uptake.

Case 5.12

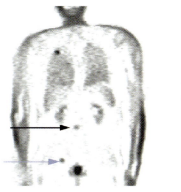

a   Coronal

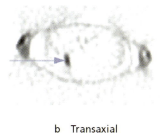

b   Transaxial

This 58 year old man with adenocarcinoma in the right lung had back pain at presentation. Both the CT and bone scan suggested the presence of a metastasis within the lumbar spine at L3. Bone biopsy at this level was negative. The PET scan showed increased FDG uptake at the level of L3 (arrowed in black), and in addition showed focal uptake within the sacroiliac joint, (arrowed in blue) confirming the presence of bony metastases.

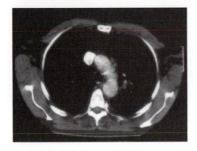

a

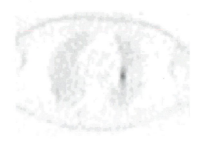

b

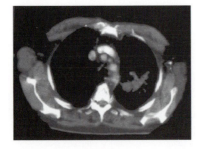

c   CT

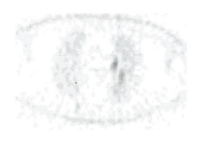

d   Transaxial

This 62 year old man with carcinoma in the left lung was referred for staging before surgery. CT scan (a,c) demonstrated a node measuring less than 1 cm just above the left hilum in addition to the primary tumour. PET was performed to assess whether the lymph node represented local spread. The PET scan confirmed uptake of FDG within this node (b) and in addition demonstrated uptake within a left paratracheal node, not visible on the CT scan (c). The CT slices are chosen to illustrate the levels at which there was nodal uptake on PET. The base of the left upper lobe tumour in the CT is seen at the level where the paratracheal node is visible on the PET. The left upper lobe tumour is not, however, visible on the PET image which was acquired during quiet breathing whereas the CT was acquired during deep inspiration.

> Small lesions are more likely to be missed in the basal lung zones, probably due to respiratory motion and due to increased normal tissue uptake in this area.

Case 5.14

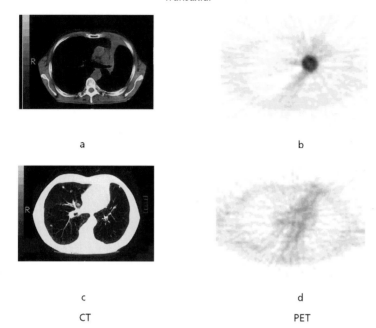

Transaxial

a   b

c   d

CT   PET

This 69 year old patient with carcinoma of the left upper lobe had a CT scan performed prior to surgery which indicated the presence of nodules in the contralateral lung. The PET scan showed intense uptake in the primary site only (CT and corresponding PET image a and b), with no uptake of FDG in the right sided lung nodules (CT and corresponding PET image c and d), suggesting disease was only within the primary site and the patient was operable.

Case 5.15

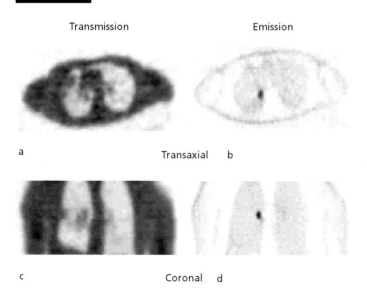

Transmission   Emission

a

Transaxial   b

c

Coronal   d

This 69 year old patient was being investigated for unresolved collapse and consolidation in the right lung. There was increased uptake of FDG within the primary tumour at the right lung hilum. Low level uptake of FDG within the region distal to the tumour which is abnormal on the transmission scan is due to low grade infection and lung collapse.

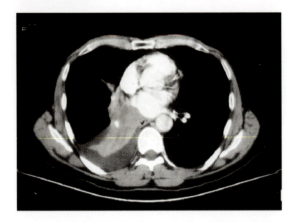

a   CT

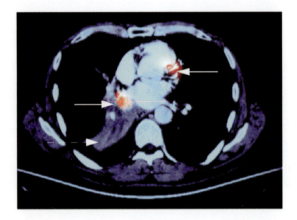

b   Registered CT/PET

From RL Wahl, LE Quint, RD Cieslak. Journal of Nuclear Medicine *1993; **34**(7), p. 1194, Fig. 3A. Reproduced with permission.*

CT (a) shows marked volume loss in the right lower lung and a localized right pleural effusion in a patient with newly diagnosed lung cancer. There was intense uptake in the anterior left chest, modest focal FDG uptake in the blood pool and the collapsed right lower lobe/effusion area. The registered CT/PET image (b) clearly demonstrates intense FDG uptake in the central portion of the collapsed right lower lung most consistent with uptake in the central tumour (solid arrows), whereas the remainder of the right lung has activity most consistent with postobstructive volume loss (dotted arrows). MRI supported this interpretation and the large central tumour was treated non-surgically.

> Uptake within consolidated lung distal to tumour is usually less intense than that in the primary tumour.

This 42 year old woman with known lung cancer and a past history of ovarian cancer was referred for PET scanning. An ultrasound examination (a) showed several small lesions within the liver, which were also seen on CT (b), the appearances of which were suggestive of haemangiomata.

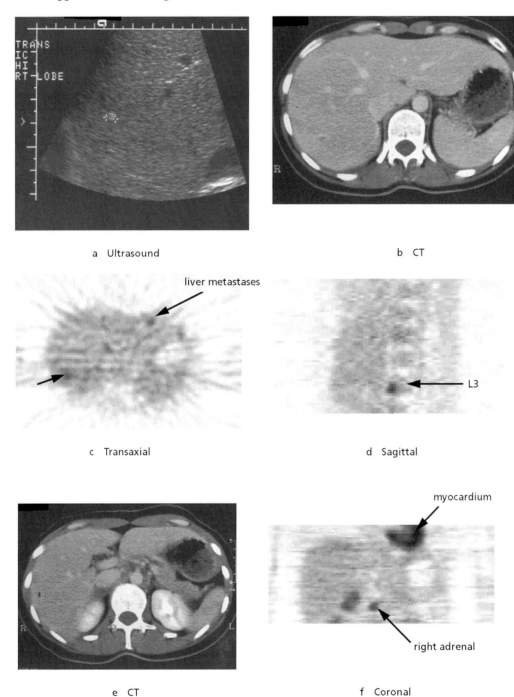

a   Ultrasound

b   CT

c   Transaxial

d   Sagittal

e   CT

f   Coronal

FDG scanning revealed uptake within the primary lung lesion and within the liver lesions, suggesting that the liver lesions were metastases rather than haemangiomata (c). There was also uptake in the bone and right adrenal gland (d, f). No abnormality is seen within the CT scan taken at the level of the right adrenal (e). PET revealed the presence of unsuspected metastases and that the tumour was inoperable.

Key issue 3 Assessment of recurrence

Case 5.18:   Local recurrence

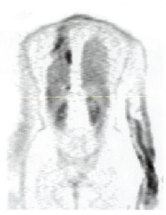

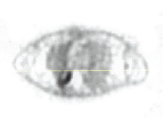

b Transaxial

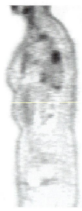

c Sagittal

a Coronal

This 51 year old woman underwent resection of the right middle and lower lobes of the lung for carcinoma in 1988. She subsequently received radiotherapy and chemotherapy at relapse in 1994 with good response. In 1996 she re-presented with superior vena cava obstruction. CT demonstrated narrowing of the junction of the right subclavian vein and superior vena cava, together with extensive pleural thickening and calcification in the paravertebral region. Bronchiectatic change in the underlying right lung and destruction of the right posterior chest wall were also seen secondary to surgery. No evidence of new lung lesions was seen on sequential CT scans performed 2 months apart. There was thus no clear evidence of recurrent disease on CT. PET was performed to establish that the cause of the SVC obstruction was fibrosis rather than recurrent disease. The PET scan shows multiple areas of increased uptake of FDG within the right chest which were predominantly pleural, indicating recurrent disease. SUV of the lower medial lesion shown on the coronal image was 5.4. Note on the coronal image in this case the injection-related uptake proximal to the injection site in the dorsum of the left hand.

> Good practice requires that the tracer should be administered contralateral to known or suspected disease where possible.

Case 5.19:   Local recurrence

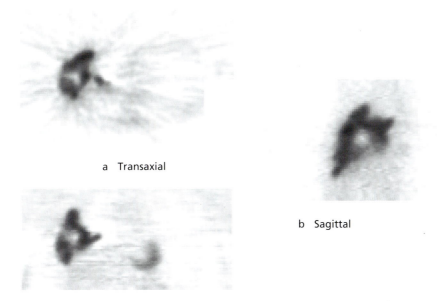

a   Transaxial

b   Sagittal

c   Coronal

This female patient with carcinoma of the lung treated with radiotherapy was known to have a radiation pneumonitis. She re-presented with clinical evidence of recurrent disease in the chest wall. PET was performed to define the extent of the chest wall tumour within the region known to be included in radiotherapy treatment and to determine whether there were other sites of disease. The PET scan shows increased uptake of FDG within the chest wall at a single site with a photopenic necrotic centre. PET confirmed the presence of recurrent disease and provided information about tumour extent.

> Mild uptake can be seen within radiation pneumonitis, but the intensity in this case indicated the presence of recurrent tumour.

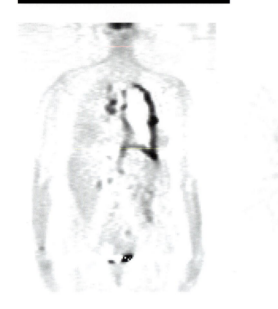

b   Transaxial

a   Coronal

This 56 year old woman had a left pneumonectomy for carcinoma of the lung. She presented within 3 months of the surgery with chest pain and lethargy associated with anaemia and leucocytosis. There was no evidence clinically of infection, and residual disease was suspected. The FDG scan shows intense uptake within the left lung cavity, the right hilum, mediastinum and bone (sites within the thoracic and lumbar spine are seen on the coronal image). The PET scan indicates residual or recurrent disease with multiple metastases. Unfortunately this patient had not been referred for PET scanning prior to surgery.

> Staging 'operable' patients with PET reduces unnecessary surgery.

Key issue 4 Monitoring therapy

Case 5.21

Transaxial

Sagittal

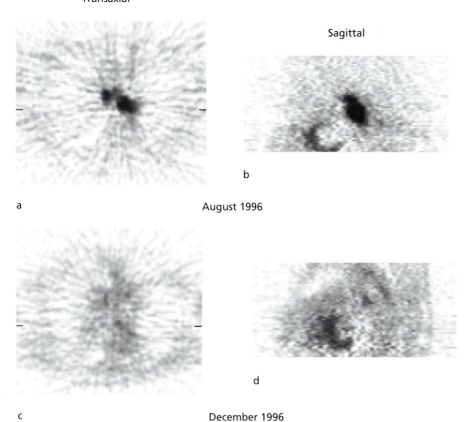

b

a   August 1996

d

c   December 1996

Corresponding transaxial and sagittal images are shown of a patient with oat cell carcinoma who underwent chemotherapy in the interval between the two PET scans in
August and December 1996. Complete resolution of FDG uptake within the tumour
is seen, indicating a good response to treatment.

FDG-SPECT imaging of lung cancer

Case 5.22 illustrates triple head SPECT; Cases 5.23–5.25 illustrate dual head SPECT with coincidence counting.

Case 5.22

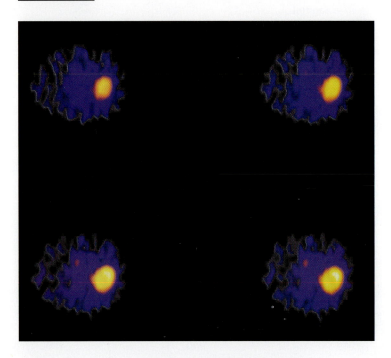

a   SPECT transaxial of thorax

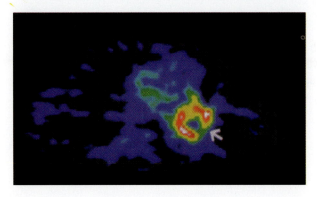

b   PET transaxial of thorax

*From DJ MacFarlane, L Cotton, RA Ackermann, H Minn, EP Ficaro, PD Shreve, RL Wahl. Radiology 1995; **194**, 426, Figs 2a,b. Reproduced with permission.*

Representative reconstructed transverse sections of FDG-PET and SPECT scans of the thorax show intense uptake of FDG within a large, cavitating squamous cell carcinoma of the left lower lobe. Note that the central cavity is clearly resolved only with PET.

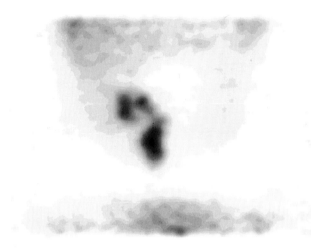

This shows a projection image of the thorax acquired using a dual head γ-camera in coincidence mode. Intense uptake of FDG is seen within a primary squamous cell lung carcinoma with mediastinal metastases.

Case 5.24

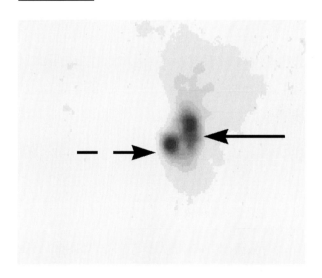

Transaxial

A transaxial image is shown of a patient imaged using a dual head γ-camera in co-incidence mode showing FDG uptake in the primary tumour (solid arrow) and within a mediastinal metastasis (broken arrow).

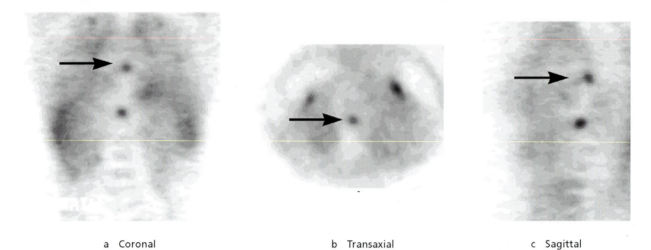

a Coronal   b Transaxial   c Sagittal

From PD Shreve, RS Stoventon, EC Deters, PV Kison, MD Gross, RL Wahl 1998. Radiology **207**, *431–7, Figs 1a and b.*

Transaxial, coronal and sagittal images are shown of a patient with recurrent squamous cell lung carcinoma imaged using a dual head γ-camera in coincidence mode. FDG uptake was seen on all the images within mediastinal metastases (arrowed) and inferiorally within a retrocrural lymph node on the coronal and sagittal images. Metastatic nodules in the upper lobes of both lungs were seen in the transaxial image.

Assessment of pleural disease

Case 5.26

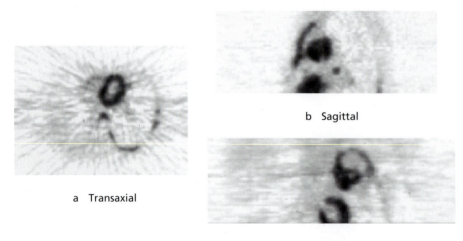

b Sagittal

a Transaxial

c Coronal

This patient with NSCLC had a CT scan showing the primary lesion only. PET scanning revealed uptake within the primary lesion, but also within pleura. Pleural biopsy confirmed the presence of pleural involvement with tumour.

> FDG-PET scanning may identify malignant pleural spread.

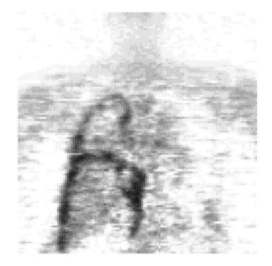

a   Coronal

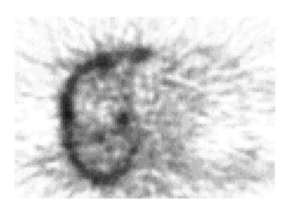

b   Transaxial

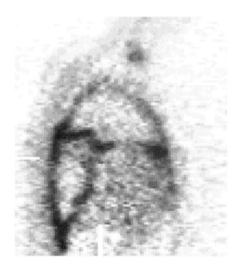

c   Sagittal

This 59 year old recipient of a renal transplant 18 years previously and a history of carcinoma of the tongue developed a blood stained pleural effusion and cervical lymphadenopathy. CT scan showed right basal collapse. PET scanning revealed FDG uptake within cervical lymph nodes and the right lung pleura. Lymph node biopsy revealed a diagnosis of tuberculosis rather than malignancy.

Conclusions

Figure 5.2 indicates a possible diagnostic pathway.

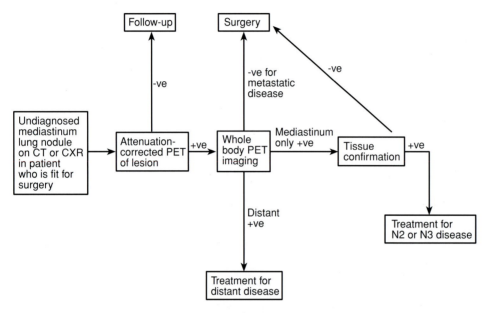

Figure 5.2 *Solitary pulmonary nodule and staging of non-small cell lung cancer: clinical algorithm.*

Further reading

Ahuja V, Coleman RE, Herndon J, Patz EF, Jr. (1998) The prognostic significance of fluorodeoxyglucose positron emission tomography imaging for patients with non small cell lung carcinoma. *Cancer* **83**, 918–24.

Bury T, Dowlati A, Paulus P *et al.* (1996) Evaluation of the solitary pulmonary nodule by positron emission tomography imaging. *Eur Respir J* **9**(3), 410–14.

Bury T, Paulus P, Dowlati A *et al.* (1996) Staging of the mediastinum: value of positron emission tomography imaging in non-small cell lung cancer. *Eur Respir J* **9**(12), 2560–4.

Bury T, Dowlati A, Paulus P, Corhay JL, Hustinx R, Ghaye B *et al.* (1997) Whole-body 18FDG positron emission tomography in the staging of non-small cell lung cancer. *European Respiratory Journal* **10**, 2529–34.

Gambhir SS, Hoh CK, Phelps ME *et al.* (1966) Decision tree sensitivity analysis for cost-effectiveness of FDG PET in the staging and management of non-small-cell carcinoma. *J Nucl Med* **37**(9), 1428–36.

Guhlmann A, Storck M, Kotzerke J *et al.* (1997) Lymph node staging in non-small cell lung cancer: evaluation by [18F]FDG positron emission tomography (PET). *Thorax* **52**, 438–41.

Gupta NC, Frank AR, Dewan NA *et al.* (1992) Solitary pulmonary nodules: Detection of malignancy with PET with 2-[¹⁸F]-fluoro-2-deoxy-D-glucose. *Radiology* **184**(2), 441–4.

Kim BT, Kim Y, Lee KS *et al.* (1998) Localized form of bronchioloalveolar carcinoma: FDG PET findings. *Am J Roentgerol* **170**(4), 935–9.

Kubota K, Matsuzawa T, Ito M *et al.* (1985) Lung tumor imaging by positron emission tomography using ¹¹C L-methionine. *J Nucl Med* **26**, 37–42.

Kubota K, Yamada S, Ishiwata K *et al.* (1993) Evaluation of the treatment response of lung cancer with positron emission tomography and L-[methyl-¹¹C] methionine: A preliminary study. *Eur J Nucl Med* **20**(6), 495–501.

Lewis P, Griffin S, Marsden P *et al.* (1994) Whole-body ¹⁸F-fluorodeoxyglucose positron emission tomography in preoperative evaluation of lung cancer. *Lancet* **344**, 1265–6.

Lowe VJ, Duhaylongsod FG, Patz EF *et al.* (1997) Pulmonary abnormalities and PET data analysis: a retrospective study. *Radiology* **202**(2), 435–9

MacFarlane DJ, Cotton L, Ackermann RA, Minn H, Ficaro EP, Shreve PD, Wahl RL (1995) *Radiology* **194**, 426.

Miyauchi T, Wahl RL (1996) Regional 2-[18F]fluoro-2-deoxy-D-glucose uptake varies in normal lung. *E J Nucl Med* **23**(5), 517–23.

Nolop KB, Rhodes CG, Brudin LH *et al.* (1987) Glucose utilization in vivo by human pulmonary neoplasms. *Cancer* **60**(11), 2682–9.

Patz EF Jr, Lowe VJ, Hoffman JM *et al.* (1993) Focal pulmonary abnormalities: Evaluation with ¹⁸F fluorodeoxyglucose PET scanning. *Radiology* **188**(2), 487–90.

Schiepers C (1997) Role of positron emission tomography in the staging of lung cancer. *Lung Cancer* **17**(Suppl 1), S29–35.

Steinert HC, Hauser M, Allemann F *et al.* (1997) Non-small cell lung cancer: nodal staging with FDG PET versus CT with correlative lymph node mapping and sampling. *Radiology* **202**(2), 441–6.

Vansteenkiste JF, Stroobants SG, De Leyn PR, Dupont PJ, Bogaert J, Maes A *et al.* (1998) Lymph node staging in non-small-cell lung cancer with FDG-PET scan: a prospective study on 690 lymph node stations from 68 patients. *Journal of Clinical Oncology* **16**, 2142–9.

Wahl RL, Quint LE, Cieslak RD (1993) Journal of Nuclear Medicine **34**(7), p. 1194.

Wahl RL, Quint LE, Greenough RL *et al.* (1994) Staging of mediastinal non small cell lung cancer with FDG-PET, CT and fusion images: Preliminary prospective evaluation. *Radiology* **191**, 371–7.

Zasadny KR, Kison PV, Quint LE *et al.* (1996) Untreated lung cancer: quantification of systematic distortion of tumor size and shape on non-attenuation-corrected 2-[fluorine-18]fluoro-2-deoxy-D-glucose PET scans. *Radiology* **201**(3), 873–6.

Chapter 6

Breast cancer

Introduction and background

Breast cancer is the commonest tumour affecting women and is the most frequent cause of death from cancer in women overall in the UK. In the US, breast cancer is now the second leading cancer killer behind lung cancer. Breast cancer is the commonest single cause of death of women in the age group 35–50 years. Early diagnosis and treatment can be curative but requires a multidisciplinary approach to the overall management. Treatment includes surgery, which has become progressively less radical than in previous years, together with chemotherapy. Chemotherapy can be therapeutic, adjuvant, neoadjuvant or palliative. Hormone therapy and radiation therapy are also key parts of the therapeutic regimes. Imaging is an important part of detection, staging and management of most patients with breast cancer.

EPIDEMIOLOGY

	UK	USA
Incidence per million (male)	7	10
Incidence per million (female)	1021	1480
All women lifetime risk	1:12	1:10
% of all cancers in women	19%	27%

Breast cancer is increasing in western industrialized countries but remains infrequent in Japan. Approximately 10% of all women will be affected in their lifetime.

PATHOLOGY

Tumour types

Carcinoma in situ

Invasive carcinoma

Infiltrating ductal	80%
Medullary	5%
Lobular	10%
Mucinous	
Infiltrating tubular	
Infiltrating comedo	~5%
Paget's disease	
Inflammatory	
Papillary	<1%

Frequency of breast tumour sites

Midline — 15% / 50% / 20% / 5% / 10% — Axilla

Most breast cancers are of the infiltrating ductal type with the upper outer quadrant and axillary tail being the most frequent site.

STAGING

T1	Tumour 2 cm or less	Stage I	T1 moveable tumours confined to breast
T2	Tumour 2–5 cm	Stage II	As stage I but with spread to lymph nodes, or tumour >2 cm without nodes
T3	Tumour >5 cm	Stage III	Locally advanced disease
T4	Tumour any size fixed to chest wall or skin or oedema, skin nodules	Stage IV	Distant metastases
N0	Nil		
N1	Ipsilateral moveable axillary nodes		
N2	Fixed ipsilateral axillary nodes		
N3	Ipsilateral internal mammary nodes		
M1	Distant metastases		

The lymph node staging of the axilla is by axillary dissection and has a key role in deciding management but probably does not itself affect outcome.

LYMPH NODE METASTATIC SITES

Lymph nodes involved	Axillary	40% +ve
	Internal mammary	
	Supraclavicular	
Frequency of axillary nodes related to tumour size	Tumour <2 cm	18% +ve
	Tumour 2–5 cm	35% +ve
	Tumour >5 cm	56% +ve
Internal mammary nodes	Tumour <5 cm	19% +ve
	Tumour >5 cm	37% +ve

Overall 30–40% of patients will have lymph node involvement at presentation. Clinical examination is poor (25% false +ve, 30% false −ve). Internal mammary nodes are less frequently involved than axillary nodes but more difficult to identify, medial breast cancers are three times more likely to involve the internal mammary nodes than the outer quadrant tumours. Internal mammary node involvement indicates a poor prognosis.

DISTANT SITES

Lung	60–70%
Liver	55–65%
Bone	45–70%
Pleura	25–50%
Adrenals	30–50%
Skin	30–35%
Brain	10–20%

PROGNOSIS

5 year survival	65%	
5 year survival in relation to axillary nodes	overall	65–80% (−ve nodes)
		25–50% (+ve nodes)
	1–3 nodes	45%
	4+ nodes	20%
20% of cancer deaths in women in the US		

The prognosis in breast cancer is highly dependent on the size of the primary lesion and involvement of axillary or internal mammary nodes and the histology of the tumour.

Key management issues

PET in breast cancer

Breast cancer can be imaged with PET using several radiopharmaceuticals including FDG, [^{11}C]L-methionine, and ^{18}F labelled oestrogen analogues. Most clinical imaging studies have been performed using FDG, owing to the increased glucose metabolism seen in breast cancers. Although early studies showed that all large primary, regionally metastatic and systemic metastases of breast cancer could be imaged with FDG (e.g. 25/25 known breast cancer lesions detected by Wahl *et al.* in 1991), and that some breast cancers could be detected by PET but not by standard imaging methods (e.g. in radiodense breasts), the exact role of PET in the management of patients with breast cancer is still in evolution. In primary lesion evaluation, one study showed 96% accuracy in characterizing lesions (27 lesions) as benign or malignant, but another study including smaller lesions showed false negative results to occur with relatively high frequency in small primaries <1 cm in size. Despite this, accuracies of over 90% in primary lesion characterization as malignant or benign are expected by PET, at least for tumours >1 cm in size.

For regional lymph node metastasis detection, the literature is varied, with one report in 20 patients showing PET to be 90% sensitive and 95% accurate. However, a follow up report in a larger series of patients showed 80% sensitivity and 95% specificity in staging, with false negatives most common in small nodal metastases and in patients with small primary tumours. Clearly, false negative studies do occur and it seems unlikely that current PET systems could ever reliably detect micrometastatic disease in the axilla. PET can show internal mammary node tumour involvement to excellent advantage, however. The role of PET in evaluating soft tissue lesions appears important, and detecting cancers in radiodense breasts such as those with silicone implants and in finding soft tissue recurrences are evolving. Whole body surveys are useful in examining for disease remote from the breast, and such surveys may be useful and rational in high risk patients.

Treatment monitoring is also an active area of clinical PET investigation, and FDG-PET studies show rapid declines in tumour SUV with effective treatments. There is a suggestion that PET can predict the response of cancers to treatment soon after it is started, but most clinical studies are performed at the conclusion of treatment in an effort to determine if residual tumour is present. A caution in such studies is marrow uptake of FDG which can rise following treatment, especially if the patient is receiving colony stimulating factors at about the time of PET. While other tracers can be used, FDG has superior diagnostic accuracy to fluoroestradiol for both primary and metastatic lesion detection, and [^{11}C]L-methionine is not clearly superior to FDG in breast tumour imaging, based on available data.

Normal appearances

Emission (attenuated and non-attenuated corrected) views of the upper chest are shown, with and without labels.

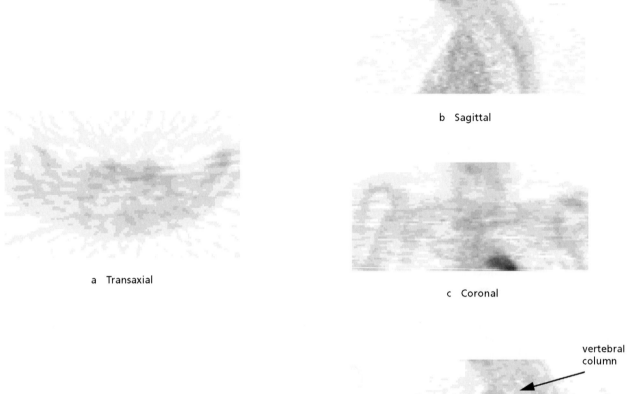

a Transaxial

b Sagittal

c Coronal

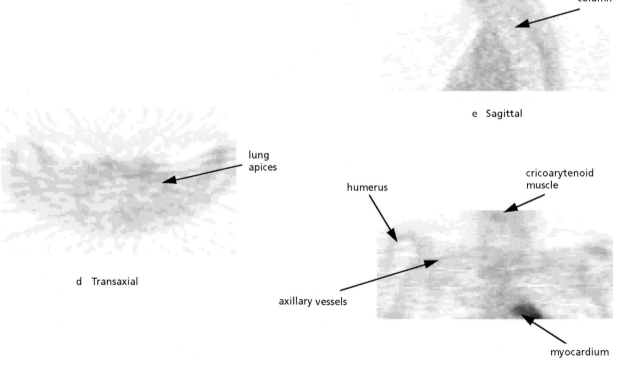

d Transaxial

e Sagittal

vertebral column

lung apices

humerus

cricoarytenoid muscle

axillary vessels

myocardium

f Coronal

Attenuation corrected emission images of the brachial plexus region.

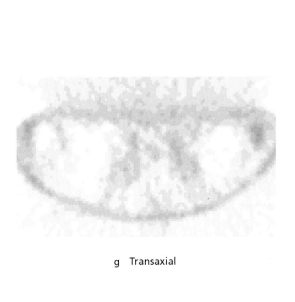

g Transaxial

h Sagittal

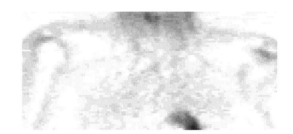

i Coronal

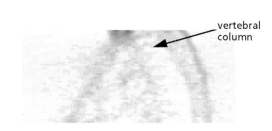

vertebral
column

k Sagittal

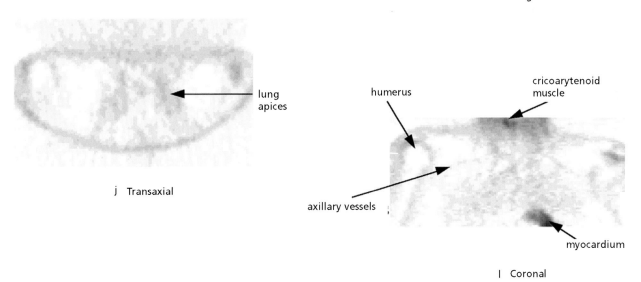

lung
apices

j Transaxial

humerus

cricoarytenoid
muscle

axillary vessels

myocardium

l Coronal

Non-attenuation corrected emission images of the upper chest and axillae.

Examples to illustrate key issues

Key issue 1 Benign vs. malignant breast masses

Case 6.1

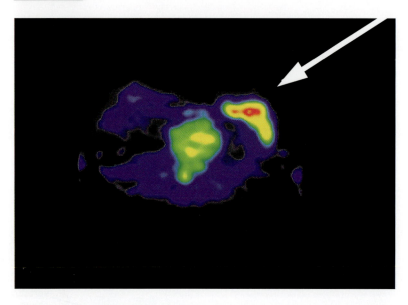

From RL Wahl, K Zasadny, GD Hutchins, B Weber, R Cody 1993. Journal of Clinical Oncology *11(11), 2104, Fig. 3b. Reproduced with permission.*

After finishing breast feeding, this patient complained that her left breast had not returned to normal. Mammography was performed but in view of the high radiographic density within a recently lactating breast, the examination was technically difficult and no tumour was seen. The patient was referred for PET which showed intense uptake of FDG within a large tumour in the left breast shown in the above transaxial emission image. Biopsy confirmed the diagnosis of breast cancer. Disease was localized to the breast without evidence of nodal or distant spread.

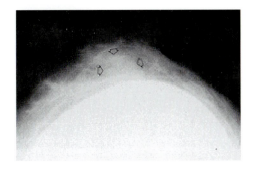

a Mammogram

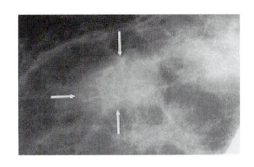

b Compression
Displacement
View

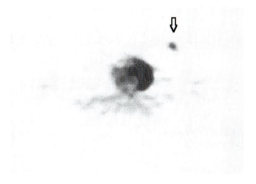

c Transaxial PET

From RL Wahl, MA Helvie, AE Chang, I Andersson. Journal of Nuclear Medicine *1994; **35**(5), p. 874, Fig. 2A–C. Reproduced with permission.*

Mammogram of the left breast shows large prosthesis and adjacent mass (arrows on a). Magnification coned compression displacement view shows a 1.5 cm x 1.0 cm mass (arrows on b) which is moderately well circumscribed and has two microcalcifications. Transverse FDG-PET scan (c) at the level of the mass demonstrates an FDG-avid nodule in the left breast (arrow) beyond the prosthesis (which does not accumulate FDG). Normal myocardial uptake is noted.

FDG-PET may be used in circumstances where mammography is technically difficult.

This includes:

- dense breasts
- breast implants
- lumpy breasts/multifocal disease
- postoperative/postbiopsy breast
- equivocal biopsy

Case 6.3: Nodal disease

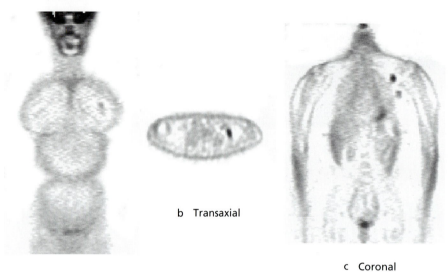

b   Transaxial

c   Coronal

a   Coronal

This young woman presented with a lump behind the left nipple. Biopsy revealed carcinoma within a small tumour seen on mammography to lie just behind the left nipple. FDG-PET showed uptake within the primary tumour (a) and in addition two large axillary lymph node metastases (b,c).

> There is normally FDG uptake in the nipple which may obscure a very small primary breast tumour. Remember to inject in the contralateral arm as false positives may occur with an extravasated injection as FDG will track rapidly to and accumulate in normal regional lymph nodes.

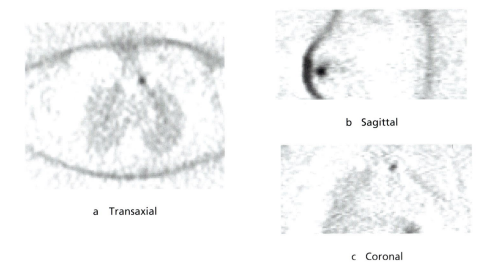

a   Transaxial

b   Sagittal

c   Coronal

This 56 year old woman had an FDG-PET scan at the time of diagnosis. FDG uptake is seen within the known cancer in the left breast on the sagittal image (b), but in addition FDG is seen within a left internal mammary lymph node shown on transaxial and coronal images (a,c).

Node dissection is largely for prognosis and management planning. PET can demonstrate positive nodes but will miss some micrometastases. The sensitivity and specificity of PET varies in published series. Some of the differences may be due to patient selection and the threshold for reading positive scans.

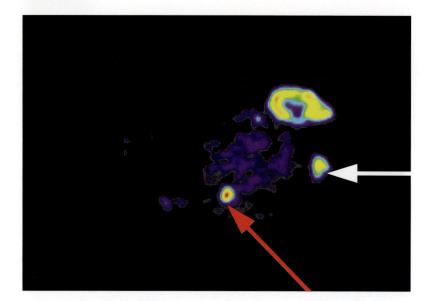

Transaxial

The FDG-PET scan done at diagnosis in this patient demonstrated uptake within the left breast mass but also showed uptake within a left axillary node (arrowed in white) and in a metastasis in the thoracic spine (arrowed in red). Thus the patient had evidence on PET of nodal and distant spread at presentation significantly changing the management plan for her.

Case 6.6: Distant metastases at presentation

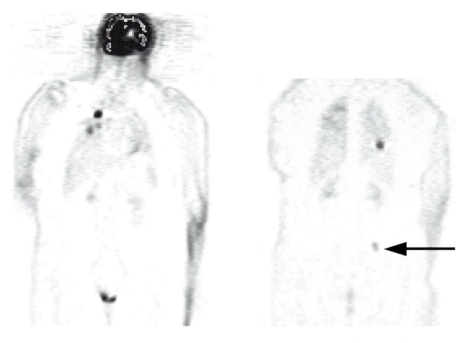

a Coronal (anterior)   b Coronal (posterior)

This 43 year old patient with carcinoma of the breast had a fracture of the right humerus at presentation. Bone scan showed uptake within the right humerus, left sacroiliac joint and right sacrum indicative of multiple bony metastases. PET scan was performed which confirmed uptake within the sites identified on the bone scan. Uptake within the left sacroiliac joint is seen on the posterior coronal image (arrowed) but PET also demonstrated abnormal uptake in soft tissue, seen within the lung fields in both coronal images.

> Whole body PET provides information with regard to metastases in soft tissue and bone at a single scanning session.

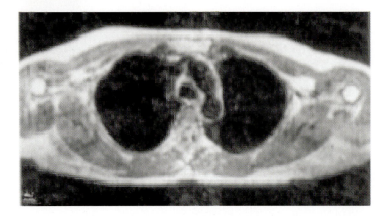

a MRI

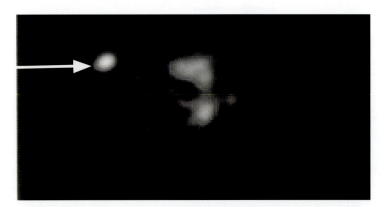

b PET

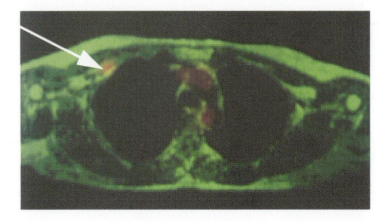

c MRI/PET registered image

From RL Wahl, LE Quint, RD Cieslak. Journal of Nuclear Medicine *1993;* **34***(7), p. 1195, Fig. 4. Reproduced with permission.*

Transaxial MRI (a) and PET (b) images are shown of the upper chest in a woman with metastatic breast cancer. The PET scan shows intense uptake of FDG (arrowed) in the right anterior chest region. The focus is difficult to localize on PET owing to the high target to background ratio and could represent either a chest wall or axillary lymph node. Proton-density MRI demonstrates focal expansion and distortion of an anterior right rib. The registered image (c) superimposes intense FDG uptake into this abnormal rib, which is an FDG-avid metastasis.

Key issue 3 Tumour response

Case 6.8

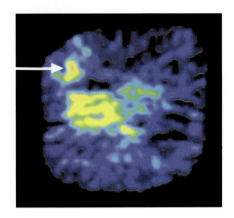

a   Baseline SUV 3.42

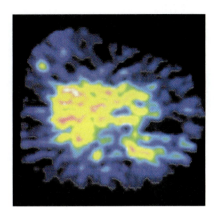

b   Day 8 SUV 2.24

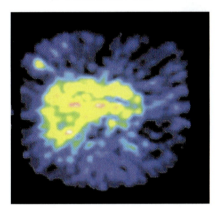

c   Day 21 SUV 2.74

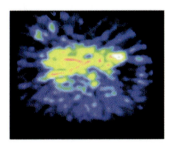

d   Day 42 SUV 1.67

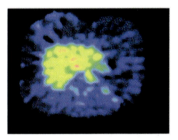

e   Day 63 SUV 1.4

Transaxial images

This 59 year old woman with invasive ductal carcinoma of the right breast was imaged with PET to monitor the effects of combined chemohormonotherapy during the first three cycles. No decrease in tumour size was observed clinically over this time course, but the transaxial images shown above clearly indicated a reduction in glucose metabolism within the tumour in response to treatment. Clinically complete remission was achieved within 6 months of commencing treatment.

> PET may give an early indication of treatment response which precedes clinical response.

Transaxial images

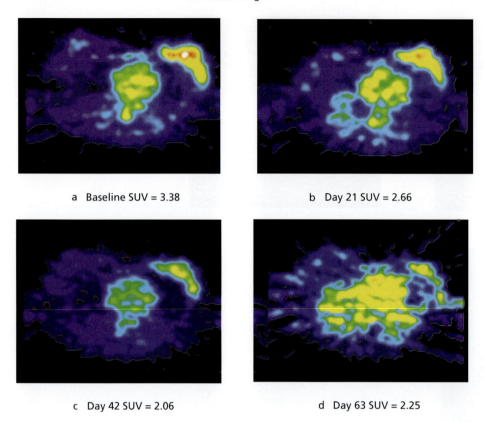

a   Baseline SUV = 3.38   b   Day 21 SUV = 2.66

c   Day 42 SUV = 2.06   d   Day 63 SUV = 2.25

From RL Wahl, K Zasadny, M Helvie, GD Hutchins, B Weber, R Cody. Journal of Clinical Oncology *1993; **11**(11), p. 2104, Fig. 3B. Reproduced with permission.*

Sequential transaxial images through a left breast tumour are shown during treatment with chemotherapy. The time interval between individual scans was 3 weeks. There was partial response to treatment with chemotherapy prior to a planned mastectomy.

Case 6.10

Transaxial images

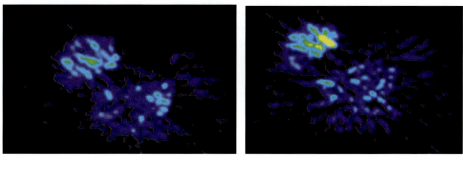

a Baseline SUV = 4.77   b Baseline SUV = 5.62

From RL Wahl, K Zasadny, M Helvie, GD Hutchins, B Weber, R Cody. Journal of Clinical Oncology 1993; 11(11), p. 2109, Fig. 8. Reproduced with permission.

In this case, activity within the breast increases, despite treatment with chemotherapy, and the patient proceeded to early mastectomy rather than possible lumpectomy after effective neoadjuvant chemotherapy as had been previously planned.

Case 6.11

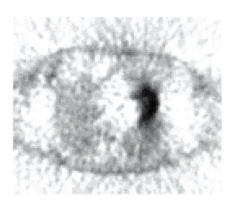

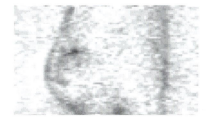

c

a

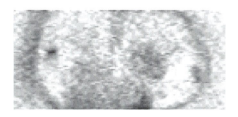

b

This 39 year old woman underwent primary chemotherapy before surgery. PET was performed to determine whether disease was sufficiently localized within the right axillary tail post-treatment to make breast conservation a surgical option. PET showed a single focus in the axillary tail of the right breast without diffuse changes permitting breast conservation to be undertaken.

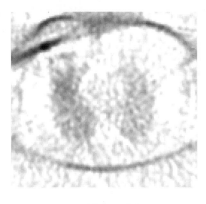

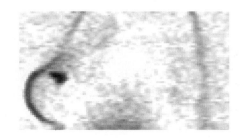

b   Sagittal

a   Transaxial

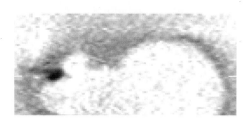

c   Coronal

This 61 year old woman was treated with chemotherapy for a local recurrence in the right breast. Residual disease was suspected and confirmed on the PET with uptake of FDG within two lesions. The SUV of the larger lesion shown here on three planes was 3.7.

> Mammographic assessment of the conserved breast following surgery may be difficult and PET can provide diagnostic information.

Case 6.13

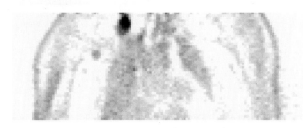

a   Pre-treatment

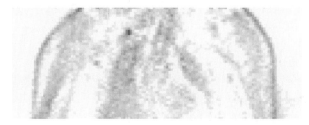

b   Post-treatment

This 40 year old woman had chemotherapy for right brachial plexopathy secondary to malignant infiltration by tumour, with a good response clinically to treatment. The PET demonstrates reduction in FDG uptake within the right brachial plexus on the second scan performed 6 weeks after completing treatment.

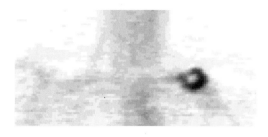
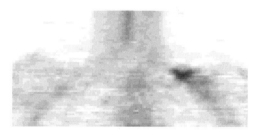

a   Coronal images June 1996   b

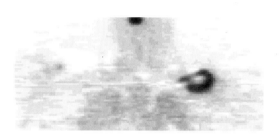
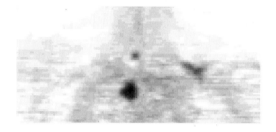

c   Coronal images August 1996   d

This 45 year old woman with breast cancer received radiotherapy to the supraclavicular and infraclavicular fossae and axillae followed by chemotherapy. She then developed a further left infraclavicular mass. MRI showed oedema around the mass with appearances suggestive of either inflammatory change or malignant disease. Fine needle aspiration of the mass was negative for malignancy. The initial PET scan in June 1996 shows intense uptake of FDG within the mass, indicating a malignant aetiology. Three courses of Taxotere were given but despite treatment the uptake of FDG within the mass remained unchanged when rescanned in August 1996 and new metastases were identified indicating progressive disease.

Case 6.15: Recurrence within soft tissue and bone

a   Transaxial

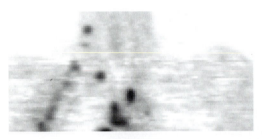

b   Coronal

This patient had carcinoma of the breast in 1994. She had a local recurrence in the right neck which was treated with radiotherapy in 1995. She re-presented with a further palpable node in the right side of the neck in 1996. Fine needle aspiration showed no suspicious cells. The clinical index of suspicion for recurrent disease remained high and the patient was referred for PET scanning. The PET scan showed FDG uptake not only within the palpable node (a, transaxial image through the neck) but in multiple nodes in the right cervical chain, both supraclavicular fossae and the mediastinum (b). The PET thus confirmed both recurrence and identified multiple rather than a single site of disease.

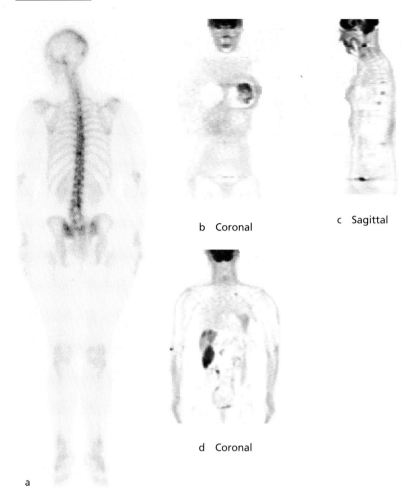

b   Coronal

c   Sagittal

d   Coronal

a

^{99m}Tc MDP Bone scan

This 48 year old woman had a known local recurrence in the left breast. Bone scans performed at this relapse showed abnormal uptake in the thoracic spine at T4 and T9 suggestive of bone metastases and uptake in the lumbar spine reported as degenerative in association with a mild scoliosis.

FDG-PET scanning confirmed the presence of disease in the left breast (b) and in bone (c) but also demonstrated unsuspected soft tissue disease in the left supraclavicular fossa, the liver and in a soft tissue mass anterior to the right kidney (d).

Case 6.17

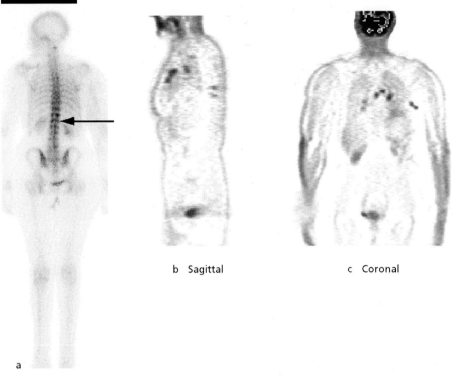

b Sagittal   c Coronal

a

^{99m}Tc MDP Bone scan

This 69 year old woman was diagnosed with carcinoma of the breast in 1988 and treated with surgery and chemotherapy. She was well until 1996 when she re-presented with back pain. Bone scan showed uptake within the cervical spine indicative of degenerative disease and uptake in the right side of T12 posteriorly, likely to be degenerative uptake within an osteophyte (a, arrowed). She was referred for PET scanning to determine whether the uptake in T12 was degenerative or metastatic. FDG-PET showed multiple metastases within the thoracic spine (b) and also within soft tissue; in lung, mediastinum and left axilla (b, c). PET confirmed there were metastases in bone and identified further sites of metastases within soft tissue.

Case 6.18: Recurrence within the brachial plexus

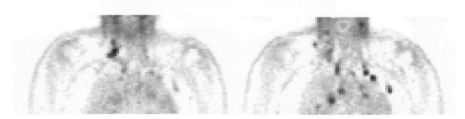

a   Coronal images   b

This 48 year old woman with carcinoma of the breast had been treated with surgery and radiotherapy. She re-presented with right arm weakness and signs suggestive of a brachial plexopathy. MR was unable to differentiate whether the plexopathy was due to fibrosis secondary to treatment or new malignant disease. PET scan showed increased FDG uptake within the right brachial plexus accounting for her symptoms (a) but also within cervical lymph nodes, lung hila, right lung, left axilla and mediastinum (b).

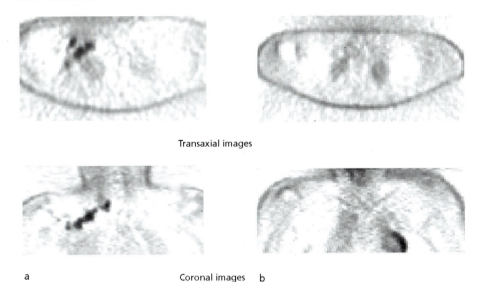

Transaxial images

a   Coronal images   b

These are contrasting cases of two women who previously had mastectomies and combination radiotherapy and chemotherapy for carcinoma of the breast. Both presented with symptoms suggestive of brachial plexopathy. MR was performed on one patient and was equivocal, the other patient underwent CT which was normal as she was unable to tolerate the MR examination. In the patient on the left (a) there is intense uptake of FDG within multiple foci in the right brachial plexus region indicating malignancy, the patient on the right (b) had no uptake of FDG within this region indicating a radiation induced plexopathy.

> PET can differentiate treatment induced from malignant brachial plexopathy. This is an area which is difficult to assess on conventional anatomical imaging.

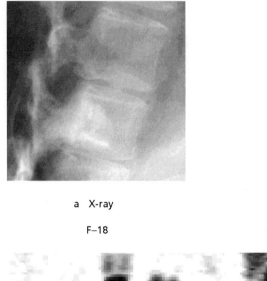

a   X-ray

F–18   FDG

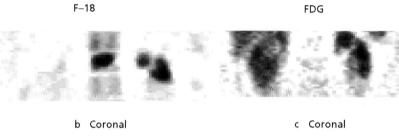

b   Coronal   c   Coronal

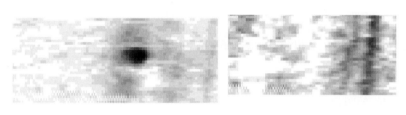

d   Sagittal   e   Sagittal

This patient with carcinoma of the breast had a new sclerotic bone metastasis at L1. The metastasis is visualized on fluoride scanning but does not accumulate FDG.

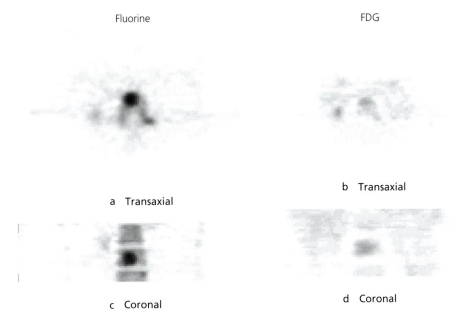

Fluorine   FDG

a Transaxial

b Transaxial

c Coronal

d Coronal

Intense uptake of fluorine and FDG are seen within this metastasis at L3 in a patient with carcinoma of the breast, which on radiography appeared to be lytic.

> Lytic or mixed lytic and sclerotic bone metastases in carcinoma of the breast usually accumulate FDG, sclerotic metastases may not. Patients with osteolytic or mixed lesions have a poorer prognosis.

Conclusion

CURRENT CLINICAL INDICATIONS (IN ORDER OF IMPORTANCE)

1 Equivocal lymph nodes

2 Brachial plexopathy

3 Recurrent disease clinical equivocal

4 Breast implants ? recurrence + conserved breast

5 Detection (bilateral, multifocal)

6 Biopsy equivocal

7 Treatment response

POSSIBLE INDICATIONS

1 Staging: axillary and internal mammary

2 Bone metastases (e.g. bone scan?)

3 Surveillance of conserved breast

4 Prediction of response

5 Risk stratification

References and further reading

Adler LP, Faulhaber PF, Schnur KC *et al.* (1997) Axillary lymph node metastases: screening with [F-18]-deoxy-fluoro-D-glucose (FDG) PET. *Radiology* **203**(2), 323–7.

Ahmad A, Barrington S, Maisey M, Rubens RD (1999) Use of positron emission tomography in evaluation of brachial plexopathy in breast cancer patients. *British J of Cancer* **79**(3/4), 478–82.

Avril N, Dose J, Janicke DF *et al.* (1996) Metabolic characterization of breast tumors with positron emission tomography using ^{18}F fluorodeoxyglucose. *J Clin Oncol* **14**, 1848–57.

Bassa PE, Kim EE, Inoue T *et al.* (1996) Evaluation of preoperative chemotherapy using PET with fluorine-18-fluorodexoyglucose in breast cancer. *J Nucl Med* **37**(6), 931–8.

Bombardieri E, Crippa F, Maffioli L, Draisma A, Chiti A, Agresti R *et al.* (1998) Nuclear medicine approaches for detection of axillary lymph node metastases. *Quarterly Journal of Nuclear Medicine* **42**, 54–65.

Brown RS, Leung JY, Fisher SJ *et al.* (1996) Intratumoral distribution of tritiated-FDG in breast carcinoma: correlation between GLUT-1 expression and FDG uptake. *J Nucl Med* **37**(6), 1042–7.

Cook G, Houston S, Maisey M *et al.* (1997) Detection of bone metastases in breast cancer by 18-FDG-PET. Differing metabolic activity in osteoblastic and osteolytic lesions. *J Nucl Med* **5**(S), 127.

Cook GJ, Houston S, Rubens R, Maisey MN, Fogelman I (1998) Detection of bone metastases in breast cancer by 18FDG PET: differing metabolic activity in osteoblastic and osteolytic lesions. *Journal of Clinical Oncology* **16**, 3375–9.

Crippa F, Agresti R, Seregni E, Greco M, Pascali C, Bogni A *et al.* (1998) Prospective evaluation of fluorine-18-FDG PET in presurgical staging of the axilla in breast cancer. *Journal of Nuclear Medicine* **39**, 4–8.

Dehdashti F, Mortimer JE, Siegel BA *et al.* (1995) Positron tomographic assessment of estrogen receptors in breast cancer. Comparison with FDG-PET and in vitro receptor assays. *J Nucl Med* **36**(10), 1766–74.

Leskinen-Kallio S, Nagren K, Lehikoinen P *et al.* (1991) Uptake of ^{11}C-methionine in breast cancer studied by PET. An association with the size of S-phase fraction. *Br J Cancer* **64**(6), 1121–4.

McGuire AH, Dehdashti F, Siegel BA *et al.* (1991) Positron tomographic assessment of 17 alpha-[^{18}F] fluoro-17 beta-estradiol uptake in metastatic breast carcinoma. *J Nucl Med* **32**(8), 1526–31.

Moon DH, Maddahi J, Silverman DH, Glaspy JA, Phelps ME, Hoh CK (1998) Accuracy of whole-body fluorine-18-FDG PET for the detection of recurrent or metastatic breast carcinoma. *Journal of Nuclear Medicine* **39**, 431–5.

Noh DY, Yun IJ, Kim JS *et al.* (1998) Diagnostic value of positron emission tomography for detecting breast cancer. *World J Surg* **22**(3), 223–7.

Petren-Mallmin M, Andreasson I, Ljunggren O *et al.* (1998). Skeletal metastases from breast cancer: uptake of 18F-fluoride measured with positron emission tomography in correlation with CT. *Skeletal Radiology* **27**(2), 72–6.

Scheidhauer K, Scharl A, Pietrzyk U *et al.* (1996) Qualitative [^{18}F]FDG positron emission tomography in primary breast cancer: clinical relevance and practicability. *Eur J Nucl Med* **23**(6), 618–23.

Utech CI, Young CS, Winter PF (1996) Prospective evaluation of fluorine-18 fluorodeoxyglucose positron emission tomography in breast cancer for staging of the axilla related to surgery and immunocytochemistry. *Eur J Nucl Med* **23**(12), 1588–93.

Wahl RL (1998) Overview of the current status of PET in breast cancer imaging. *Q J Nucl Med* **42**, 1–7.

Wahl RL, Cody R, Hutchins GD, Mudgett E (1991) Primary and metastatic breast carcinoma: Initial clinical evaluation with PET with the radiolabeled glucose analog 2-[^{19}F]-fluoro-deoxy-2-D-glucose (FDG). *Radiology* **179**, 765–70.

Wahl RL, Zasodny KR, Helvie M *et al.* (1993) Metabolic monitoring of breast cancer chemo-hormonotherapy using positron emission tomography (PET): Initial evaluation. *J Clin Oncol* **11**(11), 2101–11.

Wahl RL, Helvie MA, Chang AE, Andersson I (1994) Detection of breast cancer in women after augmentation mammoplasty using positron emission tomography: Initial clinical evaluation. *J Nucl Med* **35**, 872–5.

Wahl RL, Quint LE, Cieslak RD (1993) Journal of Nuclear Medicine **34**(7), p. 1195.

Chapter 7

Head and neck cancer

Introduction and background

Cancer of the head and neck is relatively uncommon in western countries (2–4% of all cancers) but may be extremely common (up to 40% of all cancers) in some Asian countries. The vast majority in western industrialized countries are squamous cell tumours which have a variable aggressiveness depending on the site and histological appearances. There is a strong environmental link associating their occurrence with tobacco and alcohol usage together with other factors such as chemicals, fumes and viruses. Good outcomes are dependent on patients being treated in specialized centres with experienced multidisciplinary teams including head and neck surgical oncologists, radiotherapists, imaging specialists and medical oncologists. Because of the site of the tumour, treatment is directed at maintaining form and function of the head and neck structures as well as eradicating disease. Imaging has an important role in the management of these tumours because of the need to limit surgery and because local nodal spread is the most important prognostic factor. After treatment the conventional anatomical imaging procedures are less useful because of the distortion of anatomy due to treatment. FDG-PET therefore has a particularly important role in follow-up and for suspected recurrence.

EPIDEMIOLOGY

Annual incidence	Male	15 per 100 000
	Female	5 per 100 000
Male/female ratio	3:1 (overall)	5:1 (larynx)
Deaths per year	2000 (UK)	13 000 (US)
Age	85% >50 years	
Frequency	2–4% of all malignancies	

Approximately 1 in 30 of all malignancies are tumours of the head and neck. This may rise to nearly half of the tumours in Asian countries such as Hong Kong. Men are more likely to develop this cancer than women. The incidence has fallen, particularly in men.

PATHOLOGY

Tumour types	Tumour sites
Squamous cell (90%)	Paranasal sinuses
Adenocarcinoma	Nasopharynx
Mucoepidermal	Nasal cavity
Adenoid cystic carcinoma	Oral cavity
Others	Oropharynx
	Hypopharynx
	Larynx
	Salivary glands

Nearly all the tumours are histologically squamous cell origin with only 1:10 other cell types. Nasopharygeal is most commonly undifferentiated. These tumours may arise from any of the structures in the aerodigestive tract, the most frequent sites being nasopharynx and oral cavity.

PROGNOSIS OF SQUAMOUS CELL CANCER

5 year survival

Overall	50%
Early oral	>75%
Advanced	35%
Cervical oesophagus	70%
Lip, glottic larynx	>80%

Overall there is only a 50% 5 year survival rate but this figure conceals a wide variation from small, localized, quite curable, tumours of the lip and glottic larynx with survivals in excess of 80% to highly malignant tumours of the floor of the mouth. The stage at presentation is critical to prognosis – early presentation has a much better prognosis whatever the site. Recurrence rate is very high (50%) mostly in first year.

STAGING

T	Size (Oral cavity and oropharynx)		Stage I	T1N0M0
T1	<2 cm		Stage II	T2N0M0
T2	2–4 cm		Stage III	T3N0M0
T3	>4 cm		Stage IV	(T1,T2,T3)N1M0
T4	Invasion			T4(N0N1)M0
				(Any T)(N2N3)M0
N0	No nodes			(Any T)(Any N)M1
N1	Ipsilateral node <3 cm			
N2	a Single ipsilateral node 3–6 cm			
	b Multiple ipsilateral nodes <6 cm			
	c Bilateral or contralateral node <6 cm			
N3	Lymph node >6 cm			
M1	Distant metastases			

Staging is important to the planning of treatment and prognosis. The single most important prognostic variable is the presence or absence of regional lymph node involvement and this may help determine how radical the surgical node dissection is. CT and MRI are currently the cornerstone but with a relatively low sensitivity. 1 in 5 Clinical N0 patients have pathologically involved nodes.

There is an established probability of which nodal groups will be involved from a particular tumour site (Figure 7.1). This can be helpful in defining the probability of node involvement on PET scans. These tumours usually spread locally initially, but with advanced disease they may spread to lung and elsewhere.

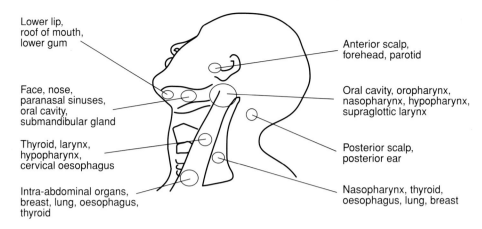

Lower lip,
roof of mouth,
lower gum

Face, nose,
paranasal sinuses,
oral cavity,
submandibular gland

Thyroid, larynx,
hypopharynx,
cervical oesophagus

Intra-abdominal organs,
breast, lung, oesophagus,
thyroid

Anterior scalp,
forehead, parotid

Oral cavity, oropharynx,
nasopharynx, hypopharynx,
supraglottic larynx

Posterior scalp,
posterior ear

Nasopharynx, thyroid,
oesophagus, lung, breast

Figure 7.1 *Loco-regional sites of metastases from head and neck cancers.*

Key management issues

PET in head and neck cancers

Head and neck carcinomas in western countries are most commonly of squamous cell origin and are generally well-imaged with PET using FDG or $[^{11}C]$L-methionine. The majority of clinical studies have been with FDG. Several studies evaluating FDG-PET imaging performance in primary lesions have shown that sensitivities from 88% to nearly 100% are seen, with failures in detection most common in very small lesions. Several studies have shown the highest levels of FDG uptake in primary lesions to be correlated with the least good prognosis. Studies with $[^{11}C]$L-methionine have shown well over 90% of primary lesions to be detected, but with methionine to a greater extent than FDG tracer, uptake in normal soft tissues like the salivary glands makes diagnosis challenging. Malignancies of the parotid are not as well imaged as those originating from the squamous mucosa, and sensitivities for parotid cancers have been <70% and worse than those reported for MRI.

The accuracy of FDG-PET for staging lymph node metastases of primary head and neck carcinoma varies in several reports. In the earliest reports, accuracy for staging comparable to that of CT or MRI were reported, however in a recent report, PET was significantly more accurate than MRI ($p < 0.05$) ± 75% accuracy for MRI, but >90% accuracy for PET. Thus, PET is at least as good as, and quite possibly somewhat better than, standard anatomic imaging for staging primary head and neck carcinoma.

PET with FDG excels at assessing treatment response and in evaluating the neck postoperatively or after radiation, which is exceedingly difficult to do by standard imaging methods after surgery. Several series have now shown FDG-PET to be more accurate than CT or MRI in detecting recurrent head and neck cancer. Indeed, some have proposed that FDG-PET should be the first imaging test ordered when evaluating for recurrent head and neck cancer, i.e. before MRI or CT is done. A caution in the interpretation of FDG-PET studies in the head and neck after treatment is that the FDG signal may decline only relatively slowly following radiotherapy, despite effective treatment. In such a situation, waiting until several months after treatment before PET imaging is recommended. Interpreting head and neck PET studies with either FDG or $[^{11}C]$L-methionine can be challenging, as there is substantial normal tissue uptake, which must be appropriately identified lest it be confused with tumour involvement. It should also be noted that FDG-SPECT imaging has also been reported to be of some clinical utility in the detection of head and neck carcinoma recurrence, although the resolution of this method is limited.

Normal appearances

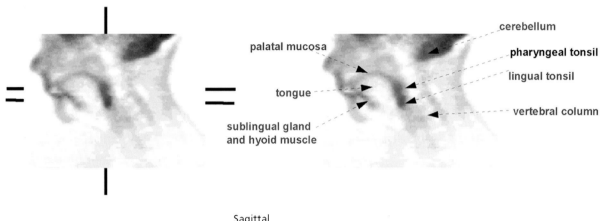

Sagittal

A sagittal image close to the midline, illustrating the physiological uptake seen within palatal mucosa, tonsillar tissue and sublingual salivary glands. Uptake within tissue sublingual salivary and overlying hyoid muscles is indistinguishable, and uptake at this site is likely to be due to a combination of uptake within both structures.

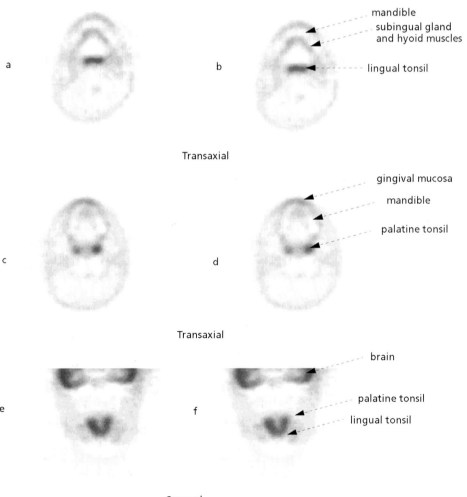

Transaxial

Transaxial

Coronal

Tonsillar uptake. Transaxial and coronal images (corresponding to the levels indicated on the sagittal image above) are shown through the level of lingual and palatine tonsils, with and without labels attached.

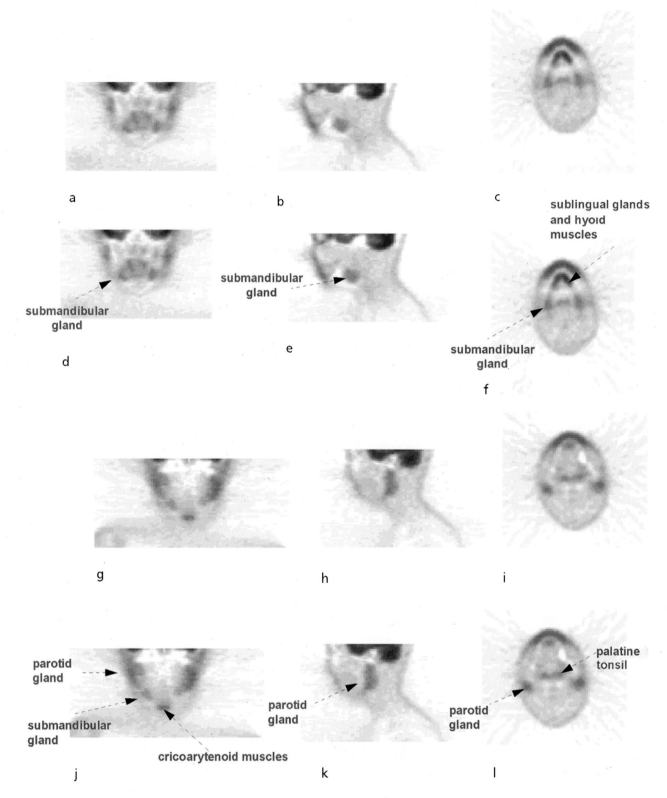

Three orthogonal views demonstrating salivary gland uptake, centred on the submandibular glands (a–f) and parotid glands (g–l). Views are shown with and without labels.

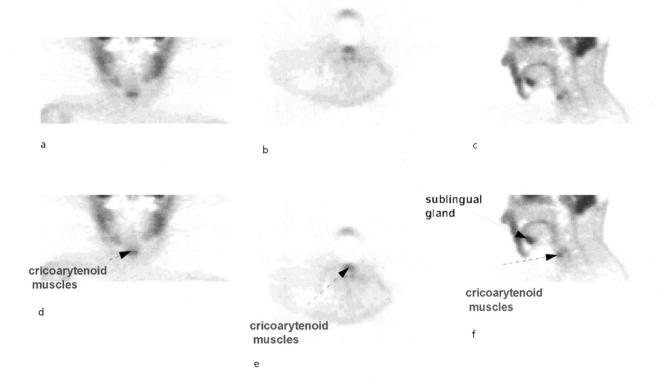

sublingual
gland

cricoarytenoid
muscles

cricoarytenoid
muscles

cricoarytenoid
muscles

a

b

c

d

e

f

Three orthogonal views illustrating the uptake within the muscles of phonation that occurs when the patient is allowed to speak during the uptake period. Patients should not speak during the period of FDG accumulation. Views are shown with and without labels.

Examples to illustrate key issues

Key issue 1 Site of primary disease

Case 7.1

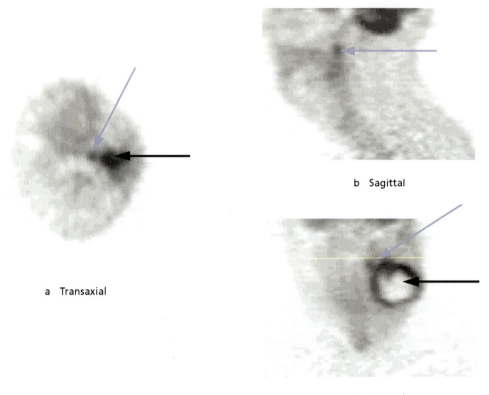

b Sagittal

a Transaxial

c Coronal

This 68 year old man presented with a mass in the left jugulodigastric region. Biopsy revealed metastatic squamous cell carcinoma. The PET was performed to find the site of the primary tumour and the extent of spread. PET scan shows uptake within the large node with a photopenic necrotic centre in the jugulodigastric region (arrowed in black) with a separate small focus in the left wall of the pharynx (arrowed in blue). SUV of the jugulodigastric node was 5.5. At surgery, the primary site was confirmed to be in the wall of the pharynx. The PET enabled accurate preoperative surgical planning.

> SCC may present with local metastasis and the primary may be tiny. PET may help identify the primary and avoid the need for multiple blind biopsies.

Key issue 2 Extent of primary disease

Case 7.2

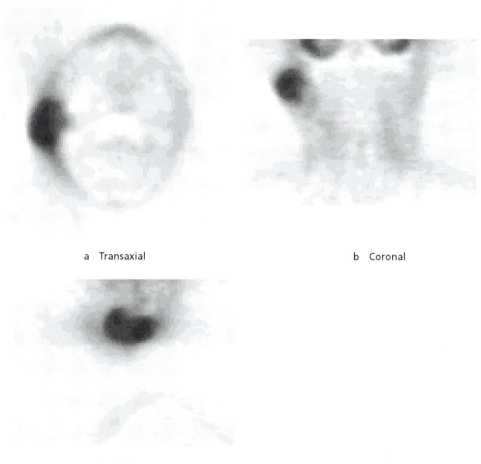

a Transaxial

b Coronal

c Sagittal

This 73 year old woman with a carcinoma in the right parotid gland was referred for PET prior to surgery to assess disease extent. PET showed intense uptake within the parotid lesion but no evidence of spread.

> In this case example, the intensity of uptake in the parotid carcinoma is high, but intensity can be variable within parotid lesions and some benign lesions may also have high uptake of FDG.

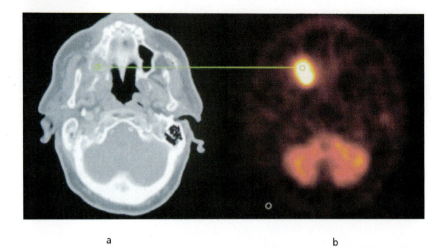

a   b

c   **Transaxial registered CT/PET**   d

This patient with a right alveolar ridge carcinoma was referred for PET scanning prior to surgery for staging purposes. The CT suggested that the tumour extended superiorly into the maxillary sinus. Registered PET and CT images show uptake of FDG within the primary site arising from the alveolar ridge (a,b) but no evidence of tumour within the sinus itself (c,d). This illustrates how the PET scan can identify extent of disease when inflammatory tissue and tumour are co-located.

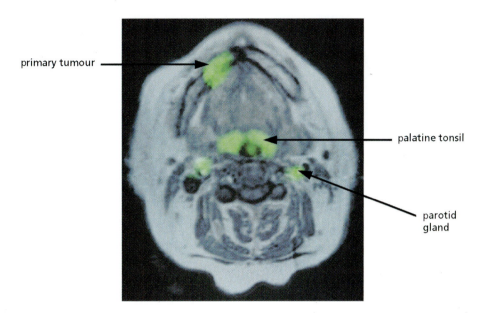

primary tumour

palatine tonsil

parotid gland

Registered MR/PET

This 70 year old woman with carcinoma of the right alveolar ridge was referred for a PET scan registered with MR prior to surgery. This PET image overlaid on the MR image demonstrated focal uptake of FDG at the primary site. The uptake was limited to the anterior mandible and did not extend to the angle of the jaw nor cross the midline, though it did extend locally into the floor of the mouth, permitting a limited mandibular resection. There was no evidence of lymph node disease on either MR or PET. Note also the physiological uptake within palatine tonsils and parotid glands.

Tumour may spread in a way that is difficult for anatomical imaging to identify but easy for PET imaging. Two examples include marrow and sheets of tumour spreading along anatomical planes.

Key issue 3 Nodal staging

Case 7.5

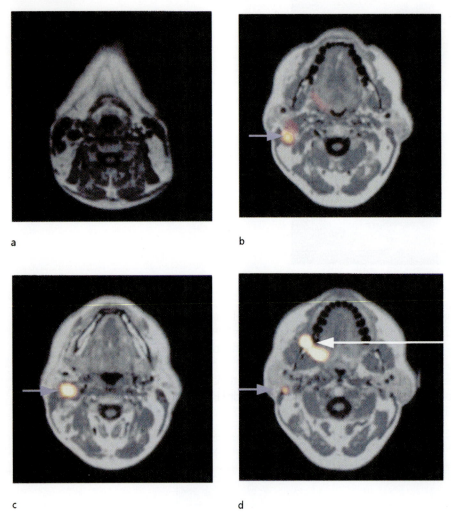

a   b

c   d

Registered MR/PET

This 48 year old man was referred for PET and MR imaging prior to surgery for staging purposes. There was uptake of FDG within the primary site in the right retromolar region extending laterally into the buccinator space and medially into the posterior third of the palate but not crossing the midline (d, arrowed in white). There was no involvement of the lateral pterygoid, maxilla or parapharyngeal space. There was accumulation of FDG within lymph nodes in the anterior and posterior triangles of the neck (b,c, arrowed in blue). The involved lymph nodes extend caudally as far as the base of the tongue, but lymph nodes seen inferior to this on MRI do not accumulate tracer, suggesting they are reactive rather than involved by tumour (d, arrowed in blue). Registered MR and PET provides accurate staging with regard to the extent of primary and nodal disease.

> Co-registration of metabolic and anatomical images may be critical in the management of head and neck tumours when the extent of surgery depends on relationship of the tumour with critical structures.

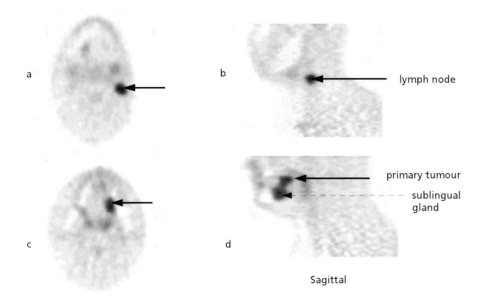

a

b ——— lymph node

c

d

primary tumour

sublingual gland

Sagittal

Transaxial

This 33 year old man with a moderately differentiated squamous cell carcinoma in the left tongue was initially treated with radiotherapy, having refused surgery. He then developed a palpable lymph node in the left side of the neck and was referred for PET, having agreed to proceed to surgery. The PET scan shows uptake within the primary tumour (c,d) and left cervical lymph node (a,b). Note also the physiological uptake seen within sublingual salivary gland. The PET scan delineated nodal spread from carcinoma of the tongue for surgical planning.

Key issue 4 Detection of recurrence

Case 7.7

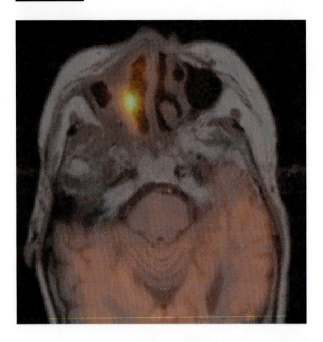

Registered MR/PET

This 73 year old woman had surgery and radiotherapy to a tumour in the right side of the nose 40 years previously. She presented with an 18 month history of increasing nasal obstruction and clinical examination showed a new squamous cell carcinoma in the anterior right side of the nose extending to the posterior choana and laterally into the right maxillary antrum but not into the side wall. CT examination confirmed the extent of disease as assessed clinically with bony changes seen within the lateral wall of the maxillary sinus ascribed to previous radiotherapy. MR was performed and suggested more extensive disease, extending posteriorly as far as the pterygopalatine fossa. The FDG-PET scan shown here, registered to the MR, revealed FDG uptake in the right nasal cavity extending towards the midline but not crossing it. FDG uptake extends into the posteriomedial aspect of the right maxillary antrum but not into the pterygopalatine fossa. No lymph node uptake was identified. In this case PET confirmed the presence of tumour in the maxillary antrum in keeping with the clinical and CT findings. The MR changes were misleading in suggesting more extensive disease.

> MRI after gadolinium contrast is given is often abnormal postoperatively or after radiation therapy. False positive examinations are less common with **FDG-PET**.

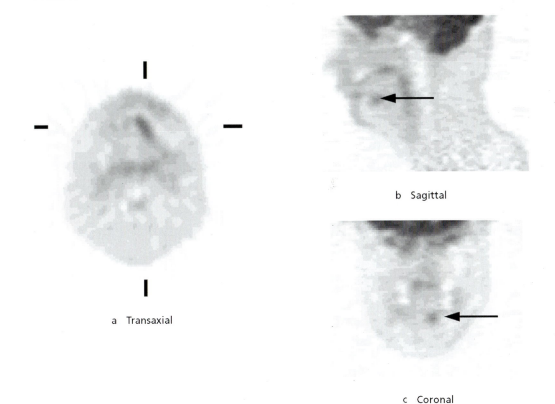

a Transaxial

b Sagittal

c Coronal

This 51 year old man was treated with surgery and radiotherapy in February 1996 for a squamous cell carcinoma of the right mandible. He re-presented with a right facial nerve palsy and was referred for a PET scan to assess whether there was recurrent disease. The PET scan showed no abnormal increased uptake of FDG. There is significant asymmetry with uptake within the left sublingual salivary gland (arrowed), but none in the right on the side of earlier surgery and radiotherapy.

> Treatment may often lead to asymmetry of normal physiological uptake within the head and neck. Correlation of FDG-PET findings with anatomical images can help avoid misinterpreting normal uptake as disease.

Case 7.9

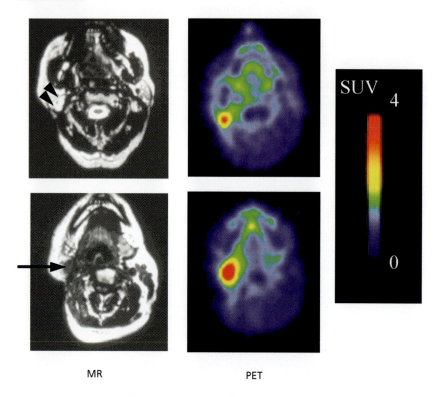

MR   PET

From Y Anzai, WR Carroll, DJ Quint, DR Bradford, S Miroshina, GT Wolf, RL Wahl. Radiology 1996; *200(1), 139, Fig. 2. Reproduced with permission.*

This patient had previously undergone radiotherapy and radical neck dissection for an unknown primary squamous cell carcinoma. He presented again with a right parotid swelling. MR images showed hyperintense signal lesions (arrowheads) in the right parotid gland (top image) and an isointense jugulodigastric node of borderline size (arrowed bottom image). PET scanning revealed abnormal uptake of FDG in both the parotid mass and the lymph node. Fine needle aspiration was performed which confirmed recurrent cancer at both sites.

Case 7.10

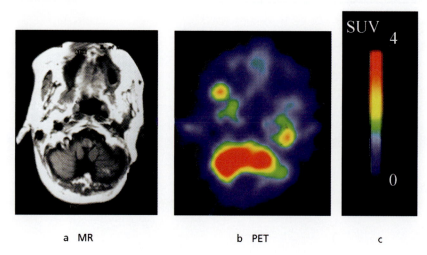

a MR   b PET   c

This patient who had undergone left parotidectomy for squamous cell carcinoma presented with recurrent nodal disease.

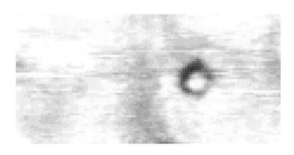

a   Coronal

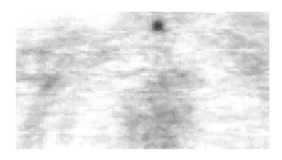

b   Coronal

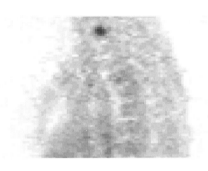

c   Sagittal

This 56 year old man had surgery for a primary squamous cell carcinoma of the larynx. He subsequently presented with recurrent disease in the left lung, which was confirmed histologically as a metastasis from the laryngeal carcinoma. He was referred for PET scanning which confirmed the presence of a metastasis in the apex of the left lung, shown here as a focus of increased FDG uptake with a photopenic centre, indicating a cystic or necrotic centre to the tumour (a). PET also demonstrated the presence of a further metastasis within the first thoracic vertebra (b, c).

Key issue 5 Response to therapy

Transaxial   Coronal

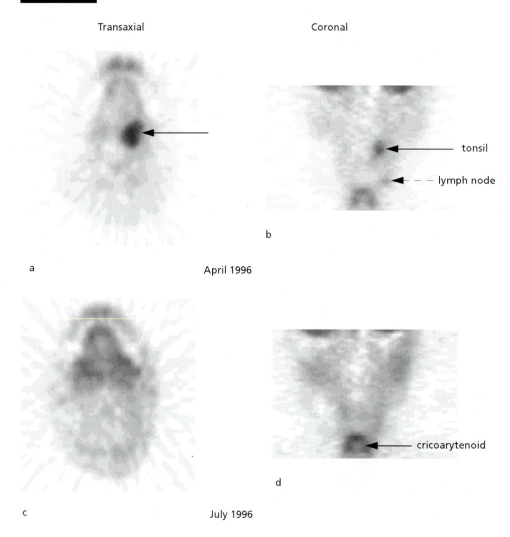

tonsil

lymph node

b

a   April 1996

cricoarytenoid

d

c   July 1996

This 61 year old male was treated for non-Hodgkin's lymphoma of the left tonsil with six cycles of chemotherapy. FDG-PET was used to assess response to treatment and to decide whether further chemotherapy was required. Uptake is seen in the first set of images (a,b) within the left tonsil and a left cervical lymph node with complete resolution in the second image set (c,d) performed 3 months later. Of note is marked uptake in the cricoarytenoid muscles, caused by the patient's speaking during the uptake period of both scans.

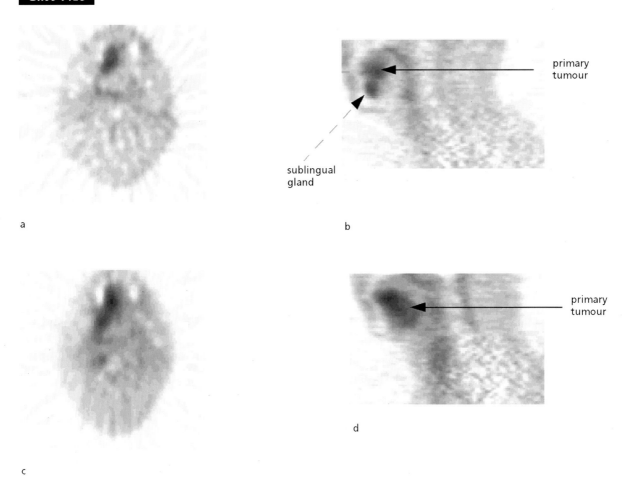

a

b

primary
tumour

sublingual
gland

c

d

primary
tumour

This 60 year old man with a squamous cell carcinoma of the right side of the tongue refused surgery at diagnosis. He underwent local radiotherapy but the disease progressed. The PET scan performed before radiotherapy shows FDG uptake in the primary tumour with physiological uptake seen in the sublingual gland at diagnosis (top images). The PET scan performed 3 months later shows increased activity within the tumour. The salivary gland uptake is no longer seen.

Conclusions

A possible algorithm for the use of FDG-PET in evaluating suspected recurrence of head and neck cancers is shown in Figure 7.2.

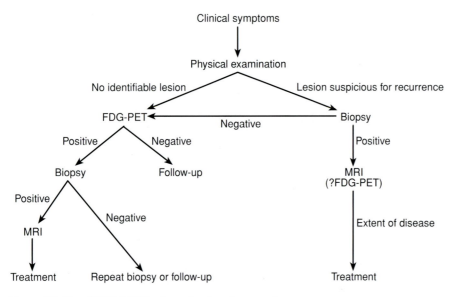

Figure 7.2 *Use of FDG-PET for the evaluation of suspected recurrence.*

Further reading

Adams S, Baum RP, Stuckensen T, Bitter K, Hor G (1998) Prospective comparison of ^{18}F-FDG PET with conventional imaging modalities (CT, MRI, US) in lymph node staging of head and neck cancer. *European Journal of Nuclear Medicine* **25**, 1255–60.

Anzai Y, Carroll WR, Quint DJ *et al.* (1996) Recurrence of head and neck cancer after surgery or irradiation: Prospective comparison of 2-deoxy-2-[F-18] fluoro-D-glucose PET and MR imaging diagnoses. *Radiology* **200**, 135–41.

Bailet JW, Abemayor E, Jabour BA *et al.* (1992) Positron emission tomography: A new, precise imaging modality for detection of primary head and neck tumours and assessment of cervical adenopathy. *Laryngoscope* **102**(3), 281–8.

Davis JP, Maisey MN, Chevretton EB (1998) Positron emission tomography – a useful imaging technique for otolaryngology, head and neck surgery. *J Laryngol Otol* **112**, 1–3.

Fischbein NJ, Assar OS, Caputo GR, Kaplan MJ, Singer MI, Price DC *et al.* (1998) Clinical utility of positron emission tomography with ^{18}F-fluorodeoxyglucose in detecting residual/recurrent squamous cell carcinoma of the head and neck. *American Journal of Neuroradiology* **19**, 1189–96.

Greven KM, Williams DW 3rd, Keyes JW Jr *et al.* (1994) Distinguishing tumor recurrence from irradiation sequelae with positron emission tomography in patients treated for larynx cancer. *Int J Radiat Oncol Biol Phys* **29**(4), 841–5.

Haberkorn U, Strauss LG, Dimitrakopoulou A *et al.* (1991) PET studies of fluorodeoxyglucose metabolism in patients with recurrent colorectal tumors receiving radiotherapy. *J Nucl Med* **32**(8), 1485–90.

Hemingway H, Wong W, Chevretton EB, McGurk M (1996) The use of positron emission tomography in the evaluation of orofacial malignancy and disease. *Br Dental J* **181**(7), 250–3.

Jabour BA, Choi Y, Hoh CK *et al.* (1993) Extracranial head and neck: PET imaging with 2-[^{18}F] fluoro-2-deoxy-D-glucose and MR imaging correlation. *Radiology* **186**(1), 27–35.

Lindholm P, Leskinen-Kallio S, Minn H *et al.* (1993) Comparison of fluorine-[18]fluorodeoxyglucose and carbon-11-methionine in head and neck cancer. *J Nucl Med* **34**, 1711–16.

Lowe VJ, Dunphy FR, Varvares M, Kim H, Wittry M, Dunphy CH *et al.* (1997) Evaluation of chemotherapy response in patients with advanced head and neck cancer using [F-18]fluorodeoxyglucose positron emission tomography. *Head & Neck* **19**, 666–74.

McGuirt WF, Greven KM, Keyes JW *et al.* (1995) Positron emission tomography in the evaluation of laryngeal carcinoma. *Ann Otol Rhinol Laryngol* **104**, 274–8.

McGuirt WF, Williams D, Keyes JW *et al.* (1995) A comparitive diagnostic study of head and neck nodal metastases using positron emission tomography. *Laryngoscope* **105**, 373–5.

McGuirt WF, Williams D, Keyes JW *et al.* (1995) Preoperative identification of benign versus malignant parotid masses: A comparative study including positron emission tomography. *Laryngoscope* **105**, 579–84.

Minn H, Lapela M, Klemi PJ *et al.* (1997) Prediction of survival with fluorine-18-fluoro-deoxyglucose and PET in head and neck cancer. *J Nucl Med* **38**, 1907–11.

Minn H, Joensuu H, Ahonen A, Klemi PI (1988) Fluorodeoxyglucose imaging: A method to assess the proliferative activity of human cancer in vivo. Comparison with DNA flow cytometry in head and neck tumors. *Cancer* **61**(9), 1776–81.

Minn H, Paul R, Ahonen A (1988) Evaluation of treatment response to radiotherapy in head and neck cancer with fluorine-18 fluorodeoxyglucose. *J Nucl Med* **29**(9), 1521–5.

Mukherji SK, Drane WE, Mancuso AA *et al.* (1996) Occult primary tumors of the head and neck: detection with 2-[F-18] fluoro-2-deoxy-D-glucose SPECT. *Radiology* **199**(3), 761–6.

Paulus P, Sambon A, Vivegnis D, Hustinx R, Moreau P, Collignon J *et al.* (1998) 18FDG-PET for the assessment of primary head and neck tumors: clinical, computed tomography, and histopathological correlation in 38 patients. *Laryngoscope* **108**, 1578–83.

Sercarz JA, Bailet JW, Abemayor E *et al.* (1998) Computer coregistration of positron emission tomography and magnetic resonance images in head and neck cancer. *Am J Otolaryng* **19**(2), 130–35.

Walsh RM, Wong WL, Chevretton EB, Beaney RP (1996) The use of PET-[18]FDG imaging in the clinical evaluation of head and neck lymphoma. *Clin Oncol* **8**(1), 51–4.

Wong W-L, Chevretton EB, McGurk M, Croft D (1995) PET-FDG imaging in the clinical evaluation of head and neck cancer. *J Roy Soc Med* **88**, 469–73.

Wong W-L, Hussain K, Chevretton EB *et al.* (1996) Validation and clinical application of computer-combined computed tomography and positron emission tomography with 2-[^{18}F]fluoro-2-deoxy-D-glucose head and neck images. *Am J Surg* **172**, 628–32.

Wong W-L, Chevretton EB, McGurk M *et al.* (1997) A prospective study of PET-FDG imaging for the assessment of head and neck squamous cell carcinoma. *Clin Otolaryngol* **22**, 209–14.

Chapter 8

Colorectal cancer

Introduction and background

Colorectal cancer is the second most common cause of death from cancer overall in western industrialized countries. There are, however, great international variations – 20-fold variations in incidence rates. Some of the highest rates are found in Connecticut in the US. Primary treatment is surgical with approximately a 50% 5 year survival rate. Adjuvant chemotherapy is widely employed but chemotherapeutic response to recurrence is poor. Follow up using serum CEA levels is valuable but is only elevated with active disease in less than 50% of the patients. Radiation therapy may be utilized for rectal carcinoma but less commonly for carcinoma of the colon. Only about 20% of patients who recur are considered suitable for further resection and of these about half relapse early due to unsuspected other metastatic sites.

EPIDEMIOLOGY

Annual incidence	Colon	350 per million
	Rectum	200 per million

Male ≅ Female

Rare under 40 years   Peak 60–69 years

1:20 persons in US will be affected

155 000 new cases per year (US)

10–15% of all cancers

Colon cancer is more frequent than rectal cancer and is increasing in frequency in all western industrialized countries. Many develop in a background of polyposis coli.

PATHOLOGY

Tumour types		Primary sites	
Adenocarcinoma	90–95%	Rectum	38%
		Sigmoid	21%
		Caecum and ascending colon	25%
		Transverse colon	5%
		Descending colon	5%

The vast majority of colorectal cancers are adenocarcinomas which may be ulcerating or fungating and cause large bowel obstruction.

PREDISPOSING FACTORS

Familial adenomatous polyposis (FAP)

Hereditary non-polyposis colorectal cancer (HNPCC)

Ulcerative colitis

Crohn's disease

Previous diagnosis of bowel cancer

High fat, low fibre diet

Although there are a number of predisposing factors the majority of colorectal cancers occur in patients with no predisposing factors.

PROGNOSIS

5 year survival	Overall	36%
	Dukes A	80–90%
	Dukes B	50–60%
	Dukes C	30%
	Dukes D	5%
	if >4 nodes involved	30%
Mortality	Colon	100 per million
	Rectum	200 per million

The prognosis in general is worse for rectal than colon cancer but varies from 90% 5 year survival for early localized disease to less than 5% when the disease presents in an advanced form. Approximately 25% of patients will have metastases at the time of presentation.

RESECTION

100 patients	70 resectable	45 cured
		25 recur
	30 advanced	

Approximately 45% of patients diagnosed as having colorectal cancer can be cured by effective surgical resection.

STAGING

T1	Submucosal invasion	**Dukes staging**	
T2	Muscularis propria	A	No nodes, not penetrated wall (10%)
T3	Through to subserosa	B	Penetration of wall (50%)
T4	Tumour directly invades other organs or perforates viscera	C	Lymph nodes (35%)
N0	Nil	D	Distant metastases (5%)
N1	1–3 peritumoral nodes		
N2	4 + peritumoral nodes		
N3	Distant nodes		
M1	Distant metastases		

Primary staging is usually surgical and pathological as most patients require resection to control local disease and prevent obstruction.

SITES OF RECURRENCE AND METASTASES

Isolated local	20%
Hepatic	30%
Other abdominal	20%
Pulmonary	20%
Retroperitoneal	10%
Ovarian	7%
Peritoneal seedlings	3–6%

Approximately 70% of patients who develop distant metastasis will also have a local recurrence.

Key management issues

PET in colorectal cancer

Colorectal cancer was the first non-CNS neoplasm to be imaged with PET (in 1982). Since then, several series have evaluated FDG-PET for detection of locally recurrent cancer following treatment or disseminated metastatic disease. Two reports showed in groups of at least 20 patients per study that FDG-PET was more accurate than CT or MRI in differentiating recurrent cancer from scar. Subsequent reports, now evaluating more than 100 patients, have shown FDG-PET to be more accurate than CT in detecting intra-abdominal metastases of colorectal cancer. The largest series, with 76 patients, reported an accuracy of 95% for FDG-PET, but only 65% for CT. Detection of liver metastases was also feasible and accurate. Instances of detecting the site of recurrent colorectal carcinoma when CEA levels are rising have also been reported. Detection of extrahepatic metastases of colorectal cancer dramatically changes management versus that planned when disease is truly isolated to the liver and changes in management in 20–30% of such patients studied by PET have been reported. These changes in patient management can result in substantial cost savings. Limited reports to date on both chemotherapy and radiotherapy support the role of PET in assessing treatment response. With radiotherapy, response assessment should be made several months or longer after treatment, as the PET signal declines only slowly, even with effective treatment. However with chemotherapy, the fall in tracer uptake occurs much more promptly. PET may be of particular utility in monitoring treatment of liver metastases of colorectal carcinoma, as it appears to be able to define responders/non-responders earlier than anatomic means. As with other parts of the body, a knowledge of the normal patterns of tracer uptake is essential, to allow differentiation of tumour uptake from that seen in normal tissues, such as colon or caecum. Overall, PET is assuming a growing role in evaluating recurrent colorectal carcinoma, although the role of PET in assessing primary tumours is, to date, limited.

Examples to illustrate key issues

Key issue 1 Suspected recurrence and restaging

Case 8.1

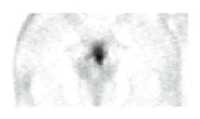
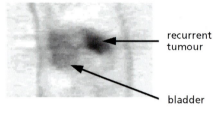

recurrent tumour

bladder

a Coronal

b Sagittal

This 57 year old man with a Duke's B carcinoma in 1994 was treated with surgery and radiotherapy. In 1996 his CEA levels increased, suggesting a possible recurrence. CT showed no definite evidence of recurrent disease, but there was a new finding of a right hydronephrosis and hydroureter. Biopsy at the anastomatic site indicated dysplasia but no recurrence. PET scanning showed FDG uptake within the presacral area indicating recurrent disease at this site. There was no evidence of distant spread.

> This patient received intravenous frusemide with injection of FDG. A large bladder is seen with dilute urine within it, enabling intense uptake within tumour tissue to be differentiated from physiological urinary activity. There are a variety of other different methods that are used to deal with the problem of urinary activity in pelvic scanning including bladder drainage and washout. With scanners allowing transmission images to be obtained after administration of FDG, post voiding images may be helpful.

Case 8.2 Liver lesions

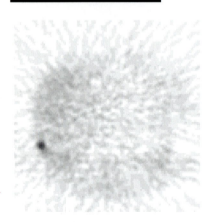

b Coronal

a Transaxial

This 67 year old man with carcinoma of the colon was treated with surgery and chemotherapy in 1993. Rising CEA levels in 1995 were due to liver metastases which were seen on CT and he underwent a wedge resection of the liver and interstitial radiotherapy. CEA levels fell to normal. He was referred for PET scanning when his CEA climbed again in September 1996. The figure shows two small metastases within the right lobe of the liver but there was no disease elsewhere.

Case 8.3

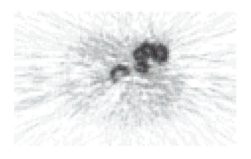

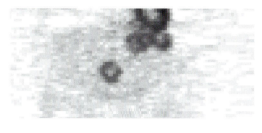

b   Coronal

a   Transaxial

This 47 year old man underwent left hemicolectomy in 1993. He subsequently underwent a wedge resection of the liver and adjuvant chemotherapy for liver metastases.
At the end of the treatment, the CEA measured 3 µg/l. He was referred for PET scanning when CEA levels rose again. Ultrasonography, chest radiography, CT and bone
scan were normal. The PET scan showed multiple liver lesions within the left lobe.

> The first of this pair of cases had potentially resectable disease with small
> metastases limited to the right lobe of the liver. Multifocal disease in the second
> patient would not be operable. PET scanning of the liver, abdomen and pelvis as
> well as the chest is advisable before surgical resection of apparently solitary
> lesions.

Case 8.4

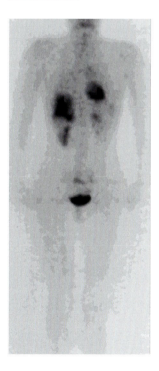

Coronal

This female with a history of treated colorectal carcinoma and rising CEA levels was
referred for PET scanning. FDG uptake is seen within recurrent tumour in the liver and
pelvis.

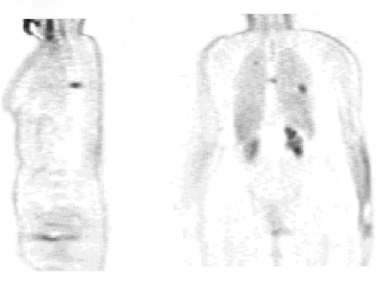

a Sagittal

b Coronal

This 45 year old woman with carcinoma of the colon was referred after a bone scan suggested the presence of a solitary metastasis at T6. FDG-PET scanning confirmed the presence of tumour within bone (uptake seen within T6 on the sagittal image (a), but also showed disease within the lungs (b).

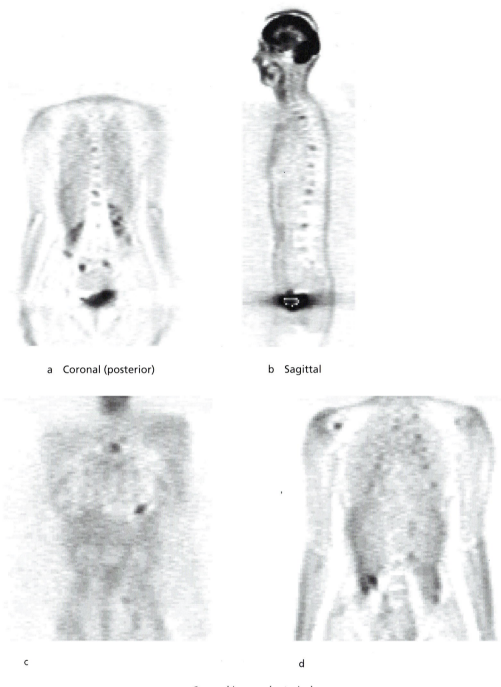

a   Coronal (posterior)   b   Sagittal

c   d

Coronal images (anterior)

This patient with carcinoma of the rectum was treated in 1992 with surgery and radio-therapy. She was referred for PET scanning with known metastases in the bone and lung prior to chemotherapy. The PET scan shows multiple metastases within the lungs and mediastinum (seen on anterior coronal images c,d), ovaries (posterior coronal image a) and bone (b).

> Whole body PET is particularly useful in assessing recurrent disease within bone and soft tissue.

Key issue 2 Response to treatment

Case 8.7

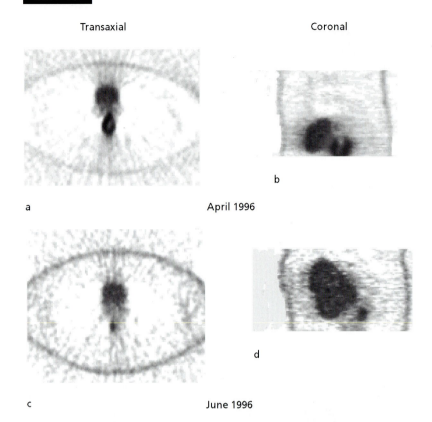

Transaxial   Coronal

b

a   April 1996

d

c   June 1996

This 46 year old patient received adjuvant radiotherapy and chemotherapy prior to surgery for carcinoma of the rectum. These scans performed 2 months apart show partial response to treatment with reduction of FDG uptake in the primary site. The measured SUV within the tumour decreased from 10.8 to 6.9.

> Residual uptake within a treated tumour does not always indicate tumour. Uptake may be seen within inflammatory tissue or within macrophages ingesting 'dead' or 'dying' tumour cells. The optimal time to scan after treatment is controversial and may differ for different tumour types and will vary based on the type of treatment. Declines in FDG uptake are probably slower following effective radiation therapy than chemotherapy. The reduction in FDG uptake may be more important than absolute uptake.

Key issue 3 Evaluating liver lesions

Case 8.8

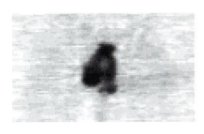

a Coronal

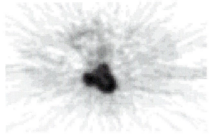

b Transaxial

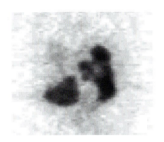

c Sagittal

This 54 year old woman with carcinoma of the rectum was scanned at disease presentation prior to radiotherapy with an equivocal lesion on CT in the liver. There was massive intense uptake within the primary tumour (SUV = 8.1) with no evidence of spread to the liver or elsewhere.

Conclusions

No role has been established for PET in the management of primary disease. Figure 8.1 shows a possible algorithm utilizing the known benefits of PET for patients with recurrent disease when surgery is contemplated.

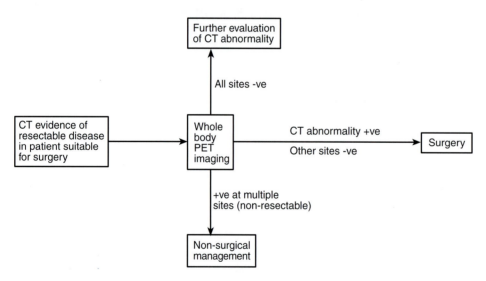

Figure 8.1 *Possible use of PET in recurrent colorectal cancer.*

Further reading

Abdel-Nabi H, Doerr RJ, Lamonica DM *et al.* (1998) Staging of primary colorectal carcinomas with fluorine-18-fluorodeoxyglucose whole-body PET: correlation with histopathologic and CT findings. *Radiology* **206**(3), 755–60.

Bohdiewicz PJ, Scott GC, Juni JE *et al.* (1995) Indium-111 Oncoscint CR/OV and ¹⁸F in colorectal and ovarian carcinoma recurrences early observations. *Clin Nucl Med* **20**(3), 230–6.

Delbeke D, Vitola JV, Sandler MP, Arildsen RC, Powers TA, Wright JK, Jr. *et al.* (1997) Staging recurrent metastatic colorectal carcinoma with PET. *Journal of Nuclear Medicine* **38**, 1196–1201.

Findlay M, Young H, Cunnigham D *et al.* (1996) Noninvasive monitoring of tumor metabolism using fluorodeoxyglucose and positron emission tomography in colorectal cancer liver metastases: correlation with tumor response to fluorouracil. *J Clin Onc* **14**(3), 700–8.

Flanagan FL, Dehdashti F, Ogunbiyi OA *et al.* (1998) Utility of FDG-PET for investigating unexplained plasma CEA elevation in patients with colorectal cancer. *Ann Surg* **227**(3), 319–23.

Gupta NC, Falk PM, Frank AL *et al.* (1993) Pre-operative staging of colorectal carcinoma using positron emission tomography. *Nebr Med J* **78**(2), 30–5.

Ito K, Kato T, Tadokoro M *et al.* (1992) Recurrent rectal cancer and scar: Differentiation with PET and MR imaging. *Radiology* **182**(2), 549–52.

Keogan MT, Lowe VJ, Baker ME, McDermott VG, Lyerly HK, Coleman RE (1997) Local recurrence of rectal cancer: evaluation with F-18 fluorodeoxyglucose PET imaging. *Abdominal Imaging* **22**, 332–7.

Lai DTM, Fulham M, Stephens MS *et al.* (1996) The role of whole-body positron emission tomography with [^{18}F] fluorodeoxyglucose in identifying operable colorectal cancer metastases to the liver. *Arch Surg* **131**, 703–7.

Meyer M (1995) Diffusely increased colonic 18F FDG uptake in acute enterocolitis. *Clin Nucl Med* **20**(5), 434–5.

Ogunbiyi OA, Flanagan FL, Dehdashti F *et al.* (1997) Detection of recurrent and metastatic colorectal cancer: comparison of positron emission tomography and computed tomography. *Ann Surg Onc* **98**(3), 373–9.

Paulus P, Hustinx R, Daenen F *et al.* (1997) Usefulness of ^{18}FDG positron emission tomography in detection and follow-up of digestive cancers. *Acta Gastroentr Belgica* **60**(4), 278–80.

Schiepers C, Penninckx F, DeVadder N *et al.* (1995) Contribution of PET in the diagnosis of recurrent colorectal cancer: comparison with conventional imaging. *Eur J Surg Oncol* **21**, 517–22.

Strauss LG, Clorius JH, Schlag P *et al.* (1989) Recurrence of colorectal tumors: PET evaluation. *Radiology* **170**(2), 329–32.

Yonkura Y, Benau RS, Brill AB *et al.* (1982) Increased accumulation of 2-deoxy-2-[^{18}F] fluoro-D-glucose in liver metastases from colon carcinoma. *J Nucl Med* **23**(12), 1133–7.

Valk PE, Pounds TR, Myers RW *et al.* (1995) Metabolic PET imaging in the diagnosis of recurrent colorectal cancer. In *Proceedings of the American Radium Society 78th Annual Meeting*, Paris, France, 29 April–3 May 1995, p. 33.

Chapter 9

Melanoma

Introduction and background

Malignant melanoma is the most rapidly increasing cancer in white populations and its incidence has been increasing at more than 5% per year since 1973, with an increasing mortality rate second only to lung cancer. Malignant melanoma is the most common cancer in young women between the age of 25 and 29 and forms 18% of all cancers in young adults between the ages of 15 and 39. It has been predicted that 1 in 75 individuals born in the year 1996 could develop malignant melanoma at the present rate of increase. Risks of melanoma include pre-existing skin lesions, but 20–50% of malignant melanomas arise *de novo*. Other risk factors include hair colour: red-haired individuals have a three times greater risk than average and fair blond individuals have a two times greater risk. The overall increase in risk is thought to be related to strong solar ultraviolet radiation.

Melanoma is one of the most metabolically active of tumours, and FDG uptake is very high in animal models and human tumour xenografts of melanoma. Melanoma is curable when diagnosed early (i.e. when thin) and completely removed by surgery from the skin. Unfortunately, thicker melanomas are more likely to metastasize to regional lymph nodes and then systemically. Disseminated melanoma is generally poorly responsive to therapy. The recent approval of recombinant interferon α for the treatment of nodal metastases to regional lymph nodes has increased the importance of early diagnosis of nodal metastases. Similarly, about 20% of patients who present with nodal metastases and no distant metastases are cured by surgical resection of the tumours. Additionally, resection of isolated metastases to brain and to lung have, in some series, been reported to improve survival. Thus, in melanoma, as in many other cancers, detecting regional lymph node involvement and detecting disseminated metastases are important. Radical surgical procedures to remove isolated metastases are rational only if disease is truly isolated. PET can play an important role in such decisions.

EPIDEMIOLOGY		
	UK	US
Incidence	≅75 per million	130 per million
Male/female ratio	1 : 1.5	
10% of all skin cancers		
18% in 15–39 year age group		
Whites ≫ blacks or Asian		

Malignant melanoma is one of the most rapidly increasing fatal cancers and is now the 14th most common in the UK and 8th in the US. The incidence is somewhat higher in women than men.

PATHOLOGY

Tumour types		Sites
Superficial spreading	70%	50% leg (women)
Nodular melanoma	20%	37% trunk (men)
Lentigo malignant melanoma	5%	
Acral lentiginines	5%	

Lentigo malignant melanoma has better prognosis, acral lentiginous higher incidence in black and Asian populations. The sites of tumour development generally reflect the distribution of skin exposed to sunlight.

PROGNOSIS

Overall 5 year survival	men	50%
	women	75%
Distant metastases 5 year survival	4%	(0% > 3 sites)
Annual mortality	25 per million	

Thickness of primary tumour (Breslow) effect

Tumour size	5 year survival
<0.75 mm	95–99%
0.76–1.49 mm	80–95%
1.5–4 mm	60–75%
>4 mm	<50%

Nodal status effect

Number of nodes involved	10 year survival
0	>80%
1	32%
2–3	21%
>4	10%

The two key prognostic factors are thickness of primary and lymph nodes. Extremity is better than trunk. Women have a better prognosis than men.

STAGING

T staging (pathological)	Breslow levels (thickness)	Clark levels	Stage	
			I	<1.5 cm; node negative
PT1	0.75 mm or less invading dermis	II	II	>1.5 cm or satellites within 2 cm of primary; node negative
PT2	0.75–1.5 mm and/or invades the papillary–reticular dermal interface	III	III	Regional nodes +ve or 'in transit' disease
PT3	1.5–4.0 mm and/or invades the reticular dermis	IV	IV	Distant metastases
PT4	>4.0 mm and/or invades subcutaneous tissue and/or satellites within 2 cm	V		
N0	Nil			
N1	3 cm or less in any regional node			
N2	Metastasis >3 cm in regional node and/or in transit metastasis			
M1	Distant metastases			

Clinical stages I and II represent 'local disease'.

In transit means >2 cm from the primary lesion. Elective lymph node dissection (ELND) shows 20% of stages I and II, i.e. localized having micrometastases.

METASTATIC SITES

	Clinical %	Autopsy %
Skin, subcutaneous and distant nodes	50	60
Lung	30	75
Liver	15	65
Brain	15	45
Bone	15	36
Gastrointestinal tract	5	40
Heart, pancreas, adrenal, thyroid	Rare	35

When regional nodes are detected clinically 70–85% of patients have distant metastases, clinical sensitivity about 80%.

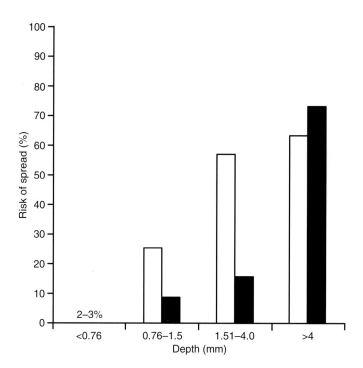

Figure 9.1 *Regional risk within 3 years of presentation (light bars) and distant metastatic risk within 5 years (dark bars).*

Key management issues

KEY MANAGEMENT ISSUES

1 Staging thick melanomas at presentation

2 Nodal spread from intermediate thickness lesions

3 Confirming recurrence

4 Surveillance

5 Monitoring response

6 Restaging before removal of isolated metastases

PET in melanoma

Gritters *et al.* (1993) demonstrated that melanoma could be imaged using PET with FDG in 12 cases. In this small study, 15/15 intra-abdominal and lymph node metastases were detected by FDG-PET. PET also identified three additional metastatic foci only noted retrospectively on CT. PET correctly identified tumour in 7/7 lymph nodes, including 3 cases where the nodes were of normal size, and excluded tumour in 6/6 nodal regions for a 13/13 accuracy in nodal disease characterization. PET was not as sensitive as CT for small lesions in the lungs, however. Of particular interest were that small bowel metastases, which are extremely difficult to identify by any method other than autopsy, were detected in several instances in this study. Macfarlane *et al.* (1995) have shown good accuracy (91%) and excellent specificity of FDG-PET for the detection of lymph node metastases of melanoma. This report suggests that a non-invasive PET scan potentially could be used to help make the decision whether or not to remove the lymph nodes draining a melanoma at the time of initial management. The results of Blessing *et al.* (1995) are less encouraging in this regard in that in 20 patients studied retrospectively, the sensitivity of PET on a per node basis was 74% and the specificity 93%, comparable to that of ultrasonography. The study results are difficult to compare to those of Macfarlane, however, as the study was performed in patients with clinically suspicious nodes; some had had treatment prior to scanning. It is clear that PET is a reasonably sensitive and highly specific test for detecting the presence or absence of lymph node metastases in patients with cutaneous malignant melanoma.

Steinert *et al.* (1995) used whole body PET imaging to survey for melanoma. Using this approach, they showed excellent lesion detection capability, with their only failures in detection using the non-attenuation corrected PET method being in cases where there were very small cutaneous lesions (3 mm). In their study of 33 patients with known melanoma, the overall sensitivity of PET was 92%. Specificity was increased by clinical knowledge of the location of biopsy sites etc., and was 77% without such clinical information and 100% with the clinical information available. Non-attenuation corrected whole body PET tends to accentuate apparent skin surface radioactivity levels, making the background higher, and it is thus harder to detect small skin lesions. Lindholm and colleagues (1995) have shown in 10 patients with 22 known foci of melanoma >1.5 cm in diameter that all tumour foci could be detected using [^{11}C]L-methionine PET. They failed to detect five smaller pulmonary lesions in the same study, possibly due to resolution or respiratory motion difficulties. Thus, FDG would appear to be the preferred PET imaging agent for melanoma. In many centres, melanoma is a leading disease indication for clinical PET referrals.

Examples to illustrate key issues

Key issue 1 Staging thick melanomas at presentation

Case 9.1

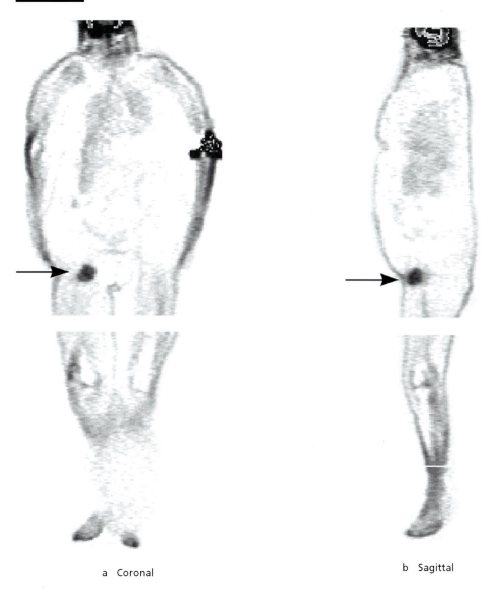

a Coronal

b Sagittal

This patient had a malignant melanoma 4.8mm thick excised from her right heel in August 1995. PET scanning performed in October indicated spread to right inguinal lymph nodes (arrowed). The uptake seen in the left antecubital fossa resulted from partially extravasated injection of tracer.

Key issue 2 Nodal spread from intermediate thickness lesions

Case 9.2

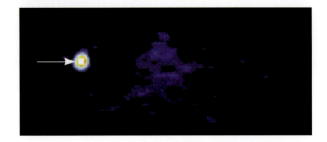

a Transaxial

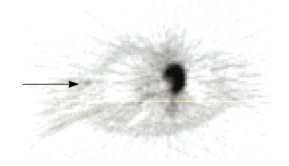

b Transaxial

The above transaxial images were acquired from two patients, the first with a melanoma on the right forearm and the second with a melanoma on the skin surface overlying the right scapula. There was intense FDG uptake within a right axillary lymph node metastasis which was non-palpable in the first case. The second patient had palpable axillary lymphadenopathy, with only moderate uptake of FDG within the right axilla, which at lymph node dissection was proven to contain tumour.

> Variable uptake may occur within lymph nodes in melanoma and may make reactive lymph nodes difficult to differentiate from nodes involved by tumour. The extent of tumour involvement in lymph nodes is important with micrometastases likely to escape detection.

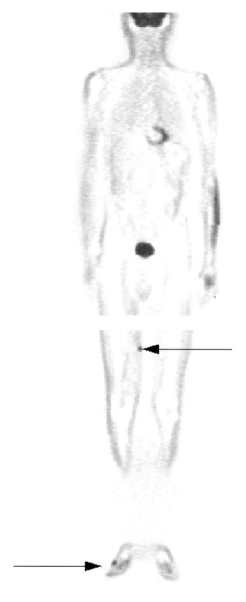

Coronal

This 56 year old patient had a malignant melanoma excised from the right foot in 1992. In 1996 he had right inguinal lymphadenopathy. Block dissection revealed nodes containing tumour. PET scanning was performed and showed further recurrence at the original site of disease (lower arrow) together with a superficial metastasis in the right thigh (arrowed), evidence of a lesion in transit.

Key issue 3 Confirming recurrence

Case 9.4

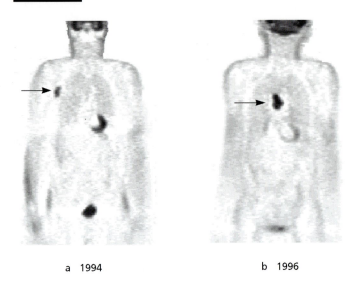

a   1994   b   1996

Coronal images

This patient had a melanoma excised from the right forearm in 1993. He re-presented with right axillary lymphadenopathy in 1994. High uptake of FDG is seen within the right axilla on the left coronal image. The presence of nodal disease increases the risk of developing visceral disease and in 1996, the patient was rescanned when he was losing weight and complaining of feeling generally unwell. PET revealed evidence of hilar and mediastinal metastases (b).

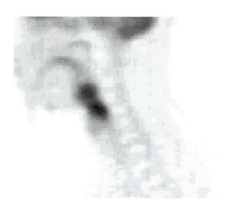

b Sagittal

a Transaxial

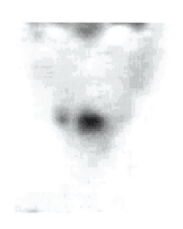

c Coronal

This 59 year old woman had a melanoma excised in 1993. In 1996 she re-presented with extensive metastatic involvement including melanoma within the larynx and pharynx. High uptake of FDG was seen within the larynx and pharynx (seen on all views) together with a right upper cervical lymph node (a,c).

Note the intense uptake within the larynx compared with the level of 'physiological' uptake that is seen in a patient speaking during the uptake period of FDG – a reminder of the need for patient silence during the uptake period when performing FDG-PET scans of the head and neck.

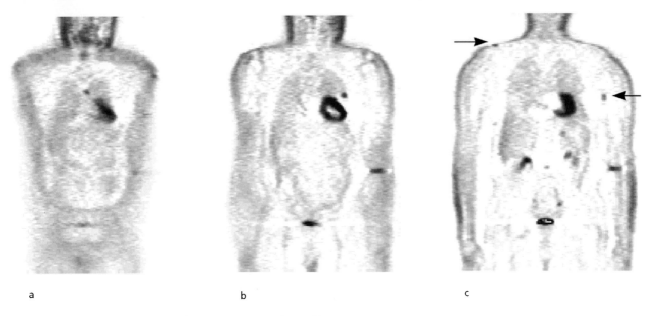

a   b   c

Coronal images

This 63 year old patient had a melanoma removed in 1995 from the skin overlying the right scapula. In July of 1995 a second metastasis was excised at the nape of the neck. Increased uptake is seen following surgery at this site on the PET scan (c, arrowed). In addition there were multiple metastases within the anterior mediastinum (a), left lung (b), left adrenal and para-aortic nodes (c). Focal increased uptake was seen within the left axilla (arrowed) which may represent a metastasis but could be secondary to nodal uptake following the injection which was administered in the left antecubital fossa.

Key issue 4 Surveillance

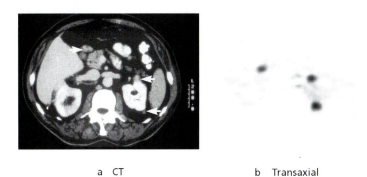

a CT   b Transaxial

From LS Gritters, IR Francis, KR Zasadny, RL Wahl. Journal of Nuclear Medicine 1993; 34(9), p. 1425, Fig. 5A,B. Reproduced with permission.

The CT scan in this case was performed for surveillance purposes. The PET scan performed concurrently showed focal increased uptake at the level of the kidneys, compatible with anterior and posterior perirenal metastases, as well as a perihepatic metastasis (a, arrowed). Small foci are seen on the CT scan at the sites that were abnormal on PET, indicative of metastatic malignant melanoma. These lesions progressed on CT, but only one of the three was prospectively identified on the CT. Note that due to the intensity of the uptake within the metastases, the expected mild liver activity and urinary FDG activity was not seen.

Case 9.8

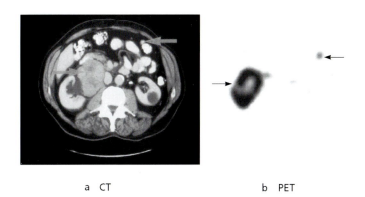

a CT   b PET

From LS Gritters, IR Francis, KR Zasadny, RL Wahl. Journal of Nuclear Medicine 1993; 34(9), p. 1423, Fig. 1A,B. Reproduced with permission.

The transaxial image here shows a large intra-abdominal metastasis from malignant melanoma with a hypometabolic centre, in the right paraspinal region (arrowed). The mass was clearly seen on CT but the small mesenteric metastasis seen to accumulate FDG was noted on CT only on retrospective review (arrowed). This small mass was subsequently shown to progress indicating it to represent metastatic melanoma. Note the presence of a simple left renal cyst, which did not accumulate FDG.

> CT has great difficulty in detecting extrahepatic abdominal lesions less than 2 cm in size where PET may be of great value and should probably be the first investigation of choice for suspected malignant melanoma.

Conclusions

Figure 9.2 shows a possible management algorithm for metastatic melanoma.

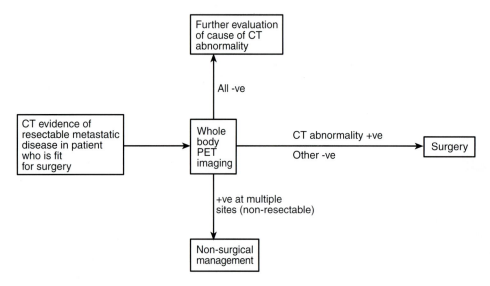

Figure 9.2 *Management algorithm for metastatic melanoma.*

References and further reading

Blessing C, Feine U, Geiger L *et al.* (1995) Positron emission tomography and ultrasonography. *Arch Dermatol* **131**, 1394–8.

Boni R, Huch-Boni RA, Steinert H, von Schulthess GK, Burg G (1996) Early detection of melanoma metastasis using fluorodeoxyglucose F 18 positron emission tomography. *Archives of Dermatology* **132**, 875–6.

Gritters LS, Francis IR, Zasadny KR, Wahl RL (1993) Initial assessment of positron emission tomography using 2-fluorine-18–fluoro-2-deoxy-D-glucose in the imaging of malignant melanoma. *J Nucl Med* **34**(9), 1420–7.

Holder WD, Jr., White RL, Jr., Zuger JH, Easton EJ, Jr., Greene FL (1998) Effectiveness of positron emission tomography for the detection of melanoma metastases. *Annals of Surgery* **227**, 764–9; discussion 769–71.

Johnson TM, Smith JW, Nelson BR *et al.* (1995) Current therapy for cutaneous melanoma. *Dermatology* **32**(5), 689–707.

Lindholm P, Leskinen S, Nagren K *et al.* (1995) Carbon-11-methionine PET imaging of malignant melanoma. *J Nucl Med* **36**, 1806–10.

Lucignani G, Paganelli G, Modorati *et al.* (1992) MRI, antibody-guided scintigraphy, and glucose metabolism in uveal melanoma. *J Comp Assist Tomogr* **16**(1), 77–83.

Macfarlane DJ, Sondak V, Wahl RL (1995) Initial prospective evaluation of FDG-PET in staging regional lymph nodes in patients with cutaneous malignant melanoma (CMM.) *J Nucl Med* **36**(5), 116.

Macfarlane DJ, Sondak V, Johnson T *et al.* (1998) Prospective evaluation of 2-[18F]-2-deoxy-D-glucose positron emission tomography in staging of regional lymph nodes in patients with cutaneous malignant melanoma. *J Clin Onc* **16**(5), 1770–76.

Rinne D, Baum RP, Hor G *et al.* (1998) Primary staging and follow-up of high risk melanoma patients with whole-body 18F-fluorodeoxyglucose positron emission tomography: results of a prospective study of 100 patients. *Cancer* **82**(9), 1664–71.

Rivers JK (1996) Melanoma. *Lancet* **347**, 803–7.

Steinert HC, Huch Boni RA, Buck A *et al.* (1995) Malignant melanoma: staging with whole-body positron emission tomography and 2-[18F]-fluoro-2-deoxy-D-glucose. *Radiology* **195**, 705–9.

Wagner JD, Schauwecker D, Hutchins G *et al.* (1997) Initial assessment of positron emission tomography for detection of nonpalpable regional lymphatic metastases in melanoma. *J Surg Oncol* **64**(3), 181–9.

Chapter 10

Primary brain tumour

Introduction and background

Primary brain tumours have an incidence of approximately 11:100 000 of the population, although overall metastatic brain disease is more common. Usually when a space-occupying lesion is the presenting clinical feature a primary brain tumour rather than a metastasis is the cause, and more than 50% of the patients present with some form of epilepsy. Primary brain tumours are the most prevalent solid tumour of children, for whom the spectrum is quite different from adults. New treatments are being introduced, with little overall improvement in outcome. These include stereotactic biopsy and stereotactic surgery which is frequently image guided, conformal radiotherapy, chemotherapy (more recently using agents which enhance the transit of the agents across the blood–brain barrier) and radioactive seed implantation. The outlook remains poor, however, with the survival less than 1 year for high grade tumours. Imaging is increasingly required to detect disease, particularly recurrent disease, and in planning and guiding therapy and biopsy. Probably the biggest imaging difficulty at present is the failure of anatomical imaging methods to clearly differentiate recurrent tumour from scar and postradiation effects.

PATHOLOGY	
Glioblastoma multiforme	30%
Astrocytoma (low to high grade)	20%
Medulloblastoma	
Ependymoma	7%
Oligodendroglioma	
Meningioma	18%
Nerve sheath tumours	10%
Pituitary tumours	5%
Other	10%

Glioblastoma multiforme is the most malignant of the astrocytomas. Astrocytomas may also be divided into grades I–IV of malignancy with worsening prognosis. Spinal cord tumours are 10 times less frequent than brain tumours.

EPIDEMIOLOGY

		UK	US
Incidence		72 per million	45 per million
New cases per year		3500	11 000
Male/female ratio	M > F		
Most patients >45 years			
Over 45 years		85% astrocytoma	(50% glioblastoma multiforme)
Children and young people		60% astrocytoma	(10% glioblastoma multiforme)
		20% medulloblastoma	
		10% ependymoma	
		10% rest	
Incidence rises with age	age 0–4	3 per 100 000	
	age >65	20 per 100 000	

It is important to appreciate the changes in tumour distribution with age.

PROGNOSIS

Overall 5 year survival	≅30%	
Deaths per year	3000 (UK)	11 000 (US)
Median survival Grade III and IV	9–10 months	
Low grade astrocytoma 5 year survival	50–75%	

Primary brain tumours generally have a poor prognosis and the higher grades, e.g. glioblastoma multiforme, are essentially incurable.

Key management issues

PET in primary brain tumours

Brain tumours are infrequent, but have been well studied by PET over the past 15 years. DiChiro and colleagues first recognized the potential of FDG for imaging brain tumours and reported on this approach (DiChiro *et al.* 1982).

Based on this experience, several settings exist for the use of PET in brain tumour management. FDG is the most commonly used tracer, despite the limitation of its high uptake into normal brain tissue, which means background activity levels are high.

Since the initial report from the NIH group, many subsequent studies have examined the ability of FDG and PET to separate between histologically aggressive (high FDG uptake) and less aggressive (low FDG uptake) brain tumours, as well as to separate viable tumour (persistent FDG uptake) from scar or necrosis post-treatment (low or absent FDG uptake). While one study did not show a separation between high and low grade gliomas, on average, the general trend of high FDG uptake substantially associated with more aggressive tumours seems true, though a great deal of overlap exists. Elevated FDG uptake in a brain tumour is generally associated with a poorer prognosis than seen in brain tumours with lower levels of FDG uptake (Alavi *et al.* 1988). Delbeke and colleagues (1995) investigated which FDG-PET criteria should be used to separate high grade from low grade brain tumours before they received any treatment. They observed the best separating index to be a tumour/white matter uptake ratio of 1.5. At this cut-off level, the sensitivity and specificity of FDG-PET for high grade tumours was 94% and 77% respectively.

There are several situations in which PET can be useful in brain tumour imaging. In actual practice, the post-treatment monitoring of brain tumours is the most common application in many medical centres. FDG allows for detection of high grade tumours, despite the fact that it has high uptake into normal brain tissue. Following the completion of radiation therapy, contrast enhancement on CT or MRI in the area of previous tumour mass may represent viable tumour or radiation necrosis, as both can have mass effect and both can have contrast enhancement. FDG uptake into such a contrast-enhancing lesion strongly suggests the presence of viable tumour, whereas absence of FDG uptake suggests that necrosis is present (particularly if the tumour is of a higher grade and was visible on PET before the treatment). This emphasizes the importance of having a baseline FDG-PET study, especially for lower grade brain tumours, to be sure they are positive before treatment (i.e. have higher FDG uptake than white matter). Alternatively, as is shown in the case examples below, the use of $[^{11}C]$L-methionine can be very helpful in delineating the location of lower grade brain tumours not well seen on PET with FDG. To date, qualitative visual analysis, in which FDG uptake is compared to normal white or grey matter is generally used for analysis, in preference to quantitative analysis. This approach generally means that any focus of activity which is more intense in tracer uptake than normal brain white matter is considered to represent viable tumour. The reason FDG uptake appears to correlate with survival and tumour grade is not yet fully clear, but may be related to the increased cellular density seen in high grade tumours, or may be related to increased FDG uptake in the more rapidly proliferating tumour cells.

Representative studies comparing FDG-PET and histology/outcome after brain tumour therapy include those of Di Chiro et al. (1987), who reported that PET with FDG appropriately diagnosed necrosis present in all 10 of the 10 patients with necrosis from a group of 95 suspected of having necrosis post brain tumour therapy. Valk et al. (1988) reported an 84% accuracy of PET in determining if necrosis was present or absent following interstitial brachytherapy for brain tumours and pointed out that PET scan results were more reliable predictors of outcome than were histology, which often showed some 'viable' cells after treatment, of questionable 'viability' clinically.

Some low grade tumours have low FDG uptake, but in other cases high uptake of FDG can be seen in tumours which have evidence of contrast enhancement on CT, but which are associated with a good prognosis – as in juvenile pilocytic astrocytomas (Fulham et al. 1993). In the situation of low grade gliomas, other tracers, such as [^{11}C]L-methionine, [^{11}C]thymidine or [^{11}C]putrescine, may potentially represent reasonable choices for PET tumour imaging in the brain in contrast to the use of FDG only (Bergstrom et al. 1987). These latter tracers have only a low level of uptake into normal brain and thus often allow for higher tumour/background uptake ratios than FDG. [^{11}C]L-methionine has been shown not to accumulate into focal radiation necrosis in the relatively small number of patients studied to date, and to accumulate in many low grade gliomas. Bergstrom et al. (1987) reported that 7/11 low grade gliomas had increased uptake of [^{11}C]L-methionine vs. normal brain. It has been shown by Roelcke and colleagues (1996) that [^{11}C]L-methionine uptake is correlated with ^{11}Rb uptake across a wide range of histologies. This is not the case with FDG. This observation suggests that a significant component of [^{11}C]L-methionine uptake into higher grade tumours may be due to blood–brain barrier alteration, as opposed to incorporation into protein tumour. This, coupled with a report by Ogawa et al. (1995) indicating that there is some [^{11}C]L-methionine uptake into intracerebral haematomas not caused by tumours, shows that some caution must still be exercised when attempting to determine if a focus of residual contrast enhancement after brain tumour therapy is due to necrosis or viable tumour, at least when using [^{11}C]L-methionine. Thus, FDG remains better established in this specific clinical setting.

Untreated CNS lymphomas are well imaged by FDG-PET, with FDG uptake into the lymphomas similar to that seen in high grade gliomas. There is higher FDG uptake into CNS lymphoma than into CNS infections, as well – a situation which may be useful in diagnosis in the HIV positive patient.

While FDG is clearly valuable in imaging primary brain tumours, especially high grade tumours, data on imaging intra-axial metastases to brain is much more limited. Griffeth et al. (1993) reported that FDG uptake into untreated metastases from a variety of cancers can, in a significant fraction of cases (up to 1/3 of patients in their study), be inadequate to produce satisfactory images of the metastases. This is particularly the case when small lesions are located in very close proximity to grey matter folds in the brain. This has also been reported by our group from Guy's and St Thomas' PET centre, where several instances of failure to detect metastatic lung cancer to brain were reported.

Meningiomas can also be imaged with PET. Di Chiro et al. (1987) reported, on a series of 17 patients, that those with the highest FDG uptake appeared to have the most aggressive histological appearance, while those with low FDG uptake appeared to have a less aggressive histology. Tumours with the lowest FDG uptake were found to have the greatest long term likelihood for survival. It is uncertain if low FDG uptake in a meningioma would suggest that surgery could be delayed, but such metabolic information may be a useful adjunct in such challenging cases.

Two other clinical issues in brain tumour management are well addressed by PET:

- The localization of active tumour for biopsy is more accurate with PET than CT in some cases.
- ^{15}O water activation PET can also define areas of the cerebral cortex which are activated during motor or visual stimulation by performing [^{11}O]water blood flow studies at rest and during a task that activates the cerebral cortex.

These data on the exact location of functional cortical areas can then be superimposed on MRI structural data to assist in planning surgical procedures, the goal being to excise all the tumour but spare normal tissue as much as possible.

Monitoring brain tumour treatment using PET is quite commonly performed if there is a difficult diagnostic question after treatment. A decline in FDG uptake in a tumour at several weeks to months after the conclusion of therapy suggests a good response of the tumour to treatment. By contrast, increased FDG uptake versus the basal level, or persistent FDG uptake, would strongly suggest residual tumour being present despite treatment. Responses of glucose metabolism immediately after treatment are less clear, however, so assessing response by PET is not currently suggested if done only a few days after a treatment is given. Indeed, the optimal time to assess treatment is still under study, but would seem to be safest if done well after the treatment course is completed. Given the resolution of current PET devices, they would not be expected to detect microscopic foci of tumour, so a negative scan does not completely exclude the possibility of residual tumour being present. PET with FDG would seem to have its greatest difficulties in assessing treatment response in patients with low grade tumours. In this setting, [^{11}C]L-methionine may be preferable if available.

Examples to illustrate key issues

Key issues 1–4 Initial management

High grade malignant tumours

Case 10.1

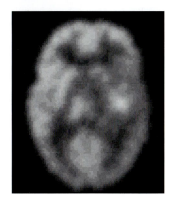 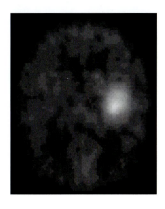

a FDG
b [^{11}C]L-methionine

Transaxial

This 10 year old child with a neuroectodermal tumour had intense uptake of tracer within the left parietal lobe extending into the temporal lobe with midline shift. The uptake within the lesion is more marked with [^{11}C]L-methionine than FDG, but the FDG uptake is still significantly greater within the lesion than normal cortex, typical of a high grade tumour. Hypometabolism of basal ganglia and the cerebral cortex adjacent to the tumour was also seen with FDG.

Case 10.2

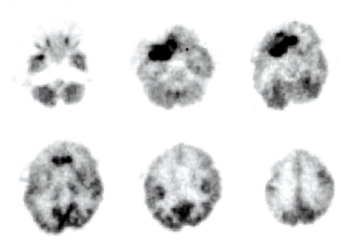

Transaxial

This is a case example of a patient scanned with a malignant 'butterfly' astrocytoma. There was intensely increased FDG uptake in the frontal subcortical region crossing the midline. This metabolic pattern predicts aggressive biological behaviour by primary neoplasms of astrocytic origin.

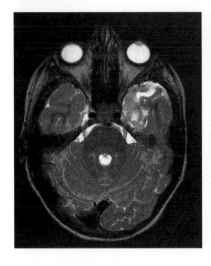

MR

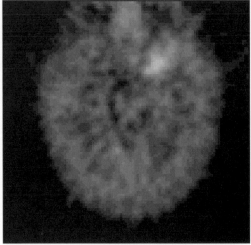

[¹¹C]L-methionine

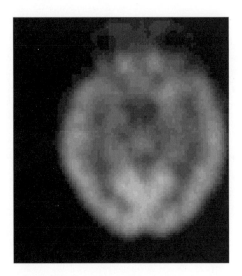

FDG

This 9 year old child presented with epilepsy. MR showed an enhancing tumour in the left mesial temporal region with thalamic infiltration. PET showed low grade uptake of FDG and moderate [¹¹C]L-methionine uptake in the region of the tumour. This suggested the tumour was low grade. Biopsy confirmed the tumour to be desmoplastic (low grade) astrocytoma.

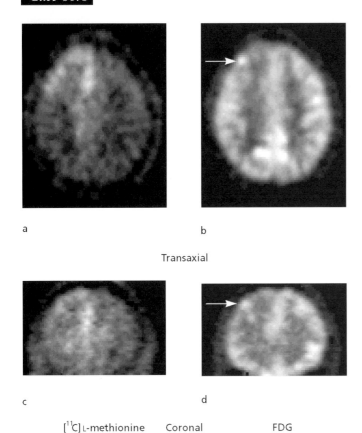

a   b

Transaxial

c   d

[¹¹C]L-methionine   Coronal   FDG

This 31 year old patient with a 2 year history of epilepsy was reported as having a low attenuation area on CT in the right frontoparietal region, suggestive of a low grade glioma. The PET scans showed diffuse low grade uptake of [¹¹C]L-methionine and FDG within the right frontal lobe and a small discrete focus of higher grade uptake (arrowed). This suggested the presence of a low grade glioma; the focus of higher uptake probably represents heterogeneity within the tumour.

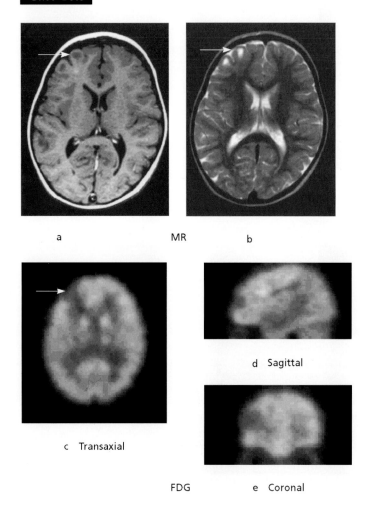

a   MR   b

c   Transaxial

d   Sagittal

e   Coronal

FDG

This 3 year old child was investigated for complex partial seizures. She was found to have a lesion on MRI (T1 and T2 weighted images are shown) in the right frontal lobe. The lesion had very low-grade uptake of FDG (arrowed), suggestive of a benign aetiology. At surgery this proved to be a benign hamartoma.

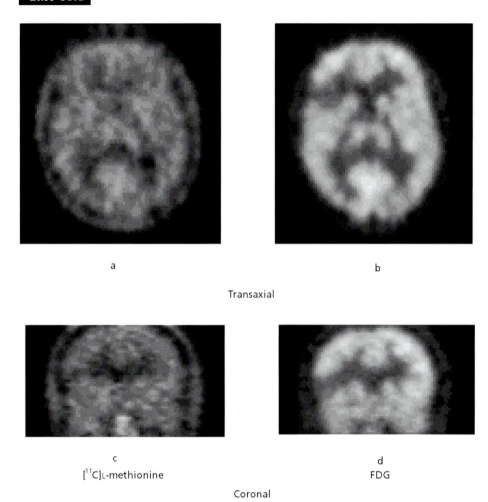

a

b

Transaxial

c

[¹¹C]L-methionine

d

FDG

Coronal

This is a further example of a hamartoma with low-grade uptake of FDG and [¹¹C]L-methionine.

The poor structural information of the [¹¹C]L-methionine image is due to the fact that there is low uptake of [¹¹C]L-methionine in normal brain. This is the type of scan in which image fusion can be very useful.

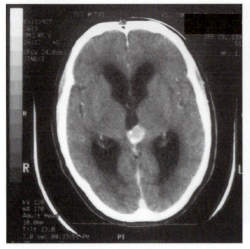

a CT

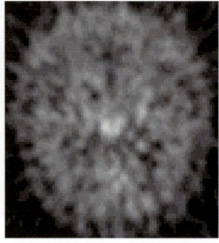

b [¹¹C]L-methionine

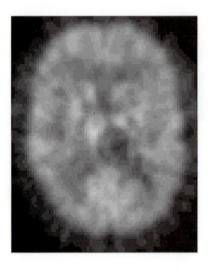

c FDG

This 73 year old patient with a pineal tumour was investigated with PET because of an enlargement in tumour size on CT. The FDG uptake was low grade with some methionine uptake within it, suggestive of a low-grade pinealoma.

> There may be significant uptake of [¹¹C]L-methionine in benign tumours. FDG gives more important prognostic information with regard to grading than [¹¹C]L-methionine, while [¹¹C]L-methionine is more useful for defining tumour extent. This is of particular use in recurrent brain tumours and the use of the two tracers is complementary especially for low grade tumours.

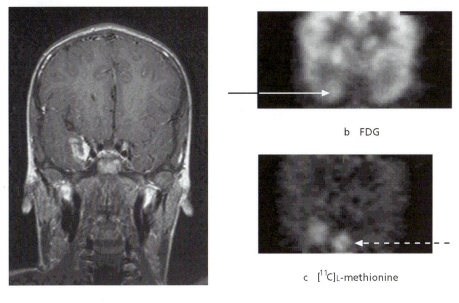

b FDG

c [^{11}C]L-methionine

a MR

This 6 year old child with complex partial seizures had a right temporal mass on MRI which had increased in size over the period of a year, raising the possibility of a glioma. Very low grade uptake of FDG and [^{11}C]L-methionine were seen within the lesion (arrowed), suggestive of a low grade lesion. Surgery was performed subsequently to remove the mass to control epilepsy rather than because of any malignant potential. The histology revealed a low grade ganglioneuroma.

There may be relatively high uptake of [^{11}C]L-methionine in the normal brain stem in some patients (dashed arrow). This is particularly marked in children and is well illustrated in the above case.

Case 10.9

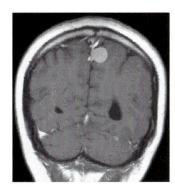

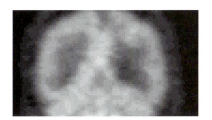

b FDG

a MR

This 50 year old woman was under investigation for recurrent low grade glioma. She also had a meningioma, which can be seen on MRI. There was low grade uptake of FDG in the meningioma, which was less than the uptake within normal cortex (shown here).

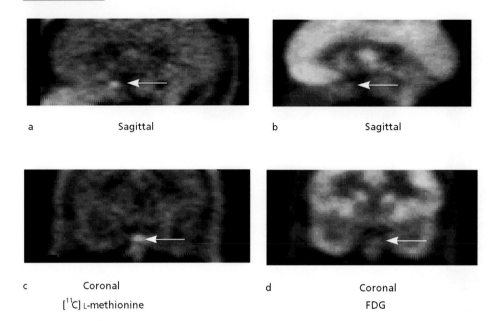

a   Sagittal   b   Sagittal

c   Coronal   d   Coronal

[^{11}C] L-methionine   FDG

This patient with persistently raised growth hormone following trans-sphenoidal adenectomy was referred for PET scanning. An octreotide study had previously failed to reveal a site of residual tumour. The PET scan showed increased uptake of [^{11}C]L-methionine and low grade uptake of FDG in the region of the pituitary indicative of a residual functioning adenoma (arrowed).

Key issue 5 Functional assessment of perilesion cortex

Case 10.11

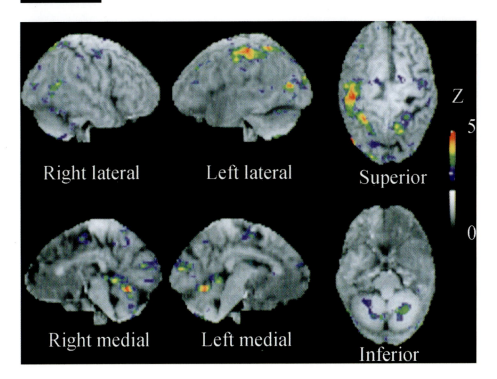

Right lateral   Left lateral   Superior

Right medial   Left medial   Inferior

This is an example of an activation study performed to establish the proximity of tumour to important functional brain areas to determine the feasibility of surgery. The study was performed while the patient was tapping his finger. Due to the mass lesions normal brain may be significantly displaced. The colour bar (Z score) refers to the number of standard deviations by which uptake differs from a normal database.

Key issues 6–8

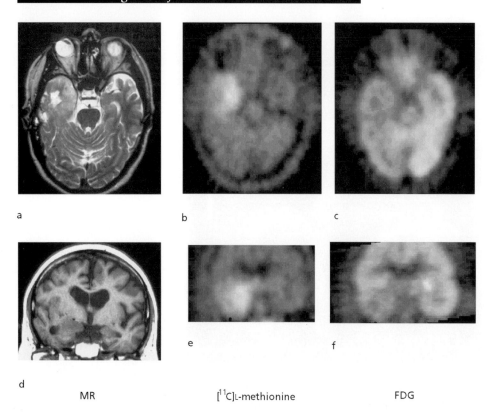

a   b   c

d

e   f

MR   [^{11}C]L-methionine   FDG

This 48 year old man had been treated in 1988 with radiotherapy for a low grade glioma. He remained well until 1995 when he re-presented with increased frequency of epileptic seizures. Increased uptake of [^{11}C]L-methionine associated with low grade uptake of FDG was present within the site of the mass on MRI, indicative of recurrent tumour. Note that there was diffuse reduction in the surrounding right temporal lobe with FDG secondary either to treatment or epilepsy.

Case 10.13

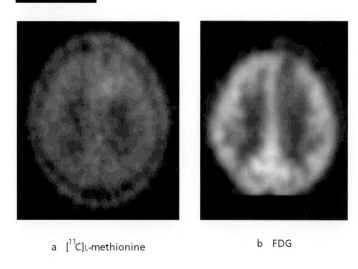

a   [^{11}C]L-methionine   b   FDG

This 38 year old patient had low grade uptake of FDG and [^{11}C]L-methionine in the left frontal lobe due to recurrent low grade glioma.

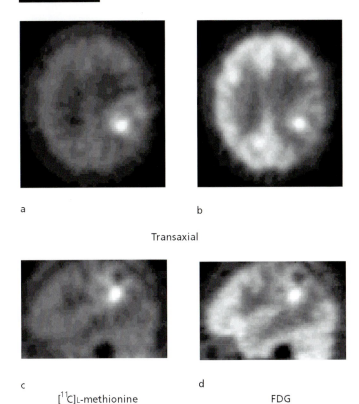

a   b

Transaxial

c   d

[^{11}C]L-methionine   FDG

Coronal

This 54 year old woman with a recurrent left parietal lobe glioma had high focal uptake of FDG and [^{11}C]L-methionine within a large diffuse area of low grade uptake, typical of recurrence within a treated brain area.

- The uptake of FDG soon after therapy is a less reliable indicator of tumour grade than at presentation.
- Low grade [^{11}C]L-methionine uptake probably occurs early in postinflammatory radionecrosis as well as tumour.
- Where there is low grade uptake of FDG, particularly within a site which has been previously treated, the presence of increased [^{11}C]L-methionine within that area, may be helpful. Both tracers may be needed, though, as [^{11}C]L-methionine does not provide the same prognostic information as FDG.

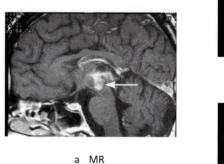

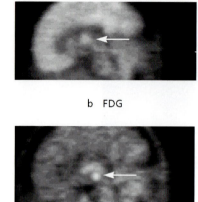

b FDG

c [¹¹C]ʟ-methionine

a MR

This 37 year old patient had a pineal lesion treated initially with craniospinal irradiation in 1992. She re-presented in 1996. MR (a) showed an enhancing lesion in the region of the pineal which had uptake of [¹¹C]ʟ-methionine and FDG within it indicative of recurrent disease. The site of recurrent disease appeared to be arising inferior and posterior to the usual position of the pineal gland, with the anatomy distorted following treatment with radiotherapy.

Case 10.16

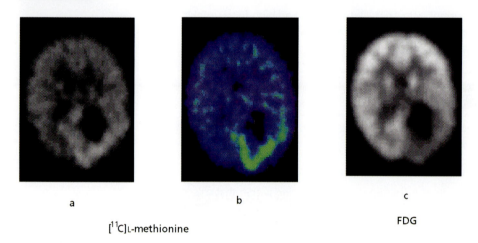

a

b

c

[¹¹C]ʟ-methionine

FDG

Transaxial

This 4 year old child with a posterior fossa primitive neuroectodermal tumour underwent surgery and was treated postoperatively with chemotherapy for known residual disease. PET was performed to assess whether residual disease remained after chemotherapy. There was reduced uptake in the left posterior parietal and occipital lobes due to treatment but a rim of increased [¹¹C]ʟ-methionine uptake along the photon deficient area suggestive of recurrence (seen in best in the colour image). There was uptake of FDG within this rim of [¹¹C]ʟ-methionine activity, suggestive of low grade recurrent disease. MR at this stage did not show evidence of recurrent disease, although within 3 months of the PET scan there was clear evidence of recurrent tumour at this site.

Case 10.17

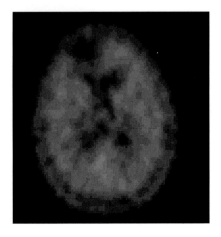

a [¹¹C]ʟ-methionine

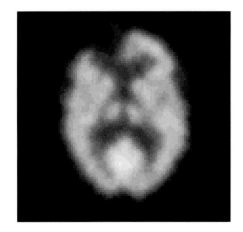

b FDG

Transaxial

This 12 year old child with a primitive neuroectodermal tumour was treated with surgery and craniospinal irradiation. The MRI showed a small area of enhancement inferior and medial to the anterior horn of the right lateral ventricle. PET was performed to determine whether this represented active tumour. [¹¹C]ʟ-methionine and FDG brain scans were normal, indicating the MR abnormality was likely to be due to radionecrosis rather than active tumour. Follow up of this patient suggests no clinical recurrence.

Case 10.18

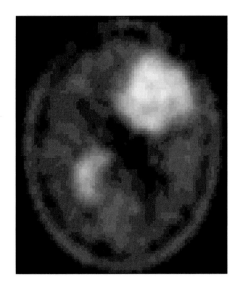

a [¹¹C]ʟ-methionine

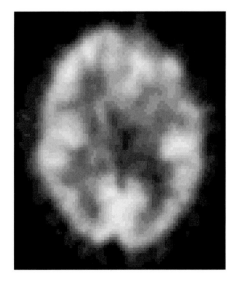

b FDG

Transaxial

This 46 year old patient had massive irregular uptake of FDG and [¹¹C]ʟ-methionine within the left frontal and right parietal lobes, typical of a high grade recurrent glioma. The uptake of methionine was greater relative to the FDG in this case, seen particularly in the right parietal lobe, such that the presence of recurrent tumour can only really be appreciated with the [¹¹C]ʟ-methionine scan.

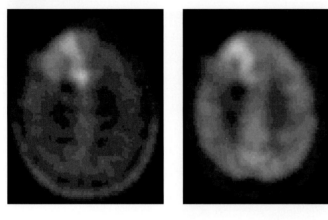

a   [¹¹C]L-methionine   b   FDG

Transaxial

This 48 year old man with a recurrent left frontal glioma had high uptake of FDG and [¹¹C]L-methionine indicating recurrent disease. In this example the uptake of FDG and [¹¹C]L-methionine are concordant, in contrast to the former case.

Case 10.20: *Residual/recurrent astrocytoma following surgery*

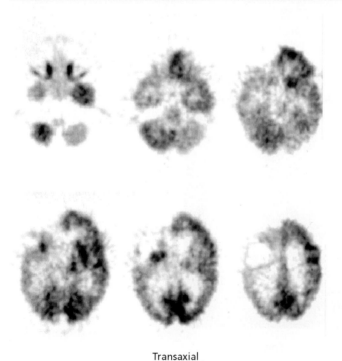

Transaxial

Intensely increased metabolism in the depth of the frontal lobe surgical defect was seen corresponding to residual astrocytoma. Note the presence of reduced metabolic activity throughout the ipsilateral cerebral cortex due to the effects of surgery and vasogenic oedema and reduced contralateral cerebellar metabolism (cross-cerebellar diaschesis).

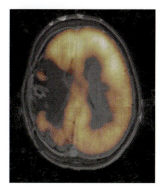 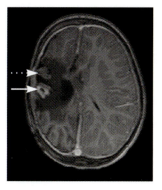

a   Registered MR/PET   b   MR

This 4 year old child had undergone multiple surgery, chemotherapy and radiotherapy for an anaplastic ependymoma. Though she was neurologically stable with a left hemiplegia, she had complained of recent new headaches. MR showed an enhancing region within the parietal lobe which was suggestive of recurrent disease. The FDG-PET scan was registered to the MR and indicated extensive right frontotemporal hypometabolism secondary to treatment. Baseline FDG scans had showed high uptake within the anaplastic tumour. The enhancing region in the right parietal lobe on MR was hypometabolic on PET and likely therefore to represent residual scar or inflammatory tissue (solid arrow). The small focus of FDG uptake in the right parietal region corresponded to an island of normal cortex on MR (dotted arrow). Therefore there was no evidence of recurrent disease. Two years later this child had no evidence of recurrence clinically.

> In this case the MR/PET registration was crucial. Where anatomy is distorted with recurrent surgery, radiotherapy and chemotherapy, registration may be necessary for interpretation.

Post-treatment management

Key issue 9 Monitoring response (surgery/radiotherapy/chemotherapy)

Case 10.22

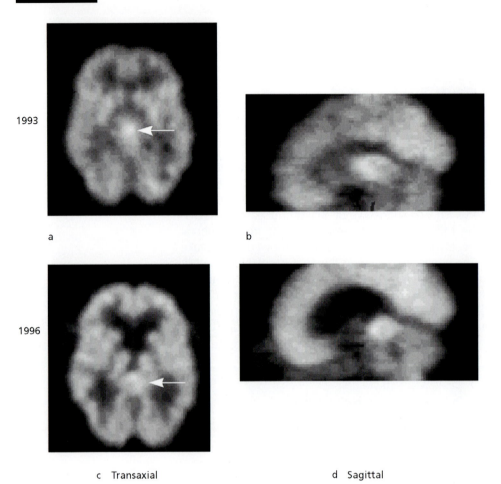

1993

a

b

1996

c Transaxial   d Sagittal

This 41 year old patient had surgery and radiotherapy for a pineal tumour in 1991. At the time of the first PET scan in 1993, a mass lesion was present on MR. There was increased uptake of FDG within this mass, suggesting the presence of active tumour rather than fibrosis (arrowed). The patient was however treated conservatively. She was re-referred in 1996 with increasing headaches and a left hemiparesis. Once again, there was evidence of FDG uptake indicative of residual tumour, but the scan showed that the patient had also developed hydrocephalus.

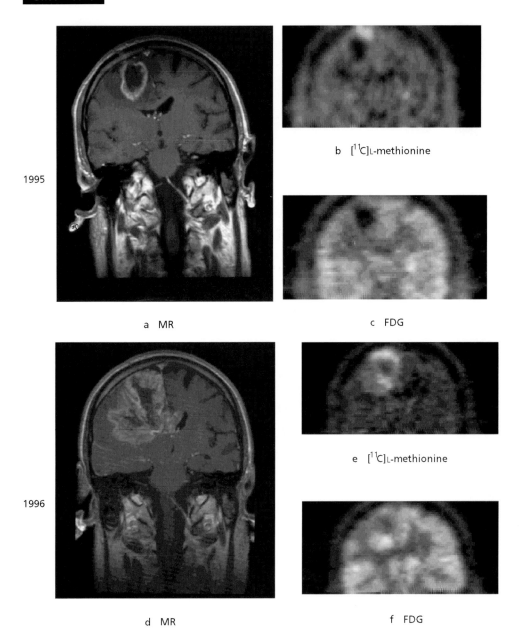

1995

a MR

b [¹¹C]L-methionine

c FDG

1996

d MR

e [¹¹C]L-methionine

f FDG

This 49 year old patient with an astrocytoma was scanned in 1995. There was low grade FDG uptake and increased uptake of [¹¹C]L-methionine corresponding to an enhancing mass seen on MR, indicative of recurrent disease. The patient was treated with radiotherapy, but despite treatment there was evidence of further enlargement of the mass on MR and increased activity of FDG and [¹¹C]L-methionine when the patient was rescanned a year later.

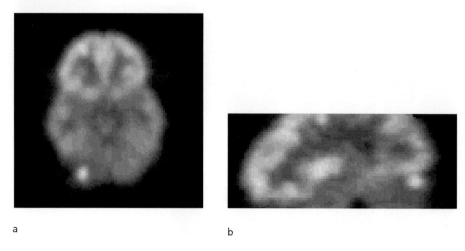

a   b

Pre-chemotherapy

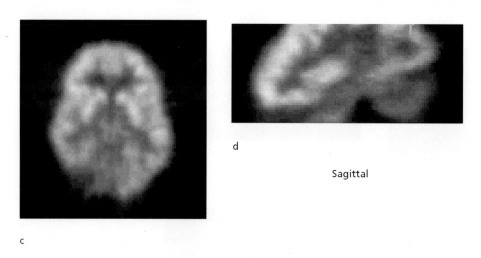

d

Sagittal

c

Transaxial   Post-chemotherapy

This 10 year old girl had an incomplete resection of a medulloblastoma in 1994. She was scanned with FDG prior to starting chemotherapy. Intense uptake within a residual focus of tumour was seen in the right posterior cerebellum. Six weeks after the completion of chemotherapy ametabolism was seen within this area, indicating complete response to treatment. She remains disease free at 2 year follow up.

Key issue 10 Adjunct to MR in spinal cord tumour management

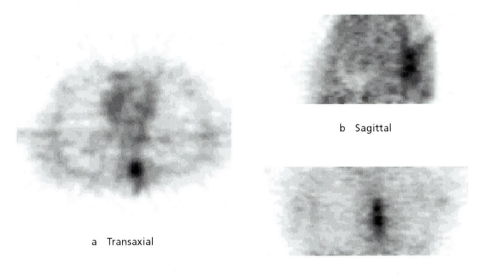

b Sagittal

a Transaxial

c Coronal

This 10 year old girl with neurofibromatosis had evidence of a cord lesion. At surgery it was found to be a low grade astrocytoma, but it was thought that the resection was incomplete. The PET scan showed residual FDG activity within T6–T8 suggestive of residual tumour.

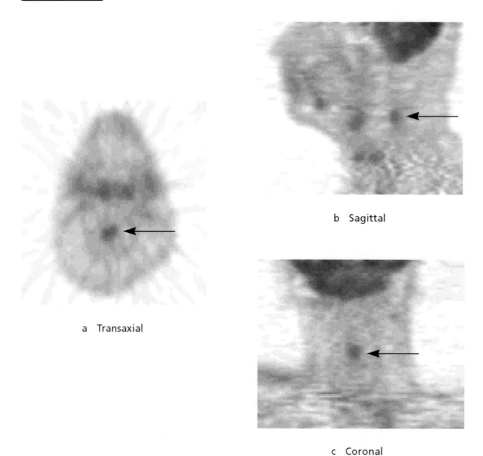

a   Transaxial

b   Sagittal

c   Coronal

This 41 year old patient with an ependymoma underwent surgery with complete excision in 1990. He re-presented in 1994 with possible recurrence. The MR was suggestive of recurrent disease and increased uptake in the mid-cervical cord with FDG also indicated active tumour (arrowed).

Physiological uptake is seen within the hyoid muscles, lingual tonsils and cricoarytenoid muscles in this case. Knowledge of the normal anatomy is important for interpretation of such images.

Conclusions

CURRENT CLINICAL INDICATIONS

1 Diagnosis of recurrence when MRI/CT is unclear in differentiating from scar/necrosis

2 Diagnosis when there is contraindication to biopsy or failed biopsy

3 Direction of biopsy where the site of tumour is unclear on MRI

4 Planning treatment when the extent of tumour is unclear on MRI

5 Monitoring response to chemotherapy/radiotherapy

6 Helping assess grade of tumour

POSSIBLE INDICATIONS

1 Prediction of chemotherapy response

2 Conformal or brachytherapy planning

3 Activation studies to locate normal functional cortical regions preoperatively

References and further reading

Alavi JB, Alavi A, Chawluk J *et al.* (1988) Positron emission tomography in patients with glioma. *Cancer* **62**, 1074–8.

Barker FG, Chang SM, Valk PE *et al.* (1997) 18-Fluorodeoxyglucose uptake and survival of patients with suspected recurrent malignant glioma. *Cancer* **79**(1), 115–26.

Bergstrom M, Lundqvist H, Ericson K *et al.* (1987) Comparison of the accumulation kinetics of L-(methyl-^{11}C)-methionine and D-(methyl-^{11}C)-methionine in brain tumors studied with positron emission tomography. *Acta Radiol* **28**(3), 225–9.

Delbeke D, Meyerowitz C, Lapidus R *et al.* (1995) Optimal cutoff levels of ^{18}F fluorodeoxyglucose uptake in the differentiation of low-grade from high-grade brain tumors with PET. *Radiology* **195**, 47–52.

Deshmukh A, Scott JA, Palmer EL, Hochberg FH, Gruber M, Fischman AJ (1996) Impact of fluorodeoxyglucose positron emission tomography on the clinical management of patients with glioma. *Clinical Nuclear Medicine* **21**, 720–25.

De Witte O, Levivier M, Violon P, Salmon I, Damhaut P, Wikler D, Jr. *et al.* (1996) Prognostic value positron emission tomography with [^{18}F]fluoro-2-deoxy-D-glucose in the low-grade glioma. *Neurosurgery* **39**, 470–76; discussion 476–7.

DiChiro G, DeLaPaz RL, Brooks RA *et al.* (1982) Glucose utilization of cerebral gliomas measured by [^{18}F] fluorodeoxyglucose and positron emission tomography. *Neurology* **32**(12), 1323–9.

DiChiro G, Hatazawa J, Katz DA *et al.* (1987) Glucose utilization by intracranial meningiomas as an index of tumor aggressivity and probability of recurrence: a PET study. *Radiology* **164**, 521–6.

Francavilla TL, Miletich RS, DiChiro G (1989) Positron emission tomography in the detection of malignant degeneration of low-grade gliomas. *Neurosurgery* **24**(1), 1–5.

Fulham MJ, Melisi JW, Nishimiya J *et al.* (1993) Neuroimaging of juvenile pilocytic astrocytomas: an enigma. *Radiology* **189**(1), 221–5.

Griffeth LK, Rich KM, Dehdashti F *et al.* (1993) Brain metastases from non-central nervous system tumors: evaluation with PET. *Radiology* **186**(1), 37–44

Hoffman JM, Waskin HA, Schifter T *et al.* (1993) FDG-PET in differentiating lymphoma from nonmalignant central nervous system lesions in patients with AIDS. *J Nucl Med* **34**, 567–75.

Ito M, Lammertsma AA, Wise RJ *et al.* (1982) Measurement of regional cerebral blood flow and oxygen utilisation in patients with cerebral tumours using ^{15}O and positron emission tomography: analytical techniques and preliminary results. *Neuroradiology* **23**, 63–74.

Lodge MA, Lucas JD, Marsden PK, Cronin BF, O'Doherty MJ (1999) A PET study of ^{18}FDG uptake in soft tissue masses. *Eur J Nucl Med* **26**, 22–30.

Lucas JD, O'Doherty MJ, Wong JC, Brigham JB, Mckee PH, Fletcher CD, Smith MA (1998) Evaluation of flurodeoxyglucose positron emission tomography in the management of soft-tissue sarcomas. *Journal of Bone and Joint Surgery* **80**(3), 441–7.

Ogawa T, Hatazawa J, Inugami A *et al.* (1995) Carbon-11-methionine PET evaluation of intracerebral hematoma: distinguishing neoplastic from non-neoplastic hematoma. *J Nucl Med* **36**, 2175–9.

Ogawa T, Inugami A, Hatazawa J, Kanno I, Murakami M, Yasui N *et al.* (1996) Clinical positron emission tomography for brain tumors: comparison of fludeoxyglucose F 18 and L-methyl-11C-methionine. *American Journal of Neuroradiology* **17**, 345–53.

Patronas NJ, DiChiro G, Brooks RA *et al.* (1982) Work in progress: [^{18}F] fluorodeoxyglucose and positron emission tomography in the evaluation of radiation necrosis of the brain. *Radiology* **144**(4), 885–9.

Pirotte B, Goldman S, Bidaut LM *et al.* (1995) Use of positron emission tomography (PET) in stereotactic conditions for brain biopsy. *Acta Neurochir* **134**, 79–82.

Roelcke U, Radu E, Ametamey S *et al.* (1996) Association of ^{82}rubidium and ^{11}C-methionine uptake in brain tumors measured by positron emission tomography. *J Neuro Oncol* **27**, 163–72.

Shinoura N, Nishijima M, Hara T *et al.* (1997) Brain tumors: detection with C-11 choline PET. *Radiology* **202**(2), 497–503.

Valk P, Budinger T, Levin V *et al.* (1988) PET of malignant cerebral tumors after interstitial brachytherapy. *J Neurosurg* **69**, 830–8.

Wong JCH, Studholme C, Hawkes DJ, Maisey MN (1997) Evaluation of the limits of visual detection of image misregistration in a brain fluorine-^{18}fluorodeoxyglucose PET-MRI study. *Eur J Nucl Med* **24**(6), 642–50.

Chapter 11

Evolving oncology applications

There are a number of cancers other than those described in the previous chapters in which PET imaging is having an impact: in some cases with very marked benefit, in others less so. At present limited information is available in the literature about many of these other tumours. In this chapter they are briefly reviewed, together with what information is available and the authors' own views of the likely role of PET.

1 Thyroid and parathyroid

Current status of PET

Many thyroid cancers can be imaged by PET, with most studies reported using FDG as the imaging agent. Some thyroid cancers accumulate FDG; others do not. It appears from the literature to date that iodine avid tumours are often the best differentiated and the least FDG avid, while more aggressive tumours which often do not accumulate radioiodine accumulate FDG. FDG-PET may be of greatest utility in locating tumour foci in patients with rising serum thyroglobulin levels and normal ^{131}I scans. FDG may also be helpful in anaplastic carcinomas and in some medullary carcinomas. Identifying non-iodine avid tumours may be important, as they may be treated by surgery if localized or by external beam radiation. The literature on FDG scanning in thyroid carcinoma is rapidly evolving. It is also clear that some thyroid cancers retain some level of responsiveness to TSH, with higher FDG uptake seen in the presence of TSH as is the case with [131]I. Some benign processes can also accumulate FDG, such as some adenomas in the thyroid.

Parathyroid tumours are less extensively studied with PET. The literature has been somewhat contradictory, with one early report suggesting a high degree of accuracy for FDG-PET imaging of these tumours. Indeed, recently, a sensitivity of 79% for adenomas and 29% for hyperplastic glands was reported for FDG, and FDG was reported to be more accurate than sestamibi in this setting. Two other reports showed a very poor sensitivity (<30%) for FDG. As one of the authors of this book, RLW, collaborated in interpreting the study by Sisson *et al.* (1994) in which poor sensitivity was found for parathyroid abnormalities with FDG, it seems clear that at least a sizable fraction of these tumours can be hard to detect with FDG-PET. [11C]L-Methionine has also been used to image parathyroid adenomas, with a sensitivity of over 80% reported. This agent appears to have substantial promise, although the literature is limited, to date. We feel that [11C]L-methionine has greater promise as a clinical PET imaging agent for the parathyroid glands than does FDG.

Examples

Thyroid

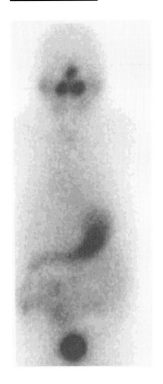

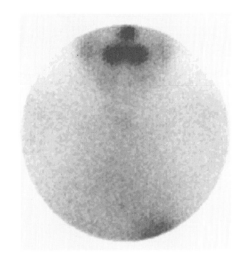

a   Anterior   b   Posterior   c   Local view of thorax

Whole body post-therapy iodine scan

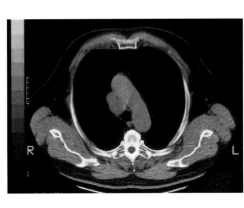
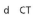

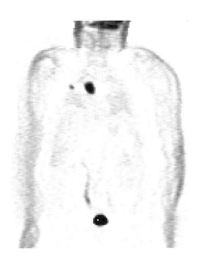

d   CT   e   Coronal

This 63 year old patient underwent left thyroid lobectomy and radioiodine ablation for papillary carcinoma of the thyroid in 1990. Following this there was no evidence of residual disease. Thyroglobulin measurements were negative until 1995 when the thyroglobulin rose to $170\,\mu g\,L^{-1}$. Thallium scanning suggested uptake in the region of the right hilum. The patient was treated with radioiodine but on the post-therapy scan no abnormal focal uptake of iodine was seen. CT scanning with contrast 3 months after treatment was reported as normal. Abnormal foci of FDG uptake were seen on PET scanning within the right hilum, periphery of the right midzone of the lung (shown on the coronal image) and in the anterior mediastinum (not shown). Note also the physiological hold up of urine within the right ureter. The CT was repeated and the presence of a single soft tissue mass was noted at the right hilum. The patient was referred for surgery. All three sites of disease identified on the PET scan were confirmed as containing tumour.

> FDG-PET scan does not invariably require discontinuing thyroid hormone and is particularly useful when tracer ^{131}I is negative with elevated Tg. SUVs may be higher, however, if the TSH is allowed to rise prior to PET scanning.

Case 11.1.2

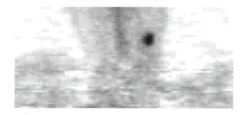

a

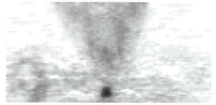

b

Coronal images

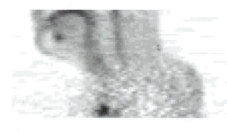

c   Sagittal

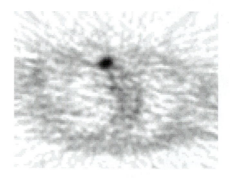

d   Transaxial

This 62 year old patient underwent left hemithyroidectomy in 1993 for medullary thyroid carcinoma. He was referred for PET scanning later that year with rising calcitonin levels. CT scan was normal. The PET showed increased uptake of FDG in the neck, SUV = 5.8 (a) and superior mediastinum, SUV = 7.0 (b,c,d) indicative of residual disease.

Case 11.1.3

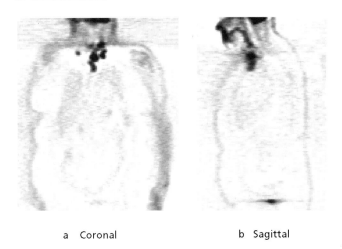

a   Coronal   b   Sagittal

This 66 year old patient was referred for PET scanning at diagnosis of an anaplastic thyroid carcinoma. PET scan shows FDG uptake within the thyroid bed, right supra-clavicular regions and superior mediastinum.

Parathyroid

Case 11.1.4

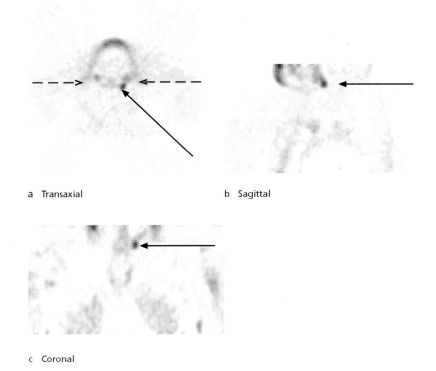

a   Transaxial   b   Sagittal

c   Coronal

This 64 year old patient with chronic renal failure had secondary hyperparathyroidism with four glands removed at surgery. The calcium and PTH level remained elevated postoperatively, and the patient was referred for PET scanning. Sestamibi scanning had shown no evidence of an adenoma. Scanning with [^{11}C]L-methionine revealed the presence of an ectopic adenoma within the left carotid sheath (solid arrows). Physiological uptake may be seen within the parotid glands on the transaxial image (dashed arrow). Removal of this adenoma resulted in normalization of serum calcium.

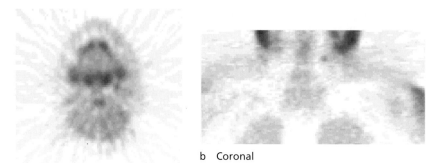

b Coronal

a Transaxial

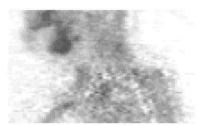

c Sagittal

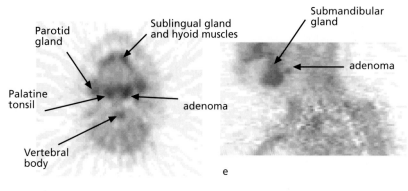

Sublingual gland
and hyoid muscles

Submandibular
gland

Parotid
gland

adenoma

Palatine
tonsil

adenoma

Vertebral
body

e

d

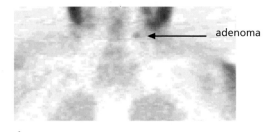

adenoma

f

This 66 year old man with primary hyperparathyroidism was referred for PET scanning after a negative sestamibi scan. Scanning with [^{11}C]L-methionine revealed a focus in the left carotid sheath, subsequently confirmed to be the site of an adenoma. Note in this case the sites of physiological uptake seen, particularly within the salivary glands, tonsils and vertebral body.

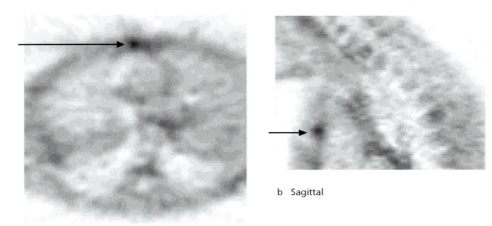

b Sagittal

a Transaxial

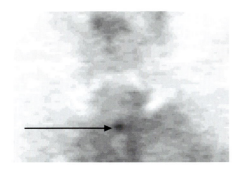

c Coronal

This patient with primary hyperparathyroidism was referred for PET scanning, which revealed a focus of [^{11}C]L-methionine uptake within the mediastinum (arrowed), suggestive of uptake within an ectopic adenoma.

Like ^{99m}Tc sestamibi, [^{11}C]L-methionine can also be seen within large thyroid nodules.

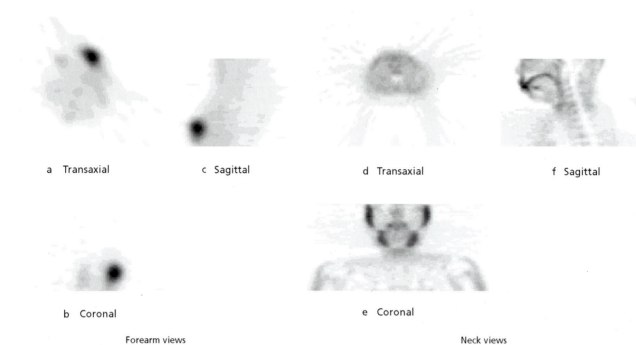

a Transaxial   c Sagittal   d Transaxial   f Sagittal

b Coronal   e Coronal

Forearm views   Neck views

This 17 year old woman with chronic renal failure developed hyperparathyroidism which was thought to be secondary to autonomous function of her left forearm parathyroid autotransplant. The PET was requested to rule out another ectopic site prior to removal of the forearm transplant. [11C]ʟ-methionine uptake was identified within the forearm (three views shown on left) but none was seen within the neck or thorax (three views shown on right).

Conclusions

EMERGING INDICATIONS

1 Negative whole body ^{131}I scan in the face of rising thyroglobulin levels (Tg) in a patient with a known differentiated thyroid cancer

2 Medullary thyroid cancer and a rising calcitonin level when a DMSA(V), octreoscan or MIBG scan is negative or is the first imaging test

3 Possibly to improve thyroid ^{131}I dosimetry by using the positron-emitting [124]I

4 To localize the site of recurrent or persistent parathyroid tissue after previous parathyroidectomy and a negative ^{99m}Tc-sestamibi scan

2 Oesophageal cancer

Current status of PET

Carcinoma of the oesophagus is increasing rapidly in frequency in the west, with the rise most apparent in patients with adenocarcinoma of the oesophagus. Much of the increase is thought to be related to reflux oesophagitis and Barrett's oesophagus, but the exact aetiology is uncertain. This tumour type appears to be very well imaged by FDG-PET. Flanagan and colleagues (1997) reported that PET was more sensitive than CT for detecting oesophageal cancer (76% vs. 45% of patients), and suggested FDG-PET could reduce the numbers of unnecessary surgical procedures by better displaying metastatic tumour foci undetected by CT, which could render surgery non-curative or non-essential. Fukunaga *et al.* (1994) reported on 42 cases and stated that all could be imaged with PET. The experience of the authors with PET is that oesophageal carcinoma represents a disease in which FDG-PET will have a growing and important role in clinical practice.

Examples

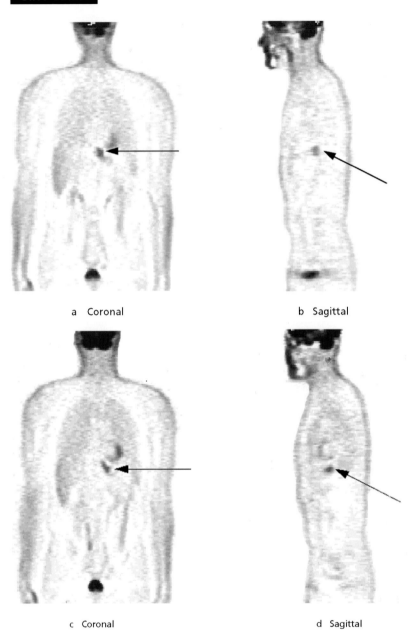

a   Coronal   b   Sagittal

c   Coronal   d   Sagittal

This 47 year old man with adenocarcinoma at the gastro-oesophageal junction was referred for PET scanning prior to surgery for staging purposes. Increased uptake of FDG was seen within the lower oesophagus (top images) and within the stomach (bottom images). There was no evidence of local or distant spread.

> FDG uptake within adenocarcinoma of the stomach may be difficult to differentiate from physiological uptake within normal stomach. Uptake within lymph nodes at the cardia may also be difficult to resolve from stomach uptake.

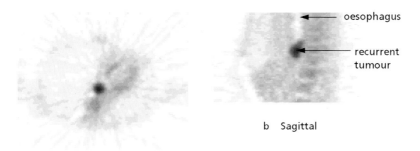

a   Transaxial

b   Sagittal

oesophagus

recurrent
tumour

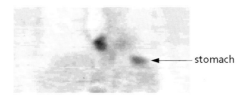

stomach

c   Coronal

This 56 year old patient had previously undergone partial oesophagectomy for carcinoma. He subsequently developed obstruction of the oesophagus. CT showed a dilated proximal oesophagus with thickening on the left side at the site of previous surgery and the patient was referred for PET scanning with the suspicion of recurrent tumour at the anastomosis. Increased FDG uptake was seen within the lower third of the oesophagus indicative of recurrent disease. Note also the photopenic fluid filled oesophagus proximal to the site of obstruction and normal stomach activity seen on the coronal image.

Case 11.2.3

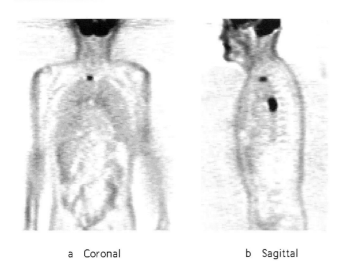

a   Coronal   b   Sagittal

This 59 year old man with known carcinoma of the oesophagus was referred for PET scanning prior to surgery. CT demonstrated the presence of a primary tumour but no nodal disease. PET showed uptake in the primary tumour (b) and a paratracheal node in addition (a,b).

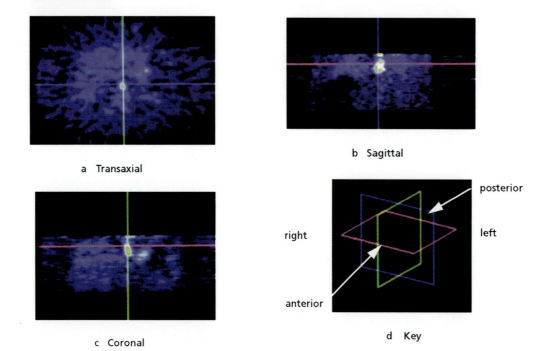

a Transaxial

b Sagittal

c Coronal

d Key

posterior

right

left

anterior

This 50 year old man presented with difficulty swallowing. Upper gastrointestinal examination revealed narrowing of the distal oesophagus. PET showed intense uptake of FDG in the distal oesophagus suggestive of oesophageal carcinoma. The lesion was proved to be adenocarcinoma.

Conclusions

EMERGING INDICATIONS

1 Primary staging in conjunction with CT

2 Treatment response

3 Neoadjuvant chemotherapy assessment

4 Suspected recurrence

3 Liver and hepatoma

Current status of PET

Hepatoma is one of the most common tumours in the world, but the role of FDG-PET in the detection and follow up of these lesions is still in evolution.

Diagnostic issues in detecting hepatoma with conventional imaging methods include separating hepatoma from cirrhosis and assessing the response of hepatomas to treatment. CT or MRI alone is sometimes not adequate for such assessments. Blood flow was first assessed by PET in these tumours, but has not been used to any great extent clinically. Imaging of hepatomas with FDG was initially performed in nine patients who then went on to therapy. In these patients, the uptake rate of FDG declined with treatment. While many hepatomas are well imaged by FDG-PET as hot spots relative to liver, up to half of the tumours cannot be detected as regions of increased tracer uptake versus the normal liver. Apparently this is due in part to a high K_4 or dephosphorylation rate. It is possible that kinetic modelling will be needed in some cases, rather than a delayed image of hepatic and tumour FDG uptake. This, of course, is very hard to implement clinically. Using kinetic modelling, K_3 was found to be correlated with tumour hexokinase content and a $K_3 > 0.025$ was consistently associated with the presence of cancer. Torizuka and colleagues (1995) showed in 17 patients with hepatoma that high K_3 values and SUV were seen in the highest grade hepatomas vs. lower grade tumours. In another series, a relatively substantial percentage of hepatic lesions showing low tracer uptake (in the range of normal liver) were hepatomas. Thus, hepatoma appears more complex to understand using FDG-PET than other tumours such as oesophageal cancer, as some large untreated tumours have lower uptake of FDG than surrounding normal tissues. FDG may, however, be helpful in following tumour response and in diagnosis if lesions are FDG avid initially. The role of amino acids in PET of hepatocellular cancers is not well explored, but the high hepatic uptake of many amino acids such as methionine means that background radioactivity levels will limit detection of small lesions.

Examples

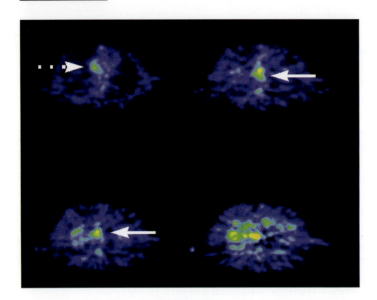

Transaxial

This patient presented with oedema of the legs and ascites. Intense uptake of FDG was seen within a hepatoma in the left lobe of the liver (shown here on the bottom right image) and within tumour extending into the inferior vena cava (solid arrows) and the right atrium (broken arrow).

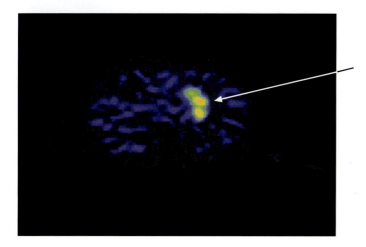

This patient with a history of alcoholism presented with a 5 cm liver mass. PET showed no uptake of FDG within the mass, but marked physiological uptake was seen within the stomach (arrowed). Subsequent biopsy revealed the mass to be a hepatoma and the PET to be a false negative scan.

> Low and intermediate grade hepatomas often have FDG uptake no greater than surrounding normal liver.

Conclusions

EMERGING INDICATIONS

1 Separating cirrhosis and hepatoma
2 Assessing response to treatment
3 Identifying multifocal lesions

4 Pancreatic cancer

Current status of PET

Pancreatic carcinoma is common in the US, with nearly 30 000 patients per year diagnosed or dying from pancreatic adenocarcinomas. Both $[^{11}C]$L-methionine, which targets to normal pancreas in preference to tumours, and FDG, which targets to tumours in preference to normal pancreas, have been used for tumour imaging in the pancreas. Most clinical imaging is done with FDG, as the normal tissue background signal is much less problematic than that of $[^{11}C]$L-methionine. Bares *et al.* (1993, 1994) reported on 40 patients with suspected pancreatic cancer, showing PET could detect 25/27 of the cancers and 11/13 benign lesions. PET could also detect many nodal and hepatic lesions. Inokuma *et al.* (1995) showed PET to detect 33/35 foci of pancreatic carcinoma, while correctly characterizing 11/13 benign lesions as benign. False positive uptake was observed in a case of chronic pancreatitis and in a cystadenoma. A large series of 73 patients with either suspected pancreatic carcinoma or benign chronic pancreatitis showed FDG-PET detected 41/43 cancers (95% sensitivity) and 27/30 (90%) benign lesions. These figures were significantly ($p < 0.05$) superior to those with CT (sensitivity 80%, specificity 74%: Stollfus *et al.* 1995). These data indicate that FDG-PET is useful in detecting pancreatic carcinoma, both localized and metastatic, and in characterizing pancreatic masses. The technique using FDG is not perfect: patients with inflammatory processes in the pancreas but no cancer can have high FDG uptake indistinguishable from cancers, and some cancers are not detected with PET. Nevertheless, FDG-PET is increasingly applied in pancreatic cancer imaging. Given the very poor prognosis of pancreatic carcinomas, PET may have its greatest role in helping to characterize masses in the pancreas, as opposed to tumour staging, though this needs additional study.

Examples

Case 11.4.1

b   Sagittal

a   Transaxial

This patient underwent PET scanning at presentation at which time liver metastases were present (a) in addition to the lesion in the head of the pancreas (b).

Case 11.4.2

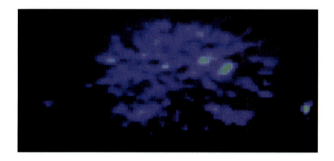

This patient with pancreatitis had markedly increased FDG uptake within the pancreas, seen on the transaxial image to be of similar intensity to renal uptake.

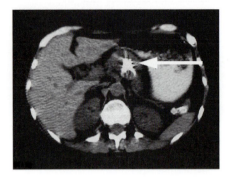

a   CT

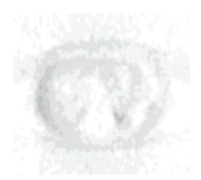

b   FDG

c   [¹¹C]ʟ-methionine

This 52 year old woman with a calcified pancreatic mass on CT (a, arrowed) was referred for PET scanning because of raised tumour markers. No uptake of FDG was seen within the mass, though there was low grade uptake of [¹¹C]ʟ-methionine (c, arrowed). [¹¹C]ʟ-methionine may, however, be seen within normal pancreas. The patient was treated conservatively with a working diagnosis of pancreatitis. CT follow up over 2 years indicated no change in mass size subsequently.

> Increased uptake of FDG may be seen within both pancreatitis and carcinoma and the two may be difficult to differentiate. Physiological uptake of [¹¹C]ʟ-methionine is normally seen within the pancreas.

Conclusions

EMERGING INDICATIONS

1   May have a role in some cases separating chronic pancreatic mass from cancer, but not as good as hoped originally

2   Staging nodal metastases, liver metastases

3   Assessment of response to chemotherapy

5 Renal cell cancer

Current status of PET

Renal cancers are relatively infrequent, but renal masses are a vexing diagnostic problem. It had been hoped that PET would clarify this difficult clinical situation. Although PET can image many renal neoplasms, we have observed several cases recently in which FDG-PET was falsely negative for primary cancers. This has been confirmed in a report by Bachor *et al.* (1996), where about 25% of renal cancers were not detected by FDG-PET. Thus, the precise role of PET in imaging this disease is still in evolution, but it seems clear that negative FDG-PET imaging of a renal mass does not exclude the presence of cancer. At present, it is not clear that FDG-PET is more useful than CT scanning. PET scanning with FDG is more likely to be valuable in the assessment of suspected recurrent disease.

Examples

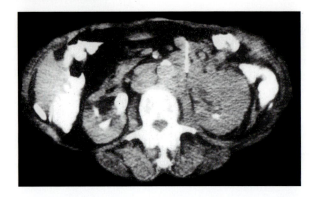

a

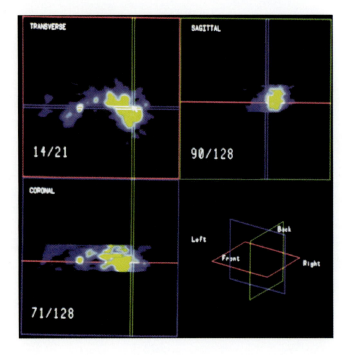

b

This 75 year old man presented with a 9 cm left renal mass. The CT image obtained during the biopsy procedure demonstrated the mass with adjacent nodes (a). Tumour within the inferior vena cava and bone metastases in the ribs and sternum were also demonstrated on multiple image planes. The PET scan shown was acquired at the same level as the CT biopsy images (b). FDG has largely cleared from the right kidney except from normal activity in the renal pelvis (as shown) but was intensely accumulated within the left renal mass, surrounding lymph nodes and inferior vena cava.

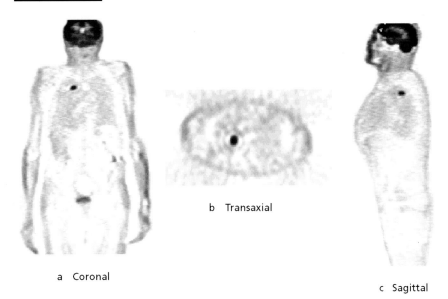

a   Coronal

b   Transaxial

c   Sagittal

This 69 year old woman was referred for PET scanning after surgery for a left hyper-nephroma. Increased uptake had been reported on a bone scan, suggestive of possible metastases. The PET scan showed no evidence of disease in bone but demonstrated a lung metastasis in the right upper lobe (a,c). Note that the left kidney is absent on the transaxial image (b).

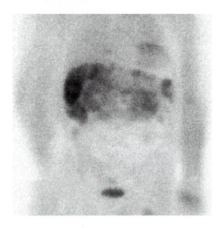

a   Coronal–projection

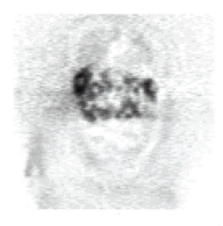

b   Coronal–volume

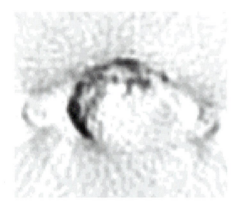

c   Transaxial

This 75 year old man with a history of hypernephroma removed in 1992 was scanned in 1997 when he was being investigated for a left parotid mass. The scan showed multiple liver metastases in addition to the left parotid mass which were both thought likely to be metastases from his original renal tumour.

Conclusions

EMERGING INDICATIONS

1   Detection of metastatic disease
2   Response of metastases to chemotherapy
3   Assessment of nature of renal masses
4   Kidney of transplant recipients

6 Cervical, uterine and ovarian cancer

Current status of PET

Accurate diagnosis of ovarian and uterine cancers at an early stage remains an elusive diagnostic goal. Staging cervical cancer at presentation is also a challenging undertaking, as treatment is highly dependent upon the extent of tumour. PET has an emerging role in these conditions, based on the available literature. In ovarian cancer, it is clear that PET can image most bulky tumours and some reports suggest that PET is more accurate than CT in imaging ovarian cancer, although small metastatic foci can elude detection. Karlan *et al.* (1993) concluded PET was best able to detect ovarian tumours ($>1\,$cm) with frequent misses of smaller tumour burden. Lapela *et al.* (1994) showed that $[^{11}C]$L-methionine uptake was increased in malignant ovarian cancer as well. Hubner *et al.* (1993) reported an 86% positive predictive value in ovarian cancer with FDG-PET. Thus, PET can image ovarian cancer and current data suggest the performance of PET to be superior to that of CT. In uterine and cervical carcinoma data are very limited, but Lapela *et al.* (1995) reported that $[^{11}C]$L-methionine could detect 8/8 known uterine carcinomas and 6/6 known cervical carcinomas. The authors' experience, though limited, is that FDG can also detect these tumours, and, in cervical carcinoma in particular, images have been strikingly positive in many cases. Certainly, FDG excretion in the bladder can make interpretation more challenging than in other parts of the body and methods to minimize FDG in the bladder are recommended for optimal tumour imaging.

Examples

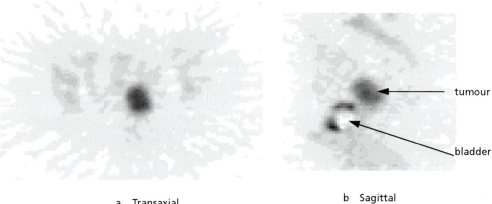

a   Transaxial

b   Sagittal

Increased FDG uptake is seen within the cervix at the site of primary disease in this 60 year old patient referred for PET scanning prior to surgery. Note the appearance of the bladder with a photon deficient centre as the patient was catheterized prior to the PET examination.

> When bladder catheterization is chosen as the method to prevent disease within the pelvis being masked by physiological urinary activity, bladder washouts are usually required. This involves a radiation dose to staff, and use of frusemide diuresis may be preferable.

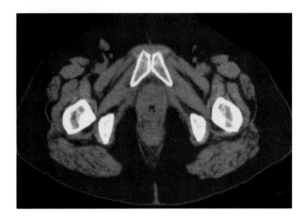

a   MR

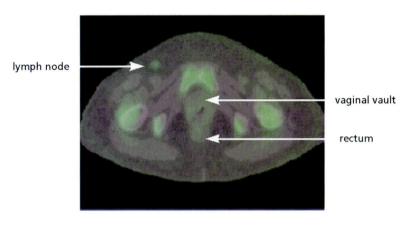

lymph node

vaginal vault

rectum

b   Registered MR/PET

This patient was scanned prior to surgery with PET and MR. The registered image showed evidence of tumour within the vaginal vault and also a right pelvic lymph node (arrowed). The PET scan was performed using a dual tracer technique (FDG together with F⁻) for the purposes of registering bony landmarks on PET to the MRI. Physiological uptake of FDG is seen within the rectum posterior to the cervix.

Teaching point: In the scan interpretation, it should be noted that high uptake of F⁻ within the bone may alter the perception of soft tissue to tumour ratio and SUV calculations.

Case 11.6.3

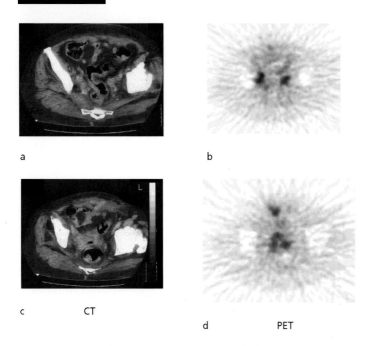

a

b

c   CT

d   PET

This woman with stage 3B carcinoma of the cervix was treated with surgery and chemotherapy. She responded well to treatment but then developed obstructive uropathy. She was referred for PET scanning to determine whether this was due to fibrosis related to treatment or active disease in the pelvis. CT and PET showed active disease within the cervix and disease within the anterior abdominal wall (c,d) and bilateral pelvic lymph nodes (a,b).

Case 11.6.4

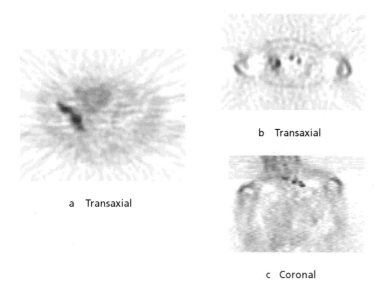

b   Transaxial

a   Transaxial

c   Coronal

This 45 year old woman with stage 4 carcinoma of the cervix at presentation was treated with chemotherapy with good response. She re-presented with right sided sciatica and underwent PET scanning. FDG scanning indicated disease within the right iliac nodes in the local emission view (a). Unsuspected disease was detected on whole body scanning, within para-aortic lymph nodes (seen anterior to the right renal activity in b) and in the supraclavicular fossa (c).

228   *Evolving oncology applications*

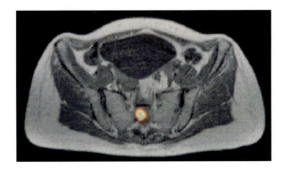

a   Overlaid display format

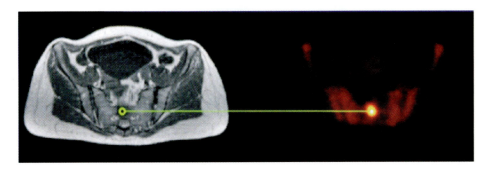

b   Adjacent display format
MR/PET Registered images

Increased uptake of FDG was seen within a sacral metastatic deposit in this patient with carcinoma of the cervix. Overlay and adjacent display formats are shown.

Case 11.6.6

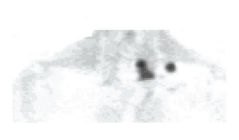

a Coronal

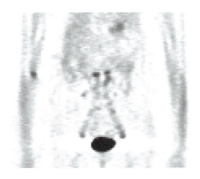

b Coronal

This patient with carcinoma of the ovary was treated with radiotherapy in 1993. She remained well until 1996 when she developed a left Horner's syndrome raising the question of recurrent nodal disease. The PET scan showed FDG uptake within nodes in the left neck in the local emission view of the neck and upper chest (a). The whole body scan also showed disease within the para-aortic and iliac lymph nodes (b).

a

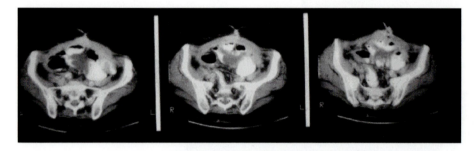

b

This woman with a previous history of ovarian carcinoma was treated with surgery and chemotherapy. She was scanned at suspected relapse. Increased uptake of FDG was seen within a peritoneal deposit (arrowed). Increased uptake seen posteriorly is within the right ureter.

Case 11.6.8

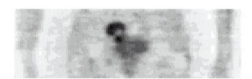

Coronal

This 59 year old woman had a history of sarcoma originating in the right broad ligament of the uterus 10 years previously. She presented with lymphoedema of the right leg and on examination was found to have a right iliac fossa mass. Intense uptake of FDG was seen within the pelvis at the site of recurrent disease.

Conclusions

EMERGING INDICATIONS

1 Staging lymph nodes

2 Identifying recurrent disease after surgery and radiotherapy

3 Response to treatment

4 Staging ovarian cancer

7 Bladder cancer

Current status of PET

Bladder cancers appear to have high FDG uptake in most instances and to have high uptake of [^{11}C]L-methionine. Thus, they can be imaged with both types of PET tracers. Clinical experience is still limited, but larger primary tumours, regional nodal metastases and pulmonary metastases can be imaged (Harney et al. 1991). The limitation of FDG-PET in patients with bladder carcinoma is dealing with the issue of excreted FDG activity in the urine. The intense FDG activity in the bladder can substantially degrade the visualization of lymph nodes in the anatomic pelvis, though this can be partly addressed through the use of a Foley catheter to drain the bladder during the conduct of the study or through the use of hydration followed by frusemide administration. Bladder cancer imaging using [^{11}C]L-methionine PET scanning has been reported, although there is variable pelvic [^{11}C]L-methionine activity as well. With careful attention to the reduction of FDG uptake in the pelvis, bladder carcinoma is a disease in which PET can be quite useful in selected cases. [^{11}C]L-Methionine, when available, may be superior owing to lower normal pelvic tracer uptake. These tumours remain under study, but PET may be useful in selected difficult situations.

Examples

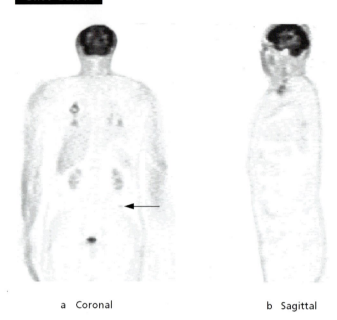

a Coronal   b Sagittal

This 49 year old patient had evidence of recurrent disease from carcinoma of the bladder on PET scanning. Increased uptake of FDG was seen within a left iliac lymph node (arrowed) and both lungs (a) and the left supraclavicular fossa (b).

Case 11.7.2

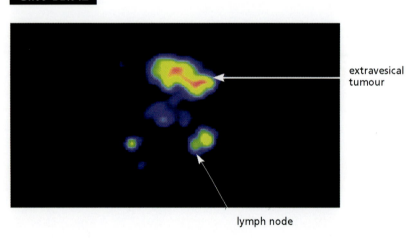

extravesical tumour

lymph node

From JV Harney, RL Wahl, M Lielbert, DE Kuhl, GD Hutchins, G Wedemeyer, HB Grossman. Journal of Urology 1991; 145, 281, Fig. 4a. Reproduced with permission.

This 63 year old woman had been treated with radiotherapy for a transitional cell carcinoma of the bladder 7 years previously. CT demonstrated thickening within the anterior wall of the bladder and soft tissue density around the bladder. Some changes were thought to be attributable to earlier radiotherapy, but recurrent tumour could not be excluded. PET showed intense uptake of FDG within the bladder extending anterior and superior to the bladder (arrowed) and into adjacent lymph nodes (arrowed) indicating recurrent tumour rather than postradiation changes. Physiological uptake can be seen within the ureters.

Case 11.7.3

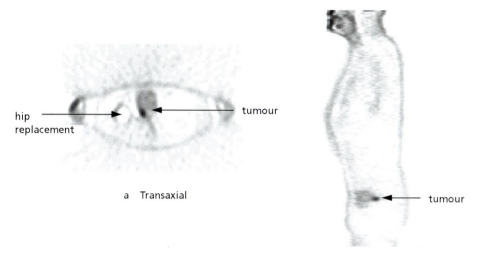

hip replacement ⟶   ⟵ tumour

a   Transaxial

⟵ tumour

b   Sagittal

This patient with carcinoma of the bladder was scanned for staging purposes. Focal increased uptake was seen within the posterior aspect of the bladder indicating primary disease only (arrowed). Accumulation of FDG was also seen around a right total hip replacement, possibly indicative of active inflammation or infection, though the patient was asymptomatic (a).

> PET cannot differentiate intravesical tumour from wall invasion in patients with bladder cancer.

Conclusions

EMERGING INDICATIONS

1   Can be used but difficult to interpret owing to high FDG in the bladder
2   [¹¹C]L-Methionine may be useful because less is excreted
3   Diagnosing systemic metastases
4   Primary nodal staging

8 Prostate cancer

Current status of PET

PET can image some prostate cancers but the overall published data on FDG-PET imaging of prostate cancer shows low sensitivity. Shreve *et al.* (1996) report that many bone metastases of prostate cancer are not detected by FDG-PET, and Yeh *et al.* (1996) report that <20% of prostate cancer metastases were detected by FDG-PET. Shreve *et al.* were able to detect some nodal metastases of prostate cancer and soft tissue lesions, but the overall SUVs were quite low relative to other cancer. PET has not been able, at least with FDG, to differentiate prostate cancer from benign prostatic hypertrophy in the prostate gland. The sensitivity of PET for detecting the primary lesion of prostate cancer or nodal metastases has not yet been rigorously determined, but there are major difficulties in imaging near the bladder with PET, as discussed previously. At present, the role of PET in prostate cancer imaging is not proven, and false negative cases appear to have been more common than in many other tumour types. Thus, prostate cancer imaging is only a small part of clinical PET. There is much room for advancement of the field of PET imaging in the area of prostate cancer through the development of new radiopharmaceuticals.

Examples

Case 11.8.1

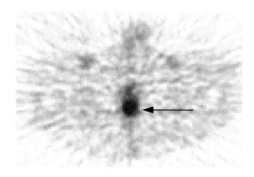

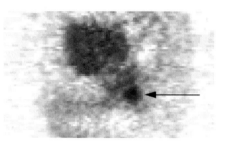

b Sagittal

a Transaxial

This patient with carcinoma of the prostate was referred at diagnosis. Small nodes were seen within the pelvis on CT and PET was performed to determine whether the nodes were reactive or neoplastic. PET shows uptake limited to the primary tumour (arrowed).

> Increased uptake of FDG may occur also within benign prostatic hypertrophy and cannot always be differentiated from carcinoma of the prostate.

Case 11.8.2

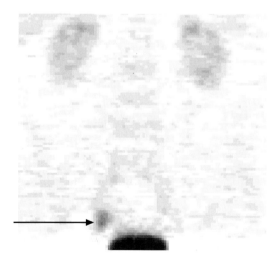

Coronal

This patient with carcinoma of the prostate was treated with surgery and radiotherapy in 1995. CT was performed because of rising PSA levels and indicated a 2 cm right iliac node. PET scanning showed FDG uptake within the node, confirming the presence of a lymph node metastasis.

Case 11.8.3

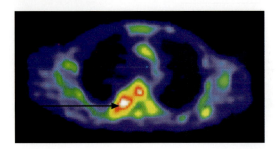

*From PD Shreve, HB Grossman, MD Gross, RL Wahl. Radiology 1996;**199**, p. 752, Fig. 1a. Reproduced with permission.*

This 74 year old man with extensive bone metastases (PSA = 4800 ng ml^{-1}) underwent bone scanning. The bone scan showed vertebral, multiple rib and sternal metastases. FDG uptake is seen within a metastasis in the right medial sixth posterior rib extending into the sixth thoracic vertebra. Other lesions seen on bone scanning did not take up FDG.

Case 11.8.4

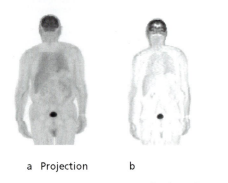

a Projection   b   c

Coronal volume images

This 73 year old man with known metastases from carcinoma of the prostate seen in the body of the first lumbar vertebra, the left sacroiliac joint and right acetabulum on bone scan, and within the first lumbar vertebra on CT scan, had no evidence of abnormal FDG uptake within bone.

Case 11.8.5

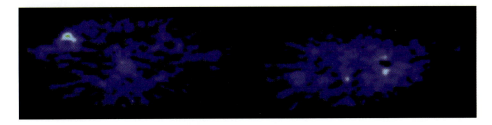

This patient with carcinoma of the prostate and bone metastases had a 'superscan' on bone scanning but no demonstrable FDG uptake on PET scanning.

> Where there is a small nidus of the tumour within bone, FDG may not detect bone metastases in carcinoma of the prostate. Bone scanning which images the osteoblastic response to metastases is often more sensitive in cases of prostate cancer.

Conclusions

EMERGING INDICATIONS

1 Equivocal bone lesion (if +ve, useful; if –ve, does not exclude)
2 Treatment response if lesion is seen in the first instance
3 Metastatic disease in soft tissue

9 Testicular cancer and teratoma

Current status of PET

Untreated malignant testicular neoplasms are generally well imaged with FDG-PET, although the available literature is very limited. Tracer uptake decreases rapidly with effective treatment, and there is only minimal FDG uptake in scar. Low tracer uptake is also seen in benign teratomas and it is so far difficult to separate scar from benign teratoma using current techniques, at least with static imaging. These tumours are infrequent, but PET appears to have a potential role in staging and follow up of treatment. Increased FDG uptake after treatment strongly suggests recurrent or residual tumour, based on the available data.

Examples

Case 11.9.1

November 1994

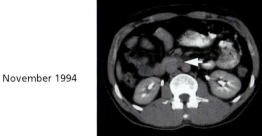

a   CT

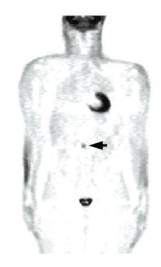

b   Coronal

January 1995

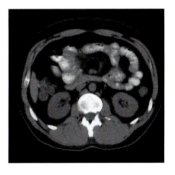

c   CT

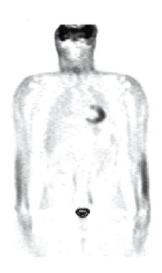

d   Coronal

A testicular teratoma was diagnosed in this 24 year old man who had a CT scan performed as part of routine staging in November 1994. The CT was reported as normal though a small node measuring less than 1 cm can be seen within the para-aortic region on the right (a, arrowed). PET showed intense uptake of FDG within a para-aortic lymph node, indicating intra-abdominal lymphatic spread (b, arrowed). The patient was therefore treated with radiotherapy with complete response on both CT and PET at the completion of treatment in January 1995.

> PET can identify malignant involvement in lymph nodes which are not enlarged by CT criteria.

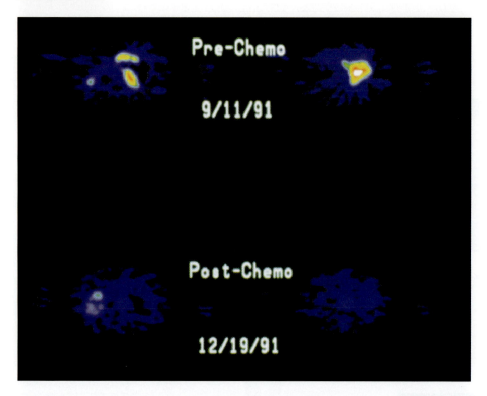

This patient with para-aortic lymphadenopathy and testicular carcinoma was treated with chemotherapy. A residual mass remained on CT, but FDG uptake diminished indicating successful response to treatment despite the persistent CT abnormality, and the patient has remained well.

Conclusions

EMERGING INDICATIONS

1 Response monitoring

2 Primary staging

3 Residual mass assessment

4 Raised markers

10 Muscle and connective tissue tumours

Current status of PET

Untreated sarcomas and primary and metastatic bone tumours are often well imaged with PET.

In several early studies the quantity of FDG uptake appeared to correlate with the grade of the sarcoma. In general, FDG uptake in patients with malignant bone tumours is greater than that in benign bone tumours. In a study of 25 patients with musculoskeletal lesions which included 6 benign lesions and 19 malignant lesions, all lesions with an SUV >1.6 were high grade while those with SUV of <1.6 were benign or of low grade. A follow up study in 20 patients with purely intraosseous lesions showed that with an SUV cut-off of 2.0, FDG-PET could detect 14/15 malignant lesions and 4/5 benign lesions. These studies suggest FDG-PET can be a useful method to help characterize soft tissue masses and intraosseous lesions non-invasively, although Nieweg et al. (1996) and others have shown some overlap between low and intermediate grade sarcomas and some benign lesions. Late imaging may improve the differentiation of benign from malignant soft tissue tumours. Using an SUV measured 4h post-injection, the sensitivity and specificity for the discrimination of high-grade sarcoma from benign tumours was 100% and 76% in a group of 29 patients presenting with soft-tissue tumours at Guy's and St Thomas' (Lodge et al. 1999). The response of sarcomas to treatment can also be assessed by PET. A rapid decline in FDG uptake is generally seen with effective treatment. Some residual FDG uptake in these tumours has been reported after treatment in foci of inflammation which remain – this is more of an issue following radiotherapy than chemotherapy. Thus, caution is necessary in assuming that FDG uptake equates to residual tumour following treatment. It is unclear whether FDG or other tracers will ultimately be the most effective in monitoring the treatment response of sarcomas.

The majority of Paget's disease cases are negative or only mildly positive on FDG-PET: this may become a way of excluding suspected malignant change. Sarcoma and bone tumour treatment monitoring is considered one of the more promising emerging areas of PET imaging.

Examples

Case 11.10.1

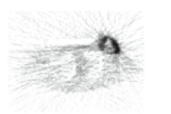
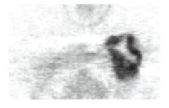

| a Transaxial | b Coronal |

Intense uptake of FDG was seen within this soft tissue sarcoma arising from the left pectoralis major muscle in this 67 year old man.

> Sarcomas are often histologically heterogeneous with variable intensity of FDG uptake in the same tumour, which can make interpretation of biopsy material problematic.

Case 11.10.2

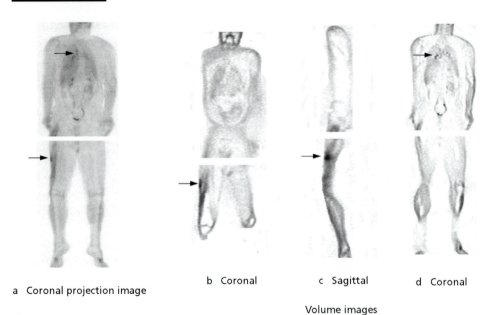

a Coronal projection image   b Coronal   c Sagittal   d Coronal

Volume images

This 41 year old patient had surgery and radiotherapy for a liposarcoma in the right thigh and a solitary metastasis in the abdomen 3 months later. He developed recurrent disease within the right thigh and was referred for PET scanning. The PET scan showed focal increased uptake within the right thigh, indicative of recurrent disease, surrounded by diffuse uptake secondary to inflammation after surgery and radiotherapy (arrowed in a–c). There was also avid uptake of FDG within lung metastases (d). The PET scan indicated that in addition to local disease there were lung and mediastinal metastases. Note the artefact seen where two scans are joined, when whole body images from skull vertex to toes are required.

> The focal uptake is often better appreciated on volume images but projection images may be better for overview.

Case 11.10.3

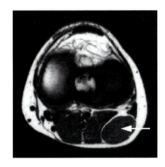

a MR

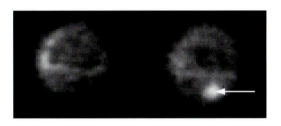

b Transaxial

c Sagittal

This child with neurofibromatosis was referred because of an enlarging fibroma in the left knee. There is intense increased uptake of FDG within the mass seen on MRI (a, arrowed). FDG can also be seen within the growth plate. Despite the intensity of uptake, this proved to be a benign fibroma at surgery.

> Neurofibromatosis may result in malignant transformation. PET can be helpful to refute this, but it must be remembered that occasionally benign lesions may have positive FDG uptake.

Paget's disease and fibrous dysplasia

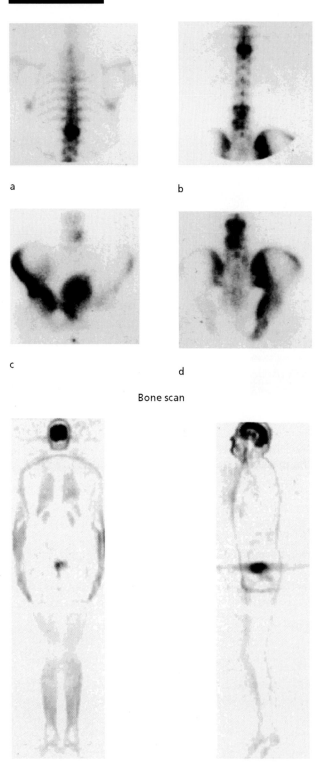

a

b

c

d

Bone scan

e Coronal   f Sagittal

This 58 year old man with Paget's disease showed no evidence of FDG uptake within the pagetic lesions demonstrated on bone scan.

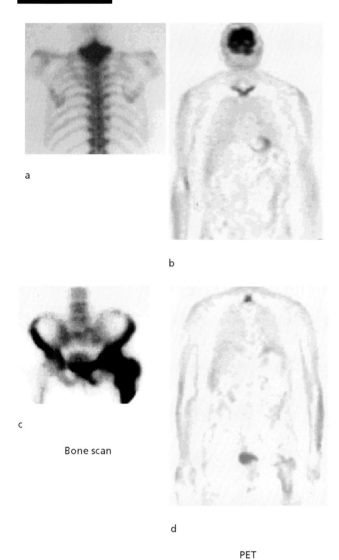

a

b

c

Bone scan

d

PET

Uptake of FDG was seen within the sites that are abnormal on bone scanning in this patient with Paget's disease, but the uptake of FDG was less extensive than the uptake on the bone scan.

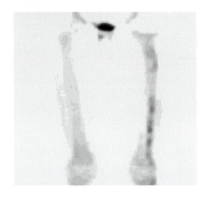

a Coronal   b Sagittal

Increased uptake of FDG occurs in fibrous dysplasia, shown here affecting the left femur.

Conclusions

EMERGING INDICATIONS
1   Follow up of sarcoma treatment
2   Grading of sarcoma
3   Separation of benign from malignant masses
4   Selection of biopsy sites
5   Assessing extent of sarcomas

11 Malignancy of unknown origin

Current status of PET

Detection of the unknown primary lesion is a very difficult situation in medicine. In many instances, patients present with obvious metastatic disease, often adenocarcinoma, and the location of the primary lesion is not easily found or may never be found. In some instances, knowledge of the site of the primary lesion is important as the type of treatment may vary (e.g. breast cancers are more responsive to some treatments than renal cancers), or the primary lesion and metastases could be resected or treated for cure, such as in head and neck cancers. The use of PET in the head and neck, which is promising, is reviewed elsewhere (see Chapter 7). Occasionally FDG-PET can locate primary tumours after metastatic disease to regional lymph nodes has appeared. PET is being increasingly applied in the search for unknown primary lesions, but the frequency with which it is successful is not yet known with certainty. The authors have had cases in which FDG-PET of the whole body was critical to identifying a previously undetected primary cancer. This area is still in evolution, but PET should be considered strongly in the work up of the unknown primary. In the authors' experience it has been rather more helpful in the paraneoplastic syndromes.

Examples

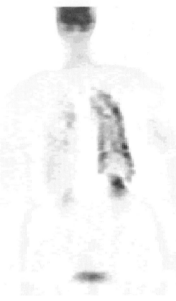

a Coronal

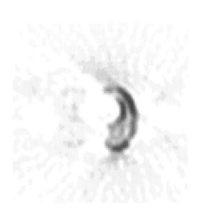

b Transaxial

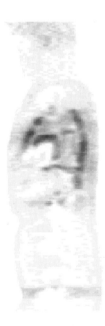

c Sagittal

This patient with adenocarcinoma of unknown origin had extensive uptake of FDG within the left lung and pleura, suggestive of a lung primary.

12 Neural crest origin tumours

Current status of PET

The role of PET in neural crest tumour imaging is not fully established, but it is clear that the neuroendocrine tumour, phaeochromocytoma, commonly accumulates FDG and can be imaged by the PET method. Indeed, two phaeochromocytomas which did not accumulate MIBG were successfully imaged with FDG in a recent report although MIBG remains the preferred agent. Phaeochromocytomas and neuroblastomas can be imaged with FDG and with [^{11}C]HED, a tracer which mimics epinephrine, although this is a research, not a clinical, endeavour at present. Neuroblastomas can also be imaged with PET in many instances, and while some neuroblastomas accumulate FDG and not MIBG, in general, MIBG uptake is superior to that of FDG in this tumour much as in phaeochromocytoma.

Examples

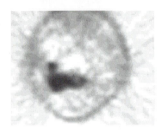

a Transaxial

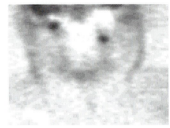

b Coronal

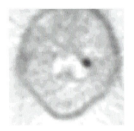

c Transaxial

Intense uptake of FDG was seen within two paragangliomas, the site and histology of which were confirmed at surgery. The left sided lesion was situated adjacent to the vertebral body of the first cervical vertebra and had an SUV of 4.5; the right sided lesion was situated close to the jugular foramen with an SUV of 4.7.

Case 11.12.2

PET   SPECT

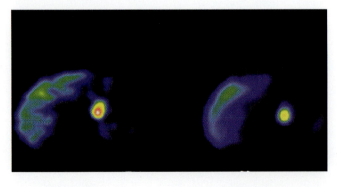

40 minutes   24 hours
p.i.^{11}C-HED   p.i.^{123}I-MIBG

Transaxial

Corresponding transaxial images are shown of a 72 year old male patient with phaeochromocytoma imaged with [^{11}C]HED-PET and [^{123}I]MIBG-SPECT.

Case 11.12.3

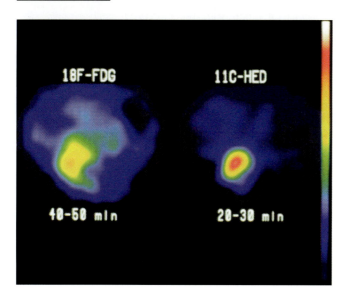

Corresponding images are shown of a 6 month old child with neuroblastoma in the pelvis imaged with FDG and [^{11}C]HED.

References and further reading

1 Thyroid and parathyroid

Adams S, Baum R, Rink T *et al.* (1998) Limited value of fluorine-18 fluorodeoxyglucose positron emission tomography for the imaging of neuroendocrine tumours. *E J N M* 25(1), 79–83.

Altenvoerde G, Lerch H, Kuwert T, Matheja P, Schafers M, Schober O (1998) Positron emission tomography with F-18-deoxyglucose in patients with differentiated thyroid carcinoma, elevated thyroglobulin levels, and negative iodine scans. Langenbecks *Archives of Surgery* 383, 160–63.

Cook GJ, Wong JC, Smellie WJ, Young AE, Maisey MN, Fogelman I (1998) [11C]Methionine positron emission tomography for patients with persistent or recurrent hyperparathyroidism after surgery. *European Journal of Endocrinology* 139, 195–7.

Grunwald F, Schomburg A, Bender H *et al.* (1996) Fluorine-18 fluorodeoxyglucose positron emission tomography in the follow-up of differentiated thyroid cancer. *Eur J Nucl Med* 23, 312–19.

Joensuu H, Ahonen A (1987) Imaging of metastases of thyroid carcinoma with fluorine-18 fluorodeoxyglucose. *J Nucl Med* 28(5), 910–14.

Joensuu H, Ahonen A, Klemi PJ (1988) 18F-fluorodeoxyglucose imaging in preoperative diagnosis of thyroid malignancy. *Eur J Nucl Med* 13(10), 502–6.

Melon P, Luxen A, Hamoir E, Meurisse M (1995) Fluorine-18-fluorodeoxyglucose positron emission tomography for preoperative parathyroid imaging in primary hyperparathyroidism. *Eur J Nucl Med* 22(6), 556–8.

Neumann DR, Esselstyn CB Jr, MacIntyre WJ *et al.* (1994) Primary hyperparathyroidism: preoperative parathyroid imaging with regional body FDG PET. *Radiology* 192(2), 509–12

Neumann DR, Esselstyn CB Jr, MacIntyre WJ *et al.* (1997) Regional body FDG-PET in postoperative recurrent hyperparathyroidism. *J Comput Assist Tomogr* 21(1), 25–8.

Sisson JC, Ackermann R, Meyer MA, Wahl RL (1993) Uptake of FDG by thyroid cancer: Implications for Diagnosis and therapy. *J Clin Endocrinol Metab* 77, 1090–4.

Sundin A, Johansson C, Hellman P *et al.* (1996) PET and parathyroid L-[carbon-11]methionine accumulation in hyperparathyroidism. *J Nucl Med* 37(11), 1766–70.

Yasuda S, Shohtsu A, Ide M *et al.* (1998) Chronic thyroiditis: diffuse uptake of FDG at PET. *Radiology* 207(3), 775–8.

2 Oesophageal cancer

Flanagan FL, Dehdashti F, Siegel B *et al.* (1997) Staging of esophageal cancer with 18F fluorodeoxyglucose positron emission tomography. *Am J Radiol* **168**, 417–24.

Fukunaga T, Enomoto K, Okazumi S *et al.* (1994) Analysis of glucose metabolism in patients with esophageal cancer by PET: estimation of hexokinase activity in the tumor and usefulness for clinical assessment using 18F-fluorodeoxyglucose. *Nippon Geka Gakkai Zasshi* **95**(5), 317–25.

Kole AC, Plukker JT, Nieweg OE, Vaalburg W (1998) Positron emission tomography for staging of oesophageal and gastroesophageal malignancy. *British Journal of Cancer* **78**, 521–7.

Luketich JD, Schauer PR, Meltzer CC *et al.* (1997) Role of positron emission tomography in staging esophageal cancer. *Ann Thor Surg* **64**(3), 765–9.

Rankin SC, Taylor H, Cook GJ, Mason R (1998) Computed tomography and positron emission tomography in the pre- operative staging of oesophageal carcinoma. *Clinical Radiology* **53**, 659–65.

3 Liver and hepatoma

Delbeke D, Martin WH, Sandler MP *et al.* (1998) Evaluation of benign vs malignant hepatic lesions with positron emission tomography. *Archives of Surgery* **133**(5), 510–15.

Hayashi N, Tamaki N, Yonekura Y *et al.* (1985) Imaging of the hepatocellular carcinoma using dynamic positron emission tomography with nitrogen-13 ammonia. *J Nucl Med* **26**(3), 254–7.

Hustinx R, Paulus P, Jacquet N, Jerusalem G, Bury T, Rigo P (1998) Clinical evaluation of whole-body 18F-fluorodeoxyglucose positron emission tomography in the detection of liver metastases. *Annals of Oncology* **9**, 397–401.

Nagata Y, Yamamoto K, Hiraoka M *et al.* (1990) Monitoring liver tumor therapy with [18F]FDG positron emission tomography. *J Comput Assist Tomogr* **14**(3), 370–4.

Torizuka T, Tamaki N, Inokuma T *et al.* (1995) In vivo assessment of glucose metabolism in hepatocellular carcinoma with FDG-PET. *J Nucl Med* **36**, 1811–17.

4 Pancreatic cancer

Bares R, Klever P, Hauptmann S *et al.* (1994) 18F fluorodeoxyglucose PET *in vivo* evaluation of pancreatic glucose metabolism for detection of pancreatic cancer. *Radiology* **192**, 79–86.

Ho C, Dehdashti F, Griffeth LK *et al.* (1996) FDG-PET evaluation of indeterminate pancreatic masses. *J Comput Assist Tomogr* **20**(3), 363–9.

Inokuma T, Tamaki N, Torizuka T *et al.* (1995) Evaluation of pancreatic tumors with positron emission tomography and F-18 fluorodeoxyglucose: comparison with CT and US. *Radiology* **195**, 345–52.

Rajput A, Stellato TA, Faulhaber PF, Vesselle HJ, Miraldi F (1998) The role of fluorodeoxyglucose and positron emission tomography in the evaluation of pancreatic disease. *Surgery* **124**, 793–7.

Stollfuss JC, Glatting G, Friess H *et al.* (1995) 2-(fluorine-18)-fluoro-2-deoxy-D-glucose PET in detection of pancreatic cancer: value of quantitative image interpretation. *Radiology* **195**, 339–44.

Zimny M, Bares R, Fass J, Adam G, Cremerius U, Dohmen B *et al.* (1997) Fluorine-18 fluorodeoxyglucose positron emission tomography in the differential diagnosis of pancreatic carcinoma: a report of 106 cases. *European Journal of Nuclear Medicine* **24**, 678–82.

5 Renal cell cancer

Hoh CK, Seltzer MA, Franklin J, deKernion JB, Phelps ME, Belldegrun *et al.* (1998) Positron emission tomography in urological oncology. *Journal of Urology* **159**, 347–56.

Goldberg MA, Mayo-Smith WW, Papanicolaou N, Fischman AJ, Lee MJ (1998) FDG PET characterization of renal masses: preliminary experience. *Clinical Radiology* **52**, 510–15.

Miyauchi RS, Brown RS, Grossman HB *et al.* (1996) Correlation between visualization of primary renal cancer by FDG-PET and histopathological findings. *J Nucl Med* **37**(5), 36.

Wahl RL, Harney J, Hutchins G, Grossman HB (1991) Imaging of renal cancer using positron emission tomography with 2-deoxy-2-(^{18}F)-fluoro-D-glucose: pilot animal and human studies. *J Urol* **146**(6), 1470–4.

6 Cervical, uterine and ovarian cancer

Casey MJ, Gupta NC, Muth CK (1994) Experience with positron emission tomography (PET) scans in patients with ovarian cancer. *Gynecol Oncol* **53**, 331–8.

Goldberg MA, Lee MJ, Fischman AJ *et al.* (1993) Fluorodeoxyglucose PET of abdominal and pelvic neoplasms: potential role in oncologic imaging. *Radiographs* **13**, 1047–62.

Hubner KF, McDonald TW, Niethammer JG *et al.* (1993) Assessment of primary and metastatic ovarian cancer by positron emission tomography (PET) using 2-[^{18}F]deoxyglucose (2-[^{18}F]FDG). *Gynecol Oncol* **51**, 197–204.

Karlan B, Hawkins R, Hoh C *et al.* (1993) Whole-body positron emission tomography with 2-[^{18}F]-fluoro-2-deoxy-D-glucose can detect recurrent ovarian carcinoma. *Gynecol Oncol* **51**, 175–81.

Lapela M, Leskinen-Kallio S, Varpula M *et al.* (1994) Imaging of uterine carcinoma by carbon-11-methionine and PET. *J Nucl Med* **35**(10), 1618–23.

Lapela M, Leskinen-Kallio S, Varpula M *et al.* (1995) Metabolic imaging of ovarian tumors with carbon-11-methionine: a PET study. *J Nucl Med* **36**, 2196–200.

Romer W, Avril N, Dose J *et al.* (1997) [Metabolic characterization of ovarian tumors with positron emission tomography and F-18 fluorodeoxyglucose]. *Rofo Forschritte auf dem Gebiete der Rontgenstrahlen und der Neuen Bildgebenden Verfahren* **166**(1), 62–8.

Wahl RL, Hutchins GD, Roberts J (1991) FDG PET imaging of ovarian cancer: Initial evaluation in patients. *J Nucl Med* **32**(5), 982.

7 Bladder cancer

Ahlstrom H, Malmstrom PU, Letocha H *et al.* (1996) Positron emission tomography in the diagnosis and staging of urinary bladder cancer. *Acta Radiol* **37**(2), 180–5.

Harney JV, Wahl RL, Liebert M *et al.* (1991) Uptake of 2-deoxy, 2-(18F) fluoro-D-glucose in bladder cancer: animal localization and initial patient positron emission tomography. *J Urol* **145**(2), 279–83.

Kosuda S, Kison PV, Greenough R *et al.* (1997) Preliminary assessment of fluorine-18 fluorodeoxyglucose positron emission tomography in patients with bladder cancer. *E J Nucl Med* **24**(6), 615–20.

Letocha H, Ahlstrom H, Malmstrom PU *et al.* (1994) Positron emission tomography with L-methyl-^{11}C-methionine in the monitoring of therapy response in muscle-invasive transitional cell carcinoma of the urinary bladder. *Br J Urol* **74**(6), 767–74.

8 Prostate cancer

Bender H, Schomburg A, Albers P *et al.* (1997) Possible role of FDG-PET in the evaluation of urologic malignancies. *Anticancer Research* **17**(3B), 1655–60.

Effert PJ, Bares R, Handt S *et al.* (1996) Metabolic imaging of untreated prostate cancer by positron emission tomography with ^{18}fluorine-labeled deoxyglucose. *J Urol* **155**(3), 994–8.

Shreve PD, Grossman BH, Gross MD, Wahl RL (1996) Metastatic prostate cancer: Initial findings of PET with 2-deoxy-2-[F-18]fluoro-D-glucose. *Radiology* **199**, 751–6.

Yeh SD, Imbriaco M, Larson SM *et al.* (1996) Detection of bony metastases of androgen-independent prostate cancer by PET-FDG. *Nucl Med Biol* **23**(6), 693–7.

9 Testicular cancer and teratoma

Nuutinen JM, Leskinen S, Elomaa I *et al.* (1997) Detection of residual tumours in postchemotherapy testicular cancer by FDG-PET. *E J Cancer* **33**(8), 1234–41.

Reinhardt MJ, Muller-Mattheis VG, Gerharz CD *et al.* (1997) FDG-PET evaluation of retroperitoneal metastases of testicular cancer before and after chemotherapy. *J Nucl Med* **38**(1), 99–101.

Stephens AW, Gonin R, Hutchins GD, Einhorn LH (1996) Positron emission tomography evaluation of residual radiographic abnormalities in postchemotherapy germ cell tumor patients. *J Clin Oncol* **14**(5), 1637–41.

Wahl RL, Greenough R, Clark MF, Grossman HB (1993) Initial evaluation of FDG/PET imaging of metastatic testicular neoplasms. *J Nucl Med* **34**(5), 6P (abstract).

Wilson CB, Young HE, Ott RJ *et al.* (1995) Imaging metastatic testicular germ cell tumours with 18FDG positron emission tomography: prospects for detection and management. *Eur J Nucl Med* **22**(6), 508–13.

10 Muscle and connective tissue tumours

Adler LP, Blair HF, Makley JT *et al.* (1991) Noninvasive grading of musculoskeletal tumors using PET. *J Nucl Med* **32**(8), 1508–12.

Cook GJR, Maisey MN, Fogelman I (1997) Fluorine-18-FDG PET in Paget's disease of bone. *J Nucl Med* **38**, 1495–7.

Eary JF, Mankoff DA (1998) Tumor metabolic rates in sarcoma using FDG PET. *J Nucl Med* **39**(2), 250–54.

Garcia R, Kim EE, Wong FC (1996) Comparison of fluorine-18-FDG PET and technetium-99m-MIBI SPECT in evaluation of musculoskeletal sarcomas. *J Nucl Med* **37**(9), 1476–9.

Griffeth LK, Dehdashti F, McGuire AH *et al.* (1992) PET evaluation of soft-tissue masses with fluorine-18fluoro-2-deoxy-D-glucose. *Radiology* **182**(1), 185–94.

Jones DN, McCowage GB, Sostman HD *et al.* (1996) Monitoring of neoadjuvant therapy response of soft-tissue and musculoskeletal sarcoma using fluorine-18-FDG PET. *J Nucl Med* **37**(9), 1438–44.

Lodge MA, Lucas JD, Marsden PK, Cronin BF, O'Doherty MJ (1999) A PET study of ^{18}FDG uptake in soft tissue masses. *Eur J Nucl Med* **26**, 22–30.

Nieweg OE, Pruim J, van Ginkel RJ *et al.* (1996) Fluorine-18-fluorodeoxyglucose PET imaging of soft-tissue sarcoma. *J Nucl Med* **37**(2), 257–61.

Shulkin BL, Mitchell DS, Ungar DR *et al.* (1995) Neoplasms in a pediatric population: 2-[F-18]-fluoro-2-deoxy-D-glucose PET studies. *Radiology* **194**(2), 495–50.

van Ginkel RJ, Hoekstra HJ, Pruim J *et al.* (1996) FDG-PET to evaluate response to hyperthermic isolated limb perfusion for locally advanced soft-tissue sarcoma. *J Nucl Med* **37**(6), 984–90.

11 Malignancy of unknown origin

Braams JW, Pruim J, Kole AC *et al.* (1997) Detection of unknown primary head and neck tumors by positron emission tomography. *Int J Oral Maxillofac Surg* **26**(2), 112–15.

Kole AC, Nieweg OE, Pruim J *et al.* (1998) Detection of unknown occult primary tumors using positron emission tomography. *Cancer* **82**(6), 1160–66.

Schipper JH, Schrader M, Arweiler D *et al.* (1996) Die Positronenemissionstomographie zur Primartumorsuche bei Halslymphknotenmetastasen mit unbekanntem Primartumor [Positron emission tomography for primary tumor detection in lymph node metastases with unknown primary tumor] *HNO* **44**(5), 254–7.

12 Neural crest origin tumours

Musholt TJ, Musholt PB, Dehdashti F *et al.* (1997) Evaluation of fluorodeoxyglucose-positron emission tomographic scanning and its associatoin with glucose transporter expression in medullary thyroid carcinoma and pheochromocytoma: a clinical and molecular study. *Surgery* **122**(6), 1049–60.

Neumann DR, Basile KE, Bravo EL *et al.* (1996) Malignant pheochromocytoma of the anterior mediastinum: PET findings with [18F]FDG and 82Rb. *J Comput Assist Tomogr* **20**(2), 312–16.

Shulkin BL, Hutchinson RJ, Castle VP *et al.* (1996) Neuroblastoma: positron emission tomography with 2-[fluorine-18]-fluoro-2-deoxy-D-glucose compared with metaiodobenzylguanidine scintigraphy. *Radiology* **199**(3), 743–50.

Shulkin BL, Koeppe RA, Francis IR *et al.* (1993) Pheochromocytomas that do not accumulate metaiodobenzylguanidine: localization with PET and administration of FDG. *Radiology* **186**(3), 711–15.

Shulkin BL, Wieland DM, Schwaiger M *et al.* (1992) PET scanning with hydroxyephedrine: an approach to the localization of pheochromocytoma. *J Nucl Med* **33**(6), 1125–31.

Part III

Other applications of PET

Chapter 12

Neurology and psychiatry

Introduction and background

The early research and clinical applications of PET were almost exclusively devoted to the brain. These early studies used single slice small volume PET scanners and have provided immense amounts of data which has driven forward our understanding of brain function. This has included a better understanding of changes in cerebral circulation including:

- the relationships between blood flow, blood volume and oxygen extraction using $[^{15}O]$water, $[^{15}O]$carbon monoxide and $[^{15}O]$oxygen gas tracers and variations which occur during and after stroke
- the developmental changes in regional glucose metabolism and the patterns of changes in dementias
- the sites of cerebral sensorimotor control by $[^{15}O]$water perfusion activation studies and a huge amount of information about the distribution of brain receptors (benzodiazapine, opioid, MAO-B receptors, histamine receptors and others) in normal and various psychiatric states. In spite of these spectacular advances in our understanding of basic physiology and pathophysiology that has arisen from PET studies, there are still relatively few clinical applications.

FDG is the most important tracer, because glucose is the major energy substrate for brain and much is known about the relationship between glucose and FDG. Flow studies with $[^{15}O]$water have a small role in cerebrovascular disorders and possibly activation studies but usually show a distribution similar to FDG. $[^{11}C]$L-Methionine is important in brain tumours and $[^{11}C]$flumazenil is increasingly applied to partial epilepsy.

CLINICAL APPLICATIONS OF PET IN NEUROLOGY AND PSYCHIATRY

Dementia

Brain tumours

Epilepsy

Cerebrovascular disease

HIV disease

Systemic lupus erythematosus

Normal appearances

The following images show sections of a normal brain, each using the same display format as shown in the key.

Key:

MRI   MRI co-registered   FDG
              with FDG
              (unlabelled)

              MRI co-registered
              with FDG
              (with labels)

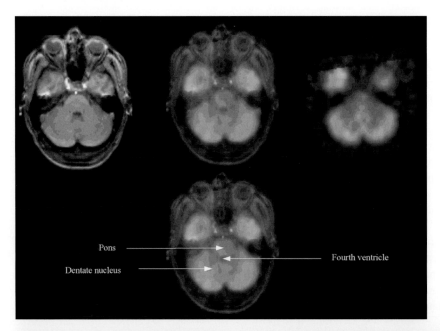

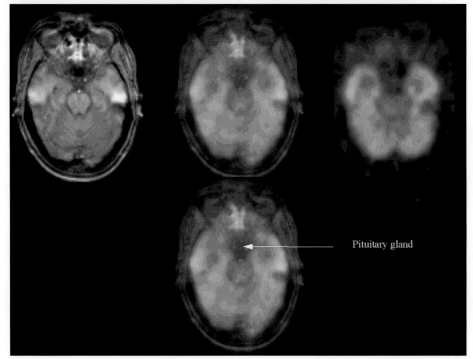

Transaxial sections: inferior to superior.

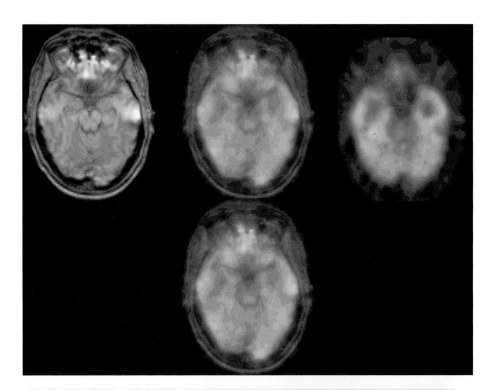

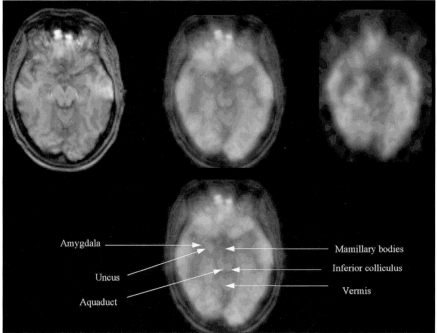

Amygdala

Uncus

Aquaduct

Mamillary bodies

Inferior colliculus

Vermis

Transaxial sections: inferior to superior (continued).

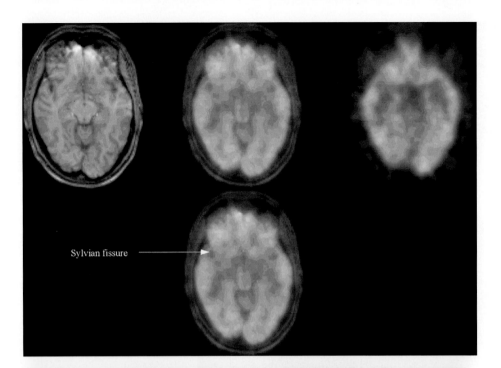

Sylvian fissure

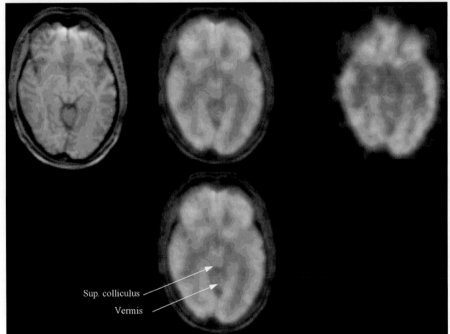

Sup. colliculus

Vermis

Transaxial sections: inferior to superior (continued).

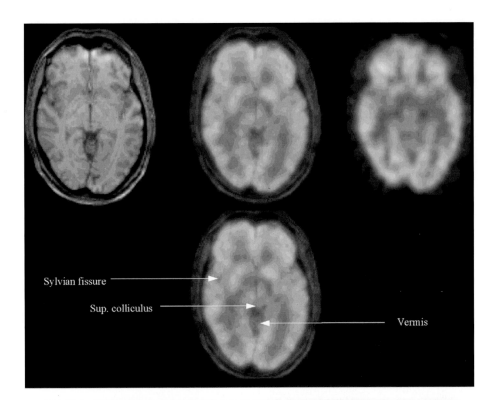

Sylvian fissure

Sup. colliculus

Vermis

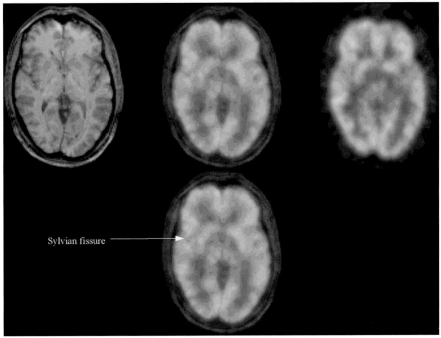

Sylvian fissure

Transaxial sections: inferior to superior (continued).

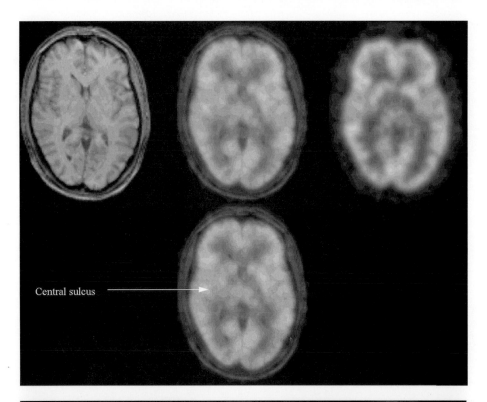

Central sulcus

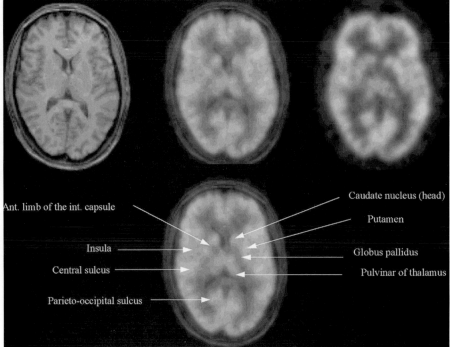

Ant. limb of the int. capsule

Insula

Central sulcus

Parieto-occipital sulcus

Caudate nucleus (head)

Putamen

Globus pallidus

Pulvinar of thalamus

Transaxial sections: inferior to superior (continued).

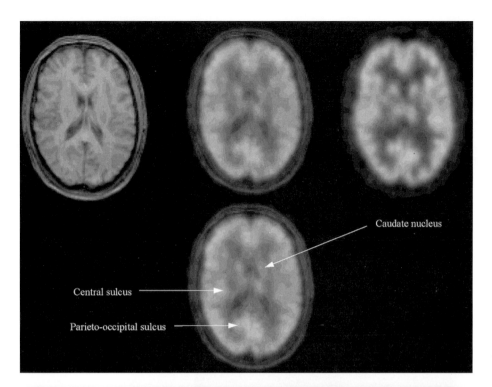

Caudate nucleus

Central sulcus

Parieto-occipital sulcus

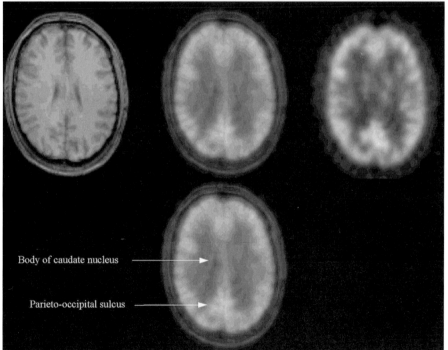

Body of caudate nucleus

Parieto-occipital sulcus

Transaxial sections: inferior to superior (continued).

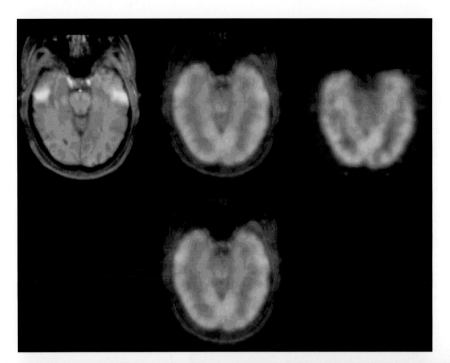

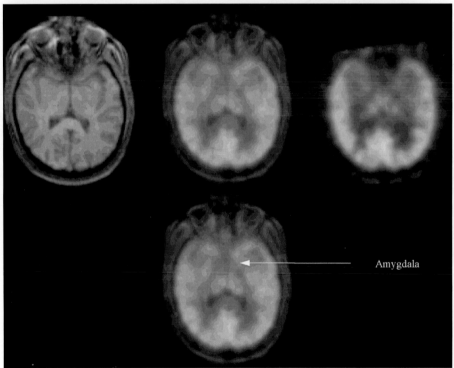

Transaxial sections aligned to the long axis of the temporal lobe: inferior to superior.

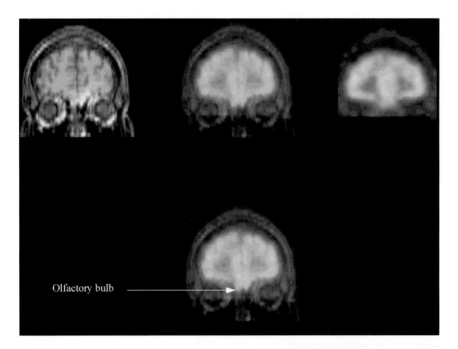

Olfactory bulb

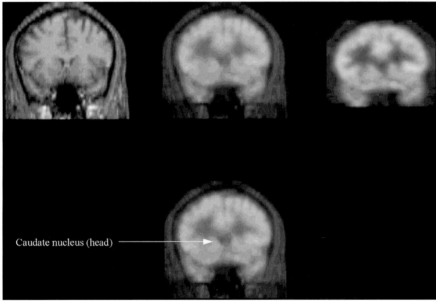

Caudate nucleus (head)

Coronal sections: anterior to posterior.

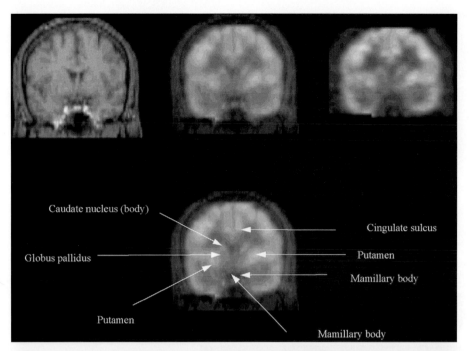

Caudate nucleus (body)

Cingulate sulcus

Globus pallidus

Putamen

Mamillary body

Putamen

Mamillary body

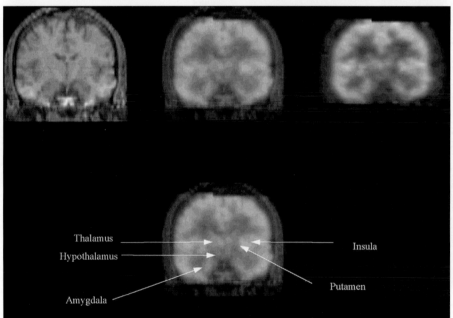

Thalamus

Insula

Hypothalamus

Putamen

Amygdala

Coronal sections: anterior to posterior (continued).

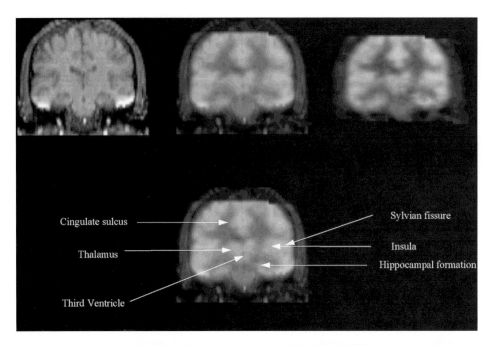

Cingulate sulcus

Thalamus

Third Ventricle

Sylvian fissure

Insula

Hippocampal formation

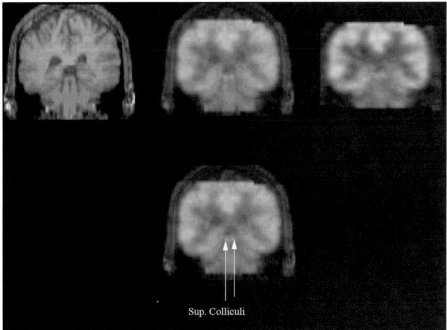

Sup. Colliculi

Coronal sections: anterior to posterior (continued).

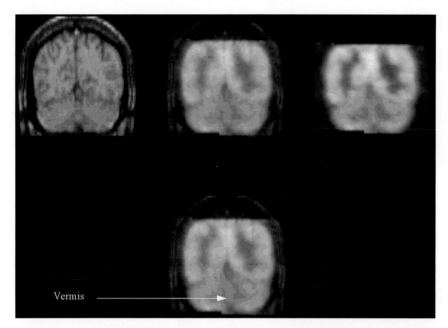

Coronal sections: anterior to posterior (continued).

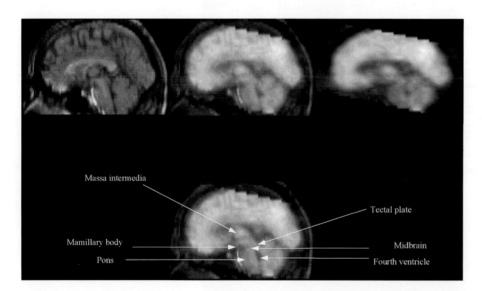

Sagittal sections: midline to lateral.

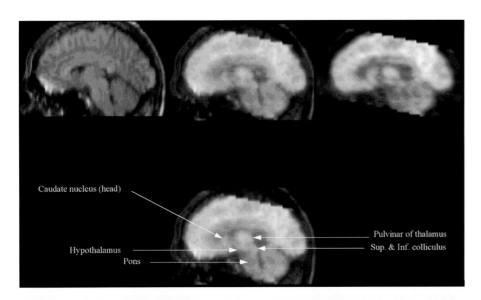

Caudate nucleus (head)

Hypothalamus

Pons

Pulvinar of thalamus

Sup. & Inf. colliculus

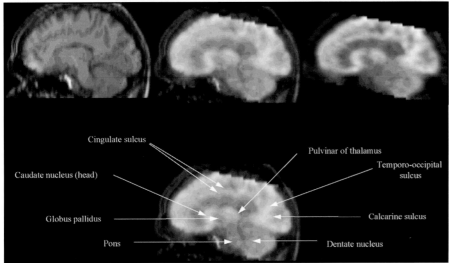

Cingulate sulcus

Pulvinar of thalamus

Temporo-occipital sulcus

Caudate nucleus (head)

Globus pallidus

Calcarine sulcus

Pons

Dentate nucleus

Sagittal sections: midline to lateral (continued).

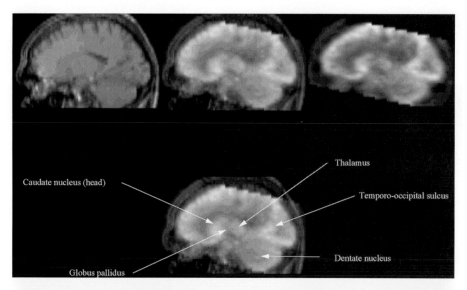

Caudate nucleus (head)

Thalamus

Temporo-occipital sulcus

Dentate nucleus

Globus pallidus

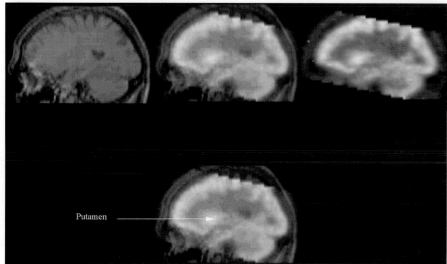

Putamen

Sagittal sections: midline to lateral (continued).

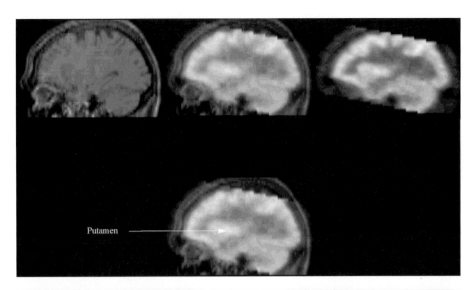

Putamen

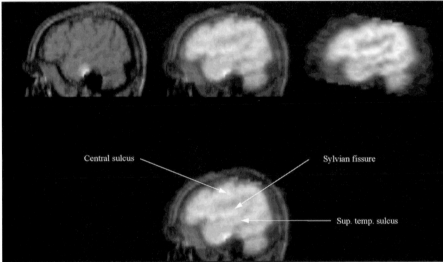

Central sulcus

Sylvian fissure

Sup. temp. sulcus

Sagittal sections: midline to lateral (continued).

1 Dementia

Dementia is defined as loss of memory and at least one other area of complex behaviour sufficient to interfere with daily life. It is an increasing problem to society and usually a personal and family tragedy. It will get worse, as it has been estimated that up to 5% of people over 65 and up to 25% of those over 80 years will have some form of dementia.

CAUSES OF DEMENTIA

Degenerative

Alzheimer's disease

Frontal lobe degeneration

Pick's disease

Olivopontocerebellar degeneration

Lewy body disease

Huntington's disease

Parkinson's disease

Vascular

Multiple infarct dementia

Small vessel (Binswanger's disease)

Trauma

Multiple

Subdural/extradural

Infective

HIV disease

Creutzfeldt–Jakob disease

Other causes

Hydrocephalus

Metabolic causes

Pseudodementia

Investigation in the first instance is to detect treatable disease, e.g. brain tumour, hypothyroidism, hydrocephalus, etc. Alzheimer's disease is responsible for approximately 50% of all cases of dementia.

Investigation is directed at excluding treatable causes and defining the likely progress of the disorder. As would be expected, metabolic changes occur before structural changes and FDG-PET abnormalities may precede structural changes by as much as 12 months. This will become much more important as treatments are designed to slow or reverse the process, as the earlier changes can be treated, the greater the likelihood of success.

IMAGING FINDINGS IN THE DEMENTIAS

MR imaging	FDG-PET imaging
Alzheimer's disease	
Early: normal or hippocampal atrophy	Temporoparietal and cingulate hypometabolism
Advanced: frontal, parietotemporal atrophy	Temporoparietal hypometabolism with sparing of subcortical structures, primary visual and sensorimotor cortex; later also frontal hypometabolism cortical atrophy and thalamic separation
Multi-infarct dementia	
White matter signals and cortical subcortical infarcts	Focal asymmetrical cortical and subcortical hypometabolic areas
Pseudodementia	
Normal	Normal or frontal hypometabolism
Fronto temporal dementias	
Early: normal	Frontal: frontal lobe hypometabolism
Late: frontal atrophy	Pick's: Frontal + temporal hypometabolism
Trauma	
Mild: normal	Focal hypometabolism
Severe: atrophy	Focal hypometabolism
HIV	
Normal	Diffuse patchy hypometabolism with sparing of deep structures
Huntington's disease	
Early: normal	Hypometabolism of caudate nucleus
Late: caudate atrophy	
Lewy body disease	
Early: nil	Alzheimer's disease-like picture but with reduced visual cortex metabolism
Late: atrophy	

Key management issues

Examples to illustrate key issues

Key issue 1 Early diagnosis of Alzheimer's disease vs. benign memory loss

Case 12.1.1

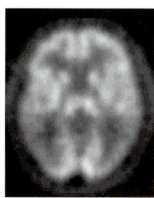

b Sagittal

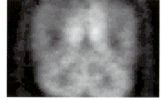

c Coronal

a Transaxial

FDG-PET scan of a 49 year old patient with early signs of memory loss being investigated for Alzheimer's disease. There is mild reduction in FDG uptake in posterior parietal lobes, typical of early Alzheimer's disease.

Case 12.1.2

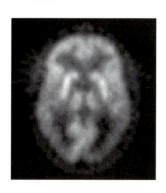

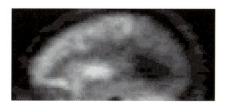

c Sagittal

a Transaxial

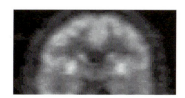

b Coronal

By contrast, this case shows florid features of Alzheimer's disease with markedly reduced FDG uptake in the posterior parietal and temporal lobes bilaterally.

Case 12.1.3

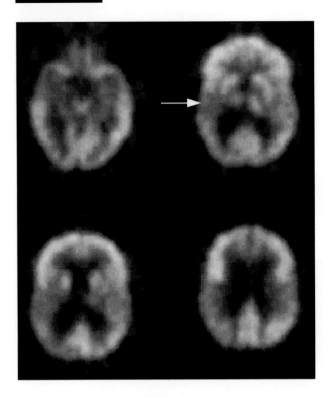

Transaxial

This 68 year old man had a history of cerebrovascular disease and depression. He had a right middle cerebral artery infarct in 1990, followed by onset of a depressive illness in 1991, which had become unresponsive to treatment. PET scanning showed evidence of his previous right middle cerebral artery infarct with reduced uptake of FDG in the right parietal lobe and posterior thalamus (arrowed). There was also widening of the sulci and separation of the thalami indicative of cortical atrophy and bilateral parietotemporal hypometabolism suggestive of Alzheimer's type dementia.

Case 12.1.4

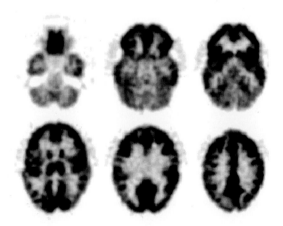

Transaxial

This demonstrates the normal distribution of FDG with 4–5-fold higher metabolic rate in grey matter than white matter.

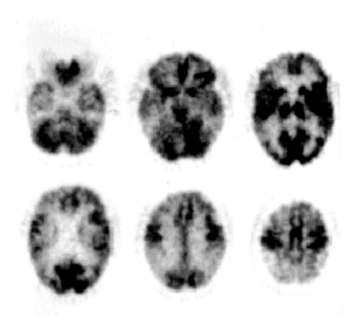

Transaxial

A case of advanced Alzheimer's disease. The metabolism is reduced bilaterally in parietal, temporal and frontal lobe cortex. Activity is preserved relatively in the motor cortices, in the anterior cingulate cortex (top left midline), the basal ganglia, thalamus and posterior fossa structures.

Case 12.1.6

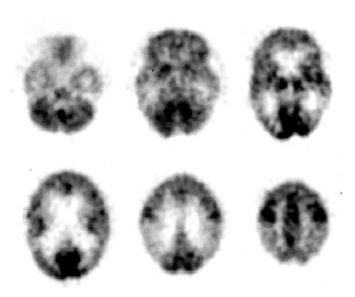

Transaxial

A case of mild Alzheimer's disease demonstrating predominant reduction of metabolism in the parietal cortex.

Case 12.1.7

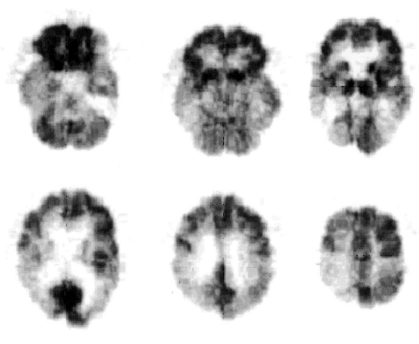

Transaxial

A case of mild Alzheimer's disease with asymmetry of metabolic reduction in parietotemporal cortices which is frequently seen.

Case 12.1.8

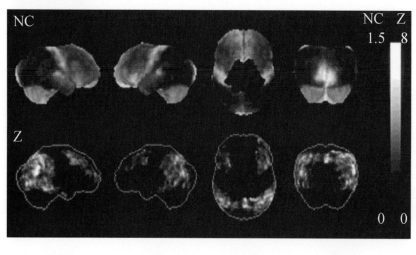

| Right lateral | Left lateral | Superior | Posterior |

A statistical stereotactic surface projection image illustrating quantitatively the reduced glucose metabolism in a patient with Alzheimer's disease compared with a normal data base. The Z score refers to the number of standard deviations by which the FDG uptake in this patient differs from the normal database.

Key issue 2 Differential diagnosis of dementia

Case 12.1.9: Pick's disease

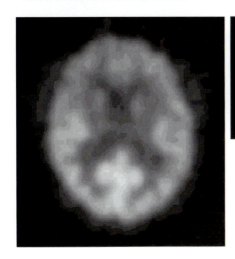

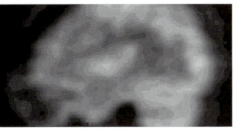

b   Sagittal

a   Transaxial

Bilateral frontal hypometabolism is seen on the FDG scan in this 50 year old dementing woman, indicating the aetiology of her dementia as Pick's disease. This is much more extensive than seen with depression.

Case 12.1.10: Huntington's disease

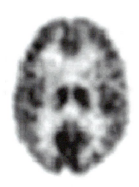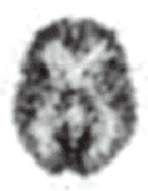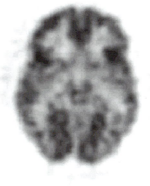

Transaxial

This FDG-PET scan is of an asymptomatic patient at risk for Huntington's disease. Metabolism in the caudate nuclei was reduced in advance of atrophy. In some instances the metabolic features on PET may occur in advance of clinical signs or symptoms.

Case 12.1.11: Olivopontocerebellar atrophy (OPCA)

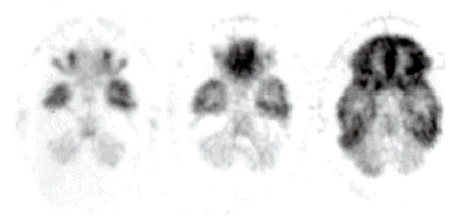

Transaxial

Cerebellar degeneration is associated with reduced metabolism to an even greater extent than is predicted by atrophy alone. Cerebral cortical metabolism is relatively preserved in multisystem atrophy including the OPCA type.

Case 12.1.12: Lewy body dementia

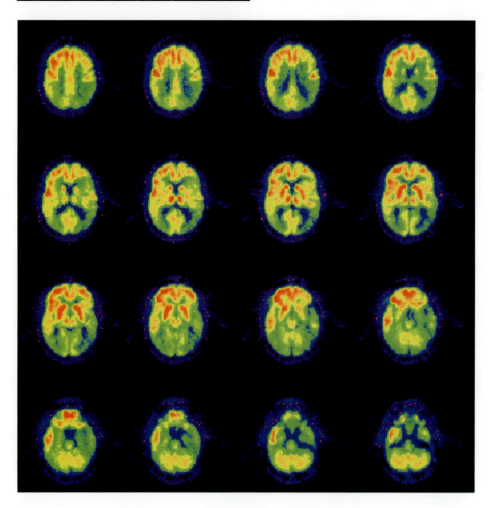

Transaxial

Multiple transverse FDG images of an elderly patient with decreasing cognitive function are shown. Images show metabolic reduction in the parietotemporal association cortices and frontal association cortex that is similar to a metabolic pattern of Alzheimer's disease. Cerebral hemispheres are involved bilaterally, but some asymmetry in the severity of hemispheric involvement is often seen (in this case more severe on the patient's left than right). In addition to the above findings, metabolic reduction involving the occipital cortex is frequently observed in Lewy body disease. Although the pathophysiology of occipital reduction is unknown, such findings may serve as a diagnostic discriminator for Lewy body disease. In both Alzheimer's disease and Lewy body disease, metabolic activity in the primary sensorimotor cortex and subcortical structures (thalamus, striatum and cerebellum) is relatively preserved.

Case 12.1.13: Multiple infarct dementia

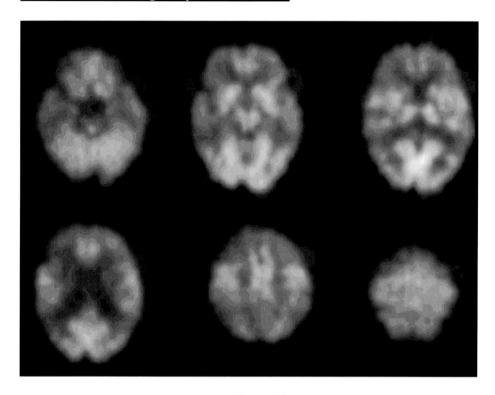

Transaxial

This 56 year old woman with recent difficulty with short-term memory was referred with a suspected clinical diagnosis of Alzheimer's type dementia. MRI had been reported as normal. The PET showed multiple cortical defects in both hemispheres, indicating multiple infarct dementia rather than Alzheimer's disease to be the aetiology of dementia.

Case 12.1.14: HIV encephalopathy

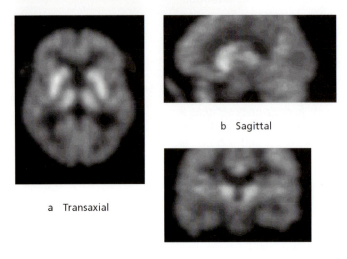

a Transaxial

b Sagittal

c Coronal

This shows the typical pattern of HIV encephalopathy, with reduced uptake in the cortex relative to basal ganglia and thalami.

> Abnormal appearances may be seen in HIV patients without clinical evidence of dementia.

Case 12.1.15

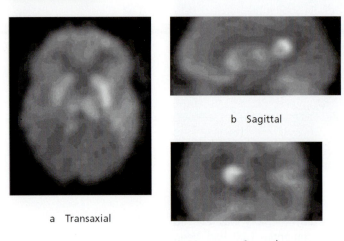

a Transaxial

b Sagittal

c Coronal

This patient demonstrated the classical features of HIV encephalopathy but in addition a focus of intensely increased uptake of FDG was seen posterior to the thalamus deep in the right parietal lobe due to lymphoma.

> FDG-PET will usually differentiate focal malignancy from focal infection in HIV patients.

Key issue 3 Differentiation from pseudodementia/depression

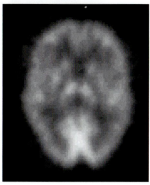

a   Transaxial

b   Sagittal

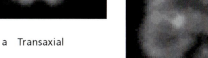

c   Coronal

This scan was performed on a 66 year old man with intractable depression and cognitive impairment. It showed a normal distribution of FDG, except for mild increase in basal ganglia compared with the cortex possibly due to phenothiazine treatment but no evidence of an Alzheimer's type dementia.

Conclusions

CURRENT CLINICAL INDICATIONS

1   Early symptoms when MRI normal

2   Parkinson's disease with dementia

3   HIV with dementia

4   Differential diagnosis when MRI is equivocal

5   Differentiating severe depression with dementia features

2 Epilepsy

Introduction and background

Epilepsy is a common condition: approximately 1 in 40 of the population will have a fit sometime in their lifetime, and there is about 1 : 200 prevalence in the population. Over the last 10 years imaging studies have generated a mass of important data increasing our understanding of the causes, pathophysiology and the treatment of this condition. MRI forms the mainstay of imaging for epilepsy, and increasingly functional MRI and MRS is playing a role. It is in the area of potentially surgically treatable partial epilepsy that PET studies have an important role. MRI will have excluded treatable mass lesions and identified the common causes of partial epilepsy: hippocampal sclerosis and malformations of cortical development, vascular malformations and acquired cortical damage. There remains a group of patients (10–40%, depending on the sophistication of the MRI techniques) where the imaging is either normal, equivocal or discrepant in lateralization with the EEG findings. It is these patients who will benefit from PET studies. An epileptogenic focus studied interictally is an area of decreased flow and decreased metabolism. These areas will usually be larger than the pathological abnormality, probably due to deafferentation of surrounding tissue which may include the ipsilateral thalamus and frontal lobes. [^{11}C]flumazenil scans may provide a more accurate delineation of the focus. Ictal scans result in increased metabolism and flow but are usually only found by accident on PET scans as PET imaging is not inherently suitable for performing ictal studies. Ictal studies often overrepresent the area of the epileptogenic focus, owing to propagation of the seizure.

Key management issues

PET in epilepsy

PET is used in both temporal and frontal lobe epilepsy.

TEMPORAL AND FRONTAL LOBE EPILEPSY

Temporal lobe epilepsy	Frontal lobe epilepsy
Hypometabolic foci in 60–90%	Hypometabolic foci in 50–60%
Hypometabolic focus larger than pathological lesion	Hypometabolic focus usually larger than lesion
Quantification is more accurate than visualization	90% with hypometabolism have MRI abnormality
No extra information when MRI definite	Useful especially when MRI normal or equivocal
Extent and severity of hypometabolism correlates with a good surgical outcome	

There are many forms of complex paediatric seizure syndromes; often they are resistant to medical therapy and being considered for surgery. PET findings may assist surgical assessment, including assessment of functional integrity of normal brain. These syndromes often show normal MRI findings, and may have single or multiple hypometabolic foci.

PAEDIATRIC SYNDROMES

West's syndrome

Lennox–Gastaut syndrome

Infantile spasms

Landau–Kleffner syndrome

Rasmussen's syndrome

Examples to illustrate key issues

Key issue 1

Cases 12.2.1–12.2.8 illustrate temporal lobe epilepsy; Cases 12.2.9–12.2.11 illustrate extra-temporal lobe epilepsy.

Case 12.2.1: Temporal lobe epilepsy

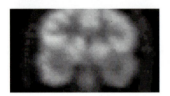

a   Coronal

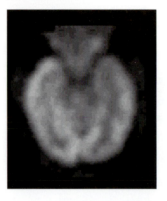

b   Transaxial

A 26 year old man with left mesial temporal hypometabolism.

Case 12.2.2

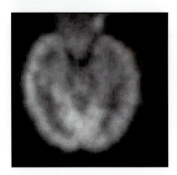

a   Transaxial

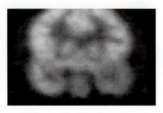

b   Coronal

This 27 year old man had complex partial seizures from the age of 20. He had an abnormal left temporal lobe on MRI and foramen ovale telemetry confirmed a left temporal origin for his seizures. PET showed left temporal hypometabolism through-out medial and lateral temporal lobe structures. He became seizure free after a left temporal lobectomy.

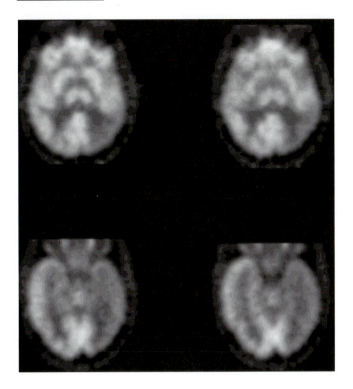

a   Transaxial

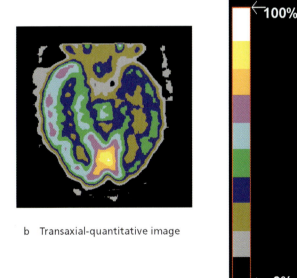

b   Transaxial-quantitative image

100%

0%

This 34 year old man developed epilepsy 3 years prior to PET scanning. MRI was normal, scalp EEG suggested a left temporal focus. Left temporal hypometabolism with adjacent parietal hypometabolism was seen with FDG, reflecting reduced metabolic activity within the temporal epileptic focus and the parietal association area. Colour scales may be used for semiquantification purposes: in this patient the left temporal lobe has 40% of the maximal FDG uptake, whereas uptake in the right temporal lobe is 60–70% of maximal.

The true focus is usually substantially smaller than the abnormality seen on both PET and MRI, indicating that the functional effects of the epileptic focus are diffuse.

Case 12.2.4

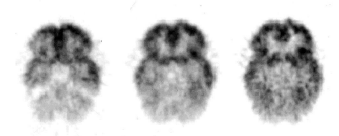

Transaxial

The scan in this patient showed mild right temporal hypometabolism and also moderately severe reduction of cerebellar activity. This is seen in up to a third of patients with medically refractory seizures and has been attributed to effects of repetitive generalized seizures or to prolonged exposure of high doses of anticonvulsants or both.

Cerebellar atrophy is observed by MRI and CT and at autopsy in many such cases, but hypometabolism may also be seen in patients who do not have evidence of structural atrophy.

Case 12.2.5

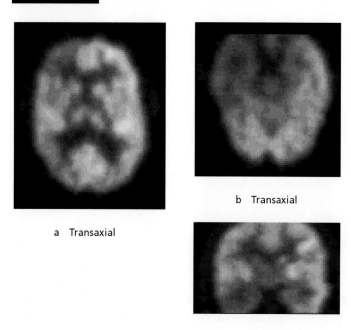

a Transaxial

b Transaxial

c Coronal

This patient had evidence of multifocal epilepsy with right frontal and temporal hypometabolism.

Case 12.2.6: Flumazenil

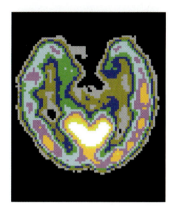

a [¹¹C]flumazenil

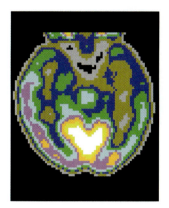

b FDG

Registered transaxial (temporal) slices

This 38 year old man was referred for PET scanning as part of a presurgical assessment. MRI suggested left mesial temporal sclerosis. Scalp EEGs showed bilateral discharges. PET was performed prior to foramen ovale telemetry. The FDG scan shows diffuse hypometabolism in the left medial and lateral temporal lobe and probable hypometabolism also in the right medial temporal lobe and tip. The [¹¹C]flumazenil scan shows a clear focus of reduced receptor density in the inferior portion of the left medial temporal lobe.

> [¹¹C]Flumazenil may be able to localize the epileptic focus more clearly than FDG as it relies on receptor density rather than glucose metabolism.

Case 12.2.7: Quantitation of metabolic changes seen in epilepsy

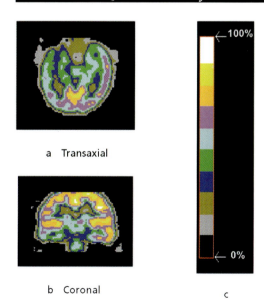

a Transaxial

b Coronal

c

This 37 year old patient had a right temporal focus for her epilepsy. There are various methods of quantitation; in this case a colour scale is used with colours chosen to represent a 10% change in counts. This can be useful as a crude method to provide asymmetry indices in disease.

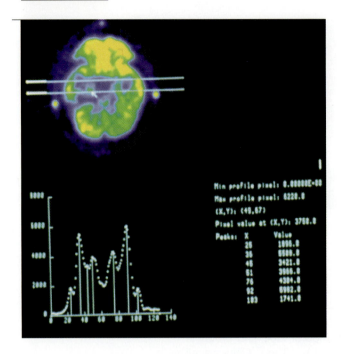

Transaxial image with line profile analysis

An alternative method of quantitation with a line profile drawn through slices within the temporal lobe to indicate asymmetry.

Case 12.2.9: Example of an occipital focus

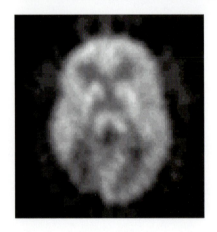

a   Transaxial

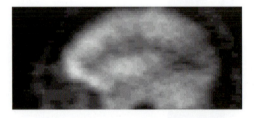

b   Coronal

This patient had complex partial seizures from the age of 3. At the time of investigation, he was 37 years of age. MR showed right occipital malformation with microgyria. Foramen ovale telemetry and scalp EEG monitoring, however, showed a bilateral synchronous onset of seizure activity. PET showed hypometabolism in the right occipital lobe. The site of seizure was subsequently confirmed with subdural telemetry and the patient underwent surgical resection with significant improvement in seizure frequency.

Case 12.2.10

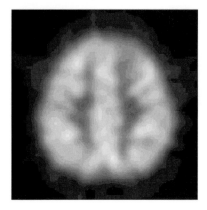

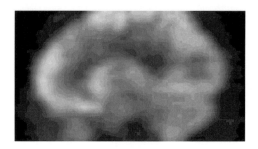

b   Sagittal

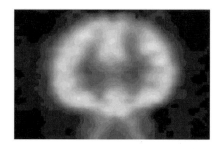

a   Transaxial

c   Coronal

This 14 year old girl with epilepsy had a normal MR and CT. Clinically and electrically, it was thought likely that the focus resided in the left temporal lobe. Left frontal hypometabolism on PET was identified and provided the impetus for further invasive investigation to confirm the focus site prior to surgery.

Case 12.2.11

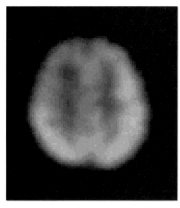

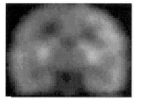

b   Coronal

a   Transaxial

This 15 month old child had intractable seizures since birth with developmental delay. The MRI was reported as normal. There were multifocal changes on surface EEG. The PET scan suggested a right frontal focus with evidence of hypometabolism. Subsequent reanalysis of the MRI raised the possibility of the presence of an abnormal right frontal gyrus. Surgery was performed and at 18 months after surgery the child remains seizure free.

Case 12.2.12: Dual pathology

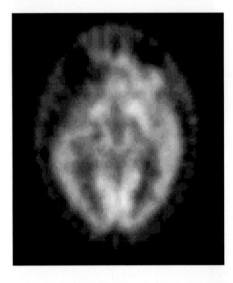

a

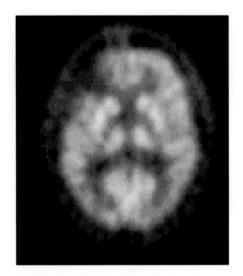

b

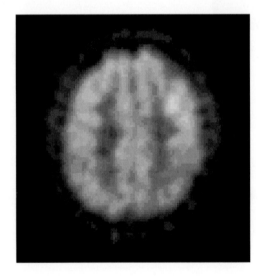

c

Transaxial slices inferior to posterior

This young patient with epilepsy and a history of a road traffic accident was investigated. The PET showed evidence of left frontal hypometabolism at the site of a frontal contusion seen on CT and MRI. There was also absent uptake within the right frontoparietal region on FDG-PET, possibly due to trauma but unusual for an epileptic focus.

When there is other organic pathology such as trauma the finding of hypometabolism may not indicate the site of the epileptogenic focus.

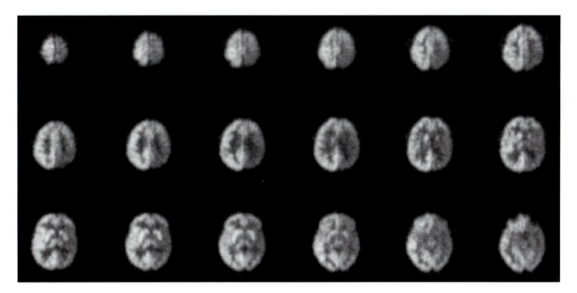

An 11 year old child had progressive right hemiparesis with diffuse changes on the MR in the left hemisphere, suggestive of a diagnosis of Rasmussen's syndrome. PET showed diffuse hypometabolism throughout the left hemisphere. The diagnosis of Rasmussen's disease was confirmed at surgery when hemispherectomy was performed.

Conclusions

CURRENT CLINICAL INDICATIONS

1 Doubt about diagnosis
2 Lateralization (localization)
3 Selection for surgery
4 Equivocal MRI

POSSIBLE INDICATIONS

1 Functional anatomy prior to surgery
2 Metabolic effects of drug treatment

3 Other neuropsychiatric applications

Cerebral infarct

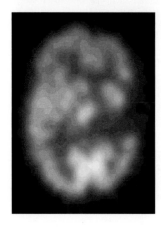

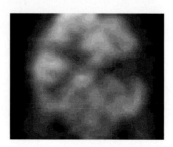

b   Coronal

a   Transaxial

This 7 year old child with intractable epilepsy was known to have intracerebral infarction in utero. The PET shows absent uptake in the left parietal hemisphere and reduced uptake in the left frontal lobe and left thalamus, secondary to infarction. There was no evidence of a separate epileptogenic focus.

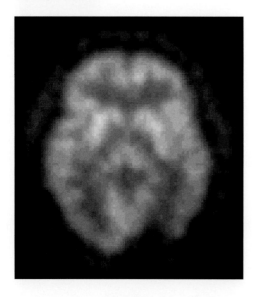

Transaxial

Absent uptake is seen within the left posterior cerebral artery territory in this 56 year old patient with a history of a cerebral infarct. On the right side focal uptake within the right frontal lobe is due to invagination of normal cortex.

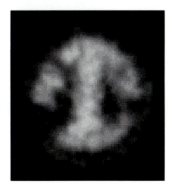
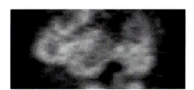
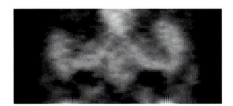

[¹⁵O] Water

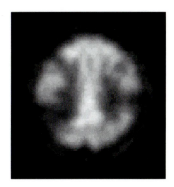
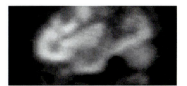
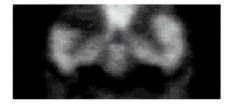

FDG

This 28 year old woman with Takayasu's disease had a history of multiple cerebral infarcts. The [¹⁵O]water and FDG scans both showed bilateral infarcts in the frontal lobes and parietal lobes. There was no alteration in distribution of the tracer on the water study with acetazolamide stress.

Perfusion and glucose metabolism are usually tightly coupled and clinically there are few circumstances in which both are required. One such circumstance would be for interventional studies.

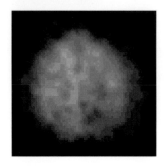
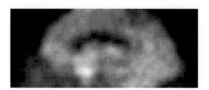

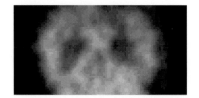

[^{15}O] Water

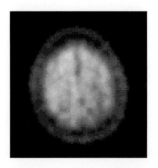
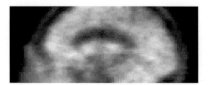

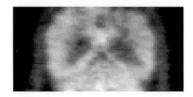

FDG

This 77 year old patient presented with a recent left parieto-occipital infarct. He had evidence of bilateral carotid artery stenoses on Doppler and angiography and was being considered for carotid surgery. PET was performed to see how extensively flow and metabolism had been affected in apparently 'unaffected' parts of the brain. There was no uptake of ^{15}O-labelled water within the area of infarct in the left parieto-occipital lobe, but the FDG uptake was relatively better, suggesting the presence of a resolving infarct. There was also evidence of some cerebral atrophy on the study, but none of cerebrovascular disease in other vascular territories.

Case 12.3.5

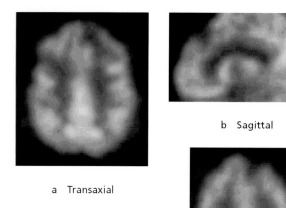

b   Sagittal

a   Transaxial

c   Coronal

This 36 year old woman with systemic lupus erythematosus and positive platelet anti-coagulant antibodies presented with malaise, headache and visual change. The PET scan was performed to assess whether this was a microvascular problem. There was no uptake of FDG within the right anterior parietal and left frontal lobes, indicative of multiple infarcts.

Neonatal encephalopathy

Case 12.3.6

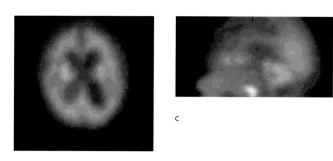

c

a

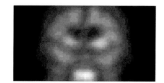

b

This 8 month old child with cortical atrophy and hydrocephalus secondary to neonatal hypoxia had evidence of reduced uptake of FDG within grey matter and features of hydrocephalus.

Moya Moya disease

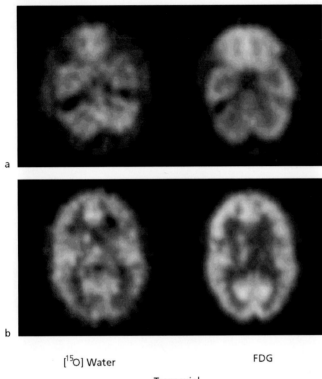

a

b

[^{15}O] Water   FDG

Transaxial

This 18 year old man presented with a right hemiparesis and fluctuating dysphasia. At cerebral angiography, the diagnosis of Moya Moya disease was made. MR had showed infarction in the left hemisphere only, but HMPAO-SPECT was reported as equivocal but with possible bilateral cortical defects. Prior to considering surgery, a PET scan was requested to determine whether there were bilateral defects in perfusion or metabolism. The [^{15}O]water (perfusion) and FDG scan showed absent uptake of tracer in the left thalamus, basal ganglia and internal capsule with evidence of crossed cerebellar diaschesis. In addition there was evidence of reduced perfusion in the left parietal cortex with normal FDG metabolism, suggestive of possible ischaemia rather than infarction at this site. There was no evidence of bilateral disease.

References and further reading

1 Dementia

Antonini A, Kazumata K, Feigin A *et al.* (1998) Differential diagnosis of parkinsonism with [18F]fluorodeoxyglucose and PET. *Movement Disorders* **13**(2), 268–74.

Burdette JH, Minoshima S, Vander Borght T *et al.* (1996) Alzheimer disease: improved visual interpretation of PET images by using three-dimensional stereotaxic surface projections. *Radiology* **198**(3), 837–43.

Imamura T, Ishii K, Sasaki M *et al.* (1997) Regional cerebral glucose metabolism in dementia with Lewy bodies and Alzheimer's disease: a comparative study using positron emission tomography. *Neurosci Letters* **235**(1), 49–52.

Mielke R, Kessler J, Szelies B *et al.* (1996) Vascular dementia: perfusional and metabolic disturbances and effects of therapy. *J Neur Trans Suppl* **47**, 183–91.

Reiman EM, Caselli RJ, Yun LS *et al.* (1996) Preclinical evidence of Alzheimer's disease in persons homozygous for the epsilon 4 allele for apolipoprotein E. *N E J Med* **334**(12), 752–8.

Rossor MN, Kennedy AM, Frackowiak RS (1996) Clinical and neuroimaging features of familial Alzheimer's disease. *Annals of the New York Academy of Sciences* **777**, 49–56.

Small GW, Leiter F (1998) Neuroimaging for the diagnosis of dementia. *J Clin Psychiatry* **59**(suppl 11), 4–7.

2 Epilepsy

Barrington SF, Koutroumanidis M, Agathonikou A *et al.* (1998) Clinical value of 'ictal' FDG-PET and the routine use of simultaneous scalp EEG studies in patients with intractable partial epilepsies. *Epilepsia* **39**(7), 753–66.

Cummings TJ, Chugani DC, Chugani HT (1995) Positron emission tomography in Pediatric Epilepsy. *Neurosurgery Clinics of North America* **6** (3), 465–72.

Duncan J (1997) Imaging and epilepsy. *Brain* **120**, 339–77.

Duncan JD, Moss SD, Bandy DJ *et al.* (1997) Use of positron emission tomography for presurgical localization of eloquent brain areas in children with seizures. *Pedr Neurosurg* **26**(3), 144–56.

Engel J Jr, Henry TR, Risinger MW, Sutherling WW, Chugani HT (1992) PET in relation to intracranial electrode evaluations. In: Theodore WH (ed.) Surgical treatment of epilepsy. *Epilepsy Research* (**suppl 5**), 111–20.

Ferrie CD, Maisey MN, Cox T *et al.* (1996) Focal abnormalities detected by [18]FDG positron emission tomography in children with epileptic encephalopathies. *Arch Dis Childh* **75**, 102–7.

Ferrie CD, Marsden PK, Maisey MN, Robinson RO (1997) Cortical and subcortical glucose metabolism in childhood epileptic encephalopathies. *J Neurol Neurosurg Psychiatr* **63**(2), 181–7.

Henry TR, Frey KA, Sackellares JC *et al.* (1993) In vivo cerebral metabolism and central benzodiazepine-receptor binding in temporal lobe epilepsy. *Neurology* **43**, 1998–2006.

Henry TR Functional imaging with positron emission tomography (1996) *Epilepsia* **37**(12), 1141–54.

Koutroumanidis M, Barrington S, Agathonikou A *et al.* (1998) Interictal regional slow activity in temporal lobe epilepsy correlates with lateral temporal hypometabolism as imaged with FDG-PET. Neurophysiologic and metabolic implications. *Journal of Neurology Neurosurgery and Psychiatry* **65**(2), 170–6.

Lamusuo S, Ruottinen HM, Knuuti J *et al.* (1997) Comparison of [18F]FDG-PET, [99mTc]-HMPAO-SPECT, and [123I]-iomazenil-SPECT in localising the epileptogenic cortex. *J Neurol Neurosurg Psychiat* **63**(6), 743–8.

Manno EM, Sperling MR, Ding X *et al.* (1994) Predictors of outcome after anterior temporal lobectomy: positron emission tomography. *Neurology* **44**, 2331–6.

Salanova V, Markand O, Worth R *et al.* (1998) FDG PET and MRI in temporal lobe epilepsy: relationship to febrile seizures, hippocampal sclerosis and outcome. *Acta Neurol Scand* **97**(3), 146–53.

Savic I, Thorell JO, Roland P (1995) 11C flumazenil positron emission tomography visualises frontal epileptogenic regions. *Epilepsia* **36**, 1225–32.

Savic I, Persson A, Roland P *et al.* (1988) In vivo demonstration of reduced benzodiazepine receptor binding in human epileptic foci. *Lancet* **2**, 863–6.

Spencer SS (1994) The relative contributions of MRI, SPECT and PET Imaging in Epilepsy *Epilepsia* **35**(suppl 6), S72–89.

3 Other neuropsychiatric applications

Baron JC (1996) Clinical use of positron emission tomography in cerebrovascular diseases. *Neurosurgery Clinics of North America* 7, 653–64.

DeReuck J, Leys D, De Keyser J (1997) Is positron emission tomography useful in stroke? *Acta Neurol Belg* **97**(3), 168–71

Chapter 13

Cardiology

Introduction and background

The frequency of coronary artery disease is increasing and it is becoming recognized also as a serious problem in women. Because of the scale of the problem and advancing sophistication of the technology available to treat the condition, coronary artery disease is placing rising demands on healthcare resources. Within the overall spectrum of coronary artery disease the patient with progressive failure of ventricular function poses particular problems and consumes an increasingly large proportion of healthcare costs devoted to cardiac disease. It also poses a challenge to diagnostic imaging with PET. The reason is that by careful selection, patients with impaired left ventricular function can gain functional improvement from revascularization, medical therapy or cardiac transplantation. It is now known that the most important determinant for functional recovery following revascularization of the failing heart is the amount of hibernating myocardium present; conversely, it appears that the amount of hibernating myocardium correlates inversely with prognosis. The importance of accurate selection for revascularization is emphasized by the high mortality and high costs associated with coronary by-pass grafting in this group of patients. Of the methods available for identifying hibernation which include ^{99m}Tc sestamibi SPECT flow studies, thallium rest/reinjection and stress echo, PET flow/metabolism studies are generally regarded as the gold standard.

Basic principles of biochemistry and physiology

SUBSTRATE METABOLISM
Fatty acid oxidation supplies >50% of myocardial fuel in fasting state
Postprandially, glucose and insulin increase GLUT4 transporter at myocardial surface and glucose oxidation increases to supply >50% of myocardial fuel
During severe exercise lactate oxidation increases and may supply >50% of myocardial fuel
Prolonged fasting may result in ketones providing significant fuel

With increasing ischaemia, glucose – first aerobic then anaerobic glycolysis – is increasingly the critical substrate. This is the basis of FDG as a PET metabolic tracer.

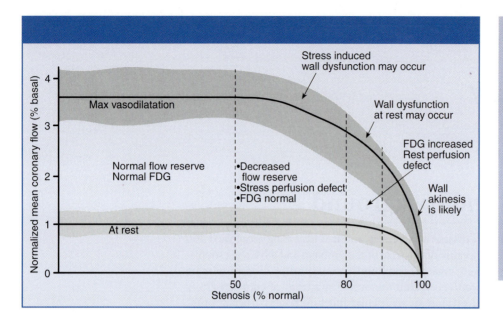

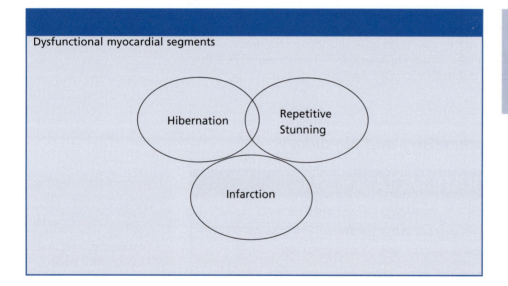

Dysfunctional myocardial segments

DEFINITIONS

Viable myocardium	Myocardium that has the ability or retains the potential to contract
Hibernating myocardium	Chronic reversible ischaemic dysfunction
Stunned myocardium	Acute reversible ischaemic dysfunction
Infarction/scar	Irreversible myocardial damage unable to contract

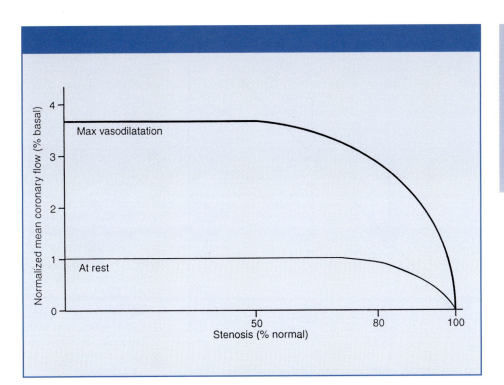

As the coronary flow decreases at stress and then rest, the myocardial contractility decreases until it ceases, when there is hibernation at low flow rates. At this point there is increasing relative FDG accumulation, indicating ischaemia and viability.

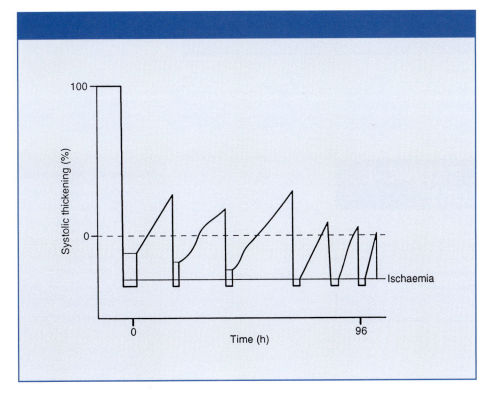

A single ischaemic event will impair myocardial contractility for a finite time before recovering. If this is repeated often enough, time for full recovery will be insufficient, and contractility will be continuously impaired – this is the effect of repetitive stunning.

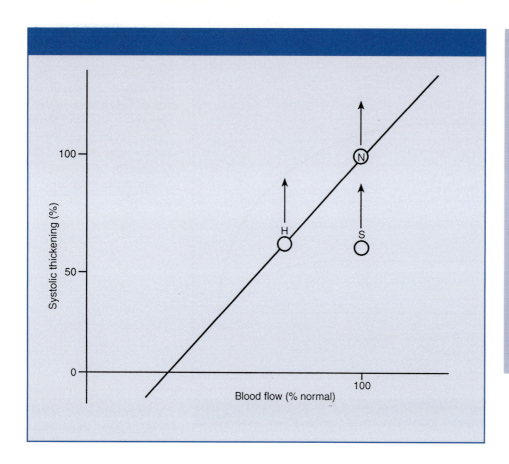

The likely relationships between hibernation, stunning and repetitive stunning are shown here. As resting blood flow falls, systolic thickening decreases until contraction ceases altogether. When stunning is repeated, full functional recovery may never take place between episodes and may be indistinguishable from hibernation although the resting blood flow may be higher. In practice it is likely that hibernation, normal, repetitively stunned and infarcted myocardial tissue will all coexist in any patient or segment of myocardium.

PET studies

PET TRACERS FOR CLINICAL CARDIOLOGY	
[18N]Ammonia	Flow
[15O]Water	
82Rb	
18FDG	Metabolism
[11C]acetate	

In perfusion studies the most widely used tracer is $^{13}NH_3$, but where a cyclotron is not available ^{82}Rb is the tracer of choice. ^{15}O-labelled water is theoretically ideal with 100% myocardial extraction but more difficult to use. ^{18}FDG is the metabolic tracer most commonly used, and can be delivered to sites without a cyclotron. ^{11}C-acetate has theoretic advantages but is not widely applied.

CHOICE OF 'STRESS'

Dipyridamole (Persantin)

Adenosine

Dobutamine

Nitrates

Pharmacological coronary vasodilatation has to be used in place of exercise because of the short half lives of the tracers used. Adenosine or dipyridamole are the vasodilators of choice for PET perfusion studies.
Dobutamine can be used in the presence of respiratory contraindications.
Nitrates are increasingly being used, but their place is yet to be established.'

PATIENT PREPARATION

Avoid caffeine-containing compounds

Glucose loading

Glucose and variable insulin doses

Euglycaemic insulin clamps

Fatty acid lowering regimes

Avoidance of all forms of caffeine is critical when dipyridamole or adenosine is used as a coronary vasodilator. Control of substrate availability is important for metabolic imaging because of the multiple sources of energy which can be utilized by cardiac muscles.

Key management issues

The use of PET in cardiology usually follows a SPECT study: the increased accuracy of PET may be helpful in diagnosis of CAD when other tests remain equivocal, in the presence of obesity and if balanced triple vessel disease is suspected. The most important role for PET is for assessing the potential for functional myocardial recovery with revascularization in high risk patients. A metabolic PET study is the 'gold standard' for myocardial viability when hibernation is suspected.

Monitoring the effect of therapy is of increasing importance particularly for aggressive medical regimes to lower lipid levels. In cardiac centres with high volumes ^{82}Rb-PET may be cost competitive with SPECT and is somewhat more accurate.

Normal appearances

Normal flow and metabolism are shown in these images, which illustrate a normal study from apex to base with rest ammonia (perfusion) and stress ammonia (perfusion) and FDG (metabolism).

Transaxial slices

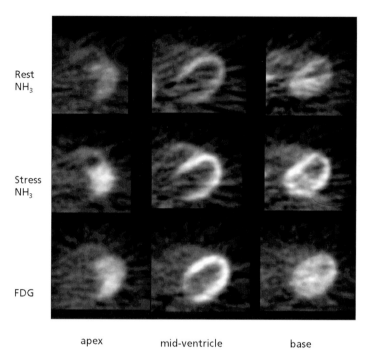

Rest
NH$_3$

Stress
NH$_3$

FDG

apex   mid-ventricle   base

Three representative transaxial slices

Short axis slices

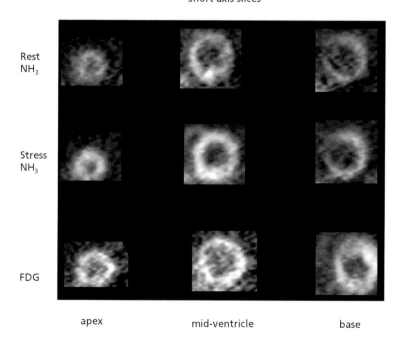

Rest
NH$_3$

Stress
NH$_3$

FDG

apex   mid-ventricle   base

Three representative short axis slices

Examples to illustrate key issues

Key issue 1 Diagnosis of coronary artery disease

Case 13.1

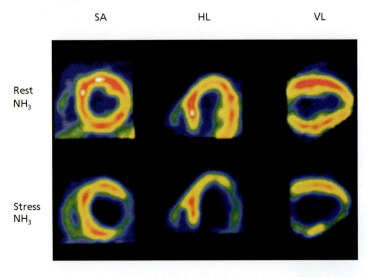

SA   HL   VL

Rest NH₃

Stress NH₃

In a patient with suspected coronary artery disease, slices are shown in three orthogonal planes of consecutive rest and stress perfusion scans, using ^{13}N-labelled ammonia. Inferolateral ischaemia (decreased coronary flow reserve) is demonstrated, confirming a diagnosis of coronary artery disease.

Case 13.2

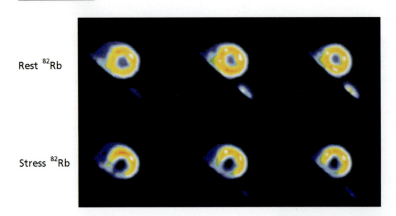

Rest ^{82}Rb

Stress ^{82}Rb

Short axis slices are shown in a patient with suspected coronary artery disease imaged with ^{82}Rb at rest and with dipyridamole stress which confirm a diagnosis of coronary artery disease with inferior ischaemia.

Key issue 2 Functional significance of coronary lesions

Case 13.3

Rest
NH₃

Stress
NH₃

FDG

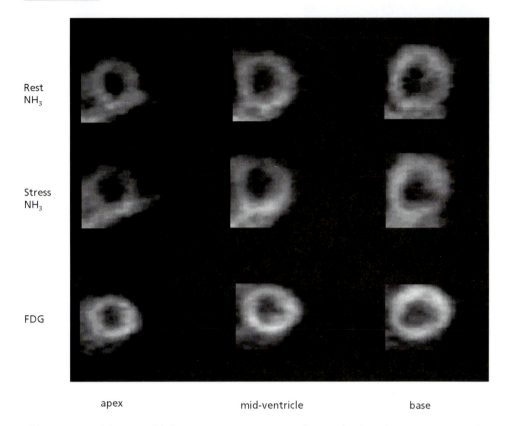

apex   mid-ventricle   base

This 59 year old man with known coronary artery disease had undergone two previous bypass operations. Repeat angiography demonstrated an occluded graft to the LAD. The PET scan was requested to determine whether angioplasty was worth attempting, if viable myocardium could be demonstrated in the LAD territory. The short axis slices demonstrate a reversible perfusion defect in the anterior wall of the left ventricle, extending into the septum and lateral wall indicative of reversible myocardial ischaemia in the LAD territory with good uptake of FDG globally. The patient proceeded to angiography.

> Where reversible ischaemia is demonstrated, the FDG usually has no added value. In order to have efficient scheduling, however, most patients will need to undergo ammonia and FDG scans at the same sitting and it is rarely possible to reconstruct the ammonia scans prior to deciding whether to proceed to FDG scanning.

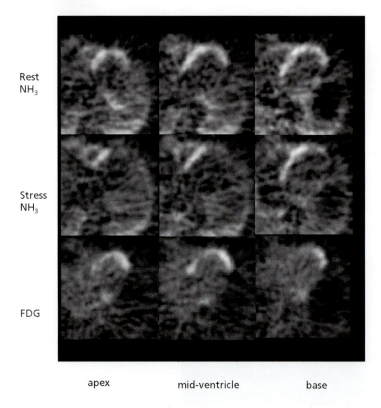

Rest
NH₃

Stress
NH₃

FDG

apex   mid-ventricle   base

This 59 year old patient with known coronary artery disease had undergone quadruple coronary bypass surgery in 1980. He developed limiting angina and breathlessness in 1991. Angiography showed an ectatic right coronary artery graft with a 60% stenosis in the native right coronary artery distally, occluded left main stem, occluded left anterior descending and two marginal grafts. Sestamibi scanning had demonstrated fixed anterior, lateral and inferior defects. Before considering repeat bypass surgery, a PET scan was performed to determine the extent of any reversible ischaemia present. Reversible ischaemia was demonstrated in the anterior wall on the rest/stress ammonia images with a fixed defect in the lateral wall which had no uptake of FDG within it indicating a true lateral myocardial infarction.

> In patients with very dilated left ventricles and large areas of myocardium which are not perfused, positioning the patient may be difficult and it may be impossible to fit the whole myocardium into the field of view. Re-alignment to produce short axis images may be misleading and viewing of the transaxial slices may be important for image interpretation.

Key issue 3 Selection of poor risk patients for revascularization

Case 13.5

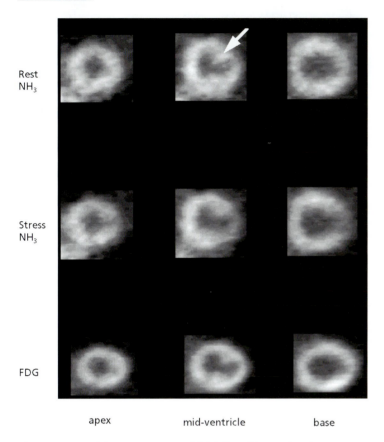

Rest NH$_3$

Stress NH$_3$

FDG

apex   mid-ventricle   base

This 65 year old man presented initially with angina in 1992. He underwent angioplasty to the circumflex artery with a good result. In 1993 his angina returned. Angiography demonstrated that the angioplasty site was still patent but there was a new stenosis within the obtuse marginal. Exercise ECG had demonstrated borderline inferolateral ST depression. The ^{99m}Tc-sestamibi scan was equivocal, with an inferolateral defect which was reported as likely to be fixed. The functional significance of the obtuse marginal stenosis was therefore in doubt and a PET scan was requested. The presence of reversible lateral ischaemia and normal uptake of FDG globally (seen on these short axis slices) indicated that the obtuse marginal lesion was functionally significant and the patient proceeded to further angioplasty.

> Uptake of ammonia and FDG is well demonstrated in this patient within the
> papillary muscle (arrowed).

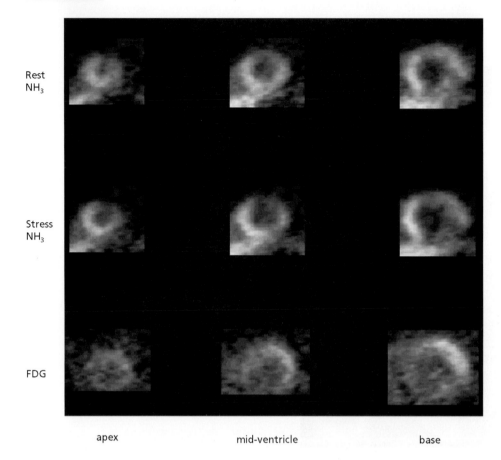

Rest
NH₃

Stress
NH₃

FDG

apex   mid-ventricle   base

This 46 year old man had undergone two previous myocardial infarctions with significant damage to the left ventricle, his ejection fraction measuring less than 30%. The thallium scan had demonstrated fixed defects only and a PET was performed to determine whether there was significant ischaemia or hibernating myocardium which would warrant revascularization. The ammonia rest and stress perfusion images demonstrated the presence of reversible ischaemia in the anterolateral wall and a small fixed anterior defect. Relatively greater uptake of FDG is seen within the area corresponding to the fixed defect on ammonia, indicating that it is viable. Relatively less uptake of FDG is seen within normal tissue in the septum. This does not indicate that the septum is non-viable, but rather that this area is metabolizing glucose at a lower rate than the ischaemic areas.

Rest
NH₃

FDG

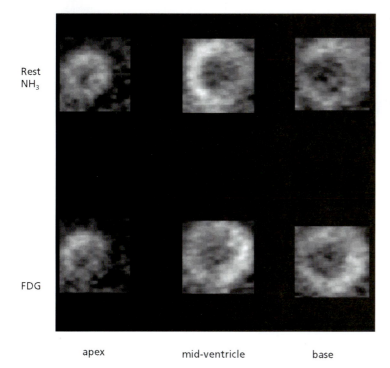

apex   mid-ventricle   base

This 50 year old man with diabetes and poor left ventricular function secondary to ischaemic heart disease underwent thallium scanning. The thallium scan demonstrated a large fixed defect in the lateral wall. PET scan was performed to determine whether this area contained viable myocardium. Increased uptake of FDG within the lateral wall is seen indicating the presence of viable myocardium and the potential for revascularization.

> Although in this patient there was reduced uptake of ammonia at rest indicating rest ischaemia, some patients with hibernating myocardium may have resting flows within the normal range.

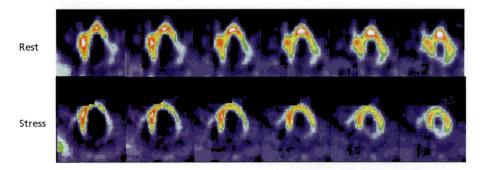

Rest

Stress

a   Sestamibi scan

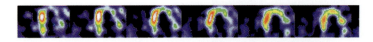

b   24 h rest redistribution thallium scan

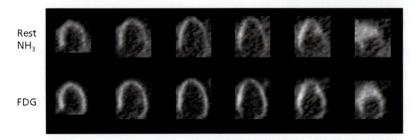

Rest
NH₃

FDG

c   PET scan

This 35 year old man with an ejection fraction of 25% was assessed for the presence of hibernating myocardium prior to revascularization. Rest/stress sestamibi indicated a fixed defect in the lateral wall of the left ventricle (seen best on the horizontal long axial images shown here) with a small area of reversible ischaemia at the apex. Twenty-four hour redistribution thallium showed uptake of less than 30% of peak uptake within the lateral wall. There was, however, significant uptake of FDG within the lateral wall which was ischaemic at rest on ammonia, indicating the potential for revascularization.

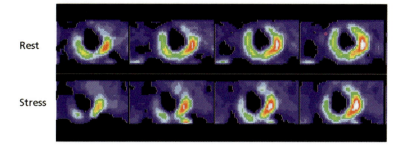

Rest

Stress

a   Sestamibi scan

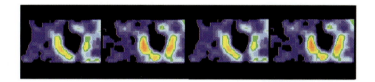

b   24h rest redistribution scan (thallium)

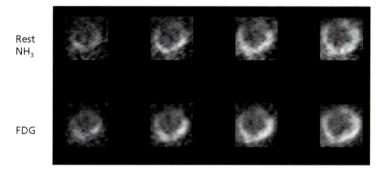

Rest NH₃

FDG

c   PET scan

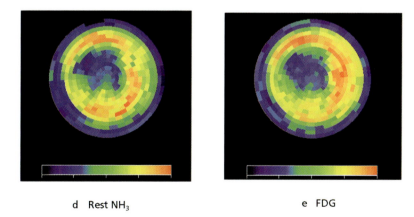

d   Rest NH₃

e   FDG

Polar maps

This 50 year old man with known coronary artery disease was assessed for revascu-larization. In this case, a large fixed defect was seen in the anterior wall on the rest/stress sestamibi scan, with only a small area of reversible ischaemia in the septum. There was no uptake of thallium in the anterior wall on 24 hour redistribution scan-ning. No uptake of ammonia nor FDG was seen within the anterior wall on PET, indica-tive of a true anterior infarction. The use of polar maps can be helpful to determine whether there is extensive hibernation, although the extent of viable myocardium and the degree of FDG uptake that is required to make revascularization worthwhile is uncertain. In this case the small area of reversible ischaemia in the septum compared with the extensive anterior infarction was thought insufficient to make revascularization worthwhile.

Case 13.10

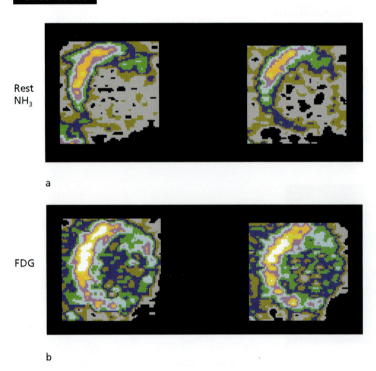

Rest
NH₃

a

FDG

b

This 71 year old man had a blocked right coronary artery and diffuse disease within the left anterior descending artery at catheterization, with inferior hypokinesia and a measured ejection fraction of 20% on echocardiography. The resting ammonia indicated that the anterior wall and septum were well perfused. Resting ischaemia was demonstrated within the inferior and the lateral walls, but there was uptake of FDG within this area, indicating potential for revascularization.

Rest
NH₃

FDG

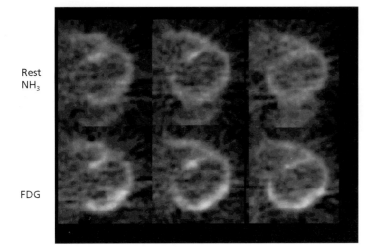

This patient with an ischaemic cardiomyopathy and ejection fraction of 20% had previously undergone bypass surgery and had re-presented with breathlessness. The Dobutamine echo had indicated widespread reversible dysfunction, but only patchy fixed perfusion defects were seen on sestamibi scanning. The ammonia scan indicated globally low flow, with FDG uptake throughout the myocardium. Relatively greater uptake of FDG was seen within the inferolateral wall. One explanation for the heterogeneity of FDG uptake is that the diffuse uptake of FDG within an area of low flow indicated true hibernation and the relatively greater uptake of FDG within the inferolateral wall indicated an area of the myocardium subject to repetitive stunning rather than hibernation.

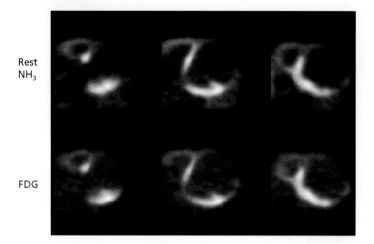

Rest
NH₃

FDG

This 59 year old woman had an anteroseptal myocardial infarction in 1991. She was re-admitted on three occasions over the ensuing two years with worsening pulmonary oedema. Coronary angiography indicated gross left ventricular dilatation with aneurysm formation, an occluded right coronary artery and left anterior descending artery, with mitral regurgitation secondary to dilatation and an ejection fraction of less than 30%. The sestamibi scan showed a fixed anteroapical defect. PET was performed to determine whether there was any significant area of hibernation that might warrant revascularization. The PET showed absent uptake of ammonia at rest, indicating resting ischaemia in the anterior and lateral wall with matched absent FDG uptake, indicating no significant area of hibernation. The patient did not proceed to revascularization.

Key issue 4 Evaluation before cardiac transplantation

Case 13.13

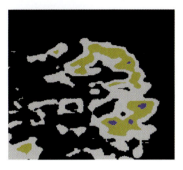

a   Rest NH$_3$

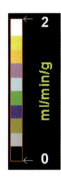

c

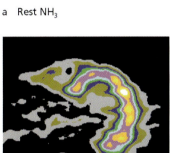

b   Stress NH$_3$

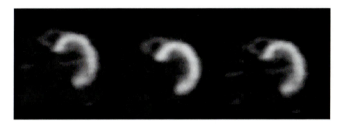

d   Rest NH$_3$ Stress NH$_3$ FDG

PET may be used to differentiate ischaemic from non-ischaemic cardiomyopathy to determine whether revascularization is worth attempting rather than bypass surgery. This 65 year old woman with a viral cardiomyopathy had uniform uptake of ammonia at rest. The calculated average perfusion in the transaxial image, as shown, was 0.6 ml min^{-1} g^{-1} myocardial tissue. After dipyridamole stress, this increased to 1.4 ml min^{-1} g^{-1} myocardial tissue. The rise in perfusion was global rather than focal as would be expected in non-ischaemic cardiomyopathy. The FDG uptake was also uniform throughout the myocardium.

> The typical appearances for a non-ischaemic dilated cardiomyopathy are uniform perfusion, normal coronary flow reserve and matching glucose metabolism.

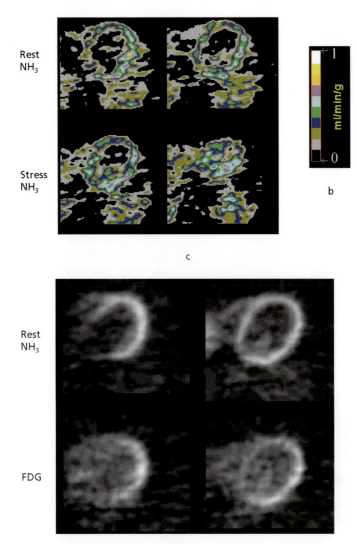

a

Rest
NH₃

Stress
NH₃

ml/min/g

b

c

Rest
NH₃

FDG

This 53 year old diabetic with left ventricular failure and an ejection fraction of 20% underwent PET scanning. Normal resting perfusion was demonstrated with an average uptake in the myocardium of $0.6\,\mathrm{ml\,min^{-1}\,g^{-1}}$ tissue. Uniform high FDG uptake is seen within the myocardium, suggesting the presence of a microvascular cardiomyopathy in a diabetic patient rather than ischaemic cardiomyopathy which might warrant revascularization.

Diabetic with glucose
loading

Diabetic with glucose
loading and insulin

Non-diabetic with
glucose loading

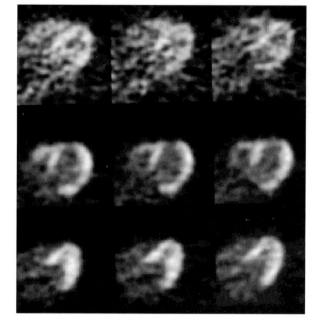

This shows transaxial slices of FDG scans performed on three patients. The top row of images are taken from a patient who was a diabetic given 25 g of glucose prior to the FDG study. The images are of poor quality, with low uptake of FDG into the myocardium and high background. The middle row of images demonstrates how intravenous injection of insulin, given according to a sliding scale, prior to administration of FDG in a glucose loaded diabetic patient improved image quality with uptake of FDG in the myocardium, comparable to that obtained in a non-diabetic patient (bottom row). This improvement in image quality was obtained without the need for a formal glucose clamp which is labour intensive for clinical studies.

Rest
NH₃

FDG

This 44 year old man with recurrent myocardial infarction had undergone successful angioplasty to the right coronary artery, but diffuse disease within the left anterior descending and circumflex arteries was not suitable for angioplasty. The siting of grafts on to the distal portion of these vessels was also likely to be problematic. The patient had therefore been accepted for cardiac transplantation. He then developed recurrent ventricular fibrillation and in view of the anticipated time for a transplant to become available, the patient was referred for PET scanning. If significant areas of hibernation were seen on PET, surgery would be attempted. The PET scan demonstrated resting ischaemia in the anterior wall, but showed good uptake of FDG globally, suggesting that there was potential for revascularization.

Emerging applications

Gated FDG scans

The following two cases illustrate gated scanning with FDG. Although in its infancy, gated FDG has the potential to give combined information about wall motion and glucose metabolism within areas of dysfuctional myocardium.

Case 13.17

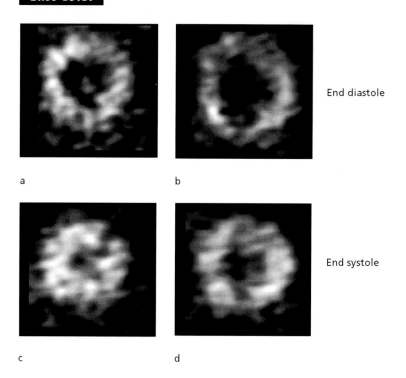

a

b

End diastole

c

d

End systole

This is an example of a normal gated cardiac scan in a 47 year old woman.

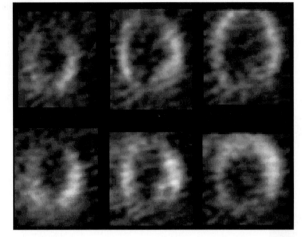

End diastole

End systole

The gated FDG scan within this 53 year old woman with an occluded left anterior descending artery and distal thrombus in the right coronary artery showed a true anteroapical infarct with no significant motion of the anteroapical wall and no uptake of FDG within it. Normal thickening of the lateral wall and septum were seen.

Paediatric studies

Case 13.19

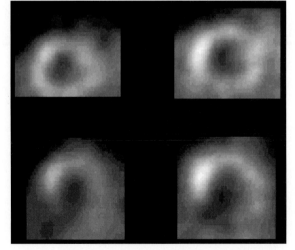

Rest NH$_3$

Stress NH$_3$

This 1 year old child with Kawasaki's disease had a suspected inferior infarction. If there was evidence of ischaemia on PET scanning, the plan was to proceed to catheterization. There was reduced uptake within the region of the inferior wall at rest, which is more extensive on stress indicating inferior ischaemia. Resting flow within the lateral wall was measured at 1 ml min^{-1} g^{-1} tissue, with no significant increase on stress, indicating impaired coronary reserve in the circumflex territory in addition.

Conclusions

CURRENT CLINICAL INDICATIONS (IN ORDER OF IMPORTANCE)

1 Assessing myocardial viability

2 Confirming myocardial ischaemia

3 Pretransplant assessment

4 Diagnosis of cardiomyopathy

POSSIBLE INDICATIONS

1 Quantitative monitoring of perfusion with lipid lowering regimes

2 Gated FDG scans

Further reading

Anonymous (1996) [Indications for clinical applications of positron emission tomography in cardiology. Position report of the PET Cardiology Study Group of the German Society of Nuclear Medicine and the Nuclear Cardiology Study Circle of the German Society of Cardiology]. *Zeitschrift fur Kardiologie* **85**(7), 453–68.

Bax JJ, Visser FC, van Lingen A, Cornel JH, Fioretti PM *et al.* (1997) Metabolic imaging using F18-fluorodeoxyglucose to assess myocardial viability. *International Journal of Cardiac Imaging* **13**, 145–55; discussion 157–6.

Beanlands RS, deKemp RA, Smith S *et al.* (1997) F-18-fluorodeoxyglucose PET imaging alters clinical decision making in patients with impaired ventricular function. *Am J Cardiol* **79**(8), 1092–5.

Beller GA (1996) Assessment of myocardial perfusion and metabolism for assessment of myocardial viability. *Qu J Nucl Med* **40**(1), 55–67.

Bonow RO (1995) The hibernating myocardium: implications for management of congestive heart failure. *Am J Cardiol* **75**(3), 17A–25A.

Depre C, Vanoverschelde JL, Gerber B, Borgers M, Melin JA, Dion R (1997) Correlation of functional recovery with myocardial blood flow, glucose uptake, and morphologic features in patients with chronic left ventricular ischemic dysfunction undergoing coronary artery bypass grafting. *Journal of Thoracic & Cardiovascular Surgery* **113**, 371–8.

Di Carli MF, Asgarzadie FM, Schebert HR *et al.* (1995) Quantitative relation between myocardial viability and improvement in heart failure symptoms after revascularisation in patients with ischaemic cardiomyopathy. *Circulation* **92**(12), 3436–44.

Fath-Ordoubadi F, Pagano D, Marinho NV *et al.* (1998) Coronary revascularization in the treatment of moderate and severe postischemic left ventricular dysfunction. *American Journal of Cardiology* **82**, 26–31.

Flameng WJ, Shivalkar B, Spiessens B, Maes A, Nuyts J, VanHaecke J *et al.* (1997) PET scan predicts recovery of left ventricular function after coronary artery bypass operation. *Annals of Thoracic Surgery* **64**, 1694–1701.

Haas F, Haehnel CJ, Picker W, Nekolla S, Martinoff S, Meisner H *et al.* (1997) Preoperative positron emission tomographic viability assessment and perioperative and postoperative risk in patients with advanced ischemic heart disease. *Journal of the American College of Cardiology* **30**, 1693–1700.

Lewis P, Nunan T, Dynes A, Maisey MN (1996) The use of intravenous low dose intravenous insulin in clinical myocardial F-18 FDG PET scanning. *Clin Nucl Med* **21**(1), 15–18.

Maddahi J, Schelbert H, Brunken R *et al.* (1994) Role of thallium-201 and PET imaging in evaluation of myocardial viability and management of patients with coronary artery disease and left ventricular dysfunction. *J Nucl Med* **35**, 707–15.

Pagano D, Townend JN, Littler WA, Horton R, Camici PG, Bonser RS (1998) Coronary artery bypass surgery as treatment for ischemic heart failure: the predictive value of viability assessment with quantitative positron emission tomography for symptomatic and functional outcome. *Journal of Thoracic & Cardiovascular Surgery* 115, 791–9.

Patterson RE, Rilcher WC (1995) Assessing myocardial viability to help select patients for revascularisation to improve left ventricular dysfunction due to coronary artery disease. *Sem Thorac Cardiovasc Surg* 7(4), 214–26.

Sand NP, Bottcher M, Madsen MM *et al.* (1998) Evaluation of regional myocardial perfusion in patients with severe left ventricular dysfunction: comparison of 13N-ammonia PET and 99mTc sestamibi SPECT. *J Nucl Cardiol* 5(1), 4–13.

Schelbert HR (1998) The usefulness of positron emission tomography. *Curr Probl Cardiol* 23(2), 69–120.

Tamaki N, Kawamoto M, Tadamura E *et al.* (1995) Predication of reversible ischaemia after revascularisation. Perfusion and metabolic studies with PET. *Circulation* 91(6), 1697–705.

Chapter 14

Problems and variants

Introduction

Because glucose acts as the basic energy substrate for so many tissues, variations in distribution of FDG can cause considerable difficulties in interpretation of clinical PET scans. Probably the most difficult thing to learn when first starting the interpretation of whole body FDG scans is to appreciate the normal variation which can occur: even experienced observers are continually learning. Perhaps the greatest cause for problematic interpretation is caused by increased glucose metabolism in different muscle groups which for a variety of reasons are under tension and hence have increased metabolism. In this chapter we have attempted to document as many of the important variations which can cause problems in interpretation as possible. It is not intended to be a totally comprehensive account, but should provide a helpful guide to those new to the field and prevent unnecessary false positive interpretations with their potential for inappropriate management.

SOME POTENTIAL PITFALLS IN SCAN INTERPRETATION
1 Muscle effects including stress
2 Tonsillar and thymic uptake in children and young adults
3 Laryngeal uptake
4 Caecum, bowel and stomach uptake
5 'Physiological' renal and urinary tract activity
6 Ovarian follicles and fibroid uterus
7 Inflammatory joint disease
8 Attenuation artefacts, e.g. pleural or lesion size/shape
9 Injection site and lymph nodes proximal to injection

Case studies

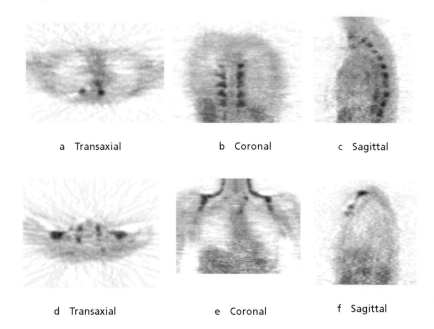

a Transaxial   b Coronal   c Sagittal

d Transaxial   e Coronal   f Sagittal

Increased uptake of FDG due to muscle tension in typical sites: the thoracic paraspinal region (a–c) and cervical region (d–f).

> Oral administration of diazepam may reduce or abolish increased FDG uptake due to muscle tension which may mask sites of true disease.

Case 14.2

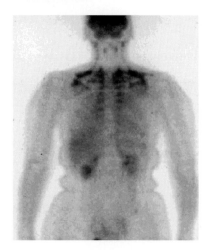

Coronal

From G Cook, I Fogelman, MN Maisey. Seminars in Nuclear Medicine 1996; 26(4), 308–14, Fig. 3. Reproduced with permission.

Increased FDG uptake in the cervical and thoracic paraspinal regions due to muscle tension.

Case 14.3

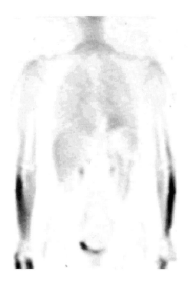

Coronal

From G Cook, I Fogelman, MN Maisey. Seminars in Nuclear Medicine 1996; 26(4), 308–14, Fig. 1. Reproduced with permission.

Increased uptake of FDG within the forearm muscles in a patient using crutches.

Case 14.4

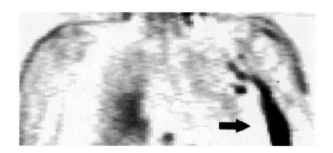

Coronal

Uptake of FDG within the biceps muscle in a patient with a known left biceps muscle tendon rupture.

Case 14.5

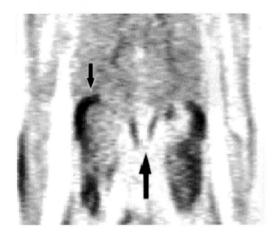

Coronal

From G Cook, I Fogelman, MN Maisey. Seminars in Nuclear Medicine 1996; 26(4), 308–14, Fig. 4. Reproduced with permission.

Increased uptake of FDG within the crura and diaphragmatic musculature in a patient due to hyperventilation.

Case 14.6

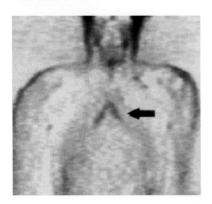

Coronal

From G Cook, I Fogelman, MN Maisey. Seminars in Nuclear Medicine 1996; 26(4), 308–14, Fig. 9. Reproduced with permission.

Normal thymic uptake in a teenager.

Case 14.7

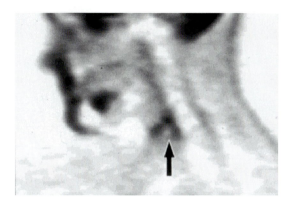

Sagittal

*From G Cook, I Fogelman, MN Maisey. Seminars in Nuclear Medicine 1996; **26**(4), 308–14, Fig. 2. Reproduced with permission.*

Laryngeal uptake.

Case 14.8

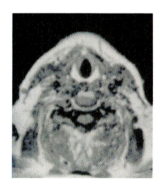

a

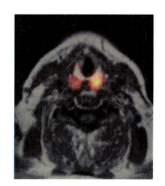

b

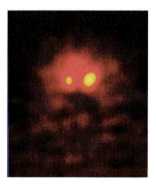

c

*From L Kostagoglu, JCH Wong, SF Barrington, BF Cronin, AM Dynes, MN Maisey. Journal of Nuclear Medicine 1996; **37**(11), p. 1772, Fig. 1A–C. Reproduced with permission.*

Increased uptake of FDG is seen within the posterior cricoarytenoid muscles which occurs during speech. Individuals vary in the site of maximal uptake of FDG within individual muscles of phonation.

Case 14.9

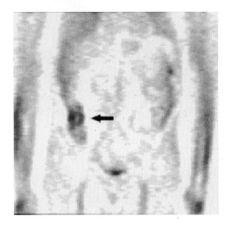

Coronal

From G Cook, I Fogelman, MN Maisey. Seminars in Nuclear Medicine *1996; 26(4), 308–14, Fig. 6.*
Reproduced with permission.

Normal FDG uptake within the region of the caecum.

Case 14.10

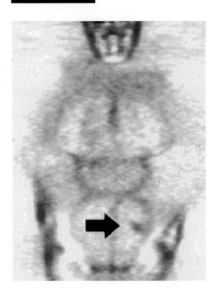

Coronal

From G Cook, I Fogelman, MN Maisey. Seminars in Nuclear Medicine *1996; 26(4), 308–14, Fig. 7.*
Reproduced with permission.

Uptake of FDG at the site of a stoma.

Case 14.11

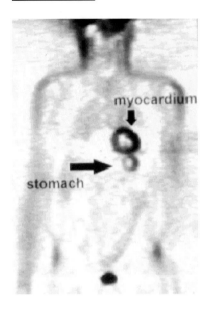

Coronal

From G Cook, I Fogelman, MN Maisey. Seminars in Nuclear Medicine 1996; 26(4), 308–14, Fig. 5A. Reproduced with permission.

High uptake of FDG within normal stomach.

Case 14.12

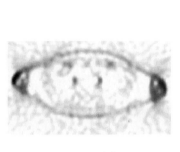

a Transaxial

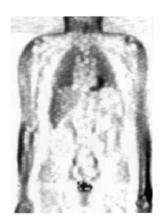

b Coronal

From G Cook, I Fogelman, MN Maisey. Seminars in Nuclear Medicine 1996; 26(4), 308–14, Fig. 8. Reproduced with permission.

Ureteric activity simulating para-aortic lymphadenopathy

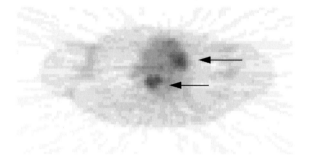

Transaxial

Uptake of FDG in a horseshoe kidney.

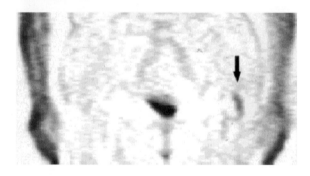

Coronal

Uptake of FDG within a trochanteric bursitis.

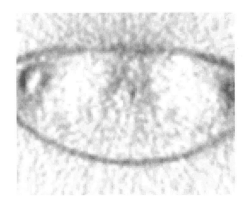

a   Transaxial

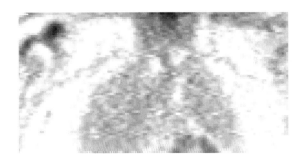

b   Coronal

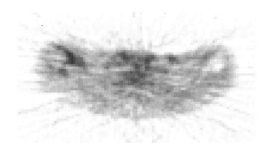

a   Transaxial

b   Coronal

Two examples of increased uptake of FDG in patients with capsulitis of the shoulder.

Case 14.17

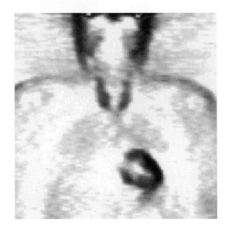

Coronal

From G Cook, I Fogelman, MN Maisey. Seminars in Nuclear Medicine *1996; 26(4), 308–14, Fig. 11. Reproduced with permission.*

Increased uptake of FDG within the thyroid gland attributed to Graves' disease.

Case 14.18

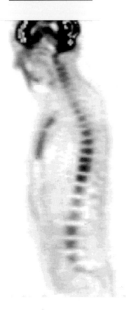

Coronal

From G Cook, I Fogelman, MN Maisey. Seminars in Nuclear Medicine *1996; 26(4), 308–14, Fig. 10. Reproduced with permission.*

Increased uptake of FDG in hyperplastic bone marrow after chemotherapy.

Case 14.19

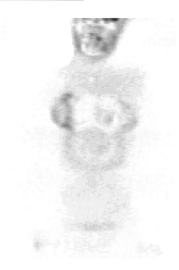

Coronal

Increased uptake of FDG within the right breast from which the patient breastfed prior to scanning.

Case 14.20

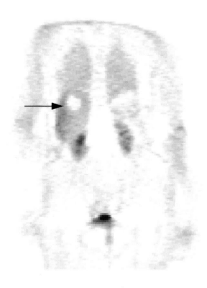

Coronal

Photopenic lesion representing a benign liver cyst.

Further reading

Barrington SF, Maisey MN (1996) Skeletal muscle uptake of F-18 FDG: effect of oral diazepam. *J Nucl Med* **37**, 1127–9.

Cook G, Fogelman I, Maisey MN (1996) Normal physiology and benign pathological variants in [18]FDG PET scanning: potential for error in interpretation. *Semin Nucl Med* **26**(4), 308–14.

Gordon BA, Flanagan FL, Dehdashti F (1997) Whole-body positron emission tomography: normal variations, pitfalls, and technical considerations. *A J Roentgen* **169**(9), 1675–80.

Kostagoglu L, Wong JCH, Barrington SF *et al.* (1996) Speech related visualisation of laryngeal muscles with F-18 FDG. *J Nucl Med* **37**, 1771–3.

Shreve PD, Anzai Y, Wahl RL (1999) Pitfalls in oncologic diagnosis with FDG PET imaging: physiologic and benign variants. *Radiographics* **19**, 61–77.

Index

Page numbers printed in **bold** type refer to figures; those in *italic* to tables. Page numbers preceded by an asterisk (*) denote case examples.

laboratories, radiochemistry 4
LAL (limulus amebocyte lysate) test 8
Landau–Kleffner syndrome 285
large cell lung cancer 75
larynx *331
Lennox–Gastaut syndrome 285
Lewy body disease 272, *280–1
  imaging findings 273
limulus amebocyte lysate (LAL) test 8
liver
  benign cyst *337
  see also hepatoma
liver metastases, in colorectal cancer 153,
  *154–5, *159
LSO (lutetium oxyorthosilicate) 10
lumped constant 15
lung cancer 75–103
  adenosarcoma 75, *89
  adrenal metastases 89
  background 75
  bronchioalveolar, false negative scans 78
  case examples *81–101
  diagnosis of a lung mass *81–4
  epidemiology 75
  FDG-SPECT imaging *98–100
  further reading 102–3
  indications, current 102
  indications, possible 102
  key management issues 78
  large cell 75
  metastatic sites 77
  monitoring therapy *97
  non-small cell 75
  non-small cell, staging *85–93, **102**
  pathology 75
  PET in 78
  pleural disease assessment *100–1
  prognosis 76
  recurrence, distant *96
  recurrence, local *94–5
  small cell 75
  spread, local 77
  spread to mediastinum 76
  squamous 75, *85, *89, *98, *100
  staging 76
  whole body staging 78
lung mass, diagnosis *81–4
lungs, lymph node drainage 77
lutetium oxyorthosilicate (LSO) 10
lymph nodes
  breast cancer metastatic sites 105
  enlarged *73, *88
  malignant melanoma 168
lymphadenopathy, generalized, mimicking
  lymphoma 73
lymphoma 51–74
  abdominal 61
  background 51
  Burkitt's lymphoma, treatment
    monitoring *61
  case examples *54–73
  cutaneous 67

differential diagnosis *69–73
FDG uptake into bone marrow 55, 58, 59
further reading 74
incidence 51
indications, current 74
indications, possible 74
intracerebral, differential diagnosis 70
key management issues 53
PET in 53
recurrence detection *64
systemic symptoms 51
see also Hodgkin's disease (HD); non-
  Hodgkin's lymphoma (NHL)

magnetic resonance imaging (MRI) 37
  after gadolinium contrast 142
malignancy of unknown origin 247–8
  case example *248
  current status of PET 247
  further reading 254
malignant melanoma 162–75
  abdominal, and computed tomography
    173
  acral lentiginous 163
  background 162
  case examples *167–73
  epidemiology 162
  further reading 174–5
  indications, current 174
  indications, possible 174
  key management issues 166
  lentigo 163
  lymph nodes 168
  metastatic melanoma, management
    algorithm **174**
  metastatic sites 164
  nodal spread from intermediate thickness
    lesions *168–9
  pathology 163
  PET in 166
  prognosis 163
  recurrence confirmation *170–2
  risk factors 162
  spread, risk of **165**
  staging 164
  staging thick melanomas at presentation
    *167
  surveillance *173
  whole body imaging 166
mammography
  assessment difficulties following surgery
    120
  conditions of technical difficulty 111
mediastinal masses, after lymphoma
  treatment *64–5
mediastinum
  enlarged lymph nodes *88
  false positive FDG uptake 78
  lung cancer spread to 76
  staging 78
melanoma *see* malignant melanoma
meningiomas 179, *187

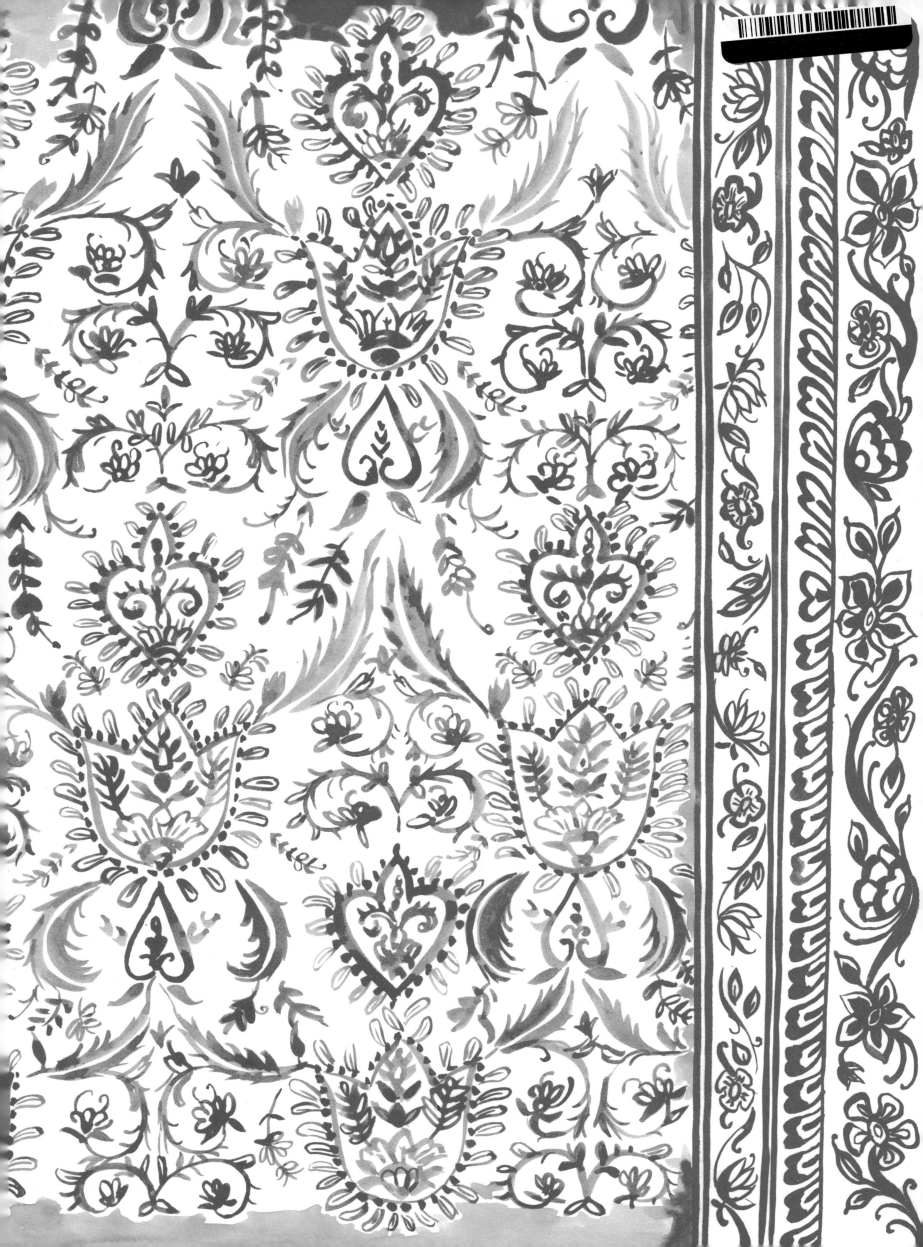

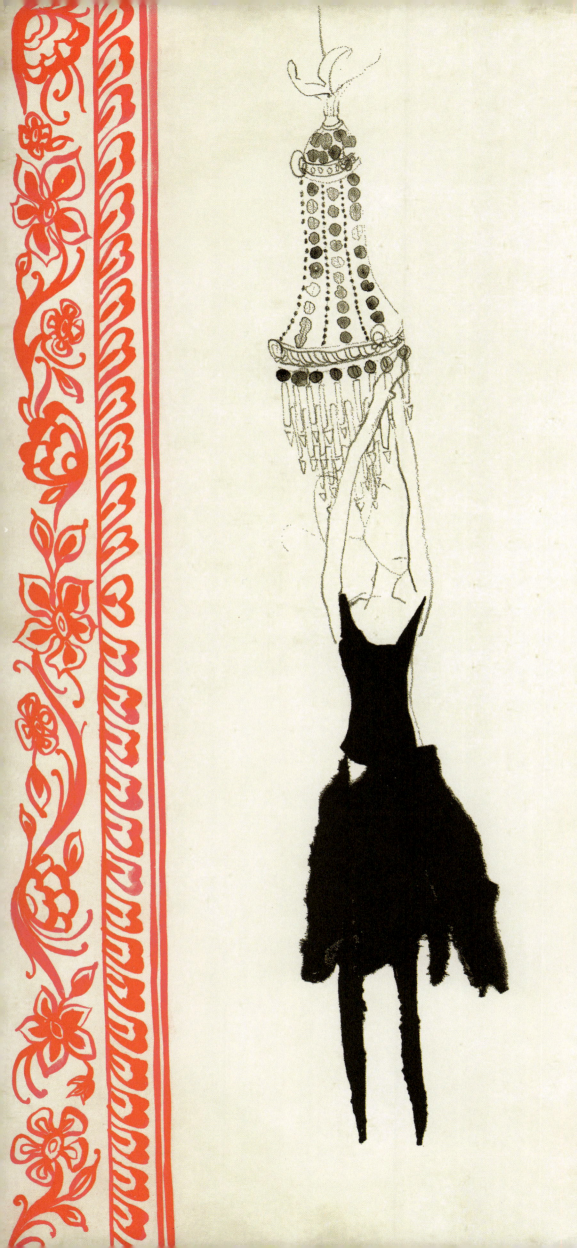
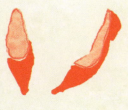

You can do anything if you have enthusiasm.   Enthusiasm
is the yeast that makes your hope rise to the stars.
Enthusiasm is the sparkle in your eye, it is the swing
in your gait, the grip of your hand, the irresistible
surge of your will and your energy to execute your ideas.
Enthusiasts are fighters.   They have fortitude, they
have staying qualities.   Enthusiasm is at the bottom
of all progress.   With it there is accomplishment.
Without it there are only alibis.

Henry Ford's Fireplace Motto.

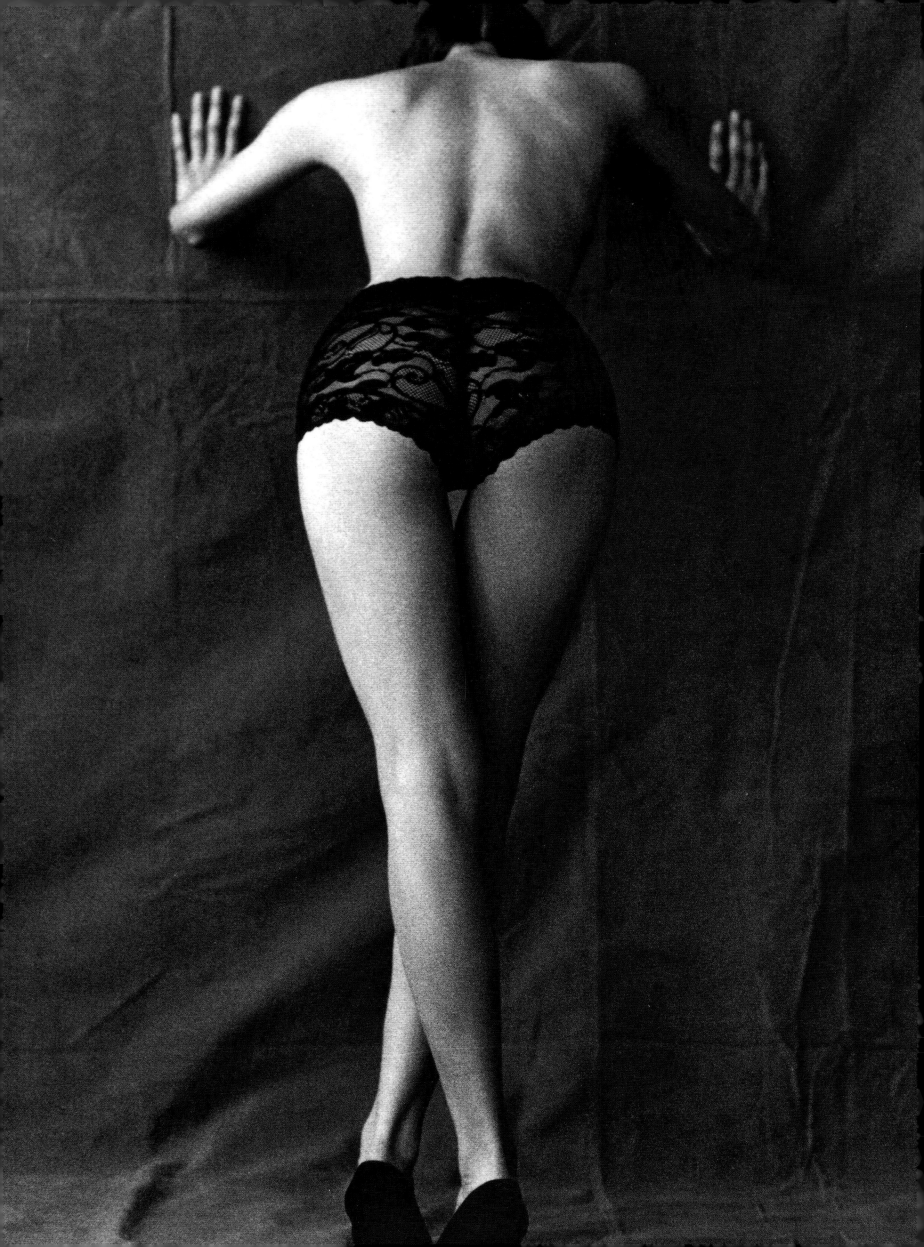

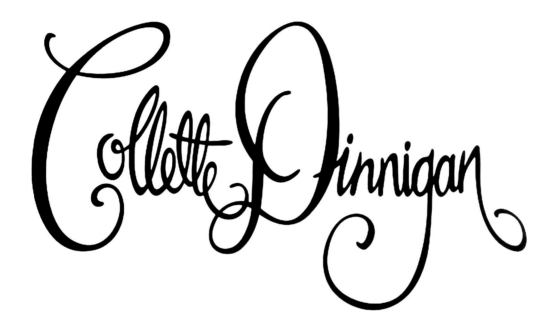

OBSESSIVE
CREATIVE

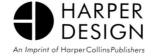

HARPER
DESIGN

An Imprint of HarperCollins Publishers

CONTENTS

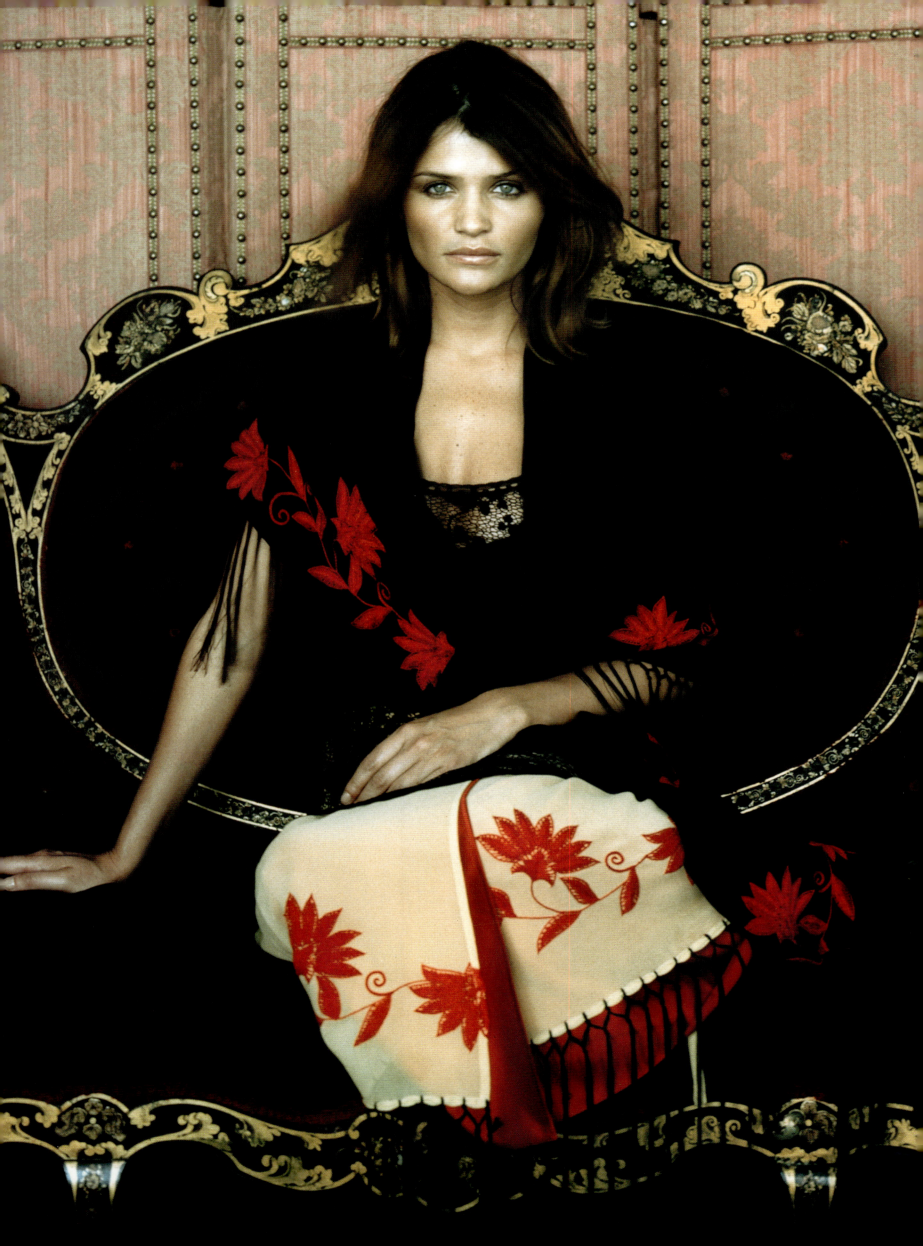

Foreword
by Helena Christensen

I first met Collette in a hotel bar in Sydney on a warm, breezy summer night about twenty years ago. She looked like someone who had stepped out of a movie from another era. Her demeanour was elegant and graceful, and her delicate features were beautifully framed by a mane of long, wild, blonde hair. She was wearing a dress with lovely lace trimmings and shiny beads that flickered in the candlelight. There was a calm, mellow vibe about her and I remember looking from across the bar and thinking, 'Wow, that girl is so incredibly gorgeous and ethereal-looking'.

Earlier that day, as I was walking around Sydney, browsing through all the exciting, sophisticated stores, I had come upon one with particularly pretty dresses. When I found out later that this vision in the bar was the woman who had created those dresses, it did not surprise me at all. Without even knowing Collette, I could sense that her designs were an extension and reflection of not only her personality and style, but also her soul and spirit. You just knew immediately that those dresses had this woman breathing through every little intricate detail.

There are many designers who make beautiful clothes, but it is very rare to come across one who so embodies every piece she designs. Someone whose spirit is embedded in every thread, every fibre of the fabric. When you wear one of Collette's dresses, you wear part of her life, her story. And you feel lucky to be part of that story. You look at her designs and touch the delicate materials, and you just know that this woman has a magical life full of wonderful dreams and adventures. All you have to do is slip into one of her dresses and you feel magical yourself.

After I got to know Collette, I learnt that my first instincts about her and her designs had been accurate. She is as elegant and beautiful as her dresses, a free-spirited soul, an interesting, fun, creative and very dedicated woman, and, more than anything, she is hugely inspiring in so many ways.

Collette and I became friends, and, when I moved to Paris to work as a model, she was one of the first people I did shows for. I would walk up and down the runway in her beautiful creations and feel like a fairy princess dancing in the mist on a dark lake in the middle of the forest. That's how wearing her pieces makes you feel. Over the years we have collaborated in so many ways. There were all the magnificent shows in Paris, and the exciting photo shoots, where I would play out silent stories in her long, flowing gowns or sexy little dresses. When Collette designed a lingerie collection, I flew to Sydney to photograph the line.

The first time I visited Collette's home, I was delighted to discover how beautifully she had put it together. Every room was full of curious objects, interesting little details and wonderful flower arrangements. There was so much attention and love in every room – yet it all looked so effortless.

Her talent is so real and honest. She is exactly what she creates and surrounds herself with. I treasure every piece I own from this lovely and inspiring woman. They are pieces that will be passed on to the young girls in my family. I want them to feel the same joy and pride I feel when I float elegantly through an exquisite ballroom, a lush, scent-filled garden or along a busy city street on my way to dinner with my beloved.

Opposite: Helena Christensen, 1998.

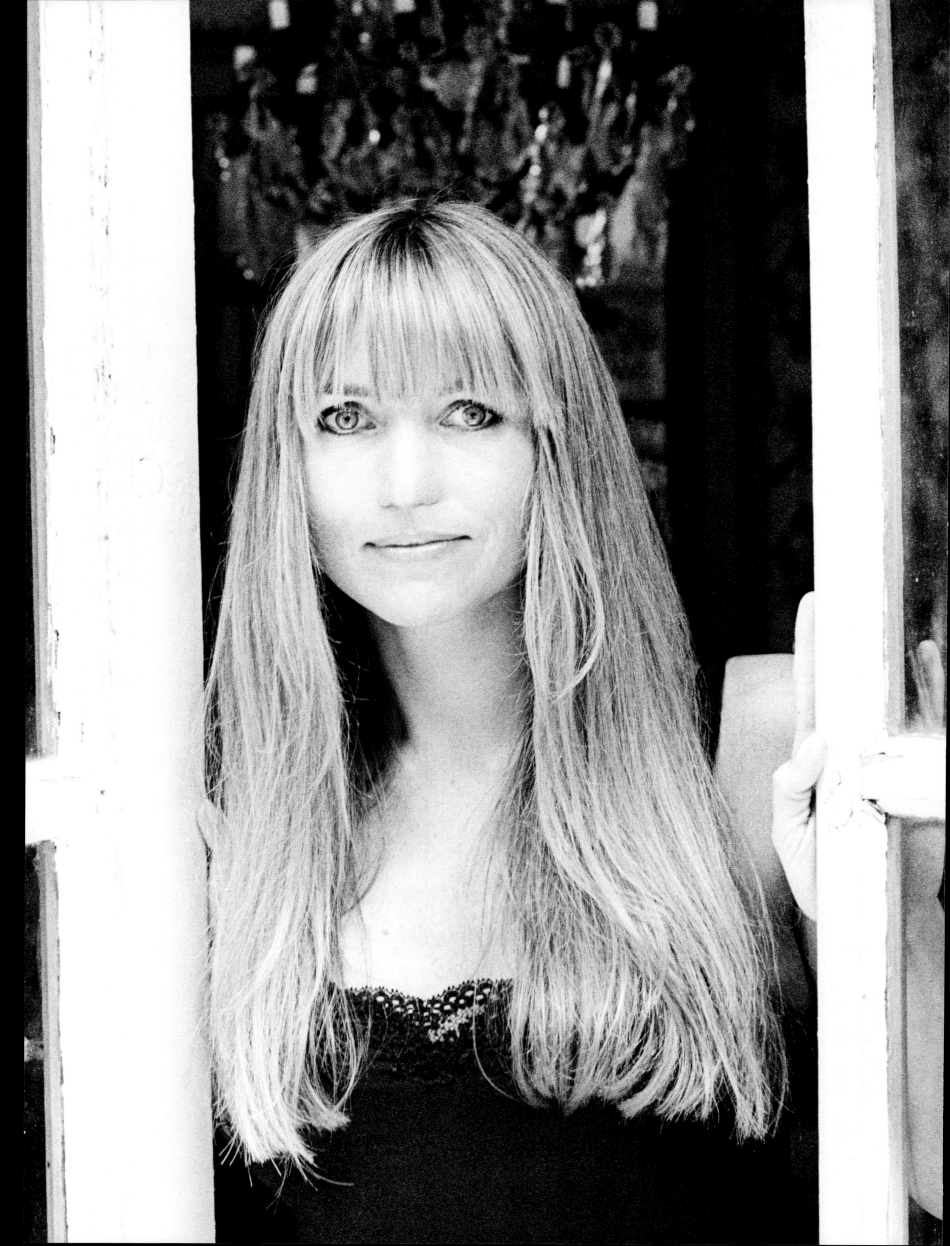

Introduction

When I started this book I wasn't sure where it would take me. I knew that it would be, in essence, a journey through my career and personal life. And I really wanted to share the tale of my nomadic, bohemian parents because it is just such a great story.

When I read through it all again now, as I write this, I can see that what I have really done is to map out the roots and foundation of my career. This book is about my first collaborations; it's about my lingerie, where I started my design journey, and it's about my early travels as part of an incredible family, across wild seas in extreme situations.

I think it shows how all of these things helped to shape my character and my design eye. From both a creative and a personal perspective, it's a good map of much of my life. And when you peel back the layers of any life, you see the richness, the hopes, the dreams, the failures, the successes and you realise that, for all of us, anything is possible.

Opposite: Photograph by Ellen von Unwerth, 2004.

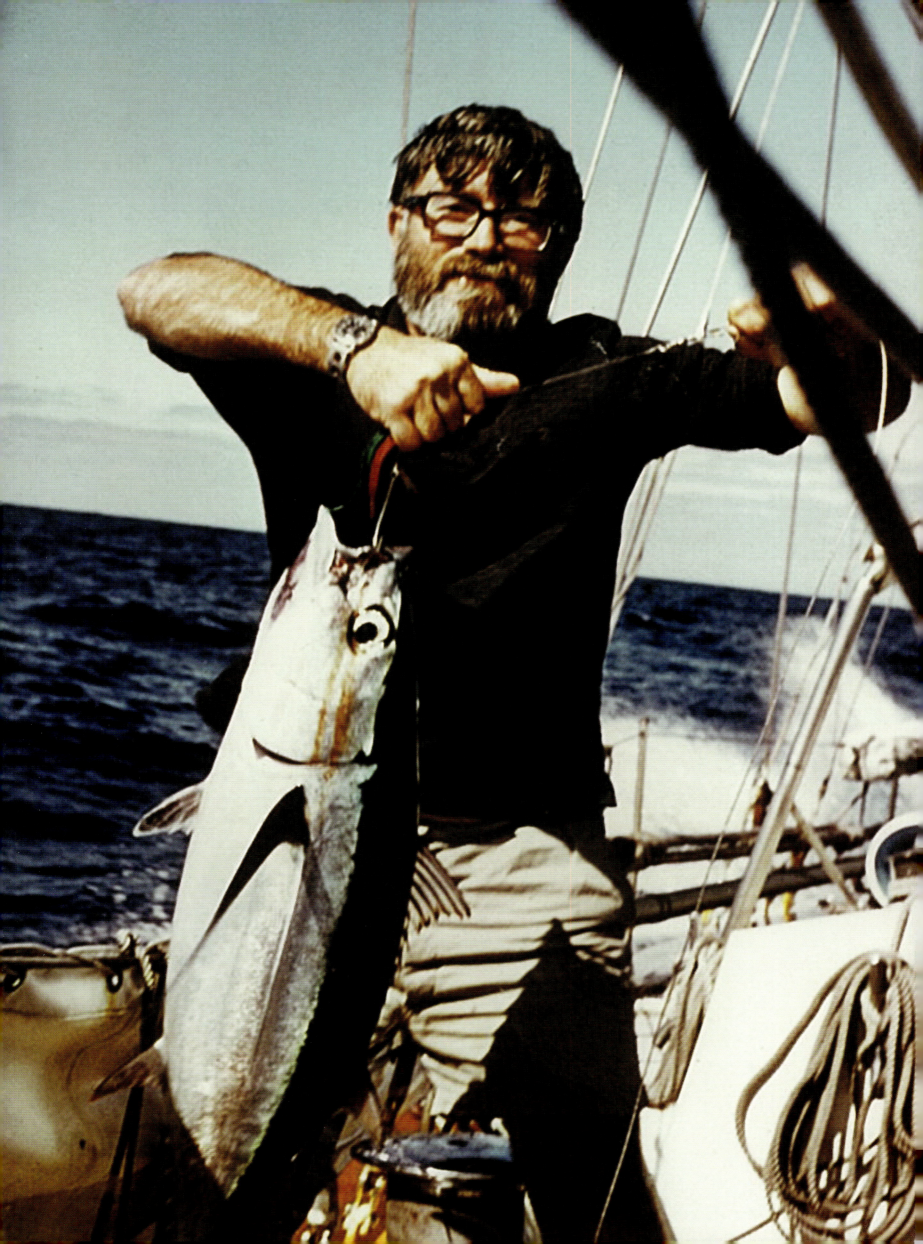

KNOW YOUR DNA

Greetings from South Africa
and New Zealand;
my dad, the last pirate;
making the tree
grow stronger.

MY CHILDHOOD

CHAPTER 1

MY IRISH FATHER, DES,
MET MY SOUTH AFRICAN
MOTHER, SHEILA,
IN THE 1960S.
Dad was an adventurer,
who had sailed the high seas for years,
CIRCUMNAVIGATING THE
WORLD THREE TIMES
(my husband Bradley calls him 'the last pirate').
ONE DAY DAD SAILED
INTO DURBAN AND MET MUM
AT A PARTY ON A YACHT
AT THE POINT YACHT CLUB.
Not long after, they married and
set up home in South Africa where
DAD GOT A JOB AS
AN ENGINEER,
working in a refinery.
I WAS BORN IN 1965
AND MY BROTHER, SEAMUS,
WAS BORN FOURTEEN
MONTHS LATER.

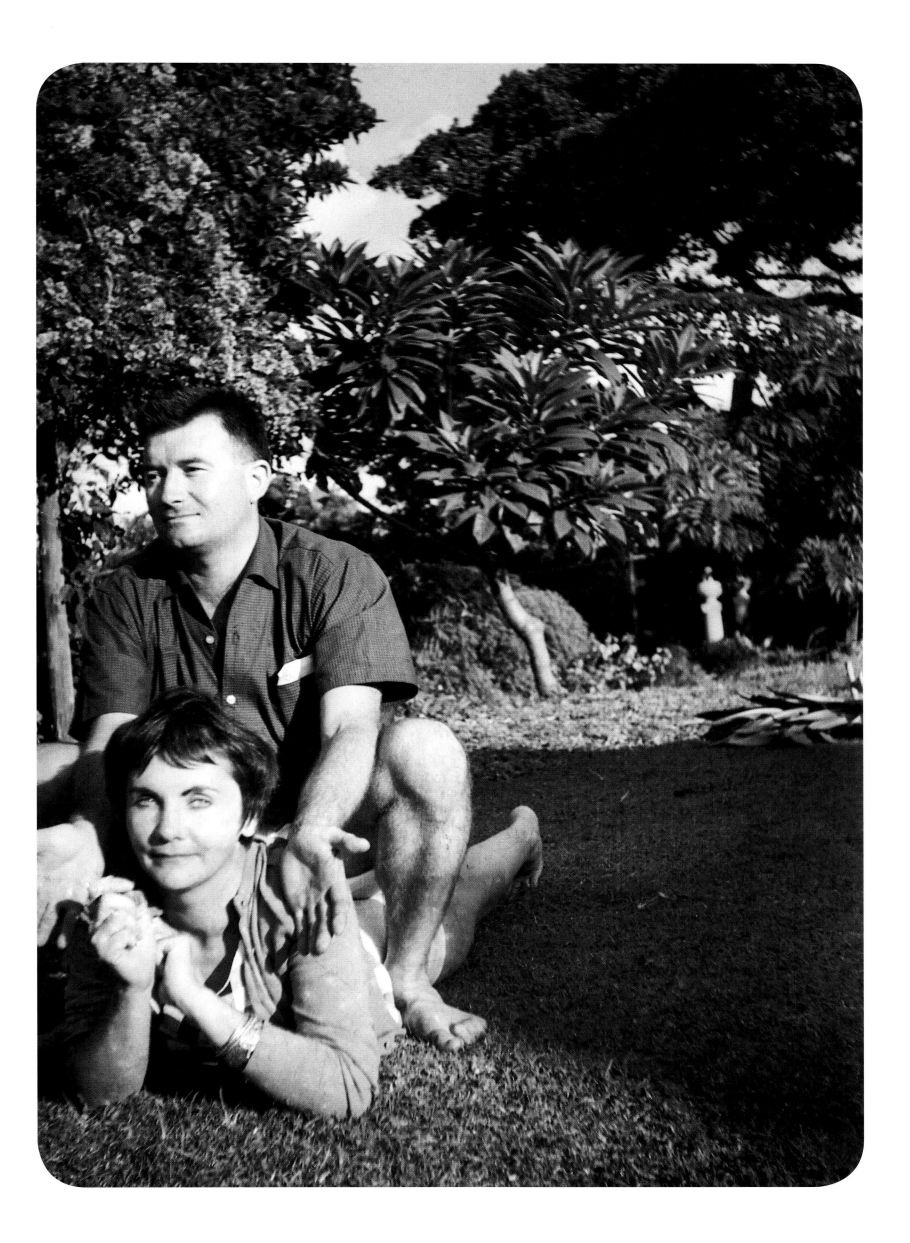

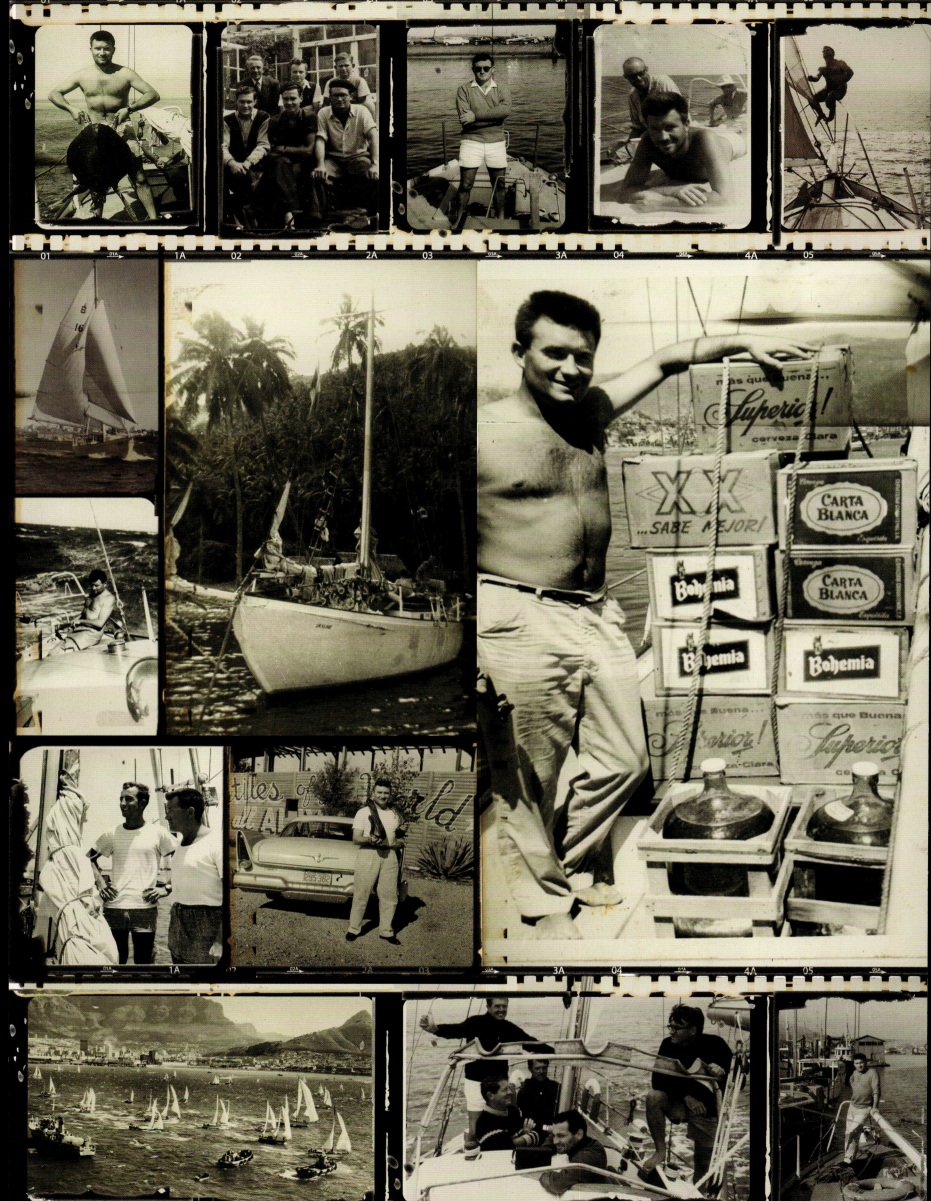

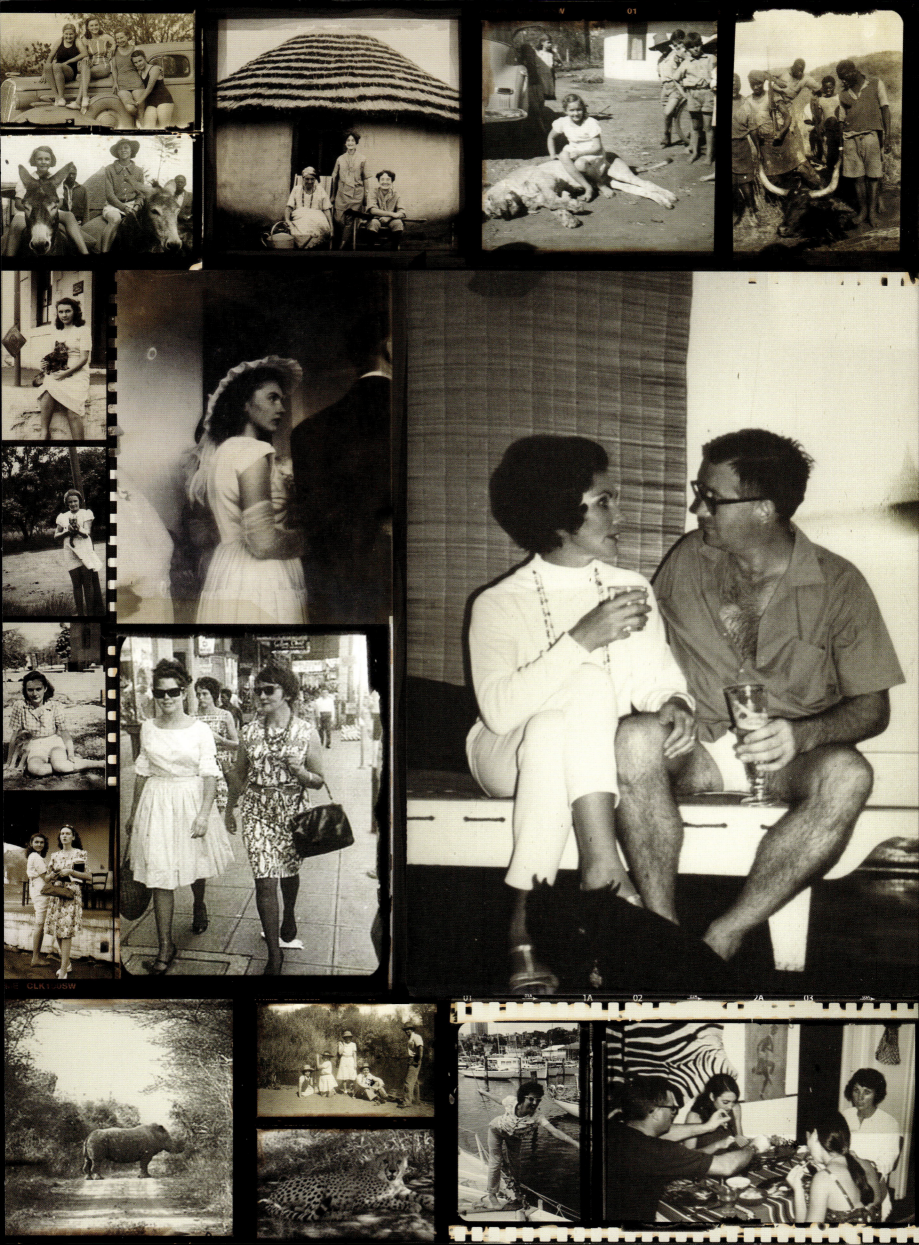

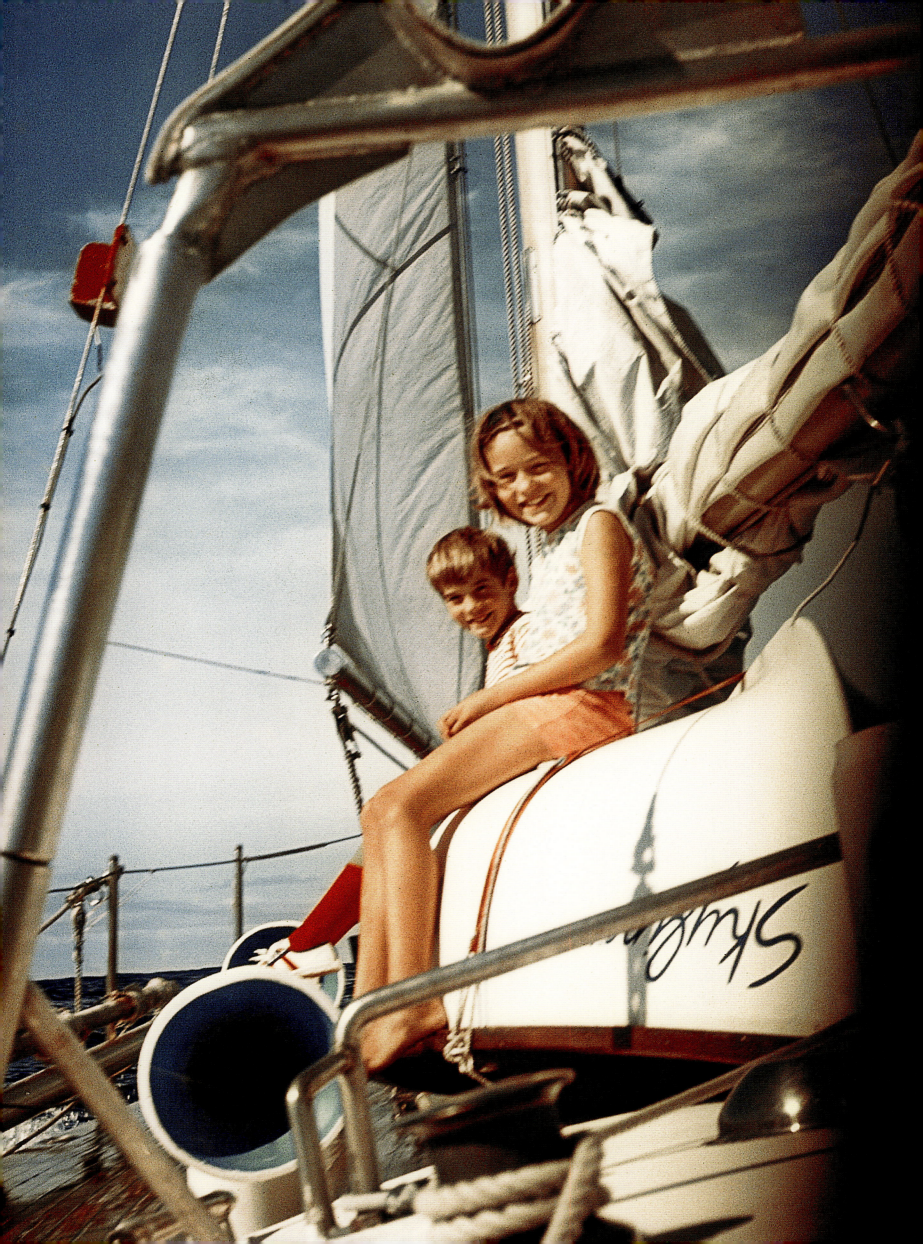

My earliest memory is of being in Dublin after my grandfather,

James Dinnigan, had died. I was about three years old and I can remember

sitting on the staircase watching my grandmother knitting.

After that, my first real memories are of when we lived on the beach in Umhlanga Rocks, just outside Durban. We had a flock of geese, who acted like watchdogs, chasing people off the property. When I was four we moved to Mandini, a small town in the middle of Zululand. My mother had lots of Zulu friends and she would often take us to spend a night with them in their villages. This was during the apartheid era, and many white South Africans did not approve. Imagine their horror when, one day, the whole tribe visited our home, dressed in animal-skin loincloths and carrying their spears and their kill, to thank Dad for making them some stainless steel pots – they called him 'Mr Stainless Steel'. They set up camp on our enormous lawns, and there was a lot of dancing. We later received threats from neighbours outraged that we were socialising with black people. They were dark, turbulent times in South Africa.

Mum was always dressed in brightly coloured clothes, and she and Dad used to hold amazing parties, where they'd invite people from all walks of life, from many different countries. Mum would play the piano, and there'd be singing and dancing – they really knew how to throw a party. Mum was such a free spirit, with friends from everywhere. We used to visit her Indian friends in their homes in the coloured areas (where white people weren't 'supposed' to go) and cook fabulous curries with them in their kitchens. It was an exciting, colourful childhood; I was always being introduced to new people and new experiences.

Mum was passionate about animals, and we grew up surrounded by them. We had two dogs, Snippy and Tess, who rescued me once when I was bowled over by a wave. Our friends had game reserves, and I have happy memories of feeding bottles of milk to baby giraffes orphaned by poachers. To this day, I feel a very strong connection to animals – we have two dogs and a cat at home.

Seamus and I knew that our parents had an adventure in mind when Dad started building a yacht, the *Skyliner*, in our back garden. It was a steel boat with fibreglass on top, which was quite innovative in those days, so it attracted a lot of attention. It was designed by an Australian, Alan Payne. Dad made all the fittings, including the blocks and cleats. He also fitted it out with beautiful teak decks and antique fixtures, including a wonderful old table rescued from a shipwreck. Although my parents never actually told us we were leaving South Africa for good, that soon became clear. They, like many others, were anxious to leave behind the increasing violence and unrest. We were bound for Canada, as Dad had lived in Vancouver before and thought it would be a good place to raise a family. What's more, true to his pioneering spirit, he was determined to get there by the quickest sailing route.

My parents had a passion for the good things in life, like food and wine. Mum was an amazing cook, and she prepared all sorts of exotic (in those days) meals for us to take on board. She had learnt how to make curries from her Indian friends, and found a cannery where they put all the curries in tins for us to take on board. Her Italian friends had taught her how to make fresh pasta, which she hung out to dry on our clothes line in preparation for the journey. Dad (as I found out many years later) made sure there was plenty of good Scotch on board. Just to be certain, he drained one of the water tanks in the bilge (it was about 80 litres!) and filled it with Scotch.

Previous pages: Dad on board the Skyliner *with a freshly-caught tuna (page 2); Mum and Dad in South Africa in the 1960s (page 5); Mum and Dad led a very cosmopolitan life (pages 6–7).*

Opposite: Seamus and me on board the Skyliner, *just before we entered Albany in Western Australia.*

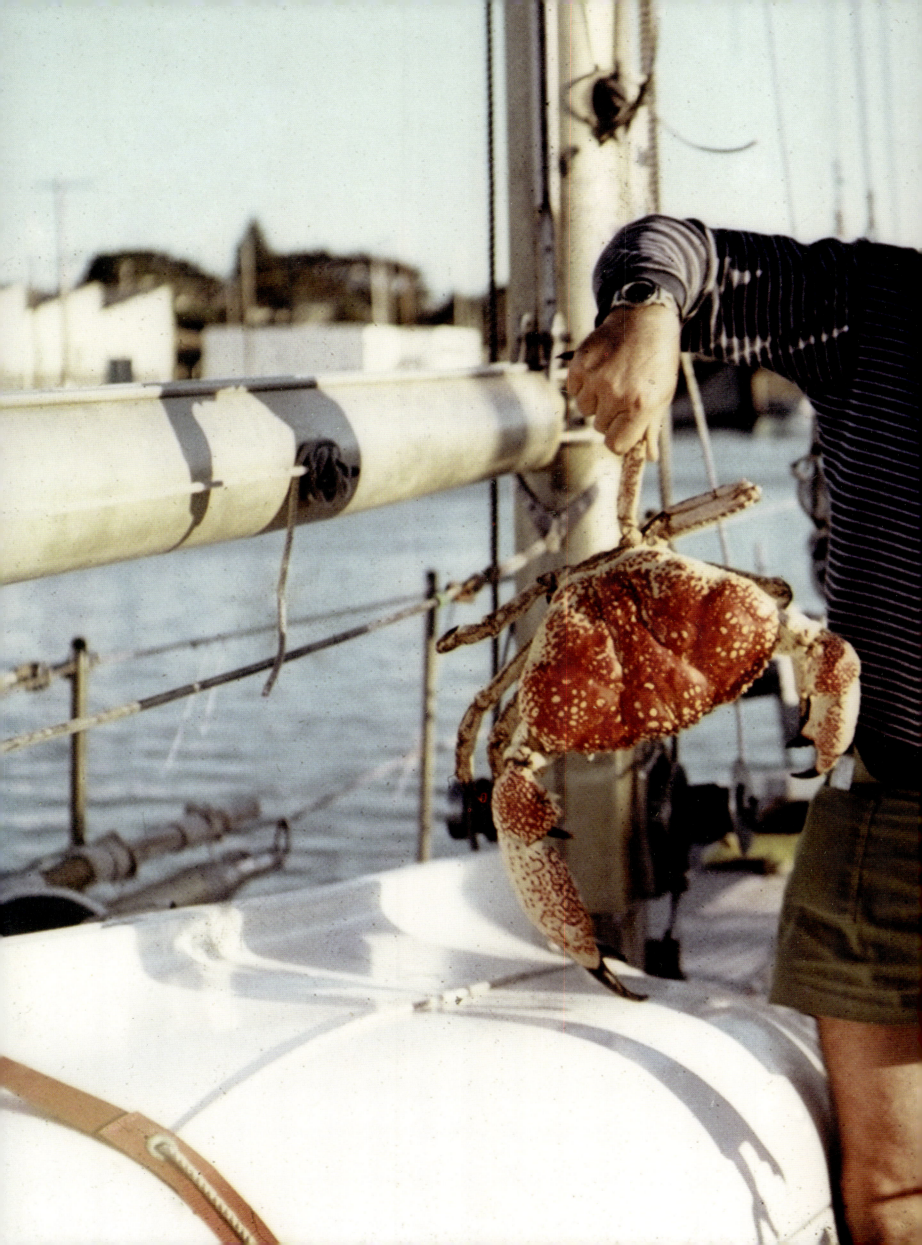

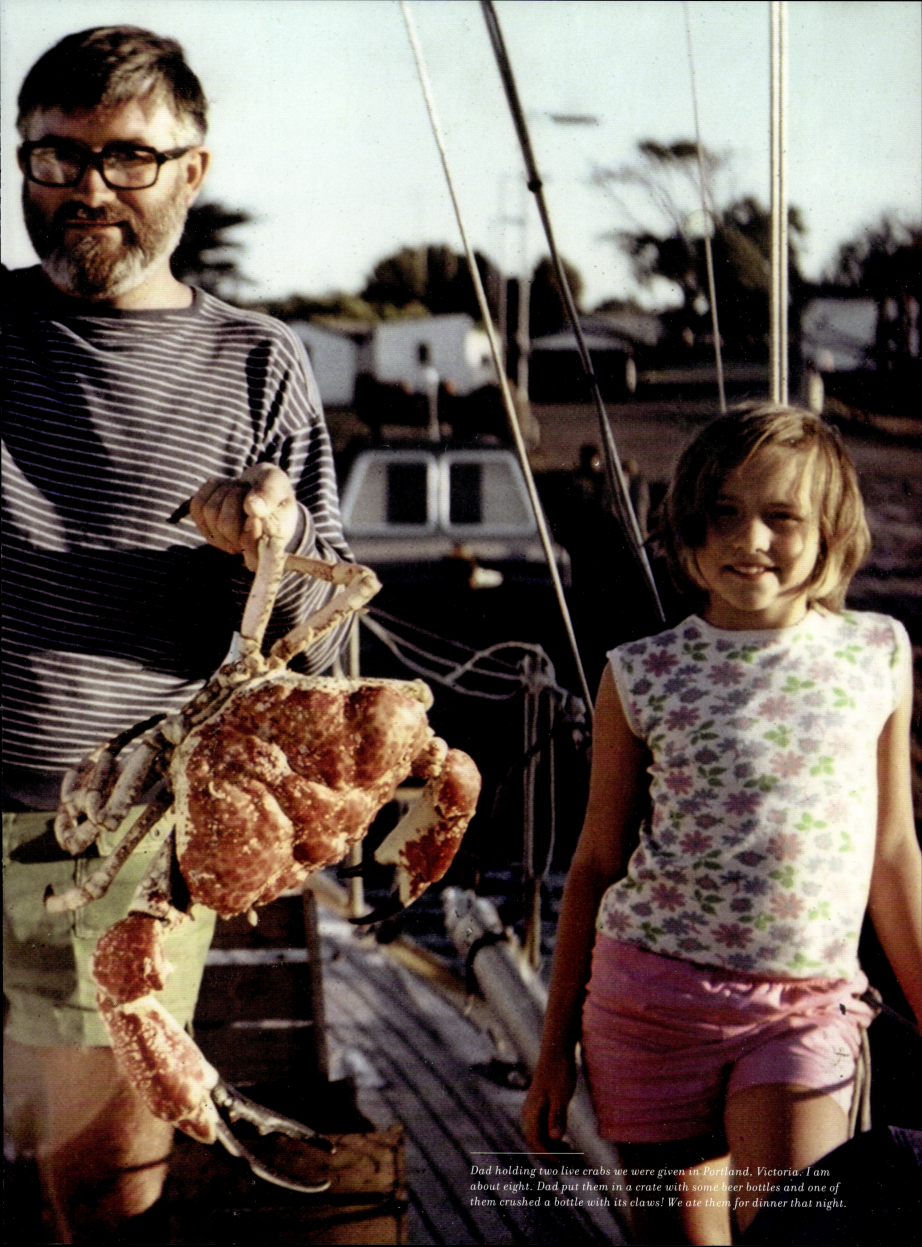

Dad holding two live crabs we were given in Portland, Victoria. I am about eight. Dad put them in a crate with some beer bottles and one of them crushed a bottle with its claws! We ate them for dinner that night.

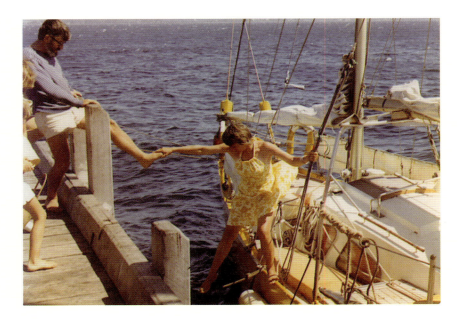

We left South Africa on Boxing Day 1973, when I was eight. Durban harbour was unusually turbulent that day, with choppy seas and gale-force winds. Aunt Theresa (Mum's sister) begged us not to sail, as it was too dangerous, but all Dad could say was: 'Amazing sailing weather; you'll never get better! This journey's going to take us half the time.' Once we left port and headed out to sea the waves were forty feet high, and the winds were so strong that we couldn't even get the sails up.

It was many weeks before we saw land again – the tiny remote islands of Île Saint-Paul and Île Amsterdam in the South Indian Ocean. Our charts were hopelessly out of date and we couldn't land because the beaches were eroded and the sea was too deep. I remember everyone on the islands running out to see us, waving enthusiastically. One of our crew paddled in on his surfboard and brought us back fresh potatoes, lobsters and crabs, so we had a real feast that night.

We were never bored at sea. Mum and Dad had planned to take a teacher on board, but when that fell through, Mum packed loads of books, with the intention of home-schooling us. I don't think those boxes were ever opened! We learnt so much else though. Dad gave us a lot of responsibility – we would give him compass readings, take the tiller if needed, and help Mum in the galley. Although our spirits were free, there was still strong discipline, as you couldn't take any chances at sea.

One of my most vivid memories is when I was nearly eaten by a shark. We were sailing far south, towards Antarctica, when we were becalmed for days. Seamus and I,

bored, convinced Dad to let us go for a swim. We couldn't just jump off the boat – Dad had to put us in harnesses and lower us down, then pull us up when we were ready to get out. Mum called out that lunch was ready, and Dad pulled Seamus up first, then, as he was pulling me up, his face went absolutely white. As I clambered onto the deck I saw a huge white pointer shark lurching out of the water, almost vertical, with its jaws wide open. It literally missed me by about a foot. Even with all Dad's knowledge of the sea he hadn't known that, despite the freezing water temperature, this was a breeding ground for great whites. To this day, much as I love the water, I am wary of going out beyond where the waves break.

We first hit dry land at Albany, in Western Australia. It wasn't exactly a quiet arrival. We were running two weeks late, so Aunt Theresa had notified the authorities that we were missing at sea. We were greeted by a large group of police, news crews and locals. Looking back, I can understand my aunt's concern, as not many families had tried to sail at forty-two degrees south. The locals were so kind – they brought us fresh fruit, meals, and, even better, they offered us hot showers. As all we had on the yacht were a bucket, salt water and saltwater soap, this was a total luxury.

We stayed in Albany for about six weeks, living on the yacht. Seamus and I went to the local school while Mum and Dad made repairs to the yacht, then we set off again. We sailed south to Portland, Victoria, then on to Eden in New South Wales, where we were hit by a terrible storm, and our boat, which was tied between two fishing boats, was battered. Undaunted, Dad set sail again, and as we

Above: Dad helping Mum disembark in Albany.

Opposite: After forty-seven days at sea,
the family touches down in Albany.

Following pages: Growing up with Seamus in
the 60s and 70s in South Africa and at sea.

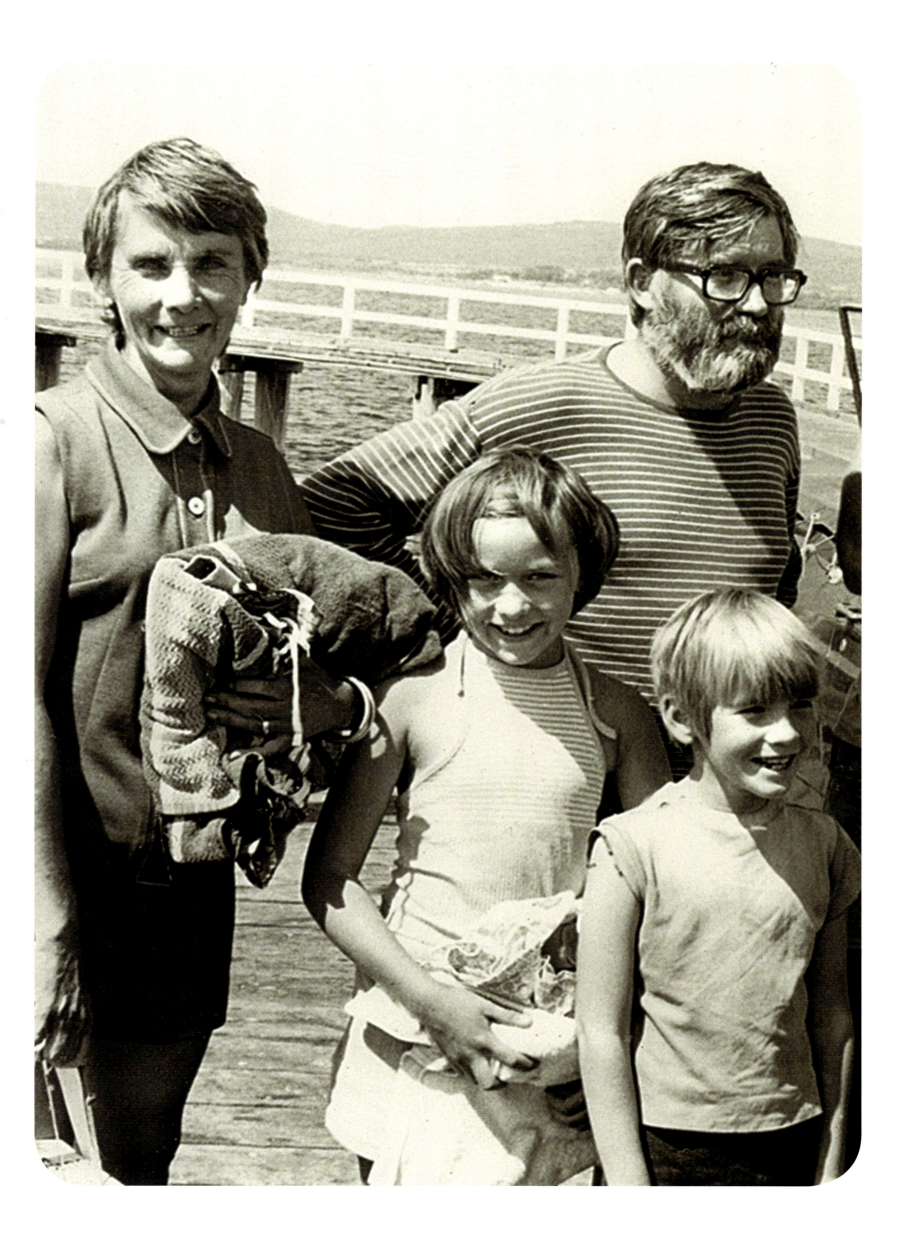

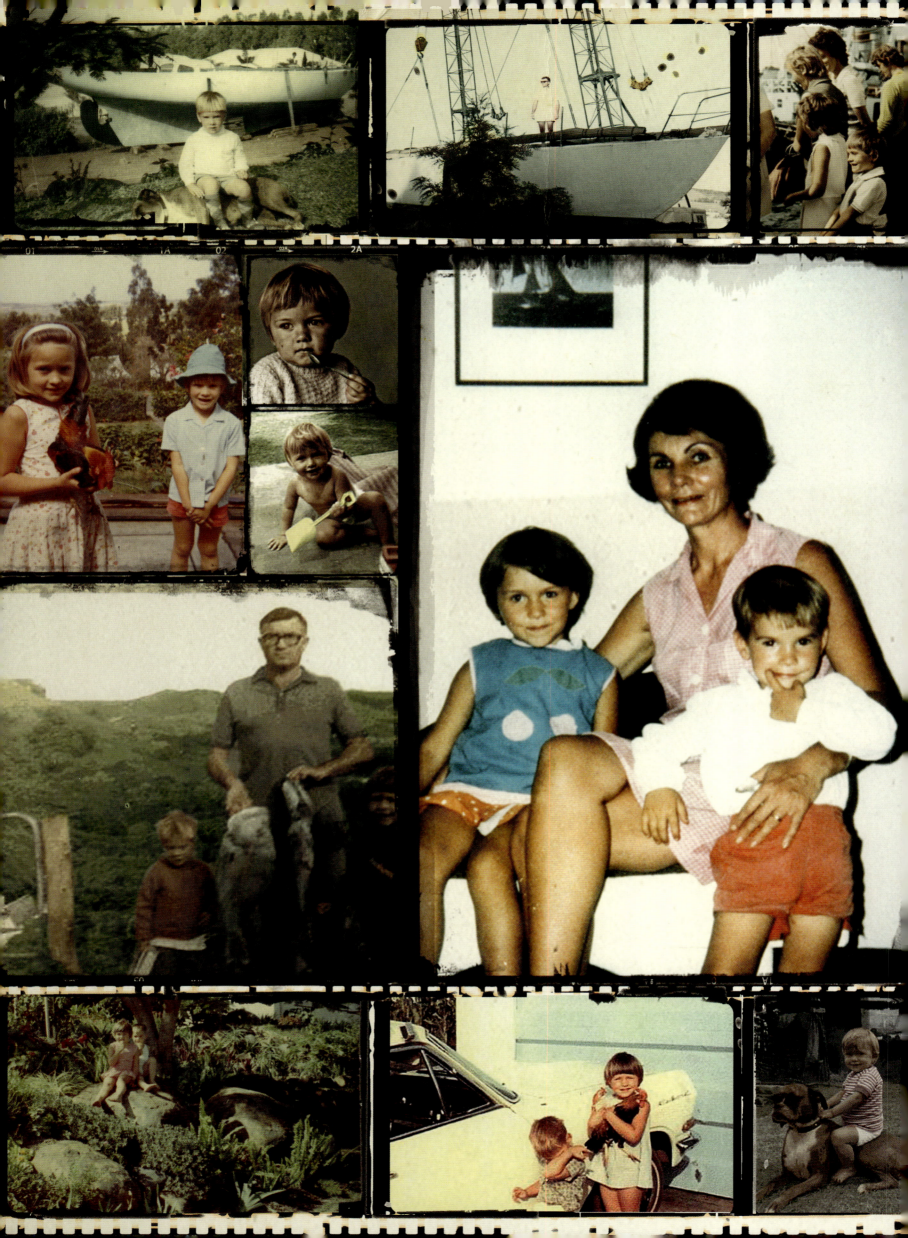

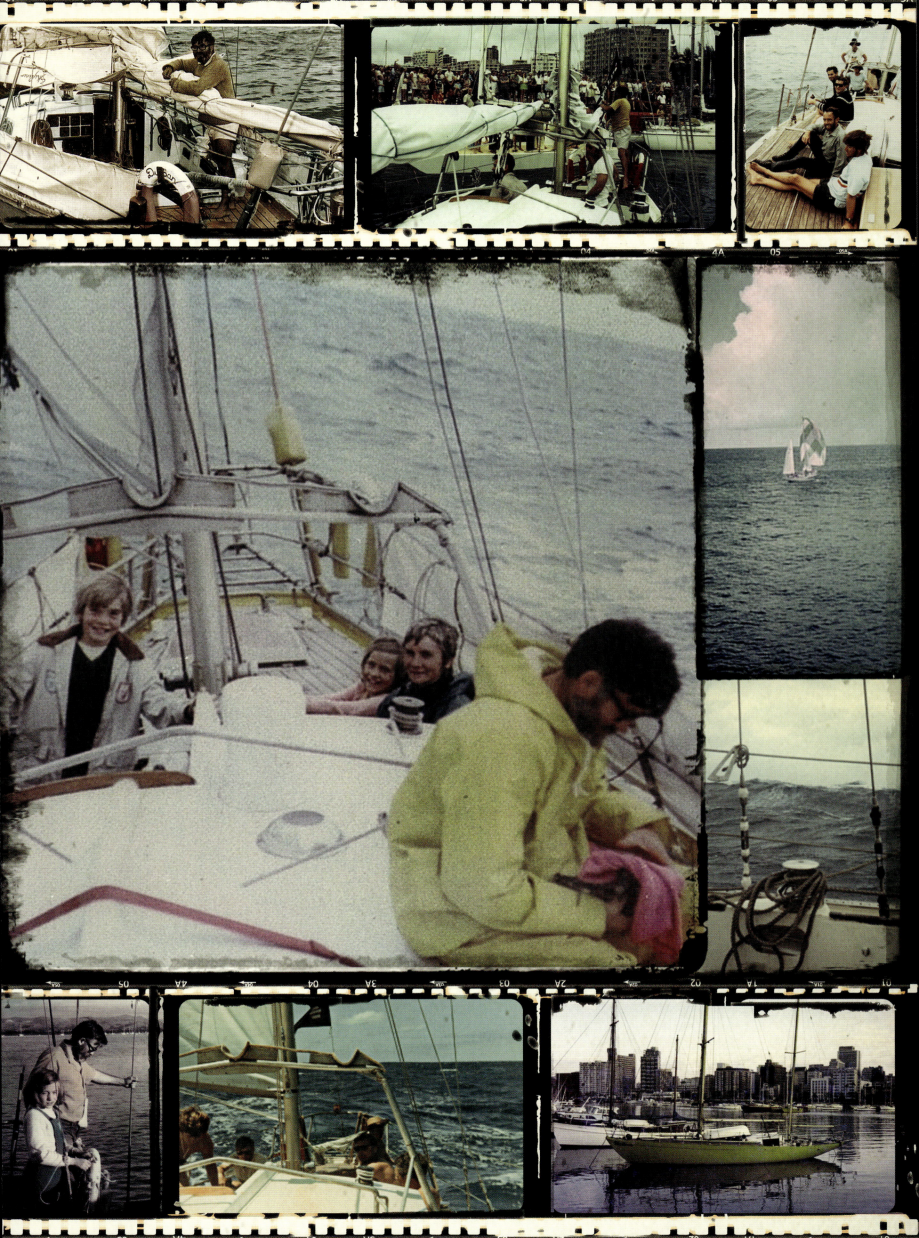

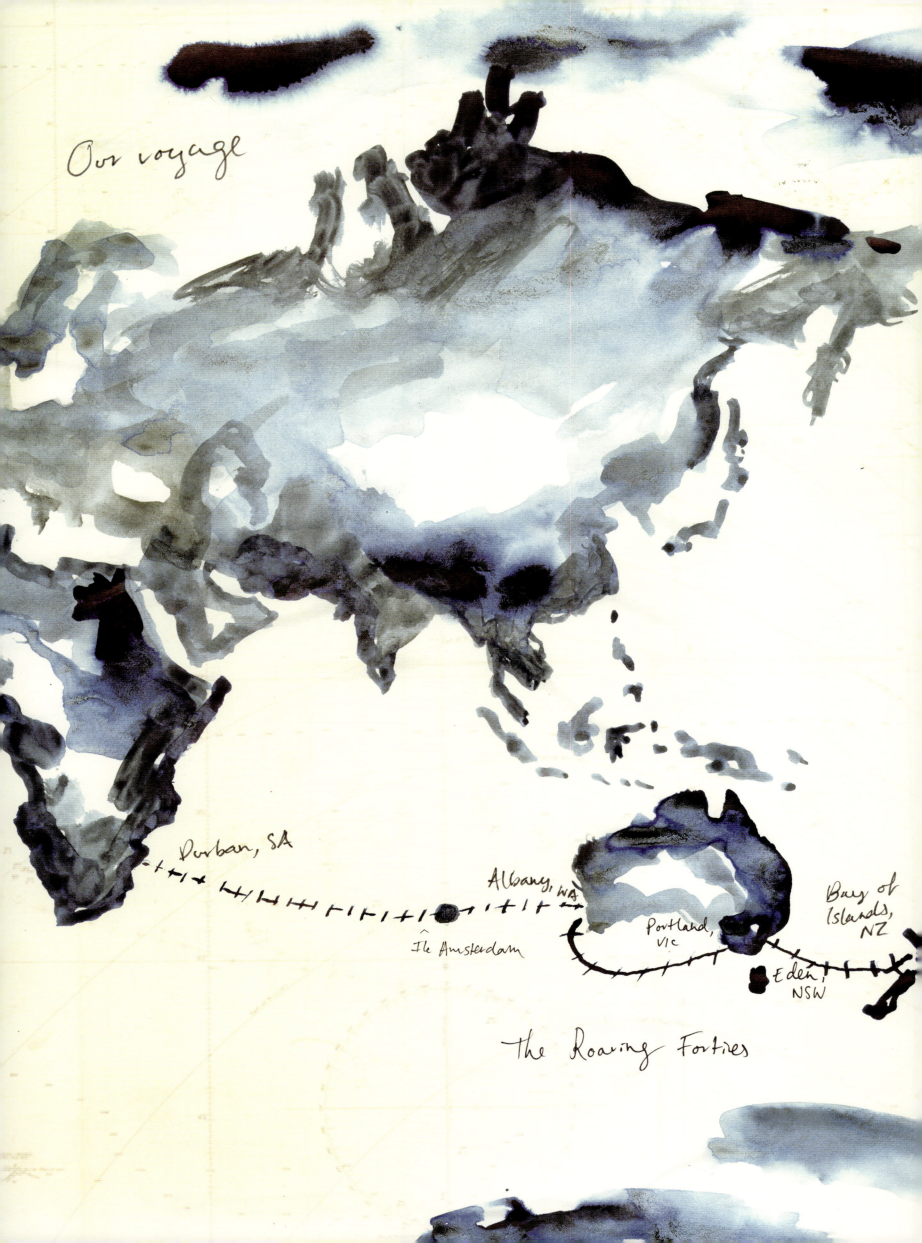

Our voyage

Durban, SA

Albany, WA

Île Amsterdam

Portland, Vic

Bay of Islands, NZ

Eden, NSW

The Roaring Forties

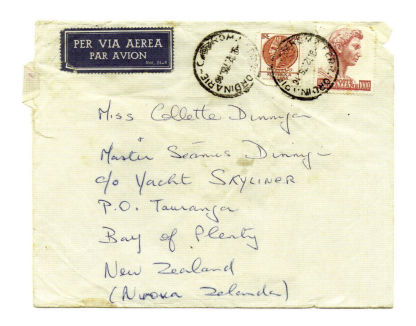

sailed into wild seas, the boat capsized. I fell from the top bunk, splitting my chin open, and my pet parrot, who had been with us all the way, died. It was all pretty intense. Somehow we got through, and sailed on to the Bay of Islands in the North Island of New Zealand.

Looking back, I think that the experience of spending a year sailing with my family at such a young age really shaped me. Living on a yacht in such close quarters, there was no room for disobedience; my relationship with my family was very real, raw even. It gave me a great sense of independence, and also, I think, the confidence to make my own decisions. Although it was pretty crowded below deck, once you were up on the deck there was infinite space. Somehow that made me feel secure. I do think that, subconsciously even, the idea of travel and a journey at sea has always inspired me. I will never forget the sight of the sky at night, the romance of the stars and the phosphorescence when the moonbeams hit the water.

Dad has always been a great storyteller, because he is such an adventurer. He sailed the high seas, and he took his family on a new, possibly dangerous, route that very few families had sailed before. When he talks about the time he ate a dozen eggs, or a dozen chops for breakfast, it's all true. Dad lived life hard; he was totally fearless. His life was rugged, and real, the life of a man conquering new frontiers. And we were there with him for some of the way.

We sailed into the Bay of Islands, New Zealand, under a big white white cloud, after about year at sea. It really was 'Aotearoa', or 'the land of the long white cloud'. On arrival, we were greeted by the worst fog they had seen in a hundred years. I was at the front of the yacht, calling out to Dad as he was moving the tiller from left to right. There were lots of rocks, making it hard to navigate, and we had to approach slowly, because you couldn't see them until you were almost on top of them. I would suddenly see a rock three feet in front of us and yell out, 'Rock to starboard . . . rock to port!' As we slowly made our way into port, we heard an American voice shouting, 'God knows who you are but you must have one hell of a captain to navigate through this fog!'

We spent a few months in Opua, then we sailed on to Tauranga. We continued living on the yacht, which was moored in the marina, and spent a lot of time swimming and fishing, taking the dinghy out to get mussels and oysters. Seamus and I started school properly for the first time. I was nine, and I found the routine and the discipline quite challenging, having led such a free, unstructured life up until then. The other kids gave us a hard time because of our accents, and it wasn't easy to make friends at first. Eventually things settled down, and I did make some good friends, some of whom I still see today, like Andrea Waters and Leeanne Richardson.

We continued living on the yacht, moored in port, for about two years, until finally Mum had had enough, and decided that it was time for us to settle down. So, we bought

Opposite: The map of our voyage from South Africa, via Australia, to New Zealand. We never made it to Canada.

Above: A letter sent to Seamus and me while the Skyliner _was moored in Tauranga, and we were living on board. We lived on the yacht for about two years!_

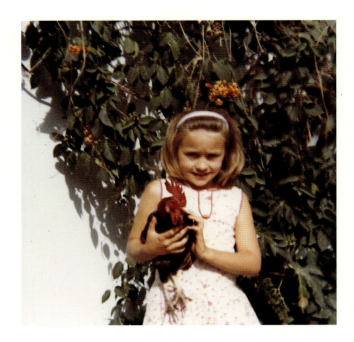

some land in the beautiful Kaimai Ranges, on the banks of the Wairoa River, and Dad started building a house out of stone and recycled timber. Just as he had built the yacht from scratch, Dad just about built the house from scratch.

Seamus and I were expected to help, and I remember the trips to rock-filled rivers sorting and looking for flat rocks to build our fireplace and hearth. The house was built on poles, as the river could rise dangerously high after heavy rains (we were asked to evacuate countless times over the years). There were floor-to-ceiling windows, and native wood flooring, and Dad used old railway sleepers to make the stairs. He was so inventive, quite ahead of his time, putting wetback systems into the fireplace to heat the whole house. No detail was too small, right down to the copper nails he used as they looked better and would weather well. Andrea Waters says that the first time she came to our house, she felt like she had entered a tree house from an exotic, far-off land.

Once we had built the house, and Dad had sold his beloved yacht, we settled down to life in New Zealand. Dad was happy enough working as an engineer, and I was happy too. I loved our home, and I loved the outdoor life. We finally had lots of animals – there was an aviary off my bedroom where I had a collection of birds, and we also had a menagerie of sheep, goats, rabbits, cats and dogs. I also had three horses, my first and favourite being Mr Chappy. I have always loved horseriding.

Mum found it more difficult to settle into life in New Zealand, which in the 1970s was quite conservative. Like me, she loved the outdoor life and the animals, but it wasn't enough for her. She had had a cosmopolitan childhood, travelling between boarding school in England and home in South Africa, meeting interesting people from all over the world. She found life in a small town in New Zealand pretty stifling. She was used to parties and playing jazz. Apart from anything else, she couldn't believe that New Zealand had no fresh coffee beans, tabasco, or even peppercorns. I am sure my love of good food came from her.

Mum was incredibly stylish, but quite unconventional. She used to ride her bike to school to pick us up, wearing flowing caftans in bright prints. She was a free spirit, creative and adventurous, and our house was always full of life, and music. She found a job working in a fabric shop, designing textiles, because she wanted to get out and meet people.

All of this was quite different from what New Zealand society expected in those days – which was that the woman would stay home and be a good wife and mother, cooking chops, mashed potato and peas for dinner every other night. Our lifestyle didn't fit into any particular box. Poor Mum must have thought, 'My God, what the hell am I doing here?', which was ironic, given that she was the one who had insisted it was time for us to put down roots. New Zealand in the 1970s was very different from how it is now. I love going back there, and I only wish Mum had lived to see how much it has changed.

I used to wish that my family was more like everyone else's – that we lived in a normal, suburban house, and ate meat and three vegetables every other night; that Mum

---

Above: Me aged five, with Tom, my pet bantam rooster.

*Opposite: Riding my first and favourite horse,
Mr Chappy, aged about thirteen.*

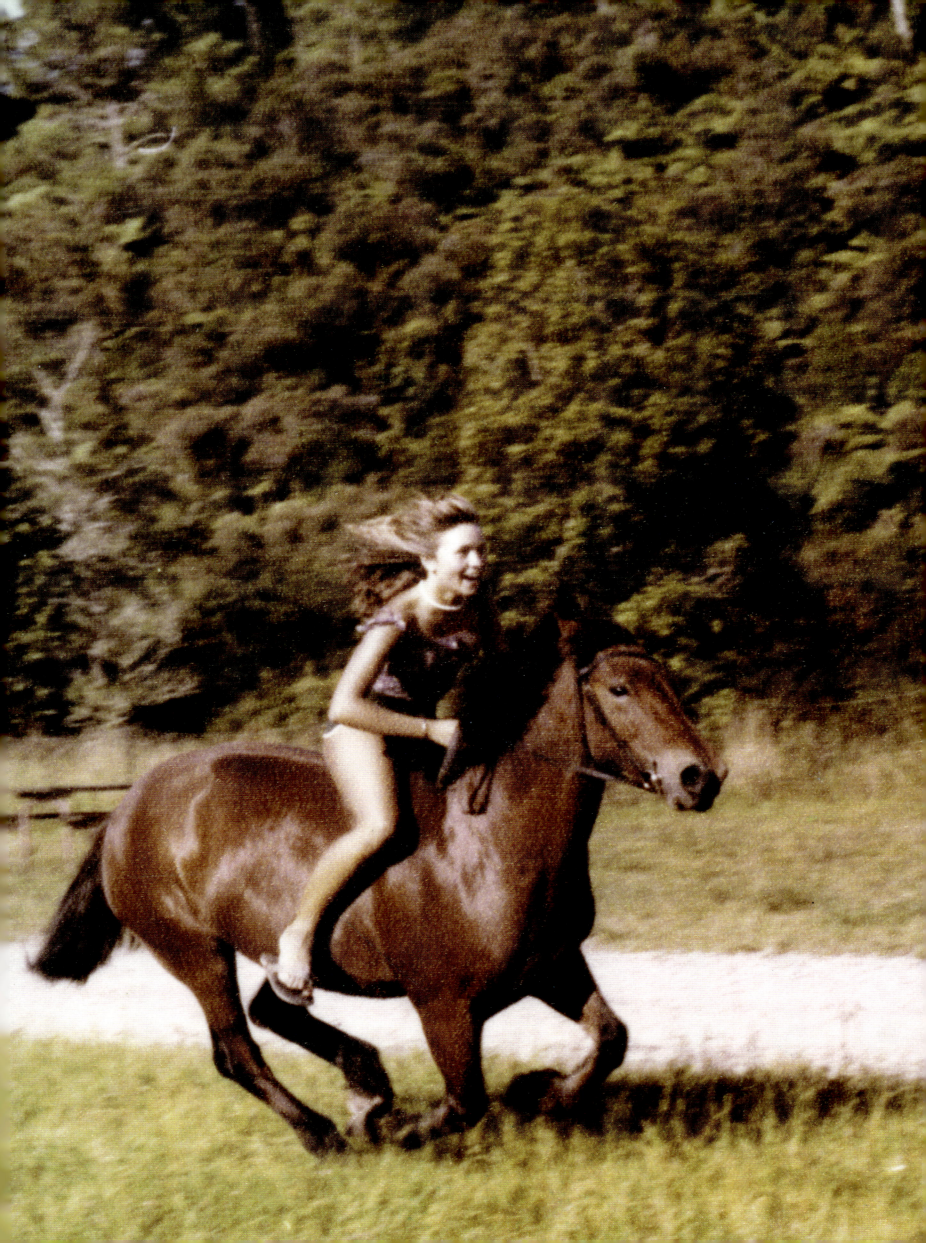

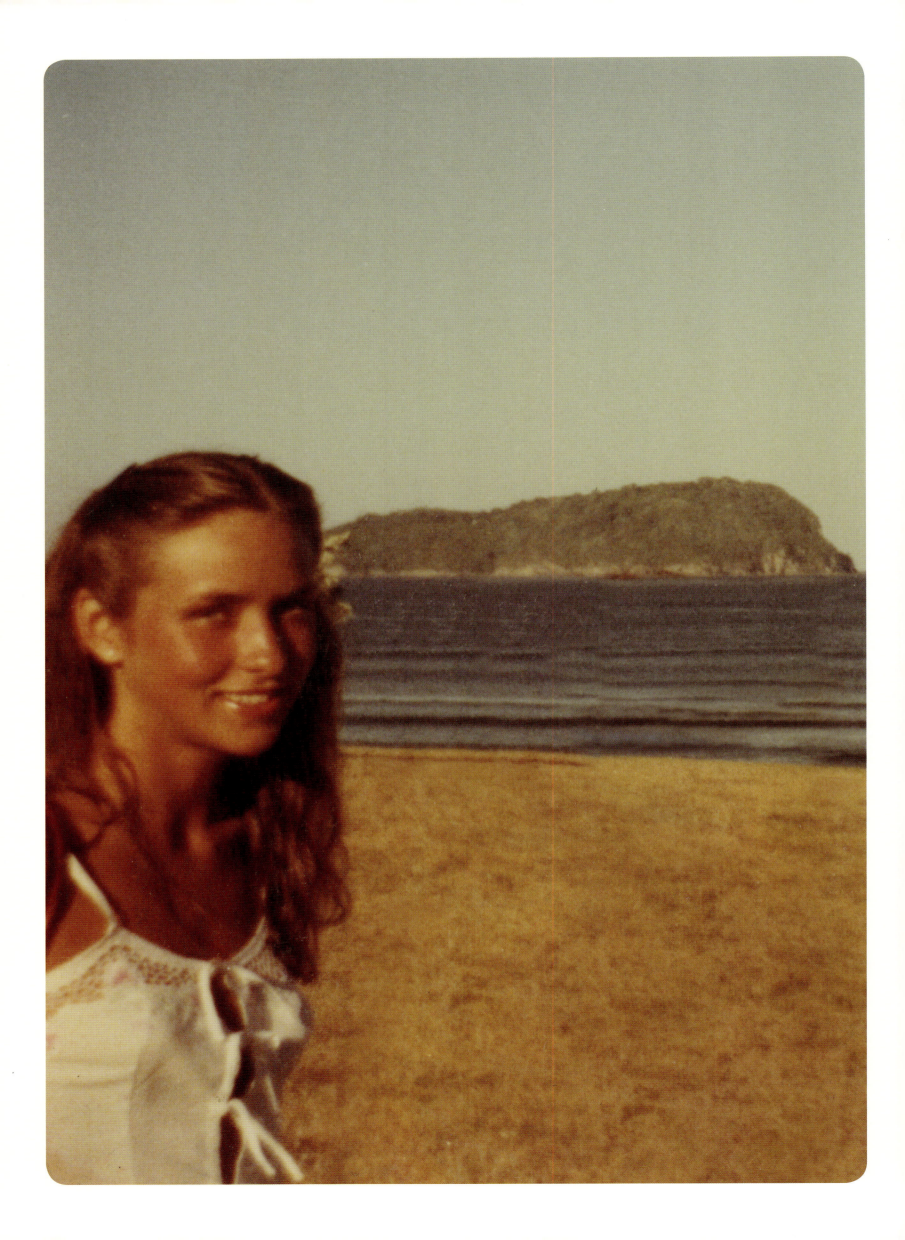

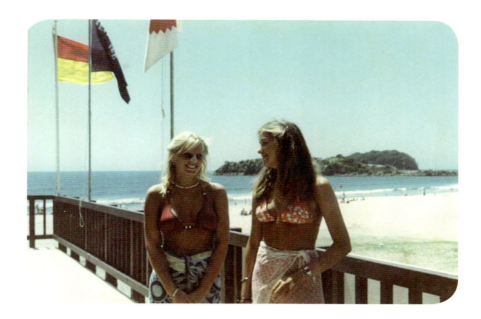

didn't wear colourful clothes, ride a bike and colour her hair, and that Dad didn't have such a strong Irish accent. It is only since Mum died (suddenly of a heart attack) nearly twenty years ago that I have realised what an impact their parenting had on me, and have started to appreciate what a unique upbringing I had. It made me very determined, and gave me the confidence to trust my instincts. As I get older, I worry sometimes that I am becoming more conservative, trusting my instincts less and relying more on other people's opinions.

My parents adored each other, but they were very different. Mum was the theatrical, gentle, free spirit who gave us unconditional love and affection, while Dad was the rugged, gruff, take-no-prisoners man. Mum was very emotional – a true romantic who always followed her heart. She wouldn't use a cookbook as she hated sticking to a formula; what was important to her was the essence of the thing. She would make the most amazing meals that no one could ever repeat. It was the same when she played the piano – she called it her 'honky tonks' and never used sheet music; she played from memory. Dad, on the other hand, was practical and down-to-earth, full of common-sense advice. He was a true intellectual, who knew about everything from weather vanes to aerodynamics, and had a special love of history.

Sadly, Dad had a funny way of showing his love for Mum. He was very critical of her, so that if, for example, she had cooked a great meal, instead of complimenting her, he was more likely to say that it wasn't as good as her last one. It is only since she died that he has become more sentimental, constantly reminiscing about their happy times together. He is critical of me, too. I know that he is proud of me because people tell me so, but he never says so himself. Just a little while ago, I asked him what he thought of my last Paris show and he said he was disappointed – 'It wasn't much of an event, really.' I don't let it bother me – I know that he is just not the type of person to hand out praise. I don't need a pat on the back from him to feel loved or to love him.

Once I had settled down, I quite enjoyed school. I was diligent and conscientious, and I especially loved art and science. I also did sewing, and found it easy, so I asked for a sewing machine for my thirteenth birthday, and it was then that I started to make my own clothes. Mum was great with handicrafts – she made me teddy bears and toys when I was small – but she was not so good with a machine, because again, she wouldn't follow a pattern. She could mend sails or make curtains if she had to, but that was about it.

Mum did know a lot about fabrics and patterns though, from working in a fabric shop. I was so lucky – she would give me scraps of designer fabrics, and, better still, at the end of each season she'd give me bundles of Butterick and Simplicity patterns. Burdas were too hard! They'd usually be size sixteens, and I'd have to cut them down to fit me – that's how I learnt to cut straight onto the fabric. I loved being able to go home on a Friday night and make myself a dress to wear to a party on Saturday night. None of my friends really sewed, it was just me, and I would end up with a fabulous new outfit each week.

Opposite: Me in Waihi, New Zealand, aged fourteen.

Above: With a friend at Mount Maunganui Surf Club.

I knew from when I was about fifteen that I wanted to leave New Zealand. It was too claustrophobic for me; I was ambitious and eager to see the world. I just had to work out the best way to make it happen. I had lots of different jobs in my last few years at school – I worked as a lifesaver, in a burger bar on the beach, picking oranges – anything to save money so that I could escape. I think my bohemian, nomadic childhood made it hard for me to stay too long in the same place. Looking back, I guess I always pushed myself. I was the first of my friends to get my drivers' licence, and the first to save up and buy my own car.

I didn't ever consciously decide to become a designer. It certainly wasn't something I had dreamed of doing all my life. In high school I had done a range of subjects, from practical arts and art history to science and languages, to keep my options open. I ended up doing well enough academically that I was 'accredited', so I was given entry to university and didn't have to sit the final exams. It basically meant that I could study any university course I chose. Dad wanted me to study law, or something equally academic.

I had always wanted to be a vet, but when it came to the crunch, I couldn't face the thought of another seven years of study. I could have done any of those degrees, but in all honesty I don't know that I would have had the patience – although I have great attention to detail when it comes to creative things, sometimes I think I have ADD in other areas; I need to be creatively stimulated.

All I knew was that I had to get some qualification, as that was my ticket out of New Zealand. I ended up applying at the last minute to Wellington Polytechnic to do a course in graphics or fashion. I knew that either would be creative, much shorter than a veterinary science degree, and would get me travelling and meeting new people. I never really thought about what would happen at the end of the course.

I actually thought I had been accepted into the graphics course, not the fashion one, until I spent my first day learning about pins and tape measures. I ended up completing what is now a three-year fashion course in two years, attending classes from eight until five every day. That was an exciting time for me. I was living in a new

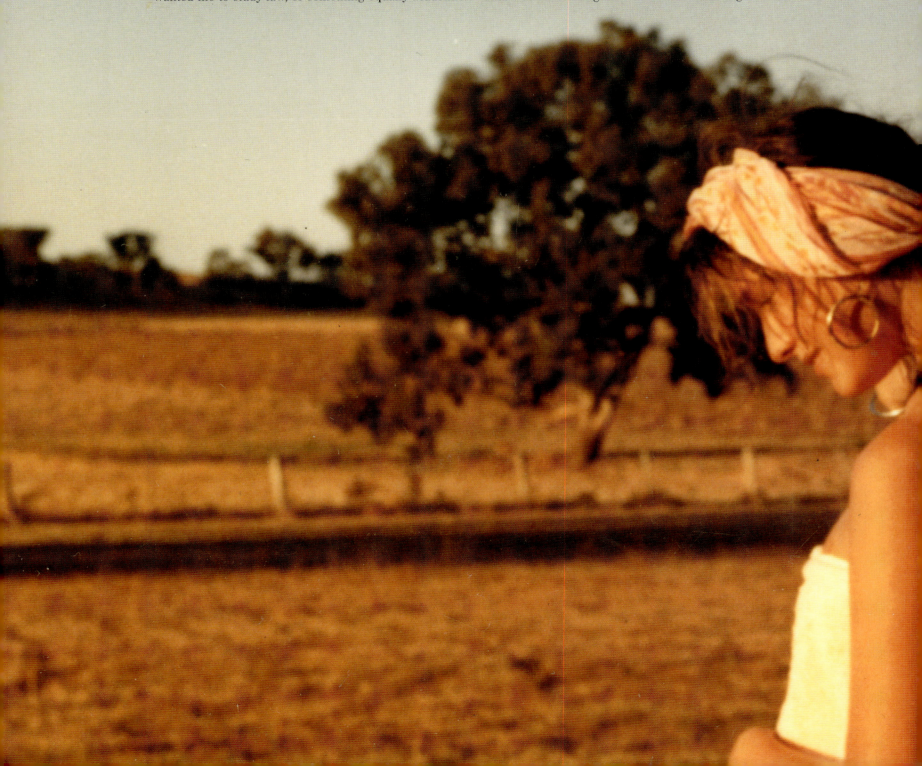

city, supporting myself with bar and waitressing jobs – it was my first real taste of independence.

The most important things I learnt at fashion school were how to cut a pattern properly, and how to tailor a garment. I learnt how to drape the fabric and saw the attention to detail that goes into making something that wears well. This gave me an appreciation of quality and bespoke tailoring, and taught me that the time invested in a good product is time well spent. I don't think that design schools today emphasise this enough. There is too much focus on marketing, and not enough on old-school crafts-manship – how to tailor a jacket, how to ease the sleeves, things which you need to understand.

I was far from the perfect student – it was a pretty intense few years for me, juggling my studies, my waitress-ing jobs and my busy social life. My tutors were quite old school, and many didn't think I had it in me to finish my degree, much less become a successful designer. It is true that my social life was pretty hectic, but I worked hard too, through the night if I had to, to get my assignments done. I never won any awards at college, and I wasn't obsessed with design – it was just one part of my life. I did love vintage clothes though. There were some great vintage shops around with dresses from the 1940s and 1950s, and I started collecting pieces I loved by designers like Yves Saint Laurent and Ossie Clark.

I do have happy memories of my days at fashion school, and was very honoured when, in 2011, Massey University (of which Wellington Polytechnic is now a part) inducted me into its Creative Arts Hall of Fame..

When I graduated, aged about nineteen, I bought a return airfare to Europe and headed to England, where I found a well-paid job in Brighton, working with fabrics and patterns. I was impatient to see the world, so I left that job to go travelling in Greece. When I returned to London, I couldn't find another job, so decided to return to New Zealand, after about eight months away.

I had booked a stopover in Sydney, where I had a few friends, including Linda McMahon, an old friend from New Zealand (now one of my managers) who was living in Sydney with her boyfriend. After a short time in Sydney I realised there were more opportunities for me there than in New Zealand, so I returned home briefly to pack up my things and say goodbye to my family, then moved to Sydney to start the next chapter of my life!

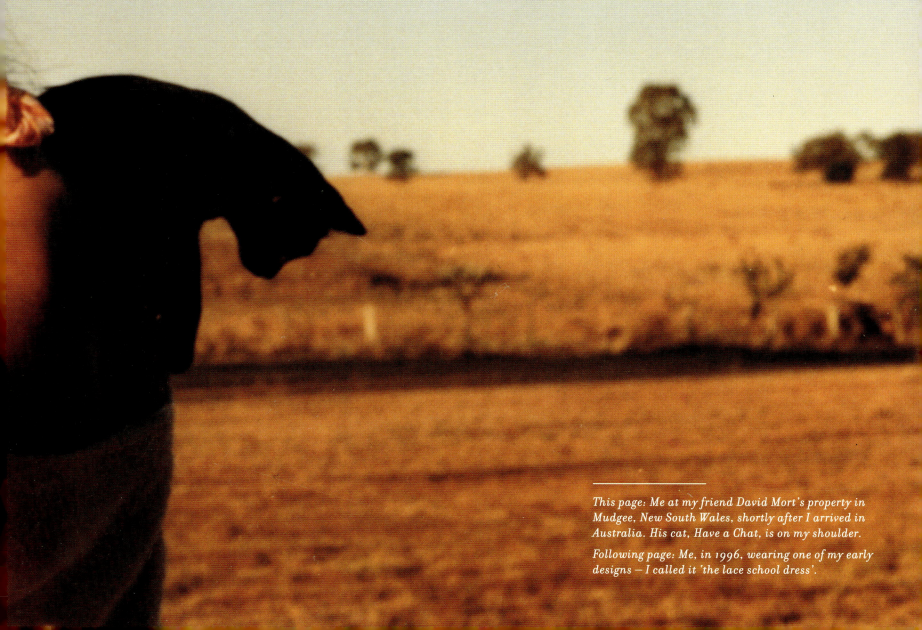

This page: Me at my friend David Mort's property in Mudgee, New South Wales, shortly after I arrived in Australia. His cat, Have a Chat, is on my shoulder.

Following page: Me, in 1996, wearing one of my early designs – I called it 'the lace school dress'.

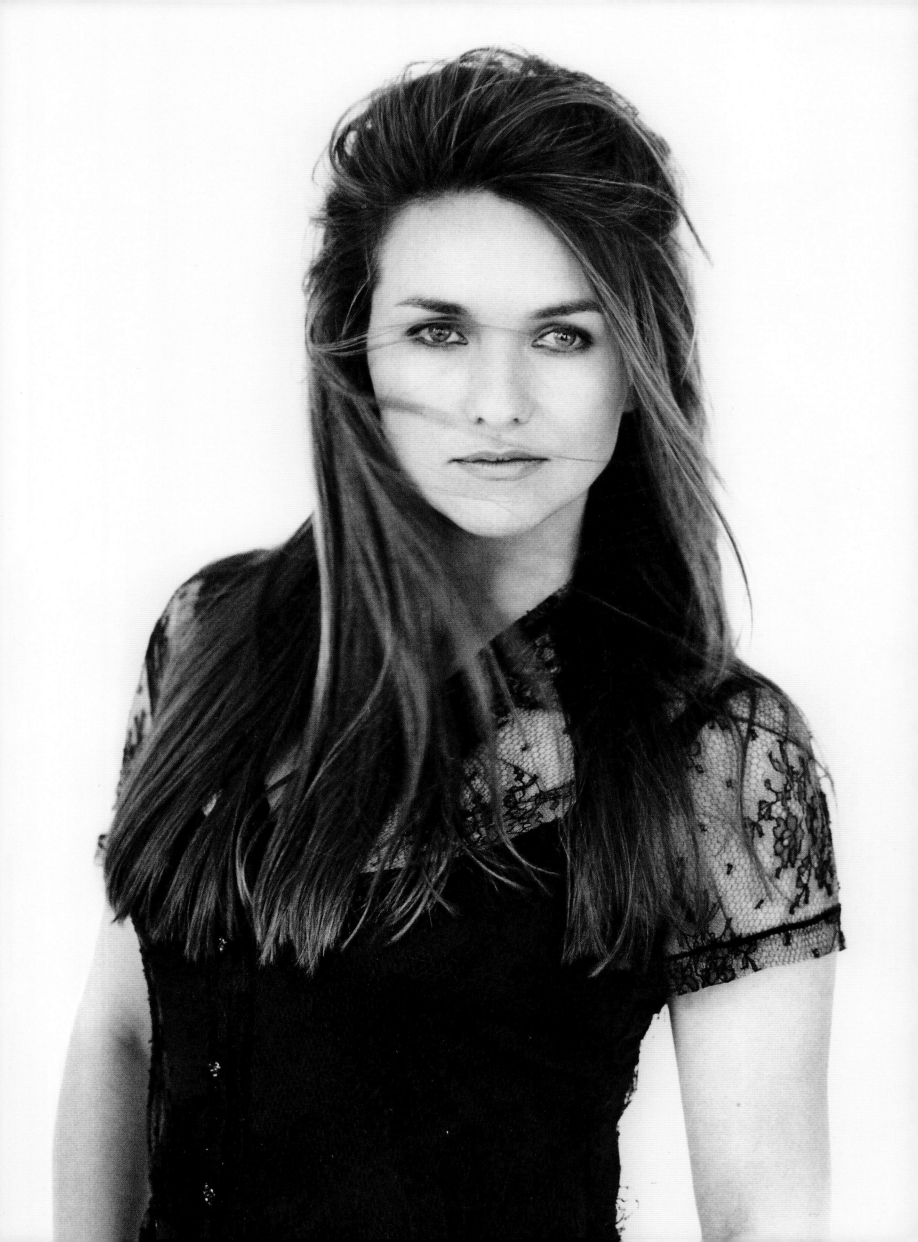

BECOMING COLLETTE DINNIGAN

The Australian Broadcasting Corporation;
period costumes and video clips;
underwear as outerwear.

REACH FOR THE STARS

CHAPTER 2

WHEN I ARRIVED IN SYDNEY

in the mid-1980s, I found a job

with the designer Anthony Bloomfield,

WORKING ON PATTERNS

IN HIS DESIGN ROOM.

His clothes were bold, bright and

eye-catching, with floral prints,

mainly hibiscus, that he also

used for deckchairs.

HE WAS FROM THE

SAME ERA AS OTHER GREAT

AUSTRALIAN DESIGNERS

such as John Macarthur of PURL HARBOUR,

STUART MEMBERY, *and the infamous*

LINDA JACKSON *and* JENNY KEE

of FLAMINGO PARK.

It wasn't couture, but it was very Australian.

After I had been there for about six months

I was ready for a change, so I approached

the Australian Broadcasting Corporation,

looking for work in THEIR

COSTUME DEPARTMENT.

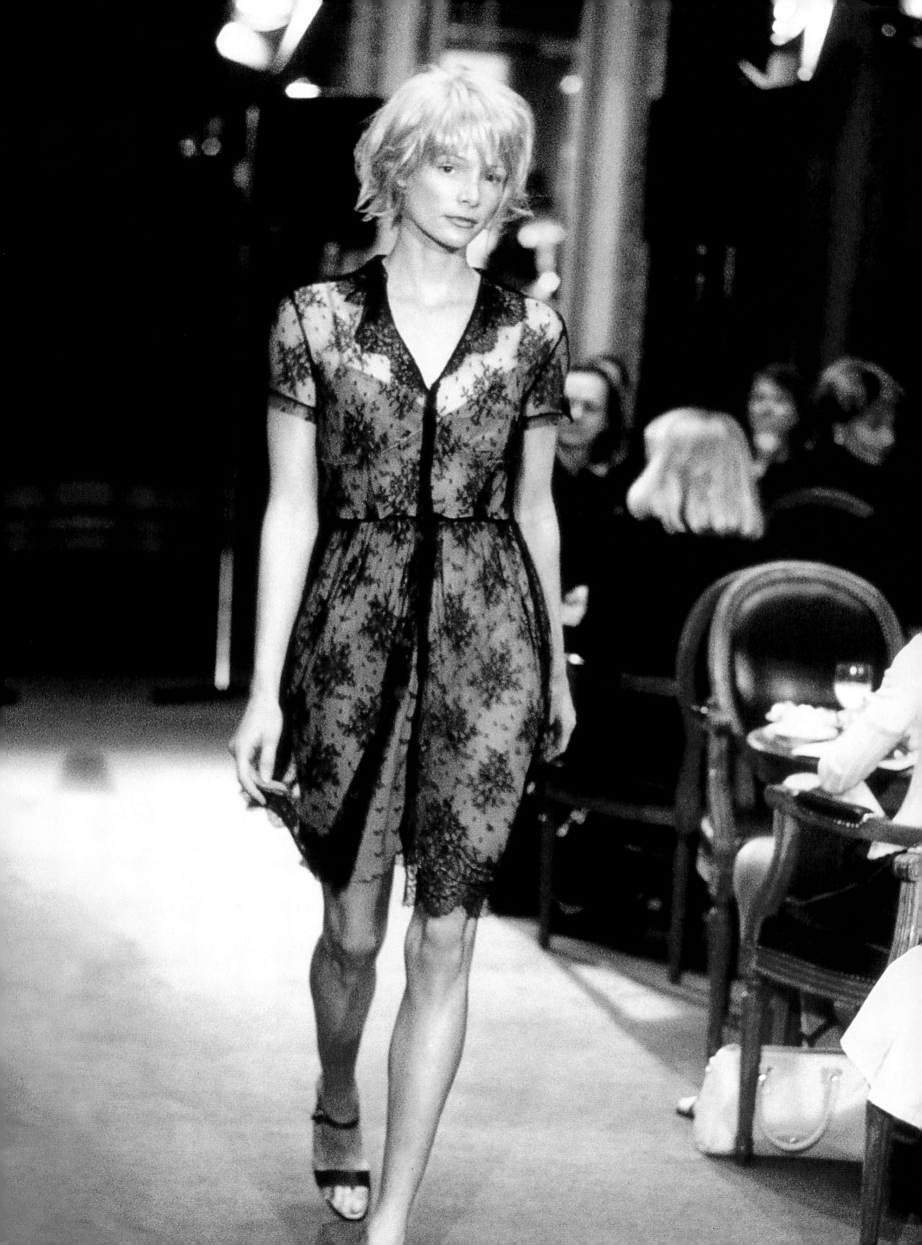

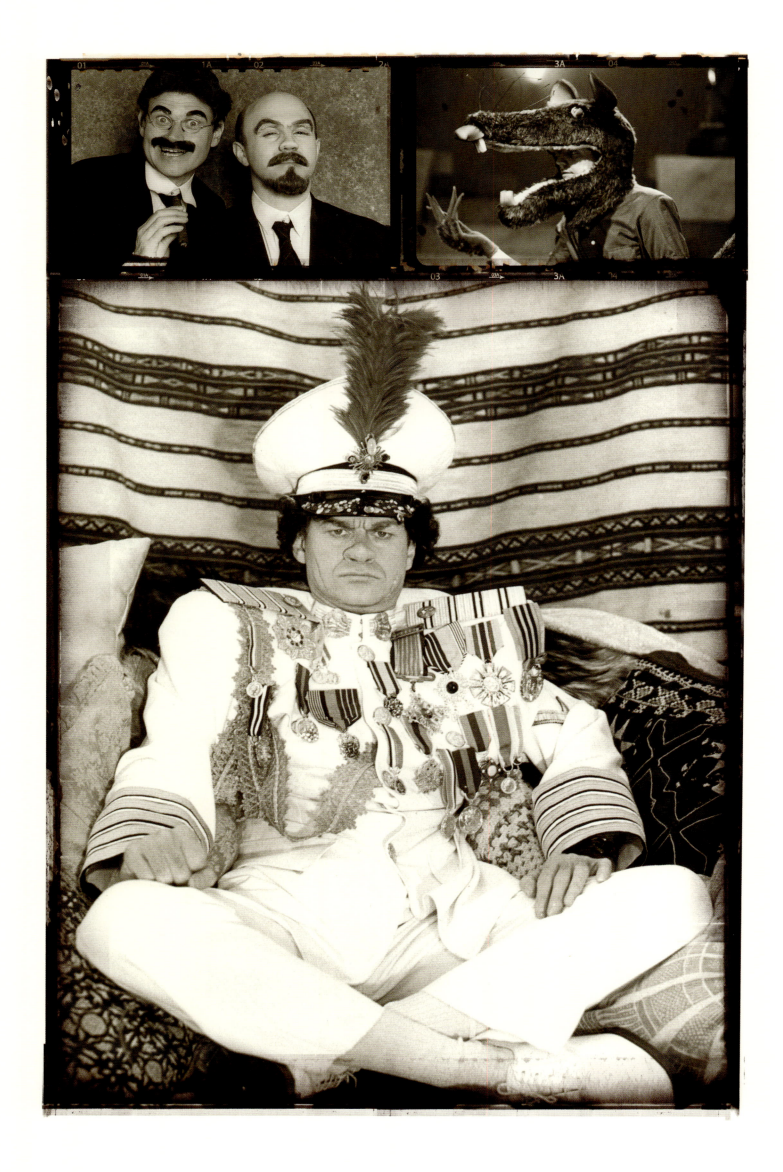

I ended up working for the ABC for a couple of years. It was such great experience, as I was designing and making costumes for everything from period dramas to comedy shows like The Dingo Principle, *a political satire featuring Jonathan Biggins, Phil Scott and Drew Forsythe.*

That was a real challenge – it wasn't so much about designing as being resourceful, as I had to make all of the costumes on a shoestring budget. The skills I learnt there, making intricate period costumes and the like, have stood me in good stead over the years.

Through my friend Joy Smithers, I also started to meet a lot of people in the music industry, and to do some freelance work designing and making costumes for rock bands. In those days, video clips could really make or break a band, and I worked with lots of well-known Australian bands, including the Eurogliders, whom Joy had joined as a backup singer. I started dating Bernie Lynch, from the band (we later married, then divorced amicably).

At that stage I had more of a connection to the music industry than to the fashion industry. They were heady days – singers were going wild on stage, and the costumes weren't just nice sparkly dresses, but real costumes, very showy. The lead singers all had an opinion about how they wanted to look, and it was really exciting working with them. I met a lot of people in the music industry, including Michael Hutchence, the late lead singer of INXS, whose then partner, Helena Christensen, has become a close friend.

I also met Kylie Minogue backstage at the Royal Bicentennial Concert at the Entertainment Centre in 1988, where the Eurogliders and others were playing for Prince Charles and Princess Diana. Joy snuck me in, as wardrobe mistress. Kylie was with her mother, wearing

a white Studibaker Hawk dress, and she had long blonde ringlets. When she found out I was a designer, she asked, 'Can you help me? Do I look okay?'

I also started to do some freelance work in the film industry. It was a very exciting, creative time. I decided to give up my job at the ABC and just focus on my freelance work. Music has always been a big influence in my life, and that early experience with music and film meant that when I staged fashion shows later on I wanted them to be theatrical, spectacular even. Unfortunately, my film work started to dry up when the Government introduced changes to the film industry, restricting the tax breaks. The film industry flagged, and lots of people found themselves looking for work – myself included.

At that time I was sharing a studio in Surry Hills with some other artists, and I started to make beautiful silk lingerie, really just because I needed something to do. I didn't consciously set out to design a lingerie collection – it was just something I gravitated towards, because I loved beautiful fabrics. I had collected vintage lace, silks and trims from the 1930s, so I started making silk chiffon knickers and crepe de Chine chemises as gifts for friends – a bit like trousseau pieces. I had a friend, Nikki Andrews at *Mode* magazine, who asked me to bring some pieces in, and before long I was taking orders from editors and other staff, then going back to my studio and making them up. I did all the sewing myself. When I first started, I was making about one piece a week. It soon grew to about five pieces, then twenty-five pieces a week, as word spread.

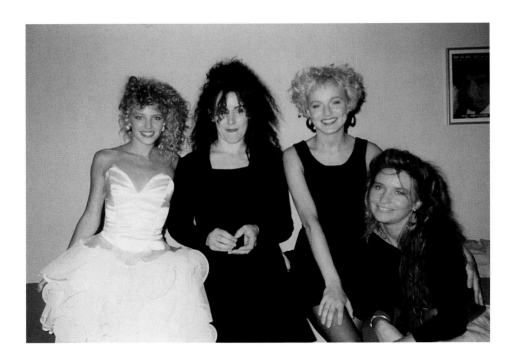

*Above: Backstage at the Royal Bicentennial Concert in 1988 with
Kylie Minogue, Grace Knight and Joy Smithers of the Eurogliders,
who had all just performed for Prince Charles and Princess Diana.*

My first real break came when Susan Owens of *The Sydney Morning Herald* wrote a piece on my lingerie. At the end of the article she said: 'If anyone is interested, please send a self-addressed envelope to receive a catalogue.' How times have changed – it's all about the database now. I received literally thousands of letters from people wanting me to custom-make lingerie pieces for them. I started trying to sell my lingerie to retailers, but there just wasn't a market for it in Australia at that time. I was trying to create luxury pieces that would last a lifetime – it was all about the cut, and mixing silk with beautiful, antique laces. I sometimes meet people today who tell me they have kept those early pieces as heirlooms as they are so beautiful.

Not long after that I went with Bernie on a trip to New York, where he had a recording deal. While I was there I visited Barneys, the famous department store on 17th Street and Seventh Avenue. It was the most beautiful store, and I could just picture my lingerie there. So, when we returned to Sydney, I started to make a lingerie collection especially for Barneys – not that they knew it!

When I was in New York I had made a note of the fax number of what I thought was the Barneys buying department, and I started sending them faxes nearly every day, trying to get an appointment. As it turned out, it was not the buyers but the doorman I was faxing! On the first Friday of the month, the Barneys buyers would meet prospective designers, who waited with suitcases full of samples in queues stretching for blocks. When I arrived back in New York, the Barneys doorman made sure that I went straight to the front of the queue.

To my delight, the buyers loved my collection, and they asked to stock it exclusively; they bought as much as I could make. After they placed their order, they told me that the doorman had admired my persistence, and thought my designs were quite good. I owe a lot to that doorman.

I remember being so excited on the day Barneys called to tell me they were running a half-page advertisement

---

Opposite: I was a keen photographer from an early age.

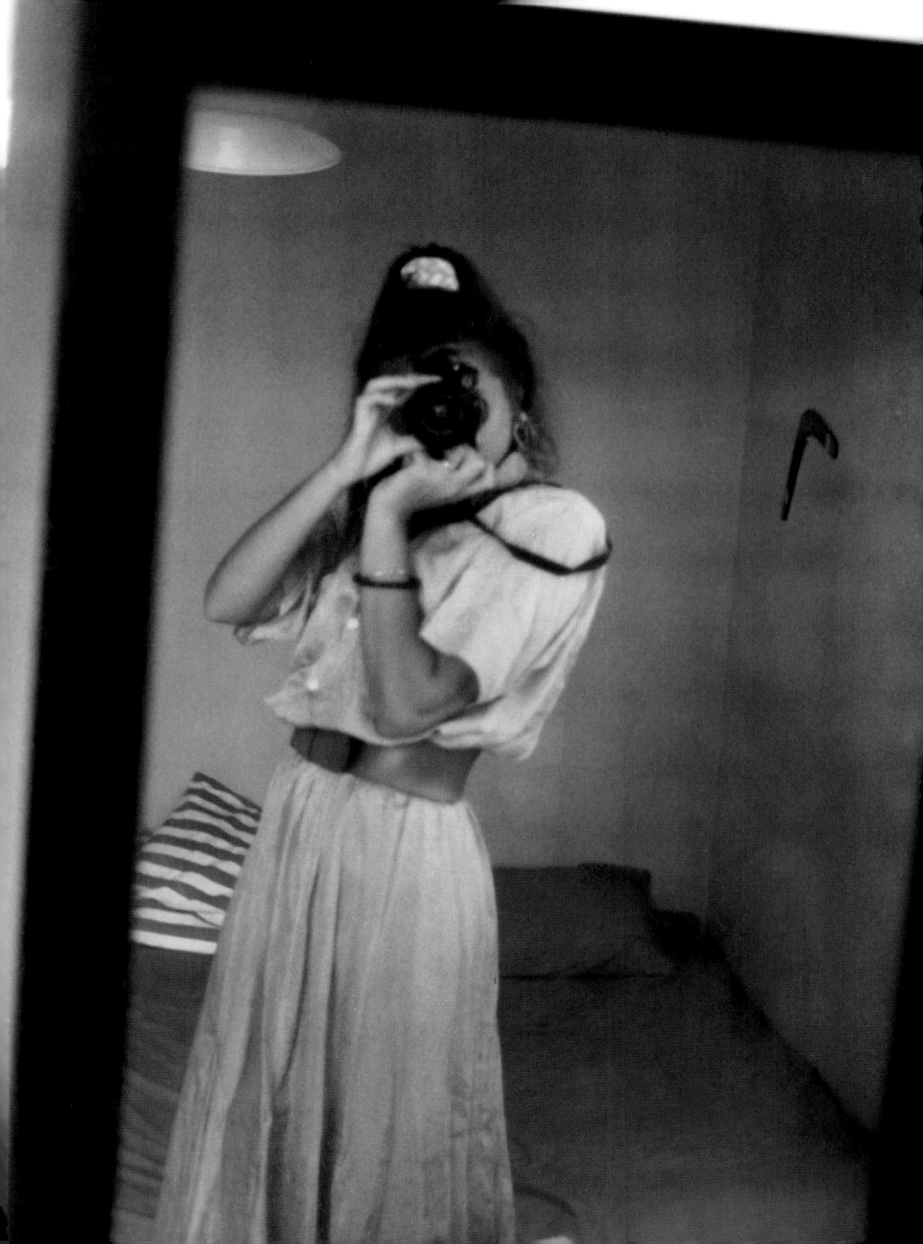

Lingerie look puts designer on Paris catwalks

By MAGGIE ALDERSON

A pair of exquisite lace knickers from Collette Dinnigan's Paddington shop cost around $100. She admits the price "makes some husbands faint", but this no ordinary underwear. It has the seal of approval from the most august of fashion institutions, the Chambre Syndicale in Paris.

This body decides which designers are good enough to be allowed to present their parades alongside the likes of Chanel, Yves Saint Laurent and Valentino, during the Paris ready-to-wear shows in March and October.

Collette Dinnigan is the first Australian designer to be accepted. So it is no surprise that one of her dresses — which she describes as a "school dress" (retailing at $520) — has been selected this year for the Powerhouse Museum-*Sydney Morning Herald* Fashion of the Year, announced last night.

Four outfits were chosen by a panel comprising two curators from the Powerhouse, *Vogue's* editor, Nancy Pilcher, and the *Herald's* fashion and style editor, Jane de Teliga.

Dinnigan's dress will join the permanent costume collection beside outfits from the Melbourne label Saba and two Italian designers: fashion's current favourite, Prada, and Giorgio Armani.

"It's amazing to be in the same selection as Armani," said Dinnigan, who has been in business for seven years. "It's like saying you are as good as him. But of course, at 30, I am much younger and I still have a long way to go. Also, it's really exciting to be in a museum collection. It's never going to go away."

Trained in New Zealand, Dinnigan hand-made exquisite lingerie for private orders before moving into outer wear. She made a big international impact in a very short time with her lacy, lingerie-inspired designs, now worth $200,000 a year in exports.

They are sold in the elite shops of New York, Los Angeles, London, Singapore and Tokyo. **GOOD LIVING 7: Designs for the archives.**

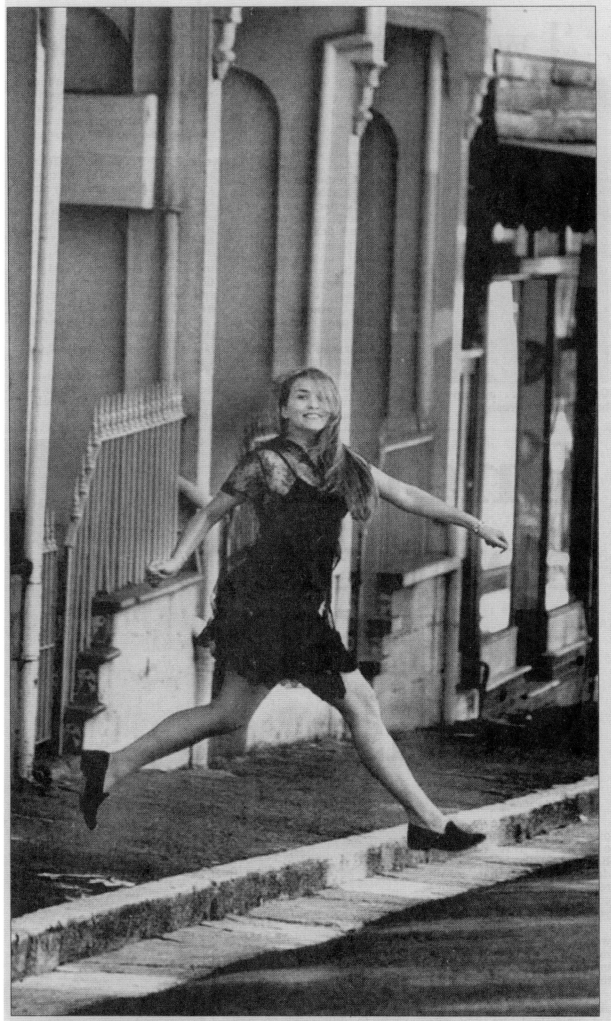

Collette Dinnigan in the $520 "school dress" on show at the Powerhouse. Photograph by GLENN SHIPLEY

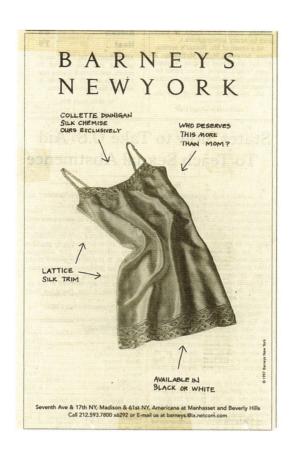

BARNEYS
NEWYORK

COLLETTE DINNIGAN
SILK CHEMISE
OURS EXCLUSIVELY

WHO DESERVES
THIS MORE
THAN MOM?

LATTICE
SILK TRIM

AVAILABLE IN
BLACK OR WHITE

Seventh Ave & 17th NY, Madison & 61st NY, Americana at Manhasset and Beverly Hills
Call 212.593.7800 x6292 or E-mail us at barneys.@ix.netcom.com

*Above: Barneys in New York was the first international store to stock my
clothes. This is an ad they ran for my lingerie in* The New York Times *in 1996.*

for my lingerie in *The New York Times* for Valentine's Day. At that stage it was just me and one machinist, helping me with the sewing. I included in the collection stretch satin corsets that could be worn under a jacket for evening. Barneys sold them in their lingerie department. The first celebrity to buy a piece was Cindy Crawford, then Madonna wore one of my corsets in a film clip. I started to branch out from lingerie, making pretty little lace skirts to wear with fitted skirts underneath, and some sheer lace tops. I was also doing slips, which looked great under the sheer bias-cut dresses in fashion at the time. Soon I started doing print dresses as well.

Before long, Mary Gallagher from Harvey Nichols in London saw my clothes in Barneys, and soon Harvey Nichols started buying them too. I had a lot of support in London in my early days from Josephine and Peter Turner, who owned the store A la Mode. They would host evenings for me where they invited influential people such as Jerry Hall, Olivia Harrison (George's wife), Kay Saatchi and Gael Boglione, the gorgeous Aussie ex-model

who knows everybody in London, and has since become a close friend. I also received a lot of support from the British press, especially Alexandra Shulman, the editor of British *Vogue*, and Hilary Alexander, the fashion editor of the *Daily Telegraph*.

Joyce Ma, owner of the legendary Joyce Boutique in Hong Kong, also started to buy my clothes. Before long I was travelling to New York, London, Paris and Hong Kong, selling. My clothes weren't part of that 1990s grunge look – what I was doing was quite different; it was fresh, and a bit complicated to wear, with all the layers. People also liked the fact that I was reinventing lace. Not everyone had the courage to wear my clothes though; the Americans especially had trouble with the concept of wearing what to them looked like underwear. A little later the great Liz Tilberis, editor of *Harper's Bazaar*, credited me with being the designer who turned underwear into outerwear. One of my proudest moments was when Bridget Foley, then editor of *Women's Wear Daily*, the fashion bible for the United States,

*Opposite: A piece by fashion editor Maggie Alderson in
the* Sydney Morning Herald *in 1996, not long after my
first show in Paris. I am on William Street, Paddington
in Sydney, where I opened my first shop on Valentine's
Day, 1992.*

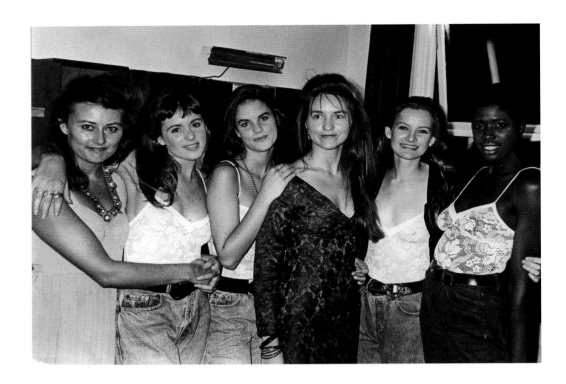

Above: My first ever show at the Alice Motel, Tamarama,
Sydney, in 1991. Jewellery designer Victoria Spring,
who helped me with the show, is on the far left.

put one of my lace dresses on its cover and gave us a double-page spread.

Meanwhile, back in Australia, I held my first show in 1991, at the Alice Motel in Tamarama. The models were from East Sydney Technical College, and I made thick clear plastic dresses for them to wear over stretch lace bodysuits. I also made 1950s-style corsetry, with embellishments, like shells and glass beads, which a friend, Victoria Spring, a talented designer of vintage-style jewellery, helped me with. I am still not sure exactly what prompted me to do a show just then, but we sent out a hundred invitations and one hundred and one people turned up. I was young, and lots of my friends came to support me. Later, many of those bodysuits were used in video clips – they were perfect for the stage.

Despite the fact that my overseas business was growing, I was still unable to persuade Australian retailers to stock my underwear and clothes. Back in the nineties, everyone wanted known labels, like Gucci, or Prada. So on Valentine's Day 1992, aged twenty-seven, I opened my own store, in William Street, Paddington, in Sydney. Victoria Spring really motivated me to do it, lending me the bond money. Bernie and I lived above the shop, and I used to dye my fabrics on the kitchen stove at night – all of our pots and pans were permanently tinted. I had no other financial backers, and no one else working for me – I did it all myself, selling in the shop by day and cutting out clothes at night. It was really hard work, seven days a week.

I would outsource some things, like bodysuits, but other than that I was making everything myself – lace dresses, silk jersey pyjama-style pants and tops – I did all the first samples and the cutting. Eventually I could afford to hire a sample machinist, then a cutter, and finally someone to help me in the shop. At night, after the shop was closed,

Opposite: Underwear as outerwear – Vogue Australia
editorial on one of my stretch-satin corsets, designed
to be worn under an evening jacket.

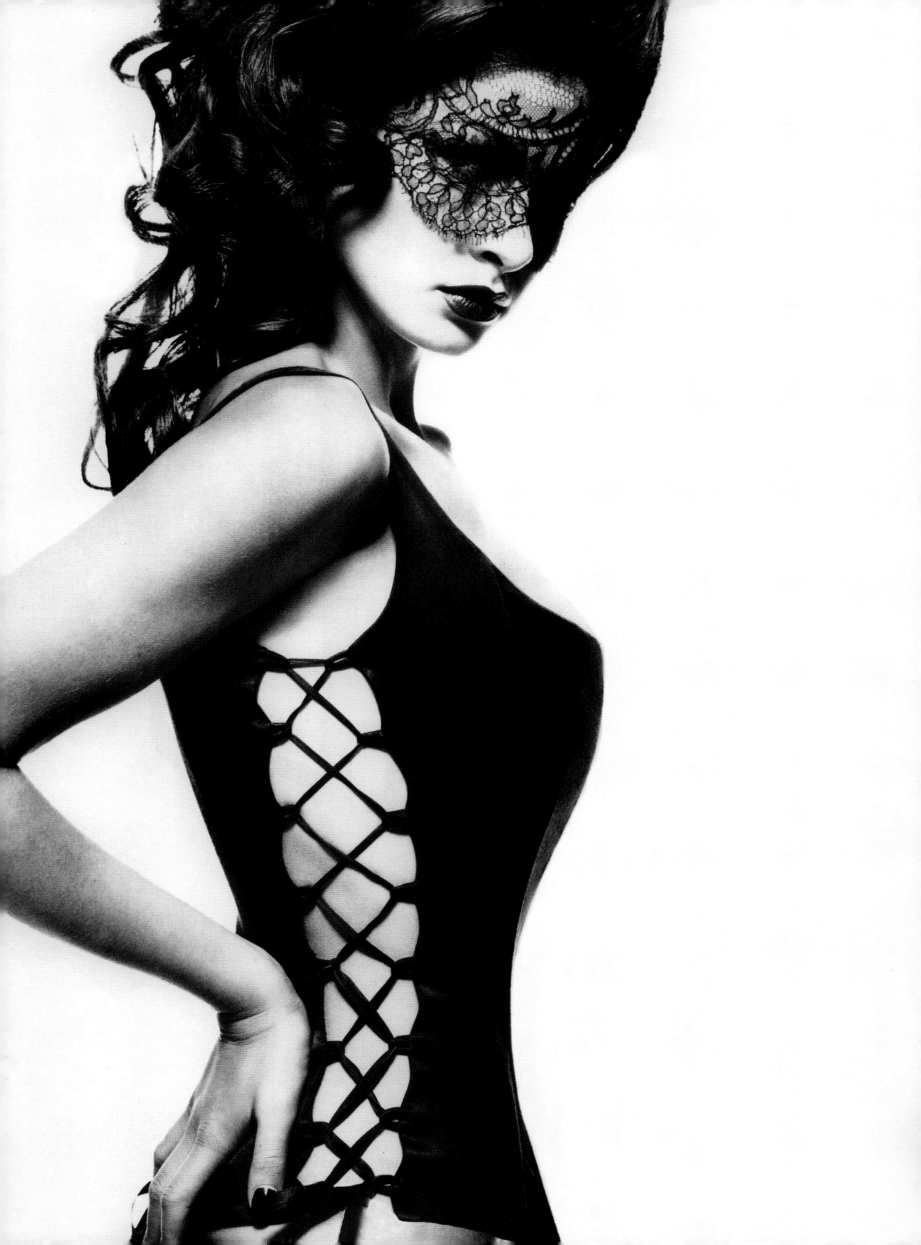

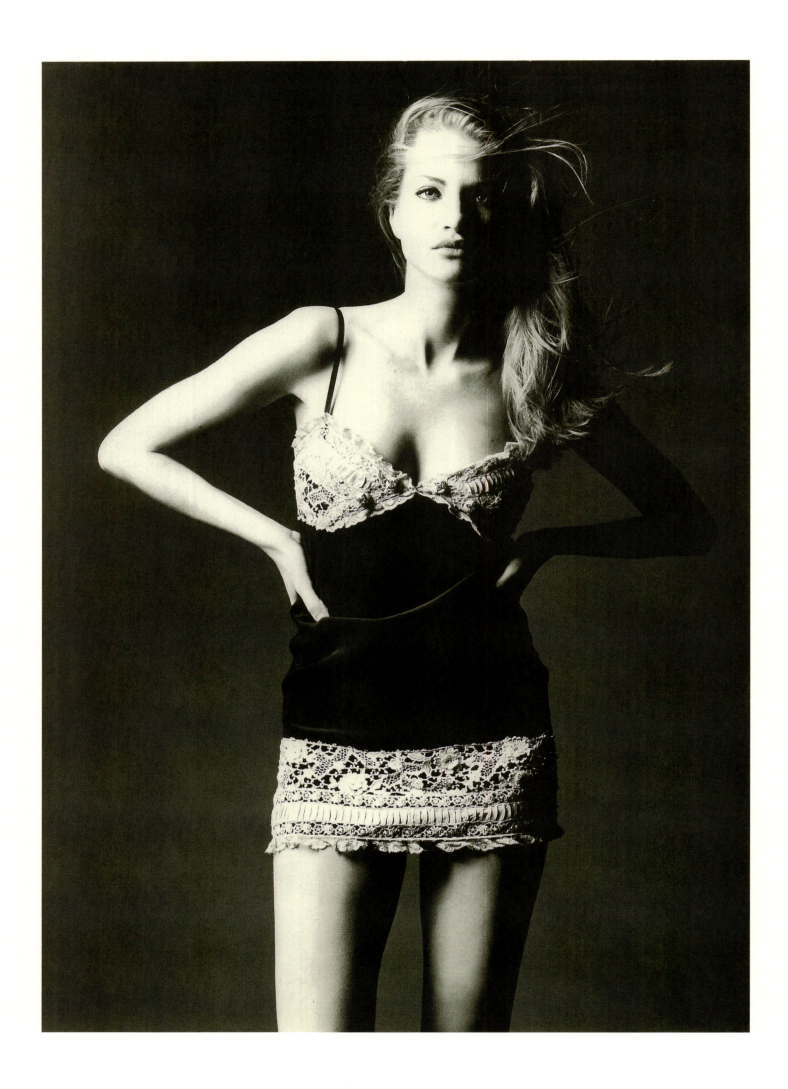

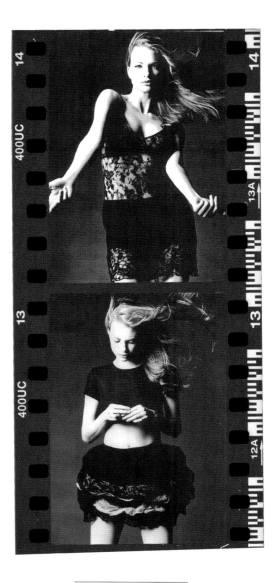

*Above and opposite: One of my first photoshoots in Paris,
in 1996, styled by Bibi Monnahan.*

we would sit around with a glass of wine and some cheese and crackers and discuss what had happened in the shop that day – the customers, what we had sold – everything about the business. How things have changed – our management meetings now have agendas and minutes!

So, that was how it all began. Today I have stores in Sydney and Melbourne, and I opened one in Chelsea in London in 2000. That was quite a milestone. I love London, and have many close friends there, and we also have a lot of English customers. My clothes are now sold in over one hundred stores around the world, including in Russia and the Middle East, both of which are growing markets, and my name appears on credit card statements the world over. Who would have thought?

One of the reasons I started my own business was that I thought it would give me the freedom and independence I had as a child. I couldn't face the prospect of a nine-to-five desk job, and thought that I wouldn't have to work so hard if I worked for myself. Ironically, as it has turned out, building my own business has been extremely hard work and I am still, today, accountable, and focussed, and across it all every minute of the day.

When I talk to other people with their own businesses, they say the same thing – we all want to make it work, to achieve something; it's instinctive. You do it because you're passionate and because you care.

Most sexy
so silky can't
get enough
Just have fun
and be adored

Collette
Dinnigan.

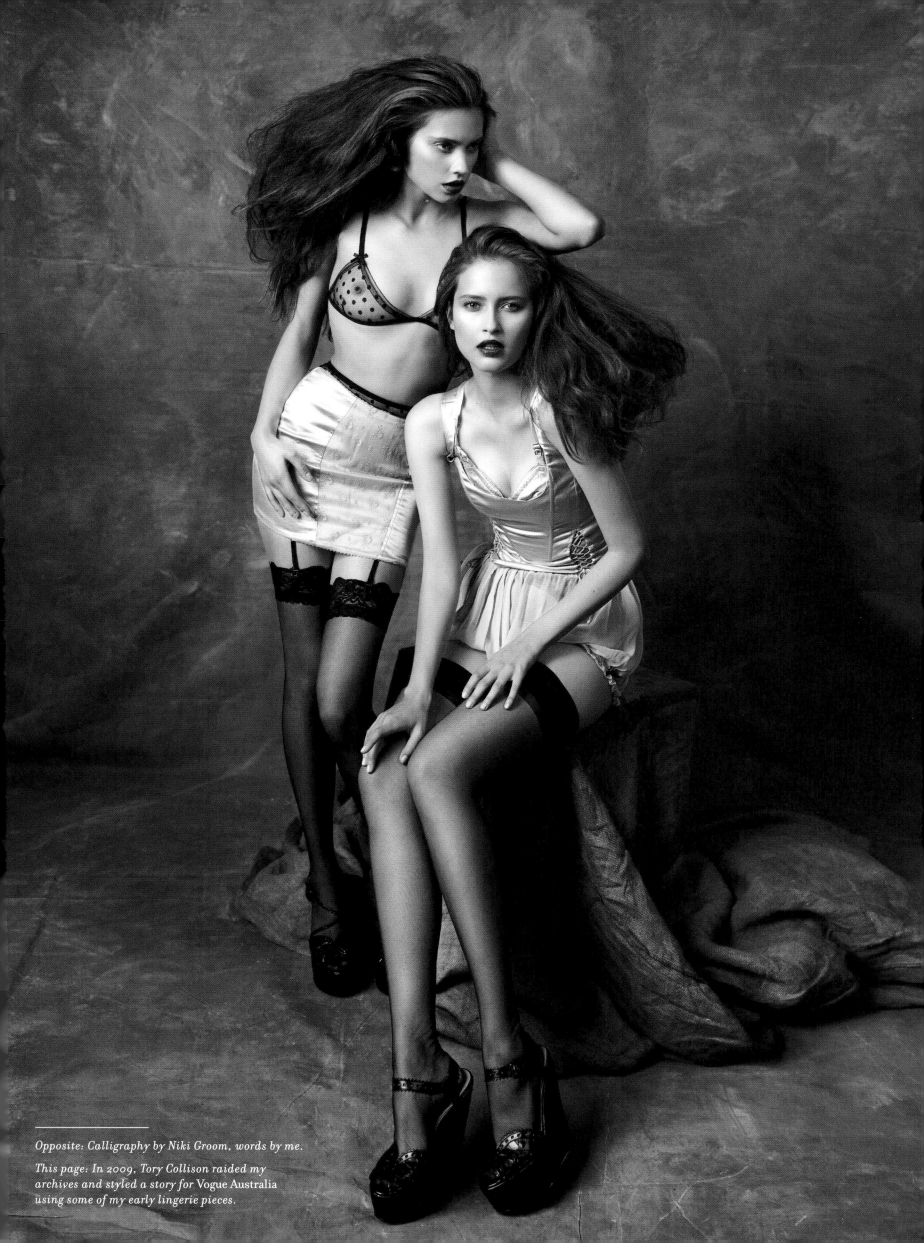

Opposite: Calligraphy by Niki Groom, words by me.

This page: In 2009, Tory Collison raided my archives and styled a story for Vogue Australia using some of my early lingerie pieces.

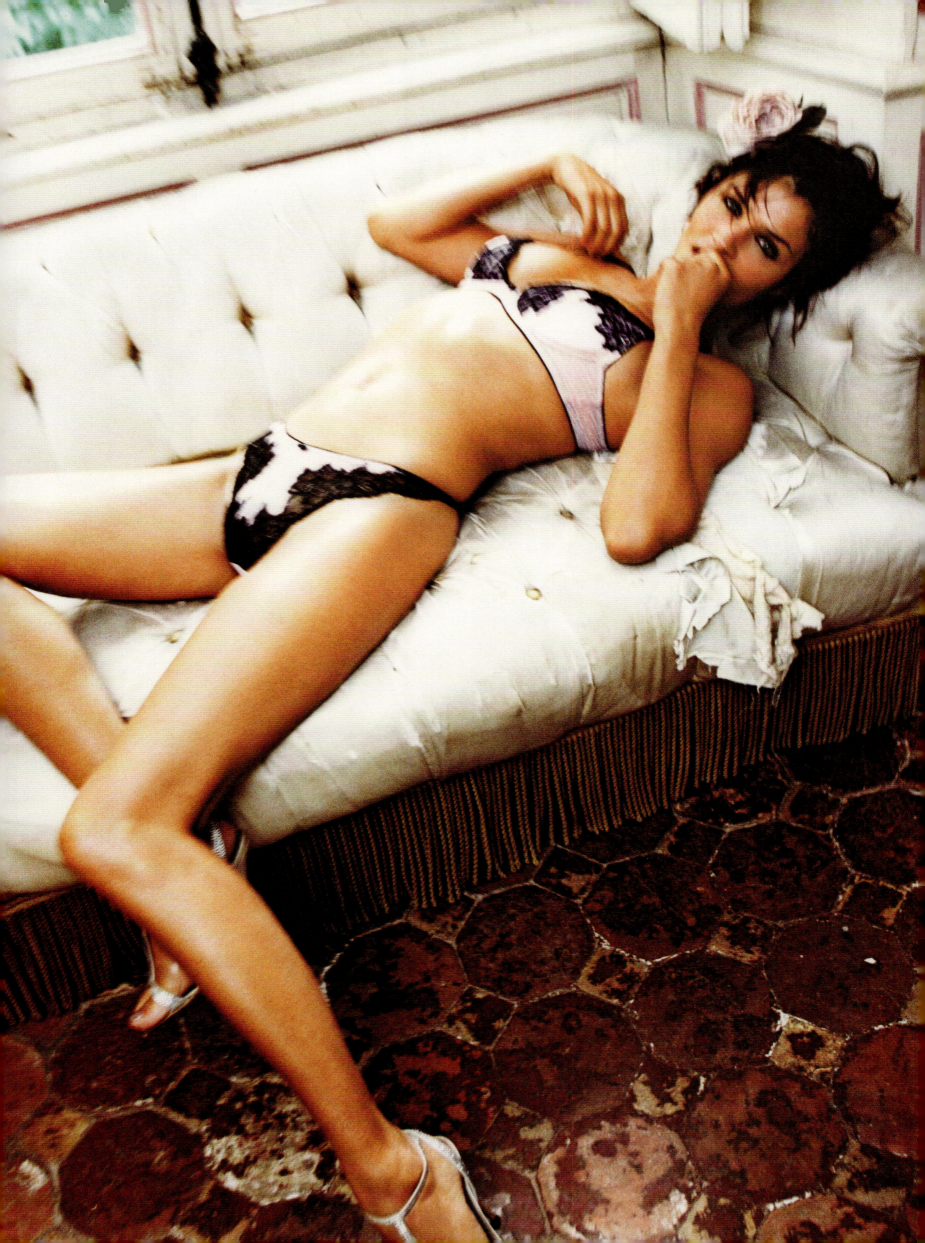

FOR YOUR EYES ONLY

Yes, dry-clean-only lingerie;

Helena Christensen;

Ellen von Unwerth.

HOW IT ALL BEGAN

CHAPTER 3

My business started almost by accident,

with me simply doing something I loved

— MAKING BEAUTIFUL,

UNIQUE PIECES OF

SILK LINGERIE BY HAND.

When you love something, you gravitate

towards it, there's a natural affinity.

I was really outdoorsy, and active,

so working with small, vintage

pieces was a kind of escapism for me.

THROUGH WORD OF MOUTH,

I STARTED TO GET COMMISSIONS,

AND IT ALL REALLY TOOK

OFF FROM THERE.

Because my lingerie was made of

FRENCH SILK AND

ANTIQUE LACE MY PIECES

ALL SAID 'DRY CLEAN ONLY'.

This caused quite a fuss, and many

people told me that it would never sell,

as it was too impractical.

I WAS DETERMINED

TO PROVE THEM WRONG.

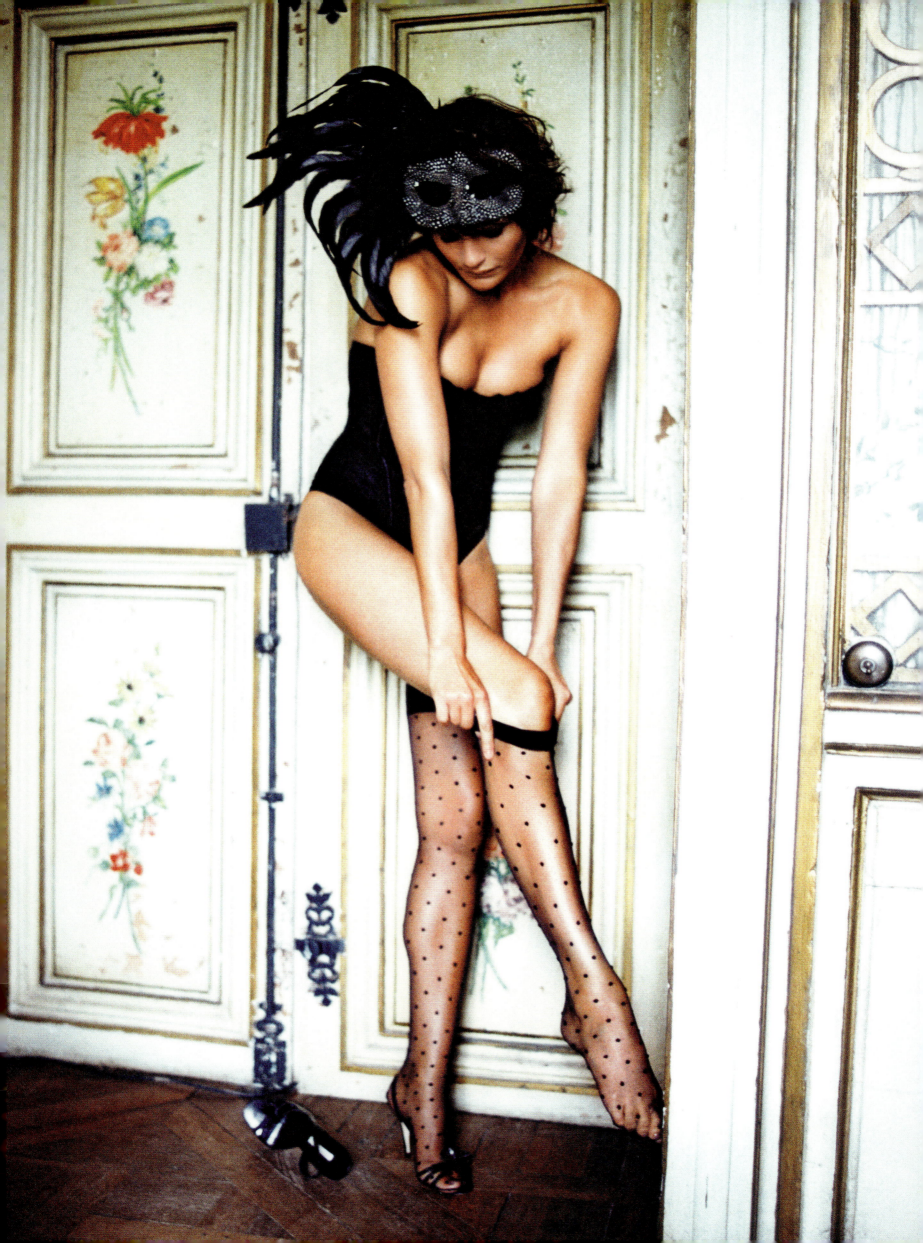

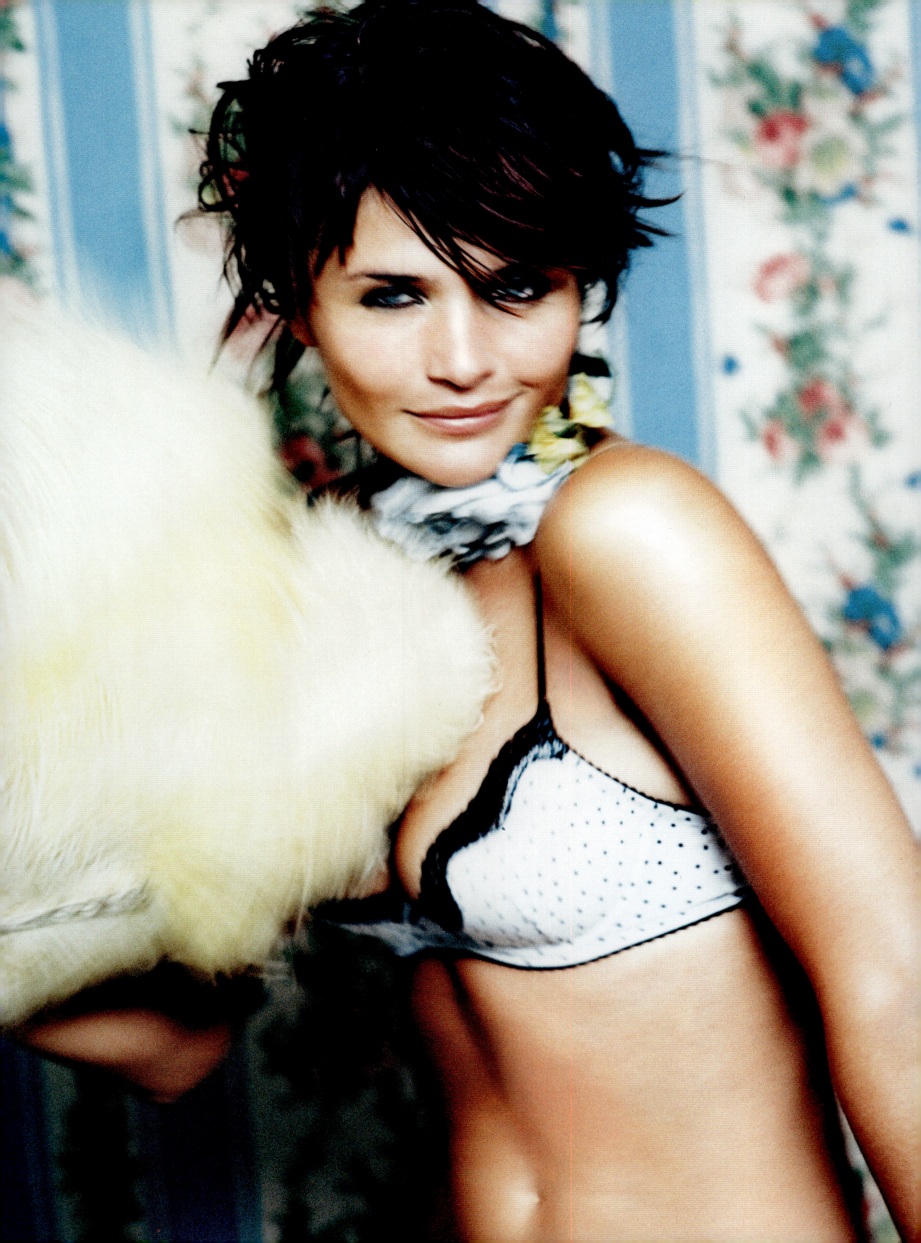

As it turned out, it was the wholesale buyers who didn't understand

what I was trying to do – the people who actually bought my pieces loved them.

It was all about the look – it wasn't meant to be functional, everyday underwear,

but more about making something which made the wearer feel gorgeous.

I remember my first ever shoot – the group I shared a studio with in Surry Hills included a graphic designer and a photographer, and together we shot a catalogue of a friend, Angie Buttrose, modelling my lingerie at my brother Seamus's apartment in Rushcutter's Bay, on the fire escape stairs. At that time, I was cutting and making all the pieces myself. It was a true labour of love, as each bra had about twenty-eight pieces, and was appliquéd by hand. As I said, it took Australian buyers a while to catch on – my lingerie had been sold in New York and London for about three years before it was available here. The more people came to know me and my work, the more the business grew, and soon people started wearing my underwear as outerwear – silk pyjamas as evening pants, silk nightdresses as dresses. Before long I was making dresses as well.

Given that I had started my business designing and making silk lingerie, it was a real thrill when Marks & Spencer asked me in 2001 to design an exclusive range of lingerie for them. As with everything I work on, I was heavily involved in the whole project, from creating the marketing and public relations strategy to designing the packaging. I have always felt that there is no

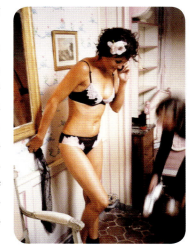

point in creating beautiful garments but having no say in how they are marketed. I worked closely with Marks & Spencer for about a year. I wanted this collection to be a knockout – for people to stop and look in the windows and think 'Wow!'. I originally planned to call it Wild Cherry, but I found out that there was a pornographic website called that, so I opted for Wild Hearts instead.

I knew immediately who I wanted to model the lingerie – the gorgeous Helena Christensen. She and I had met through Michael Hutchence years before, and she had since done many shoots and shows for me, so we had become close friends. She knew my work and trusted me. She had just the look I was after – she was seductive and feminine, and also a real woman, not too thin – she had just had her son, Mingus, six months earlier. She wasn't modelling at the time, and had told me that she didn't want to go back to it, but she agreed to do this collection for me.

There was never any doubt in my mind about who I wanted to photograph the collection – Ellen von Unwerth, who had shot my clothes before. It's difficult to photograph lingerie in a feminine, sexy and fun way; you want to see the body and the lingerie, but it shouldn't

Pages 40, 43 and opposite: Exquisite Helena Christensen, shot by Ellen von Unwerth, modelling my first Wild Hearts lingerie range for Marks & Spencer in a French château, six months after giving birth to her son, Mingus.

Above: Helena on the phone, between shots. Taken by me.

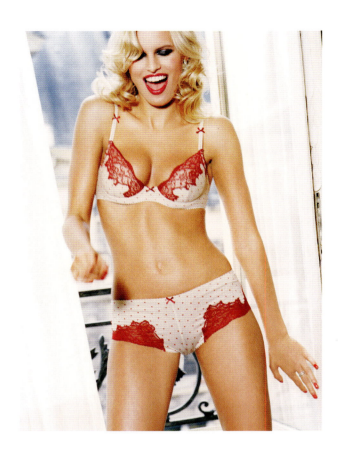

*Above: Karolina Kurkova in a shoot for a later
Wild Hearts collection for Marks & Spencer.
Photograph by Ellen von Unwerth.*

look too cheesy. When Ellen agreed to do it, I was thrilled. I had always been a fan of her work and knew that she could convey the look I wanted – sexy, confident and full of life. It took a bit of persuasion for me to convince Marks & Spencer, as they had never worked with a model or photographer of that calibre before, but eventually they agreed. The campaign became a real milestone for them.

In the end, it was a great collaboration – we all worked extremely hard, but it was worth it. The collection was a big commercial success for Marks & Spencer, and it was also great exposure for me. We got a lot of press, because it was Helena's first shoot since she'd had her baby, and also because it was something very different for Marks & Spencer. It was risky for them because it was raunchy and provocative, but in the end it changed the perception of their brand (in a good way); it made them look innovative, and it attracted a new, fashion-conscious customer. Alexandra Shulman, the editor of British *Vogue*, said at the

time, 'I might not shop for anything else at Marks & Spencer, but why not buy my sandwiches and lingerie there?'

I have since done more collections for Marks & Spencer. I have never compromised on quality – I have always tried to use silk and French laces, which they had never used in their lingerie before, and to make the cups sexy, practical and comfortable.

In 2008 I was asked by Target Australia to design a range of affordable quality lingerie for them. I called it Wild Hearts as well, and once again used my signature lace, embroidery and silk.

I keep designing lingerie because I love it. I have recently started a bridal collection; it is not overtly sexy, but it's meant to make the bride feel fabulous. I don't design lingerie to appeal to men – their idea of sexy underwear is probably a lot more red and black. I prefer to design pieces that are pretty and feminine – it is always for us.

*Opposite: Bridget Hall, in Wild Hearts.
Very distinctively Ellen von Unwerth.*

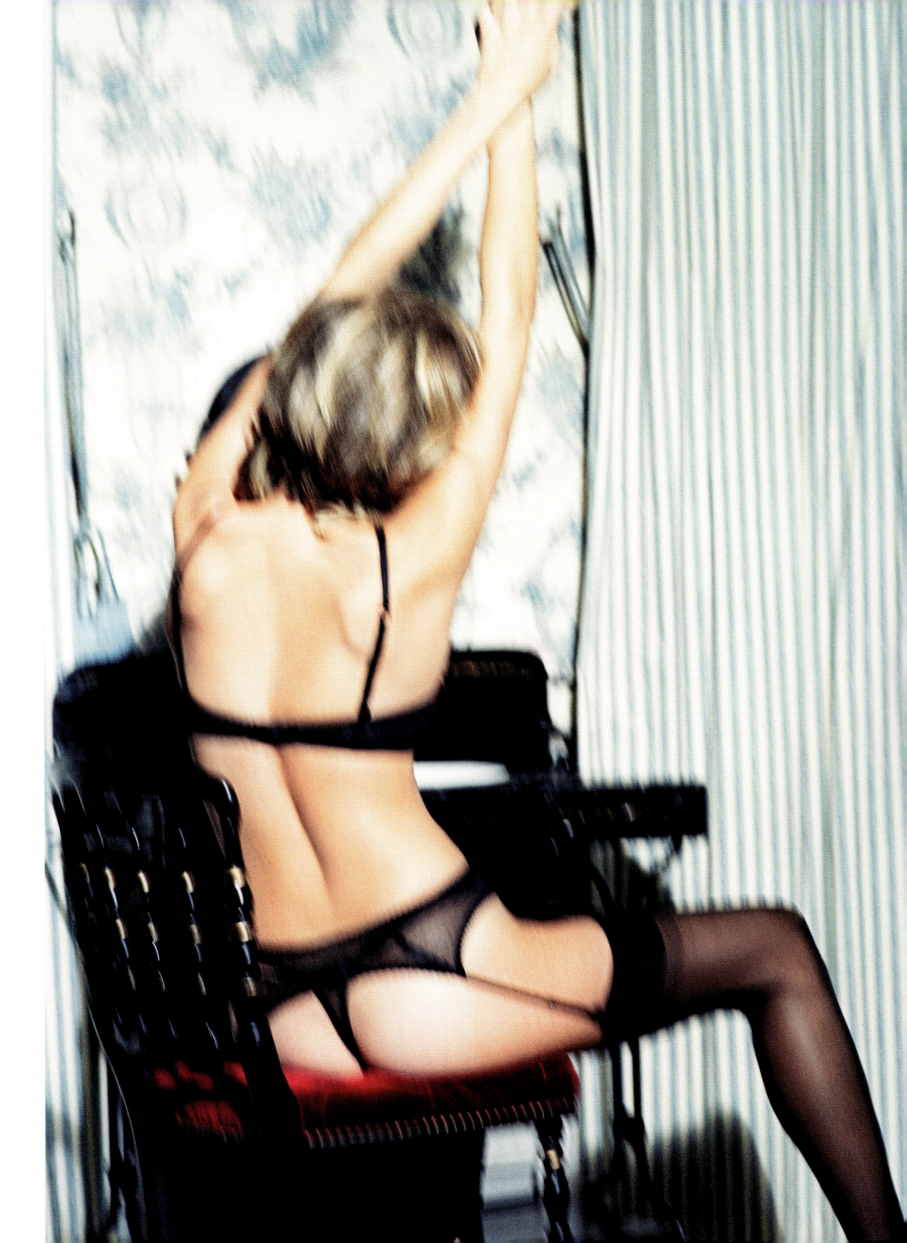

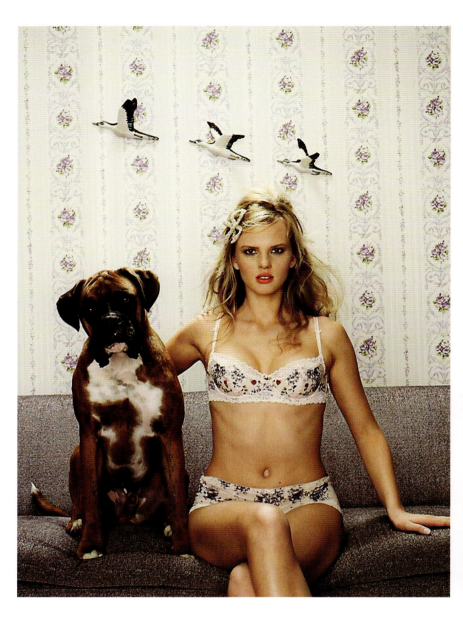

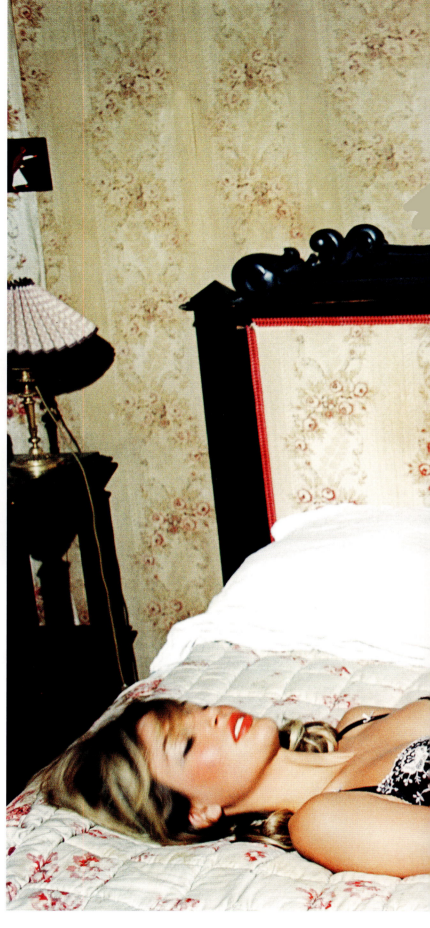

Above: Anne Vyalitsyna in Wild Hearts.

Opposite: Bridget Hall in Wild Hearts.
Photograph by Ellen von Unwerth.

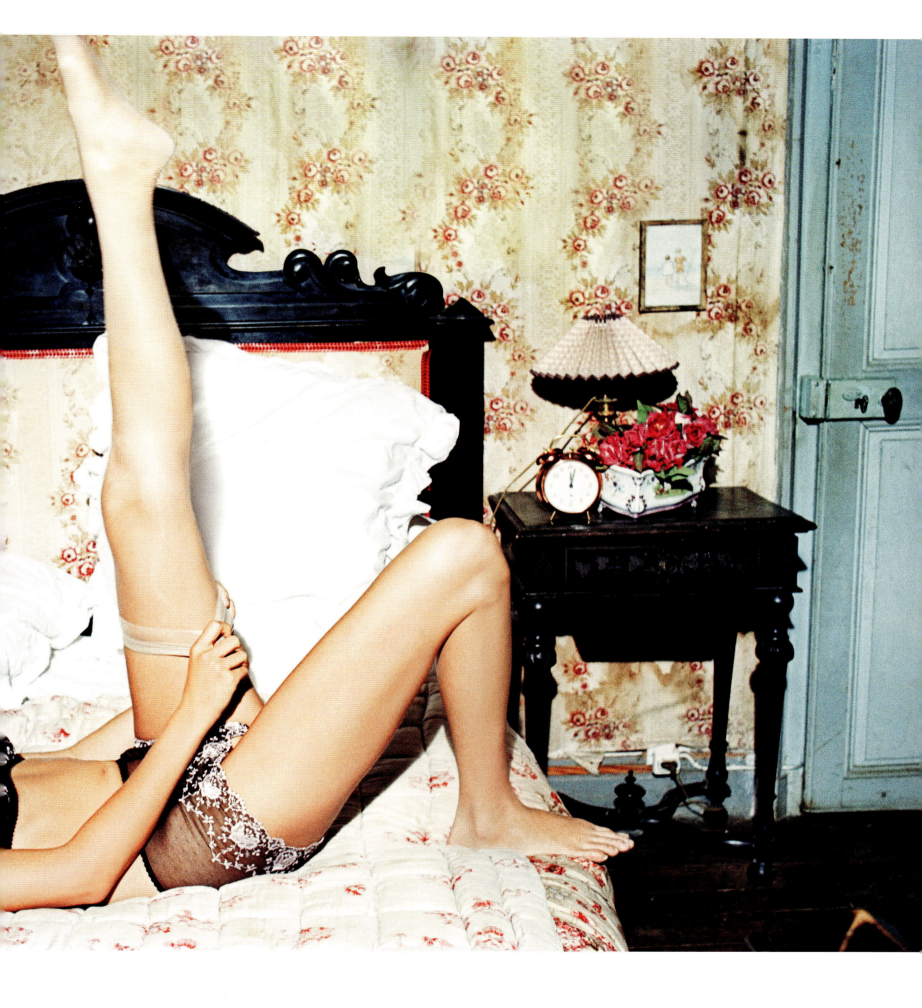

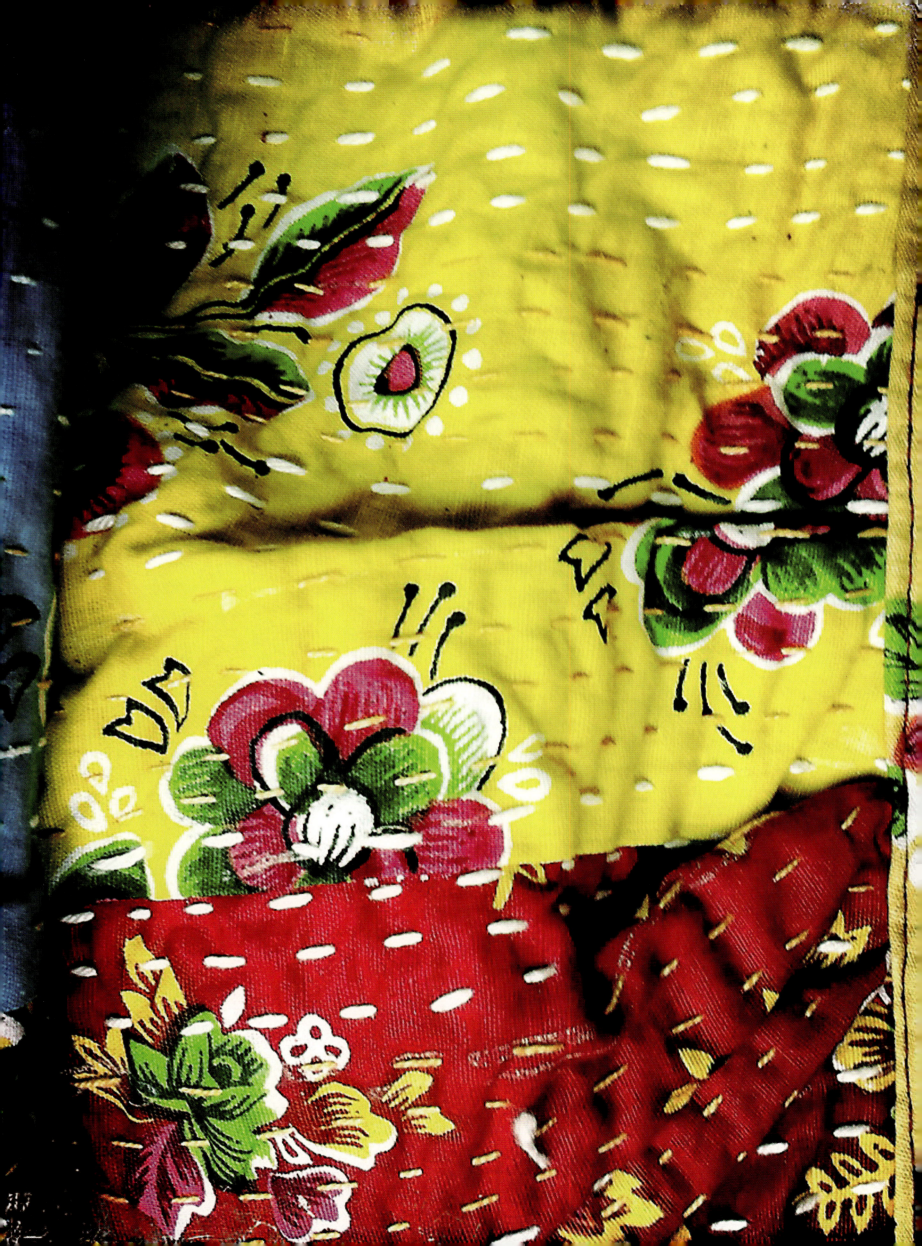

INDIA,
A
CALMING
CHAOS

Mumbai mash-up; the people,
the craft, the light; why I went
there in the beginning and
why it's still compelling.

IT'S A MAD, MAD WORLD

CHAPTER 4

I FIRST VISITED INDIA
ABOUT FIFTEEN YEARS AGO
with my friend, Tory Collison,
Vogue Australia *fashion editor,*
because Marion Hume told me about a
GREAT CRAFTSMAN CALLED
CHETAN WHO HAD A BEADING
AND EMBROIDERY FACTORY
IN MUMBAI. *It was about this time that*
I was starting to do more embellished
eveningwear, which required labour-intensive
hand-beading and embroidery,
SO I MADE AN APPOINTMENT
AND FLEW OVER TO MEET HIM.
Chetan had a small factory, WITH A
TEAM OF INCREDIBLY SKILLED
AND DEDICATED CRAFTSMEN
WORKING FOR HIM.
He and I hit it off straight away,
and that was the beginning of a long
working relationship and friendship.

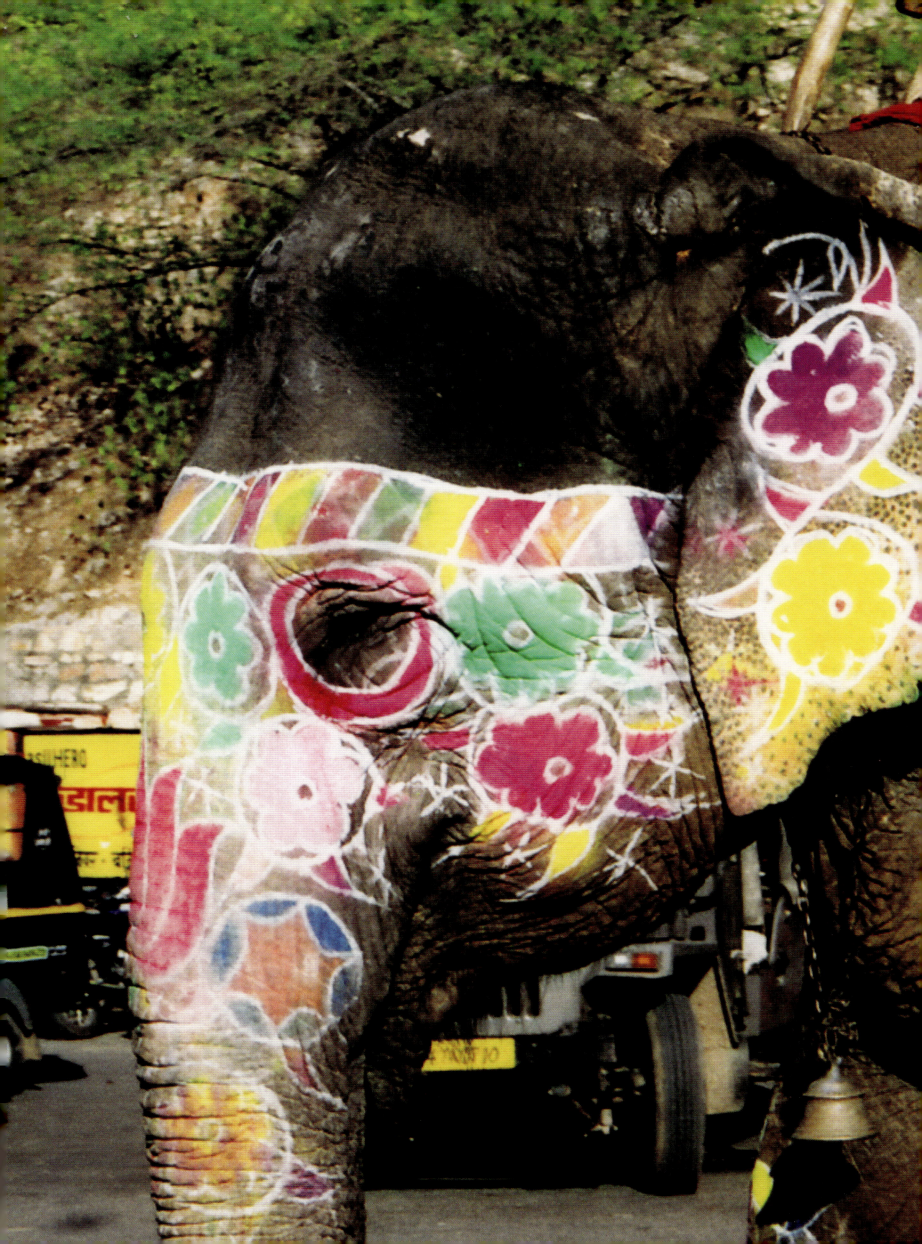

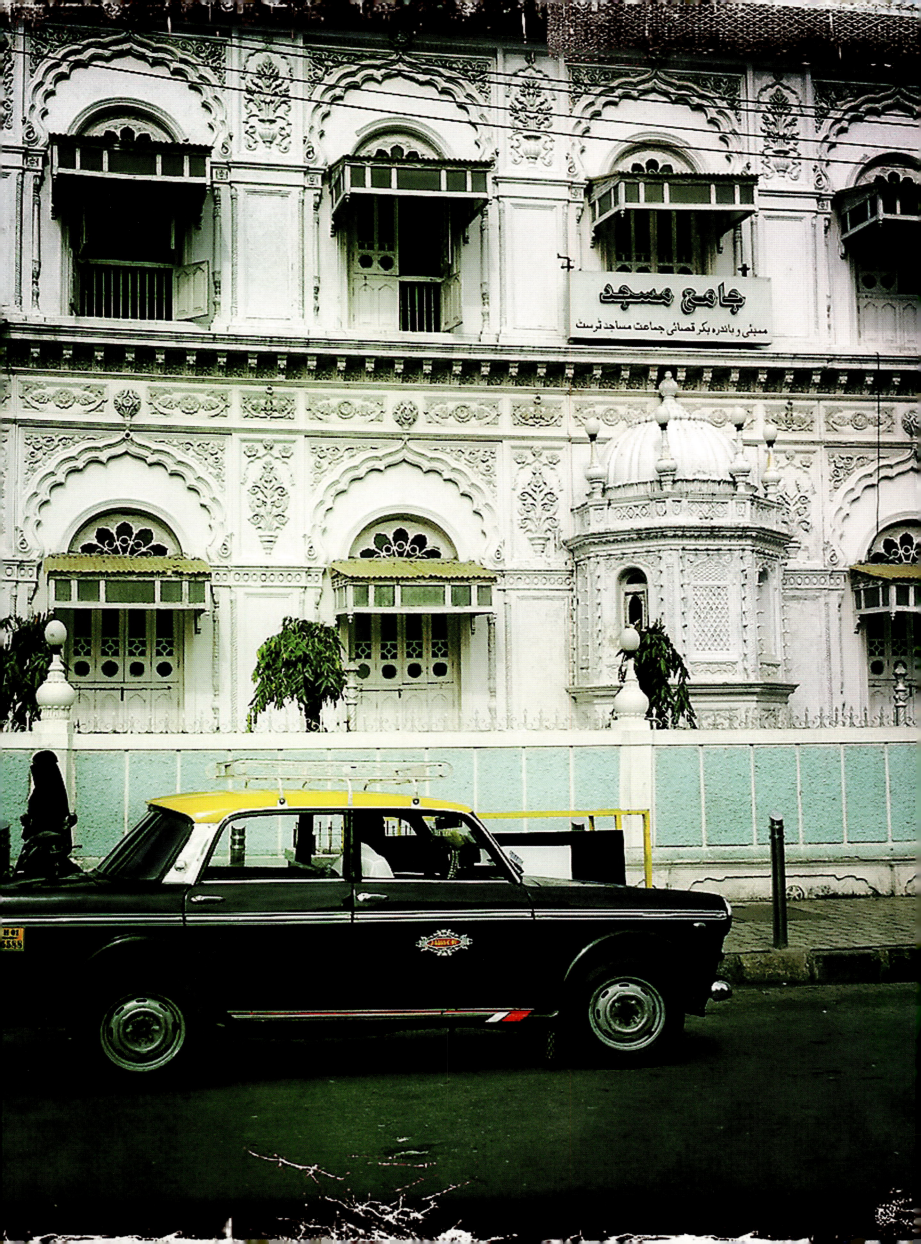

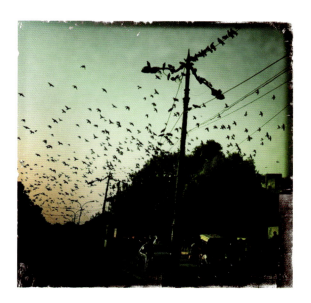

Today, Chetan's factory does most of the beading for my couture collection. We send him the fabrics, with markers to show where the beads are to go, then all the beading is done by hand. It is a long, painstaking process that takes months.

It is fascinating to watch the beaders at work. Their craftsmanship is truly unbelievable – it is passed down through the generations. You don't see beading or embroidery like it anywhere else in the world. They are absolute perfectionists. It is all quite surreal – these men travel in from their tiny villages to work in the factory, where they do amazingly ornate embroidery on luxury fabrics, then they return home to work on their farms.

When I met him, Chetan had done work for houses such as Christian Dior and Givenchy, but none of the designers had been to India to meet him – I was the first. Since then, Azzedine Alaia and others have started going over there, as they have realised how much more resourceful you can be working on the ground. Sadly though, things have changed from when I first visited, when the handcrafted work was so unique. Larger chain stores are starting to produce huge volumes of mass-market clothes, so there are more and more large factories, which rely upon machines rather than individual craftsmen. That means that some of those wonderful skills are starting to disappear. There is also the potential for exploitation – I am always very careful to try to make sure that the factories I deal with are professional and ethical, and treat their workers well.

I go to India for the craftsmanship, but also for everything else it has to offer – the saris, the markets, the ornaments, the metalwork, the buildings. I think it is the colours that inspire me the most. One of my early collections was inspired by the colours I saw at the markets in Rajasthan – the onion pinks (the late Diana Vreeland, former editor of *American Vogue*, once said that pink was the navy blue of India), and the vivid colours of the fruit and vegetables. There amid the chaos was this wonderful uniformity – everything was laid out by colour, so you would see someone selling only bananas on a green trolley, and somebody else selling only green beans or cucumbers, or lemons, with a vividly-painted blue door in the background. It was all so beautiful that it was almost poetic. The silks we had dyed later on were based on the colours of those fruits and vegetables.

Previous page: An ornately-decorated elephant on the streets of Rajasthan.

Opposite: Marine Drive, Mumbai, often referred to as 'Queen's necklace', because at night the street lights make it look a lot like a string of pearls.

Above: A flock of birds at nightfall.

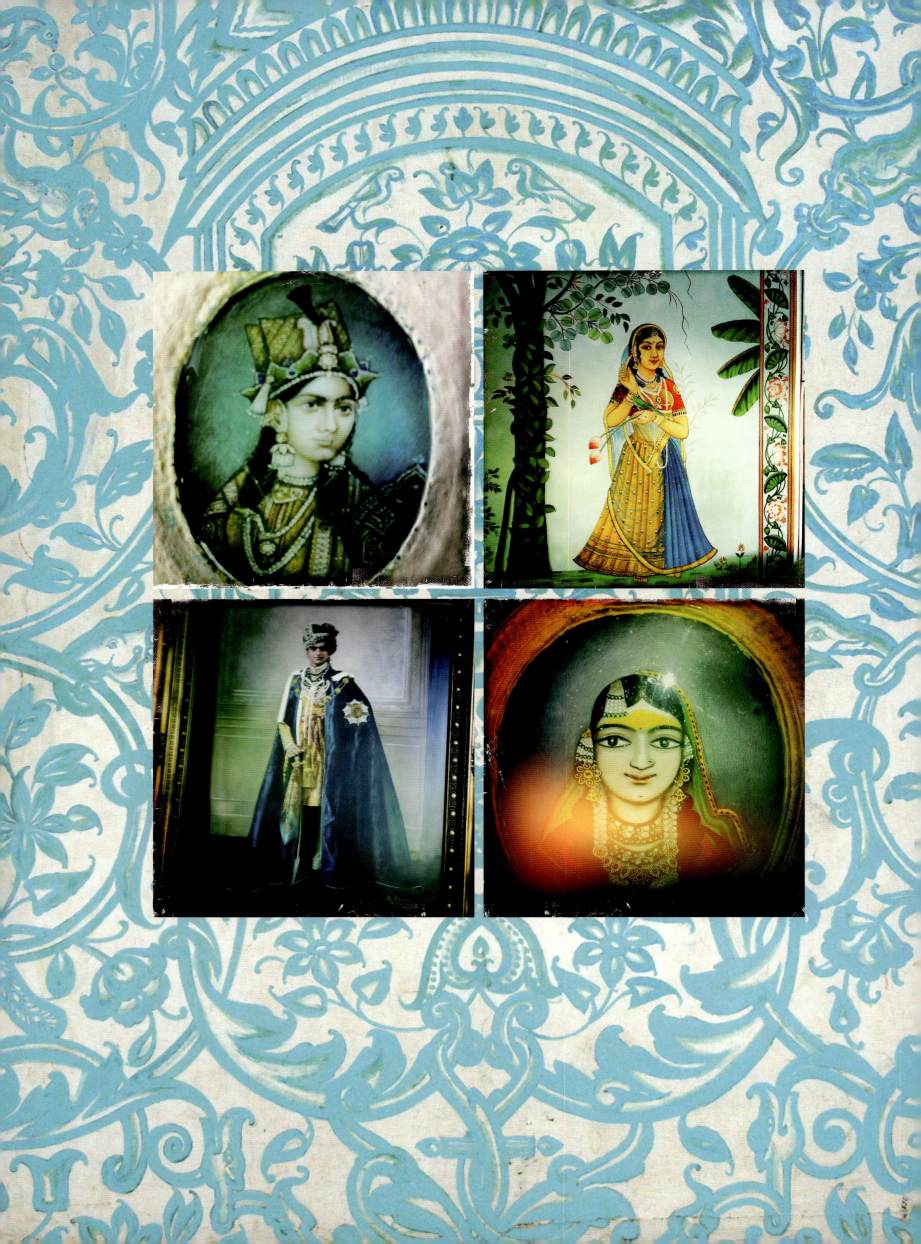

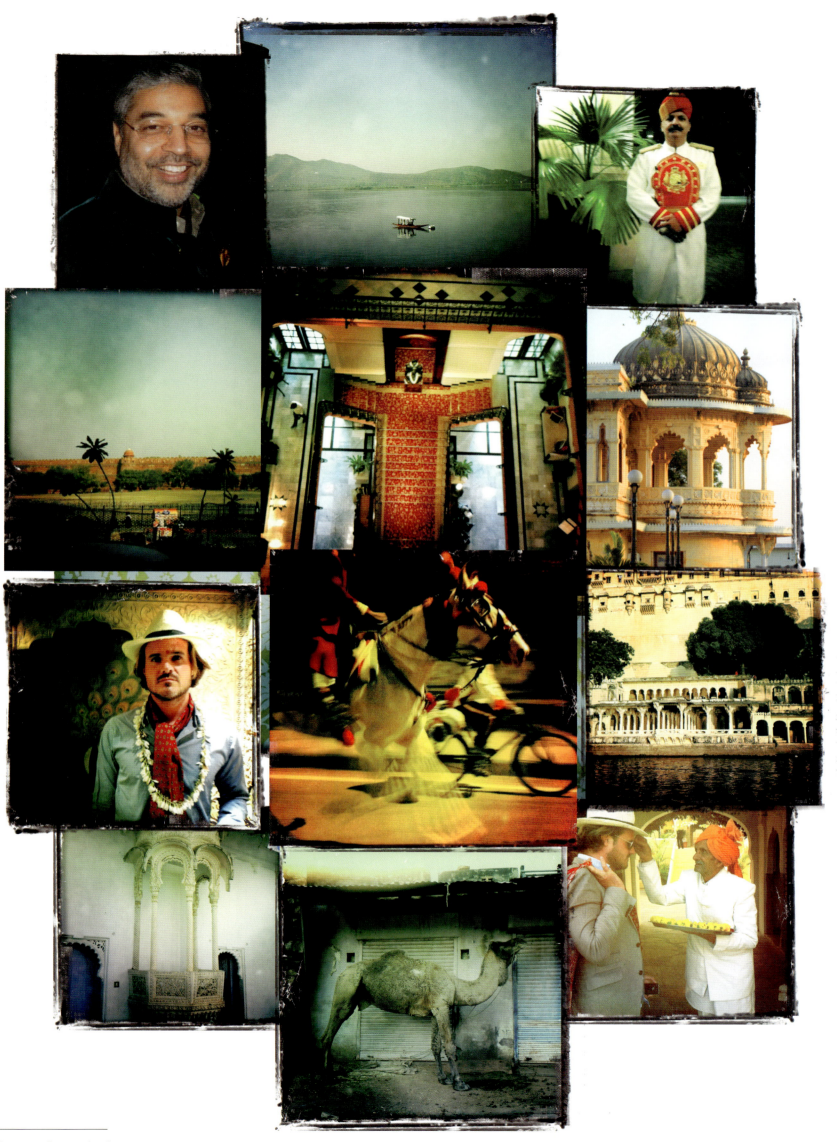

*You never know what's going
to happen next in India.*

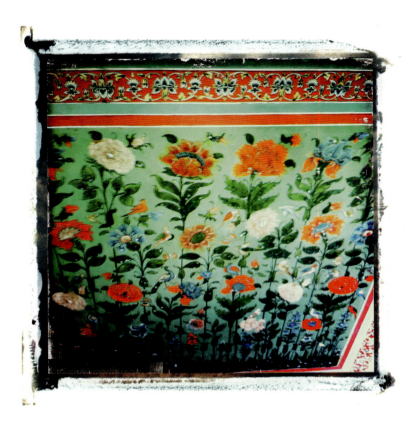

It sounds strange, but I actually find the chaos of India quite inspiring. Especially Mumbai, which is so manic and noisy – it is so frenetic that it is almost peaceful. I love the unexpected, I love symmetry, I love organised chaos – and India has all of that. People often say they have a love-hate relationship with India, and I know what they mean. There's a sense of craziness, but that brings tremendous energy. The Indian people really know how to celebrate too, whether it's a wedding, a festival in honour of Ganesha, a Hindu god, or even a funeral – there'll be masses of colours and flowers everywhere. I love that concept of celebration on a massive scale – it's something that is missing from western culture.

There is something about seeing things en masse, too, as you do in India. If you see a flock of seagulls or pigeons in Sydney, London or Paris, there aren't hundreds of them vying for the same telephone wires, as there are in India. Just as, en masse, marigolds can look amazing, but they don't have the same impact when mixed together with other flowers.

People often ask me where I get the ideas for my beading and embroidery. I get a lot of inspiration from what I see in India – it might be a repetitive mosaic pattern of some old tiles, for example. Sometimes what I remember is very different from the way it actually was, but that's okay too. Then it becomes my own version of whatever I've seen – how I see India, as opposed to how India presents itself. I also look at old beading samples and finishes, and I especially love the old crystals and beads you can find in Czechoslovakia. I love cut glass, and mirrors, and I might try to recreate fractions of reflections. There are so many different reference points that I draw on.

Another reason I love visiting India is that I have made some wonderful friends there, so I always have an amazing time. It all began in 2000 when I attended the Louis Vuitton Cup, a yacht race where competitors from around the world race each other for a place in the America's Cup Finals. It was in Auckland that year, and I met some great Indian people, such as Tikka Singh. It is through them and their friends that I have seen a very different side to life in India – a world of palaces and parties, of real-life princes and princesses, and of Bollywood stars. It is all very glamorous, and quite different from Australia. Parties start late, at ten or eleven, and the women wear the most exquisite saris, ornately decorated with embroidery and sequins. The Indian people love colour and dancing, and everything is just a celebration of life. It is mad, creative and timeless, full of colour and vigour, and I love everything about it.

You never know what's going to happen next in India – where you're going, or who you'll meet. You might meet someone who says, 'My uncle has a dyeing factory', and someone else might say, 'I know someone with a weaving factory' and somehow you just keep meeting

Above: Anything might inspire me.

Opposite: Some Indian-inspired pieces from my 1998 collection. We held the show at Government House, Sydney – the first time anyone had done an event there.

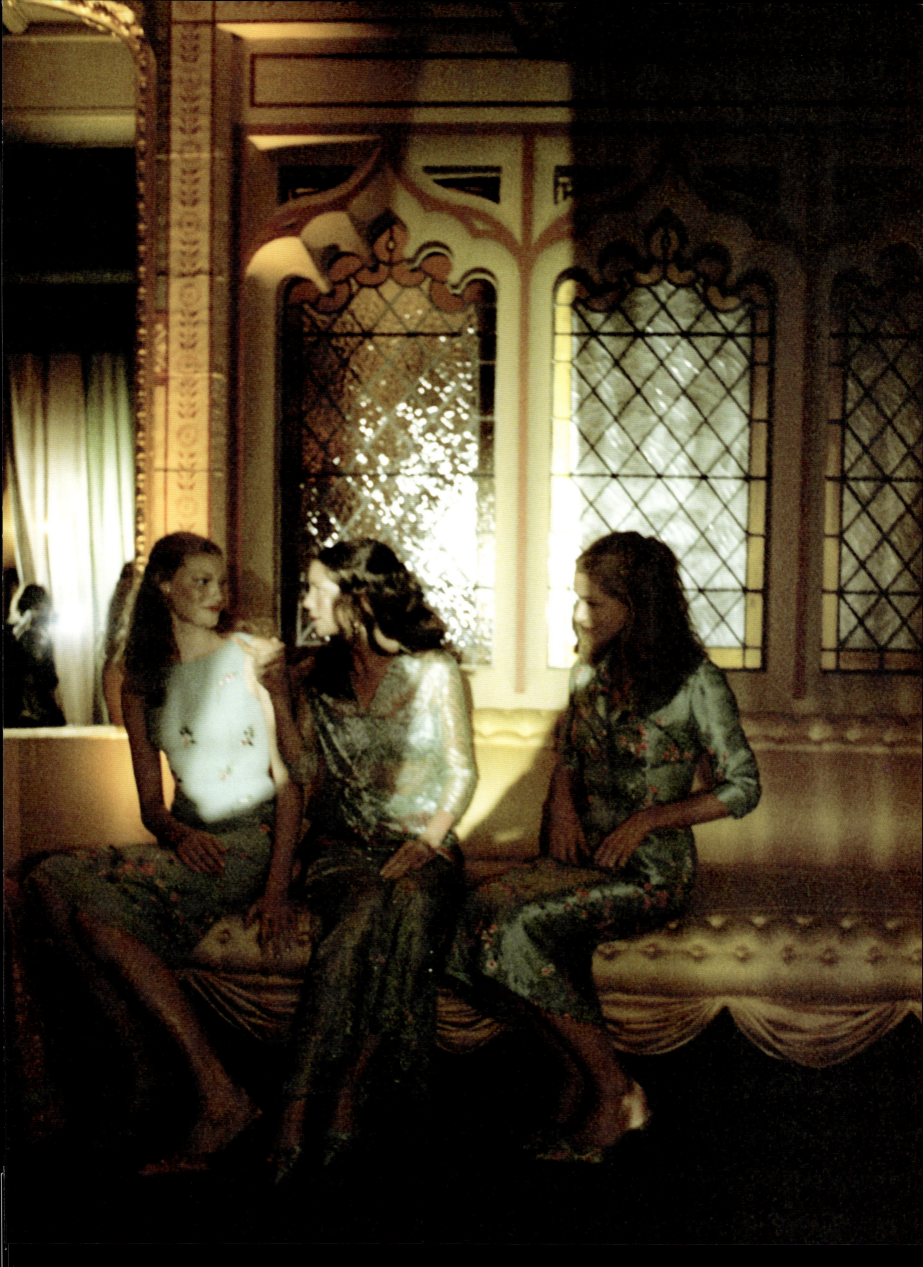

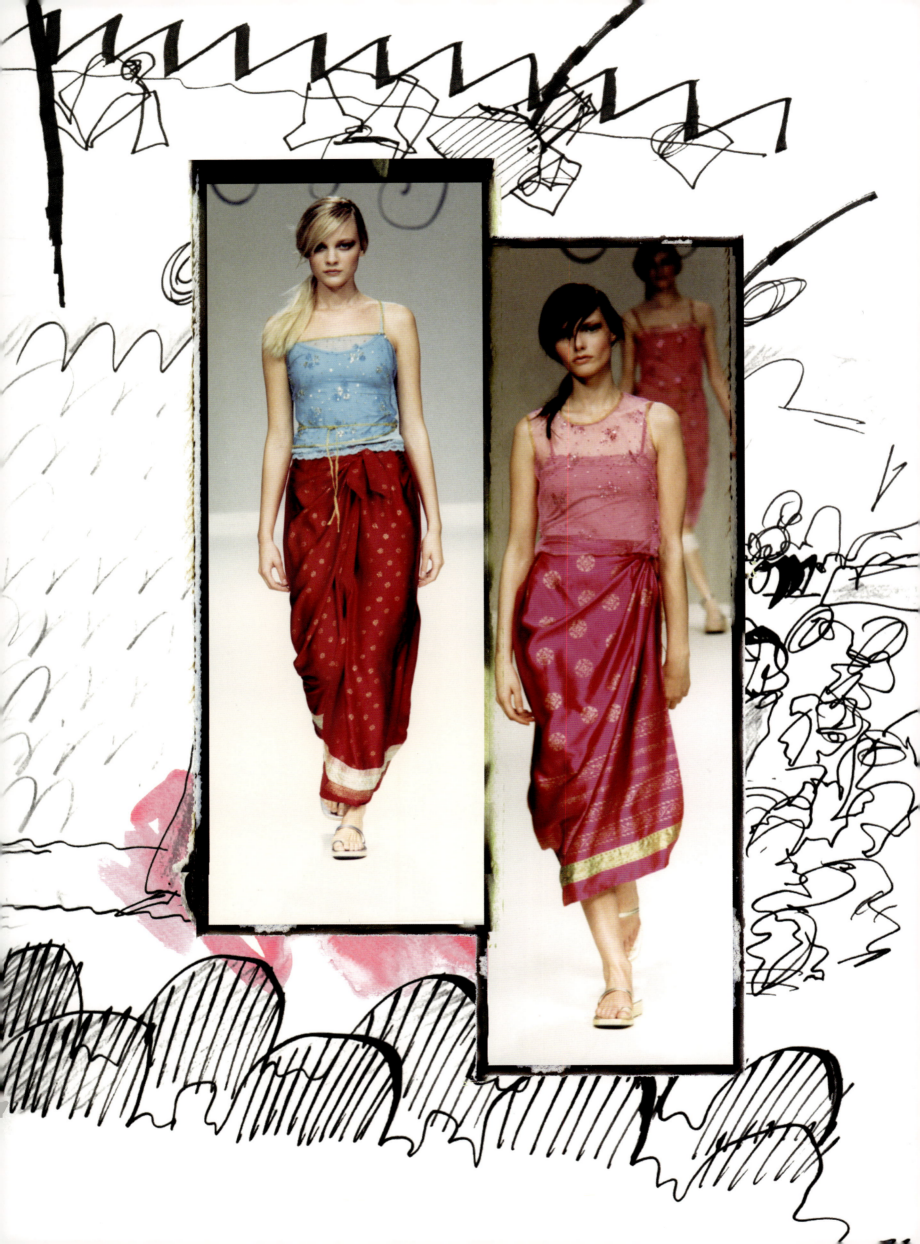

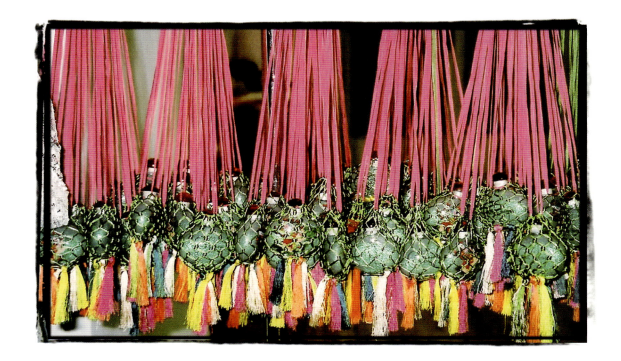

people. That is how India has evolved for me – one encounter leads to another, and you make it your business to meet as many people as you can.

Once, when I had been working in Mumbai, I decided to fly to Rajasthan for the weekend with Estella, who was still a baby. My plan was to relax with her and lie by the pool, so pretty much all I took with me was my bikini, a sarong and a t-shirt. As I was lying by the pool at the Rajvilas in Jaipur I kept seeing people I knew. Then I saw Tikka, who told me there was a wedding on that weekend, of someone we had all worked with. He insisted that I had to come, as lots of my friends would be there. I said I couldn't, because I had nothing to wear.

One of my friends offered to lend me a Nicole Miller sundress. It was too loose, so I altered it to fit me. Someone lent me some beautiful earrings and someone else lent me some sandals, which were a size too small for me. I went to the wedding, which was fabulous, and afterwards we went to a house in the middle of the desert. There was a perspex dance floor outside, and we danced the night away, under the stars. It was so romantic and so much fun.

I used to travel to India two or three times a year – it has been such a source of inspiration for me. Since the Mumbai terrorist attacks a few years ago I have stopped going so much. It is so sad – they really rocked Mumbai, which is such a tight community. It made me very wary – I don't feel comfortable leaving Estella in the hotel while I work, as I used to. I won't stop going, but I'm not as relaxed

about it as I used to be.

It also makes me sad to see how much India is changing. The first time I went there I visited Delhi, Rajasthan and then travelled down to Kerala. I was overwhelmed by the beauty of the places where we stayed, many of which were grand old palaces, wonderfully romantic. It felt almost as if we were in medieval Europe. Now, many of those places have been modernised, so have lost their charm. It breaks my heart to see grand, old buildings with beautifully patterned tiles being replaced by shopping malls and poorly constructed modern buildings. The camels and elephants are slowly disappearing from the streets, too, and there are new freeways and airports everywhere. These days you have to go deeper and deeper into parts of India that have not yet been explored to find the real heart of the country.

I would never stop visiting India, as it is such an important part of the DNA of my designs – it is so rich in ornaments, and it is inescapably influential. There are still parts of India that I haven't seen. I'd like to see Kashmir, and I'd also like to visit Varanasi, famous for its exquisite silks. The musical festivals in Rajasthan, which are said to be unbelievable, beckon me as well.

I love the Indian people – they have such a great appreciation and respect for their heritage and culture. Even though there are so many people living there, and everything is so hectic, I do find peace in India. I love the chaos – it's almost like a noise that calms you and puts you to sleep.

Opposite: I love the exquisitely beaded and embroidered saris of India – my Spring/ Summer 1998 collection paid homage to them. Illustration by Stewart Walton.

Above: One year I gave these beautiful hand-painted bottles, filled with glitter, to everyone who attended my Paris show.

Following page: Le Meurice scarf. Illustrative elements by Nina Fuga.

INDIA, A CALMING CHAOS

HOW
THE
MAGIC
HAPPENS

There's always a story;
inspiration everywhere.

THE CREATION
OF A DRESS

CHAPTER 5

When I design a collection

THERE IS ALWAYS A STORY.

I never start by thinking a particular

collection is going to be modern,

or graphic or whatever.

I BEGIN WITH A

STORY IN MIND —

I IMAGINE THE MOOD,

THE TIME, THE PLACE,

who will be wearing the clothes,

who else might be there.

I LOOK FOR SOMETHING

THAT WILL DEFINE

THE COLLECTION.

Those ideas might not always be obvious in

the final collection, but that is how it starts.

ANYTHING MIGHT INSPIRE ME —

fields of flowers, a flock of birds, old mosaics,

or even a row of striped deckchairs.

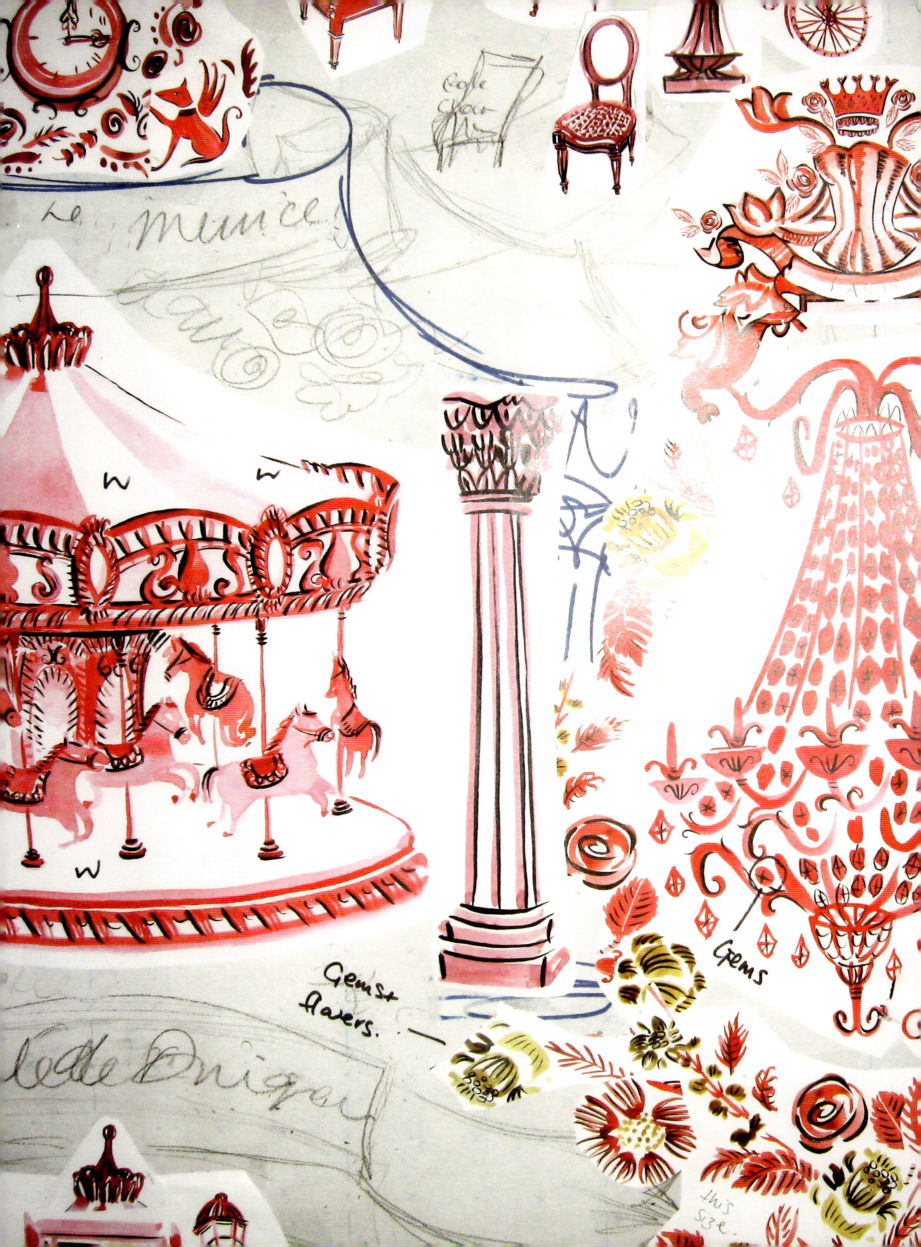

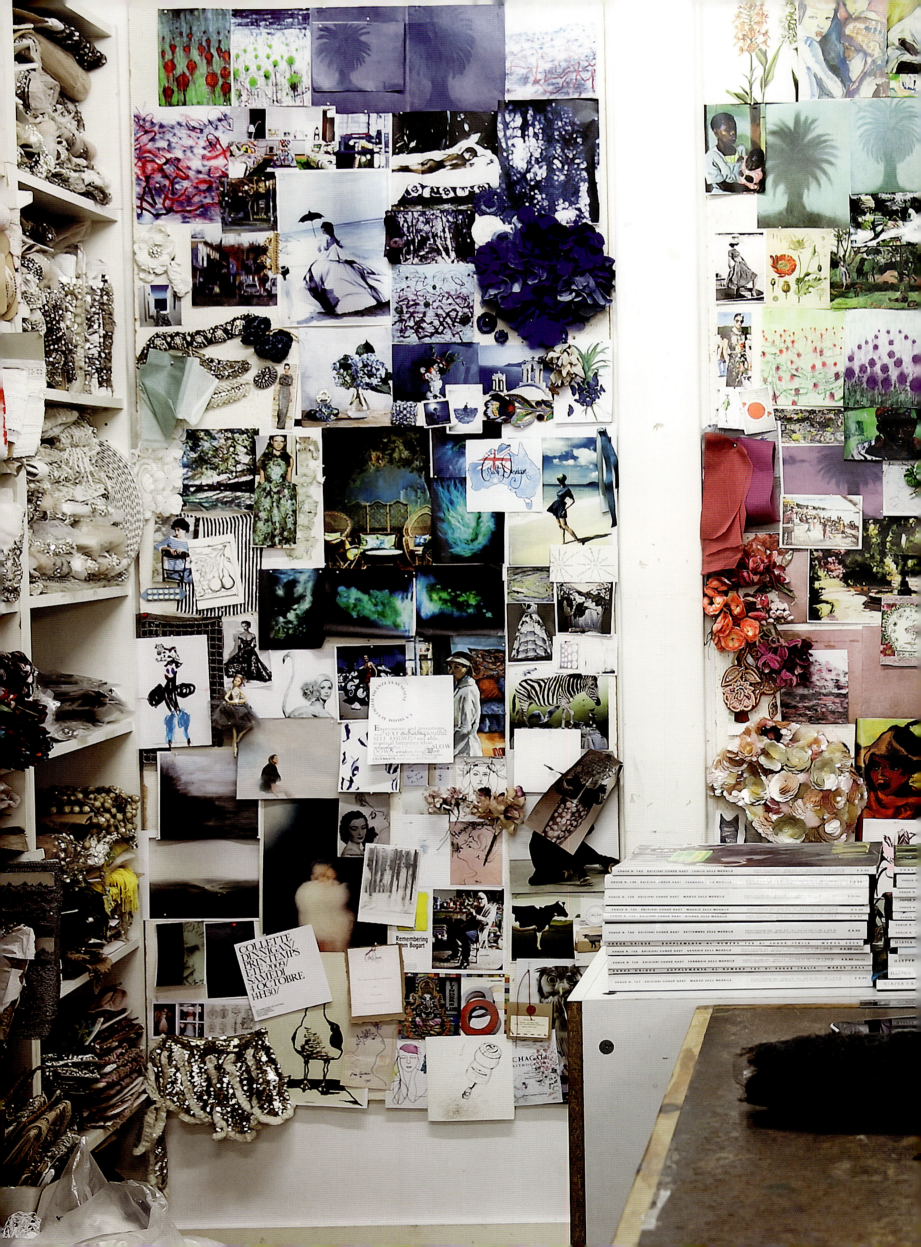

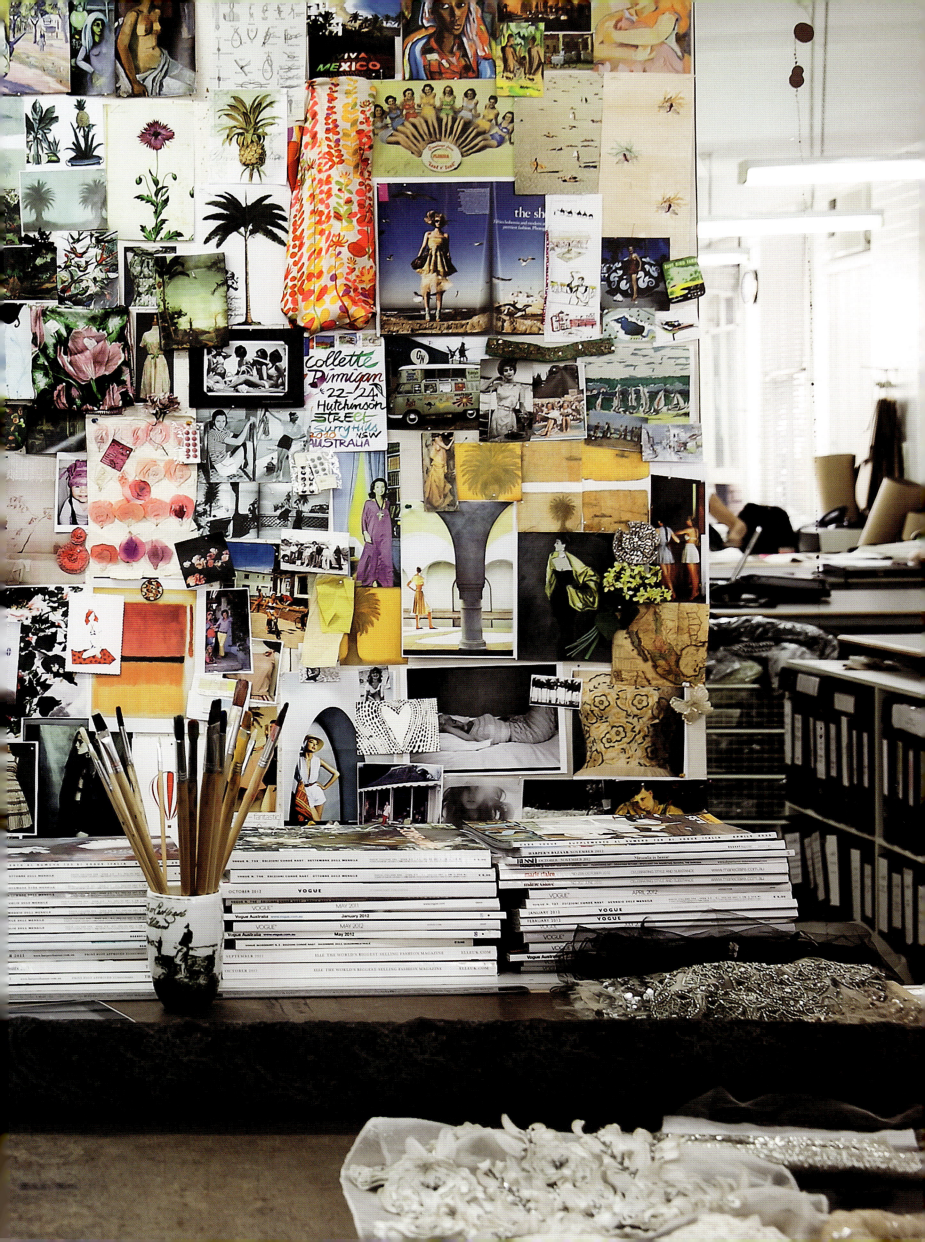

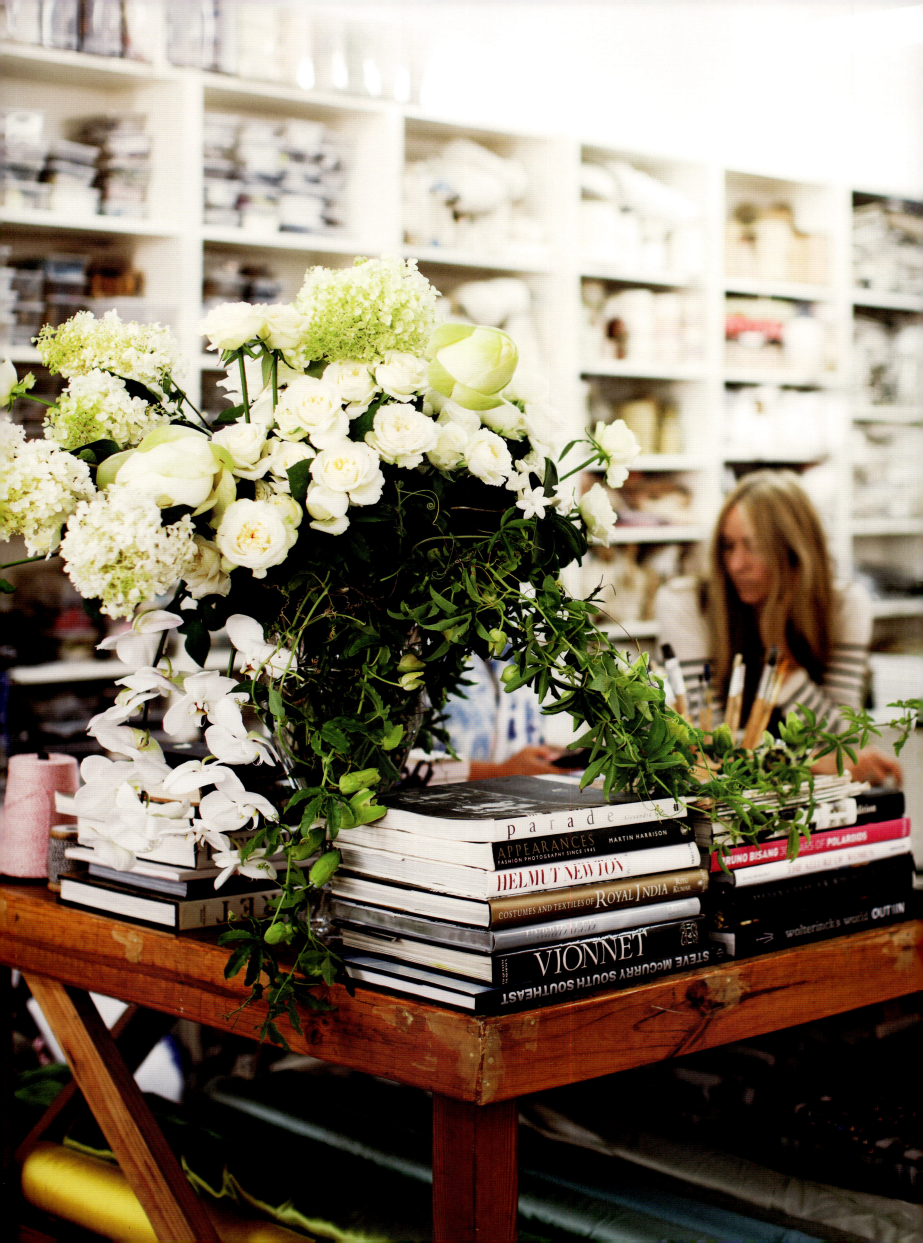

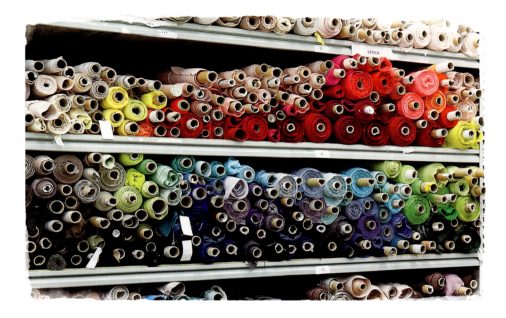

I get a lot of inspiration from travel — not because
I am consciously looking for ideas, but because I am always
aware of my surroundings, and open to new experiences.

〵〵〵

So in Italy, on the Amalfi Coast, seeing girls on Vespas wearing bright red lipstick and turquoise dresses might inspire me to design a fabric in red and turquoise, because I think that colour combination is sexy and romantic, as women's clothes should be. I design many of my fabrics myself so the design process is doubled.

Whether I am creating fabric, embroidery or beading designs, once I have an idea in my mind, I do some preliminary sketches and then work with my design team, choosing colours. I might find some vintage references, we play around with the designs and graphics, then we do a placement layout, where we fit the ornament or design to the pattern. I then decide on the best artist to work on the project – I work with different artists all the time – and together we develop the design further. When we are all happy with the final artwork, we send the design to our printing factory. I have one in Australia and one in Hong Kong. They will do a mock-up of the fabric and send it back. That becomes our exclusive print, that is never run again.

I then spend hours with that mock-up fabric, draping it in different ways over a model. My pattern-makers work with me on this, but it is essentially me, and it is very time-consuming. I do some more sketches after I have done the draping, and then I'll get the pattern-makers to cut and make it up in the final fabric. We then develop those initial pieces, and, once we are happy with the design, the pattern-makers make the necessary changes to the pattern, and the cutters and seamstresses work together to make it up. All of the cutting is done in-house, one by one with the laces. Every piece has its own unique number which refers to the collection it is part of and indicates how many have been made.

Almost all of my clothes are made in Sydney, and everything is cut in my studio. I like to drop in and keep an eye on what's happening. It's quite funny, no one likes me being in the cutting room because if I see something that doesn't look quite right, I just go straight in with the scissors and cut away. I don't need a pattern – I do it straight from my eye.

The only work that we don't do here is the beading and embroidery – that is done in India. The lace arrives from France in five-metre pieces. We check its quality, then make the first fitting sample, and make a paper marker

Previous pages: Some early sketches for the Le Meurice
scarf pictured on page 62 (page 65). Illustrative elements
by Nina Fuga; The design room at my Surry Hills studio.
It is filled with bits and pieces I have collected over the years
and which provide constant inspiration (pages 66-67).

Opposite: At work in my design room. Flowers are an
important feature in all my collections, especially my
resort and summer ones.

Above: The fabric bay in the studio.

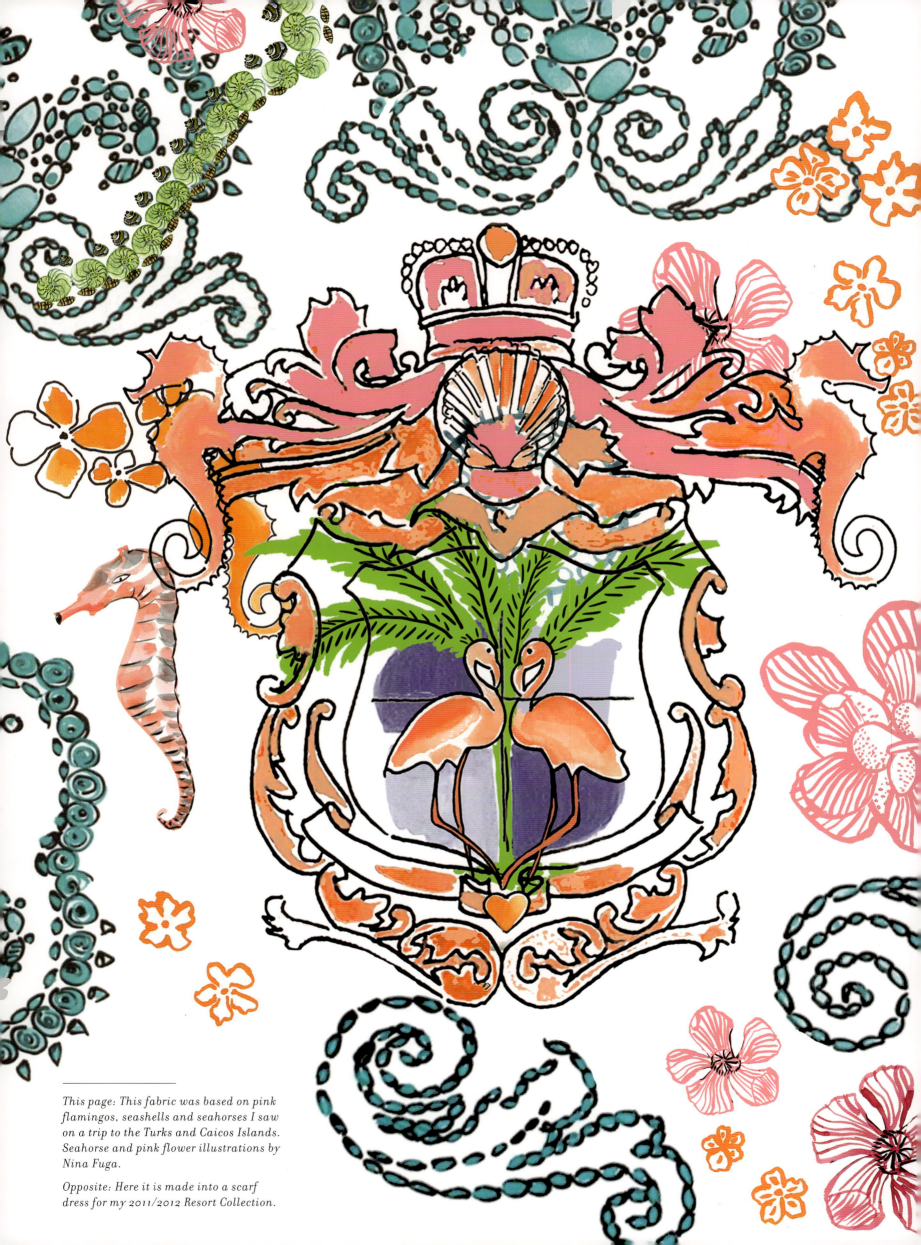

This page: This fabric was based on pink
flamingos, seashells and seahorses I saw
on a trip to the Turks and Caicos Islands.
Seahorse and pink flower illustrations by
Nina Fuga.

Opposite: Here it is made into a scarf
dress for my 2011/2012 Resort Collection.

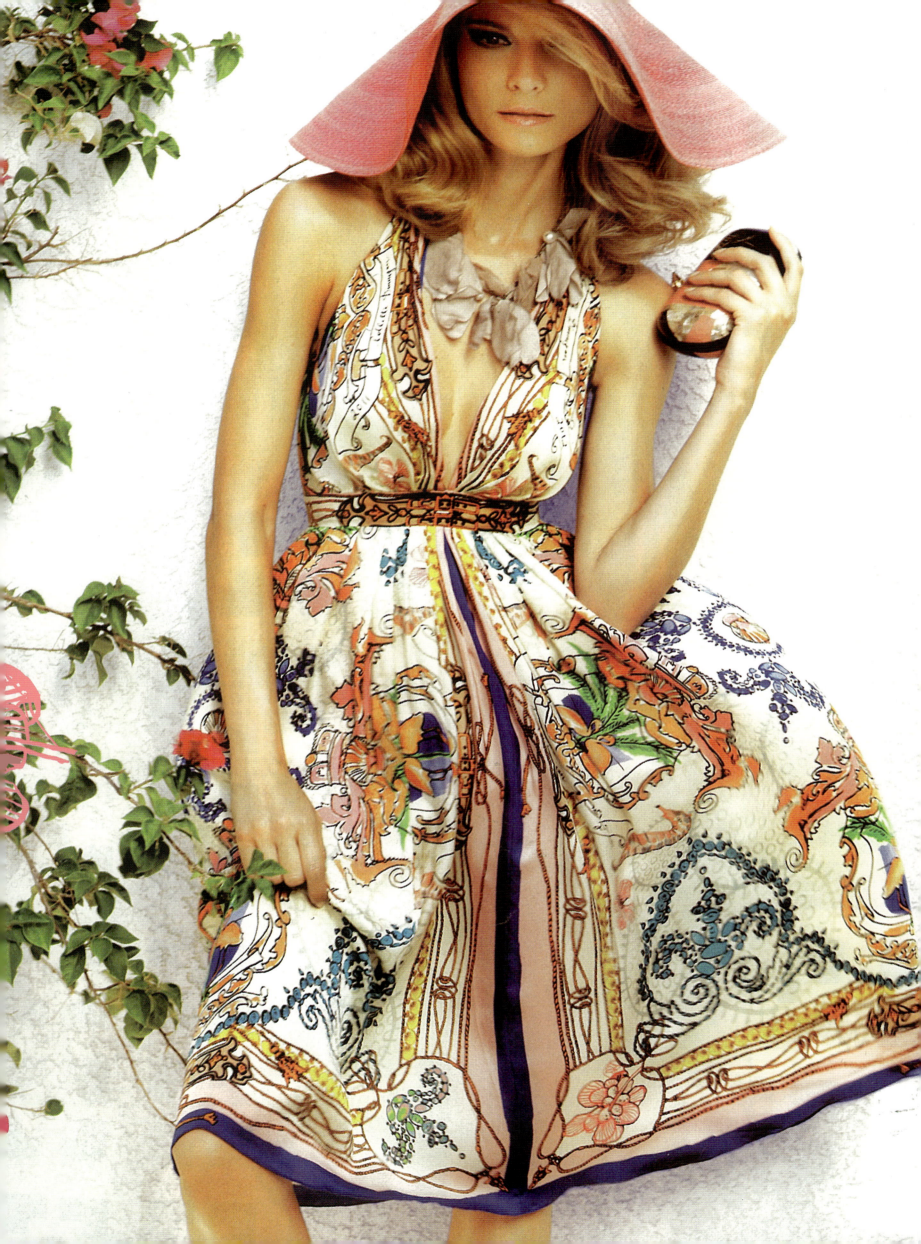

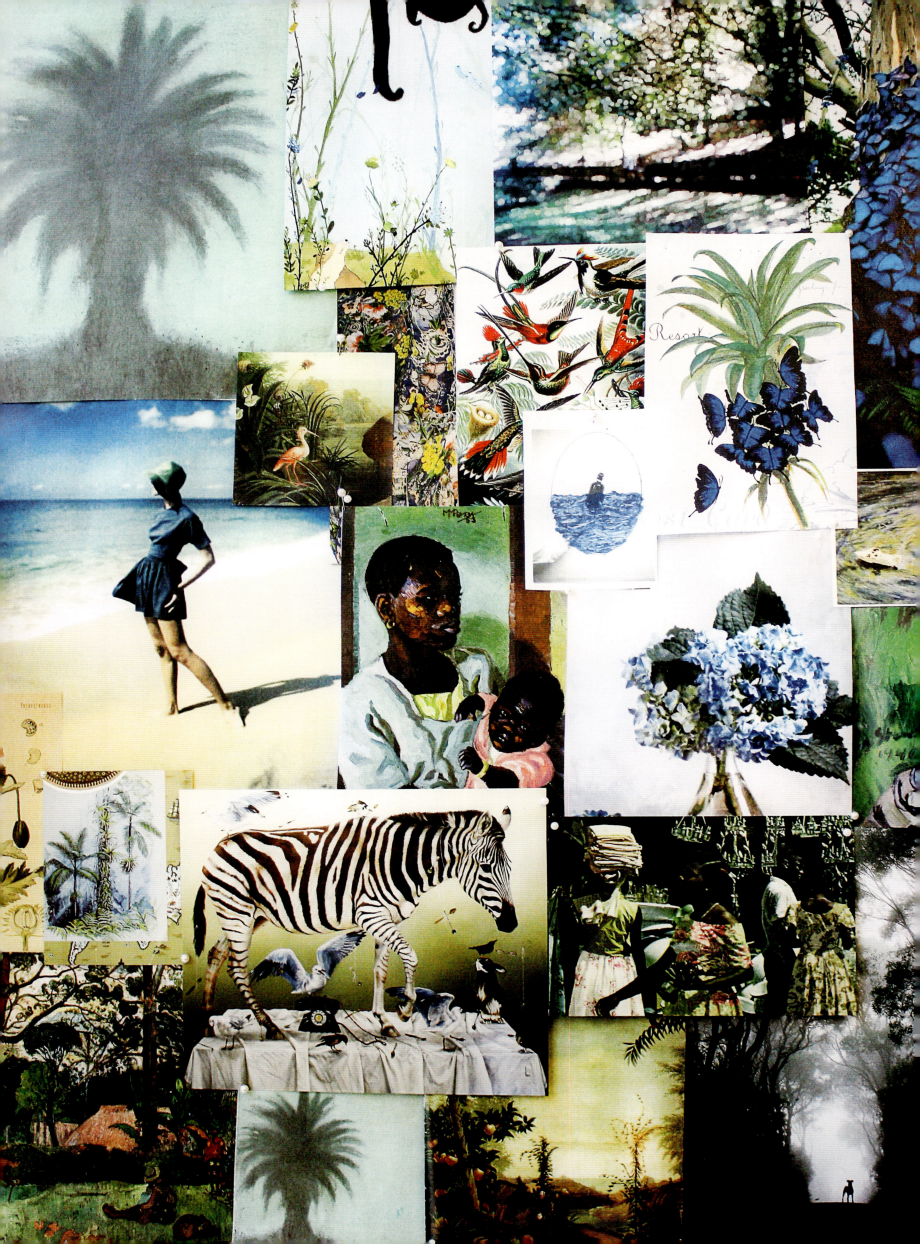

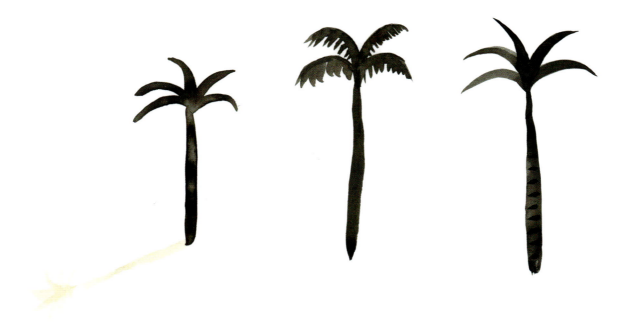

pattern showing the artwork. We then send the lace to India, where it is stretched on long frames, and they tack through the paper marker with a big running thread stitch. The embroidery and beading is finished by hand and then the lace is removed from the frames. They send the lace back here, each piece individually cut, and we put the garment back together. All of the beading is hand-knotted and then finished by hand – you can't do that fine work with a machine.

One illustration of how the whole process works is a Collette by Collette Dinnigan diffusion collection that was inspired by a blue and white tile pattern I saw on an old palace in India. It made me think of Morocco, and the Mediterranean, and I wanted to capture that lightness, that airy feel. I broke down the tile pattern visually, then blew up the elements and played around with the design until I was happy with it. Once the fabric was ready I draped it, then the pattern was cut, and finally the dress was made.

When all of the clothes for a collection are ready we shoot a look book to give people a sense of the whole collection. So something like that tile pattern, which started out on an ancient Indian palace, comes to life on a dress being modelled by Bambi on the windswept rocks of Sydney's Clovelly beach at six in the morning. She is fresh-faced, and her hair is loose and flying in the breeze, and there's an easiness about it all.

I am always involved in the photo shoots as they are so important – they set the tone for the season. I enjoy the whole process, and over the years I have worked with some wonderful stylists, photographers, hair and makeup artists and models. The right team can make or break a shoot. I love capturing the moment, being behind the camera and seeing it all come together.

One of my favourite collections is my 2011/2012 Resort Collection which was inspired by a trip Bradley and I made to the Turks and Caicos Islands in the Caribbean to celebrate a friend's fiftieth birthday. We stayed on Parrot Cay and it was like a tropical paradise. There were flocks of pink flamingos, and on the beach there were seahorses and fabulous shells called sand dollars, with lovely starry patterns. I did some rough sketches and took lots of photos, and when we got home I gave these to one of our artists and that was the birth of the season's scarf print, a beautiful fabric.

A resort collection is always bright and colourful, with a feelgood, summery theme. This one was all about pink flamingos, seahorses and starry shapes. Everything was floaty, and seamless, and nonchalant – so romantic, just like a resort holiday. Each season we do a scarf print. The scarves themselves have almost become collectable pieces, and we are often asked for them.

Because I am known for my scarf prints, I was delighted when Franka Holtmann from Le Meurice, where I have based myself for my last few Paris shows, asked me to design a scarf for the hotel. I tried to capture its essence – the chandelier, the door, the logo and the Tuileries Garden, opposite the hotel. I hope I have succeeded.

Opposite: Part of my inspiration board.

Above: Illustration by Nina Fuga.

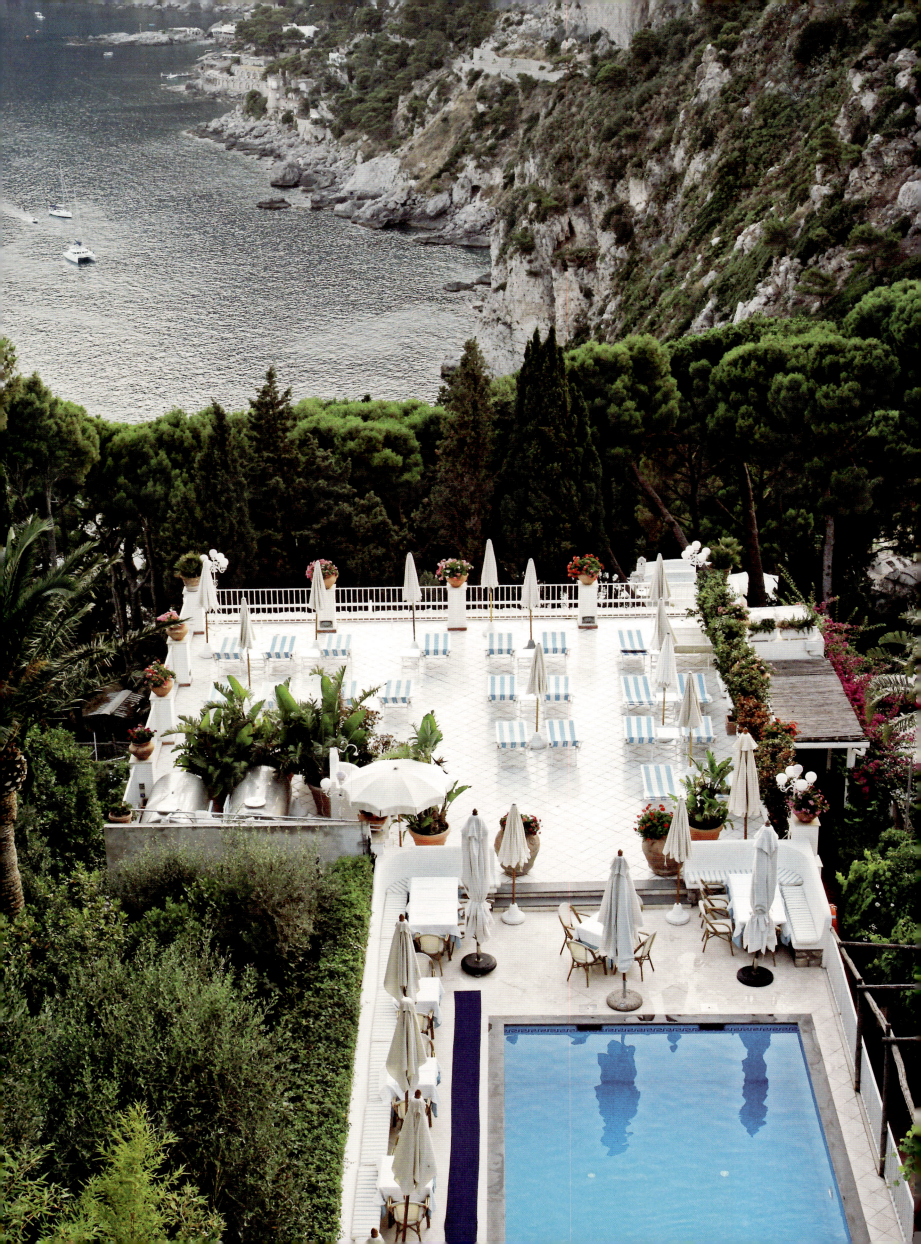

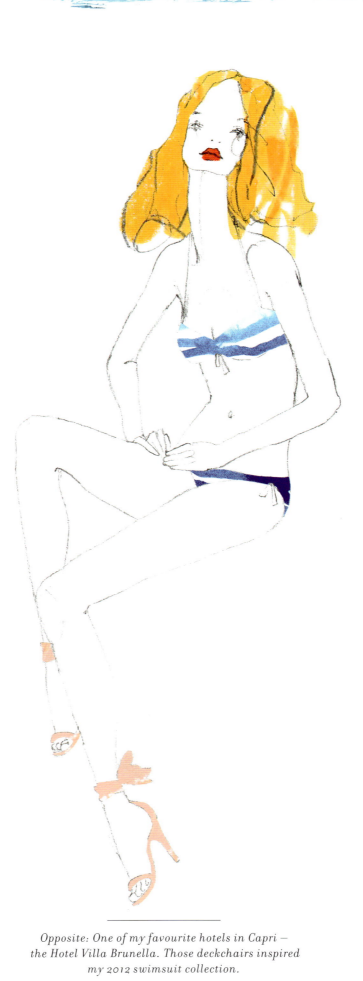

*Opposite: One of my favourite hotels in Capri —
the Hotel Villa Brunella. Those deckchairs inspired
my 2012 swimsuit collection.*

*Above: Artist Kat Macleod's sketch of one
of the bikinis from that collection.*

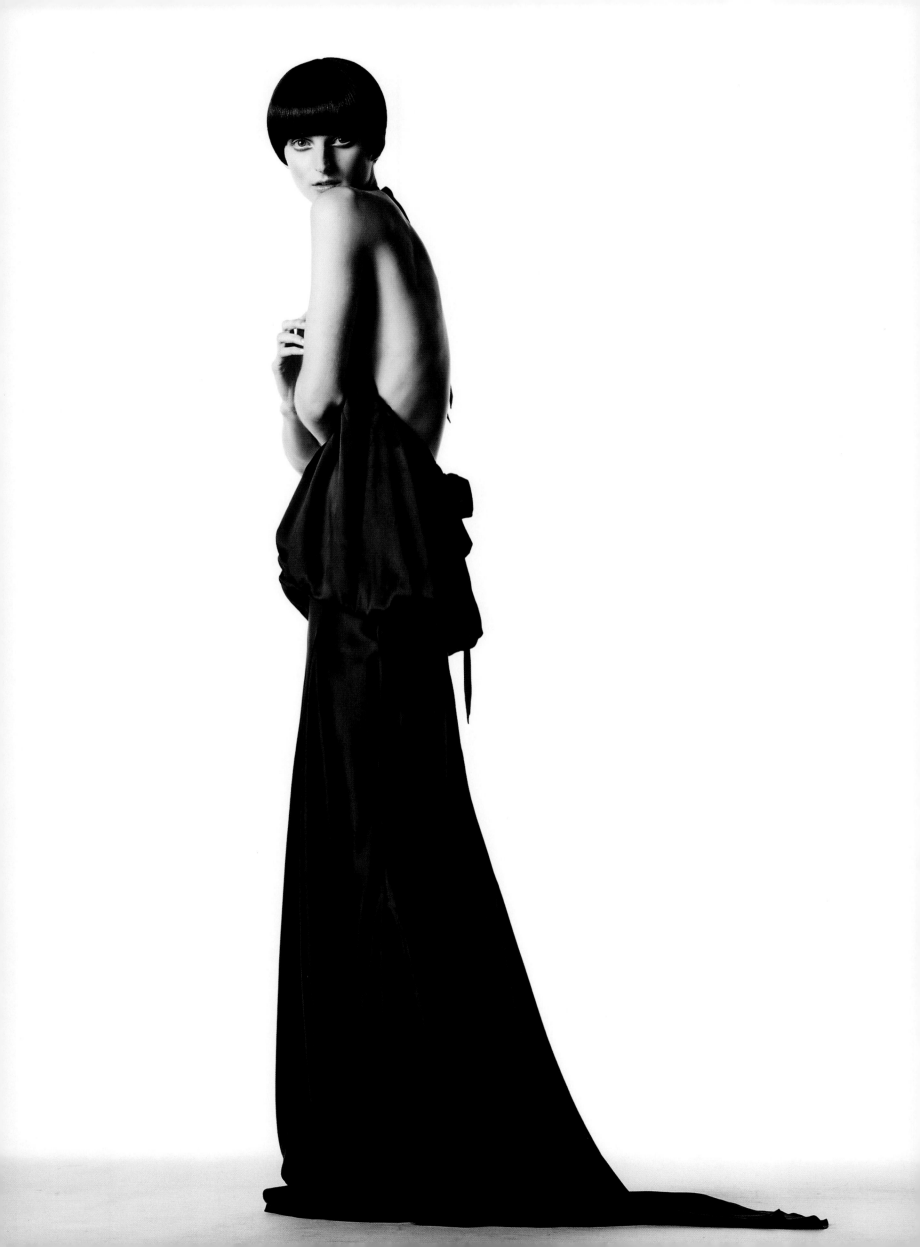

IF
ONLY

Romance with

the dresses.

THINGS I HAVE LOVED

CHAPTER 6

THE SHOTS I HAVE
CHOSEN HERE ARE
ALL VERY EMOTIVE.
They show fashion, as it is —
QUIRKY, SURPRISING
AND MODERN.
It's also about somebody
else's eye on my work.
I LOVE THAT AND
I ALSO LOVE ALL OF
THE DIFFERENT TAKES;
from futuristic, to pretty,
TO ROMANTIC,
to very Australian.

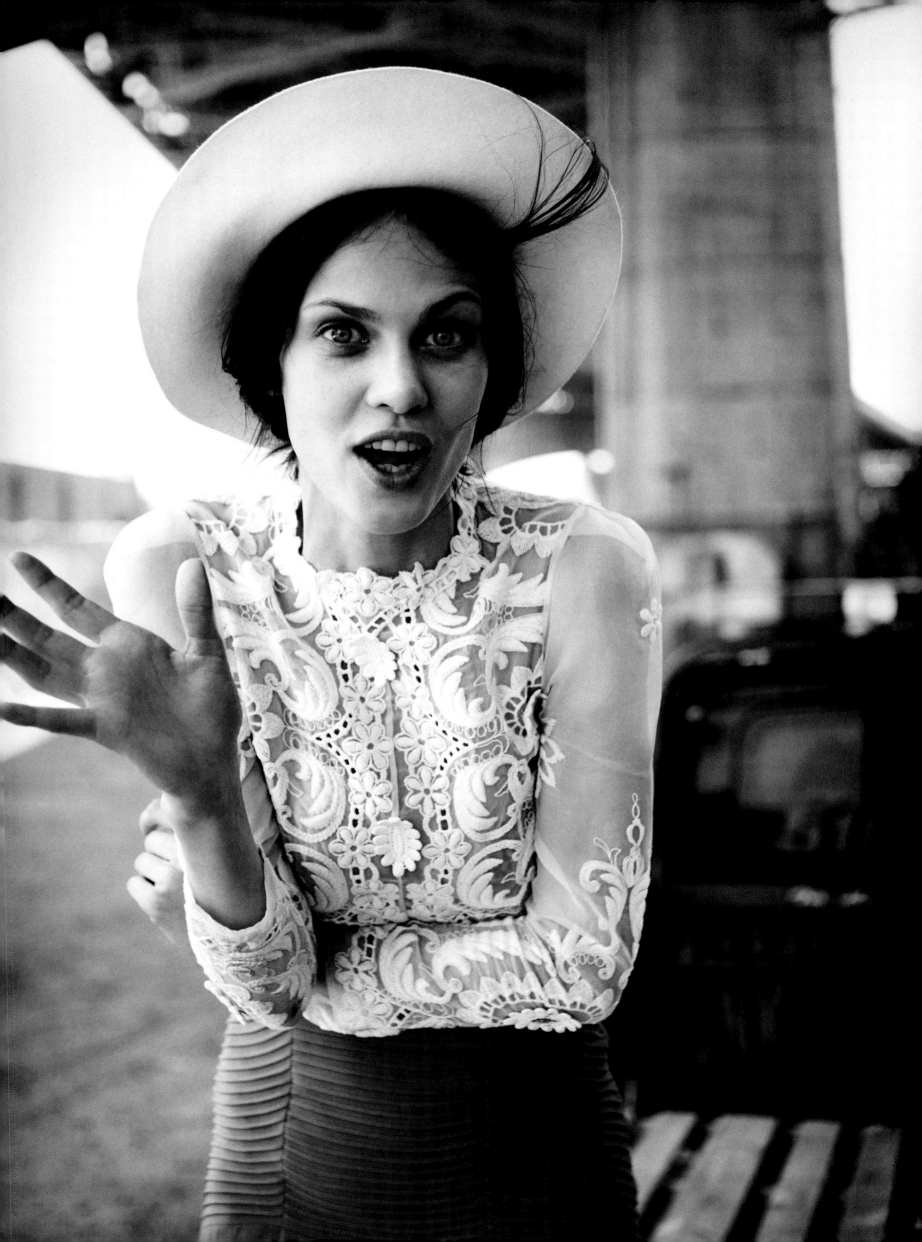

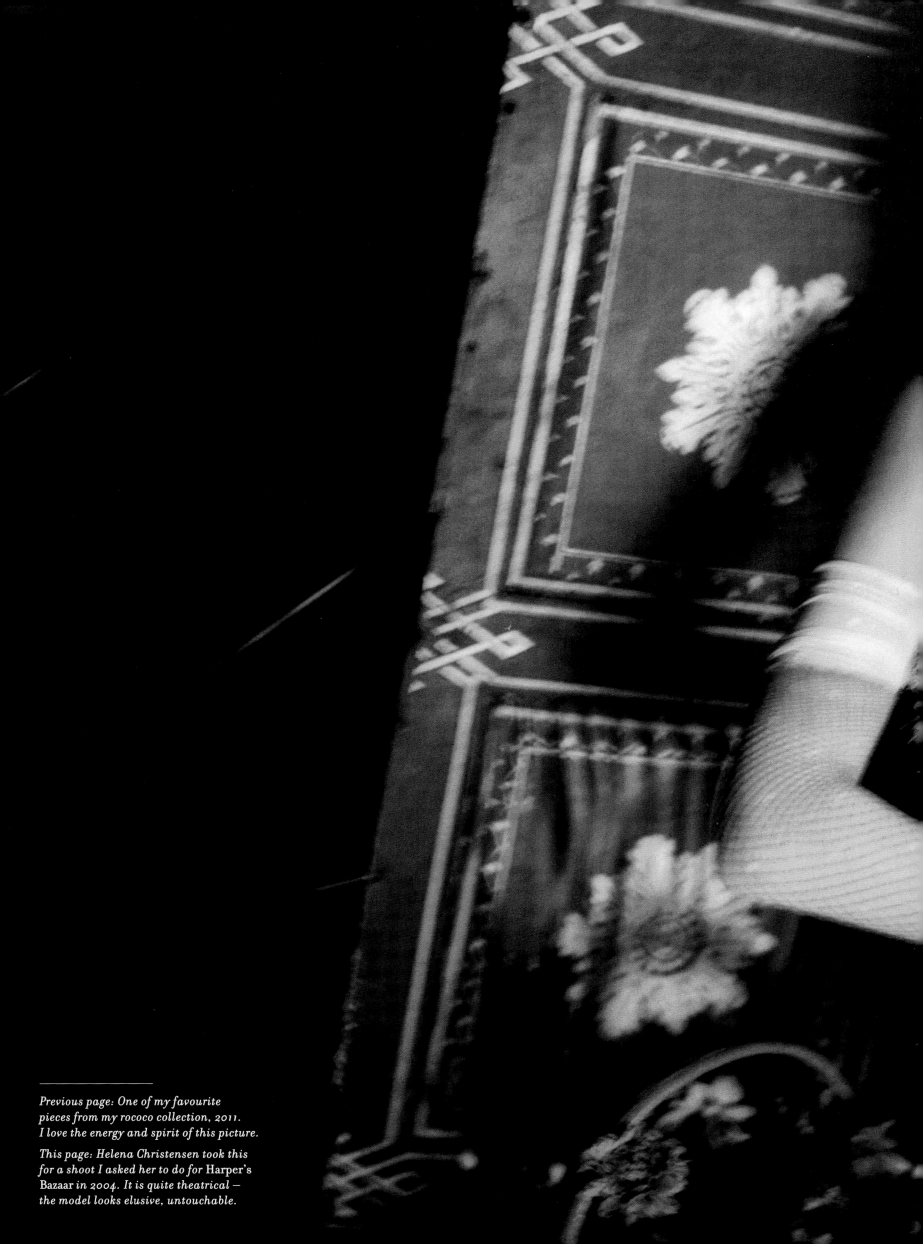

*Previous page: One of my favourite
pieces from my rococo collection, 2011.
I love the energy and spirit of this picture.*

*This page: Helena Christensen took this
for a shoot I asked her to do for Harper's
Bazaar in 2004. It is quite theatrical —
the model looks elusive, untouchable.*

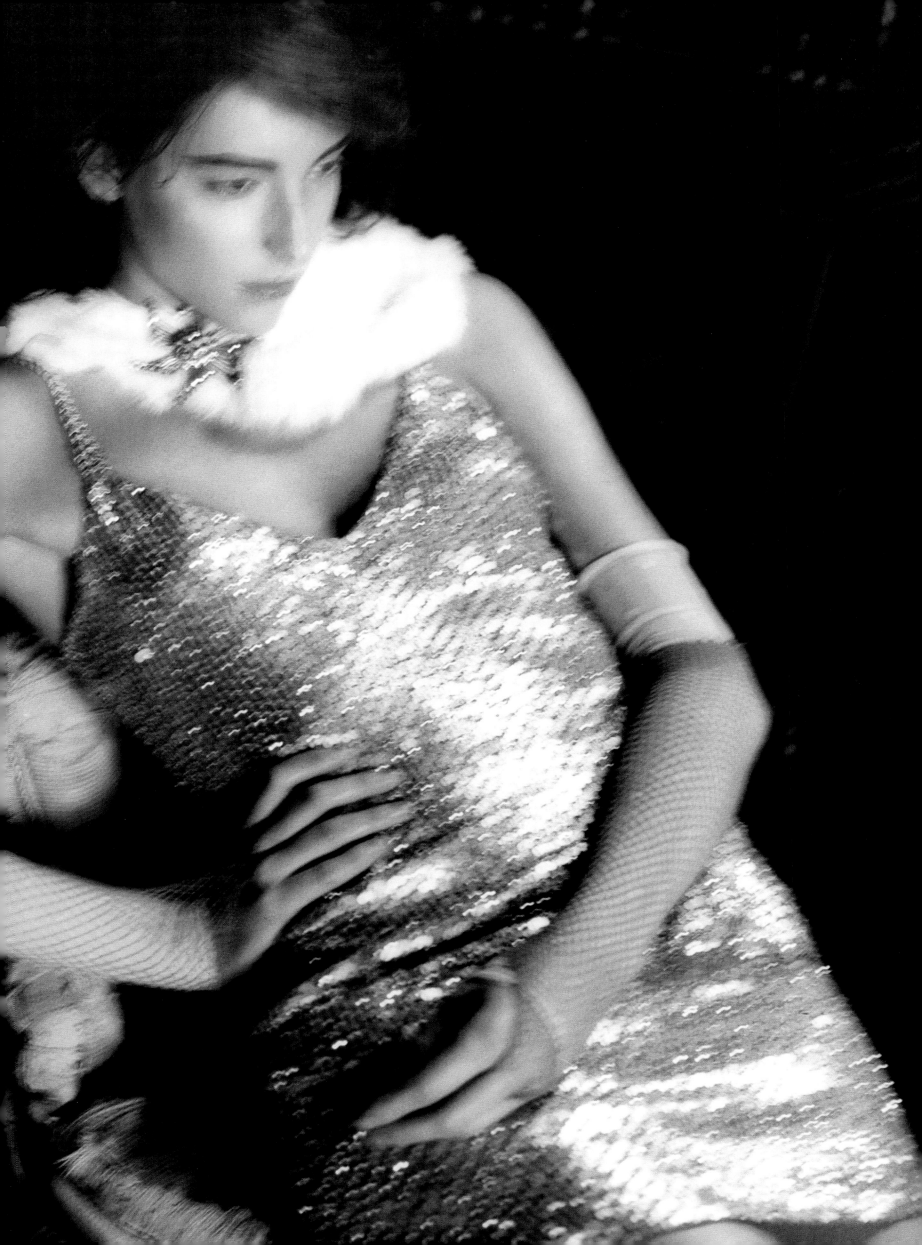

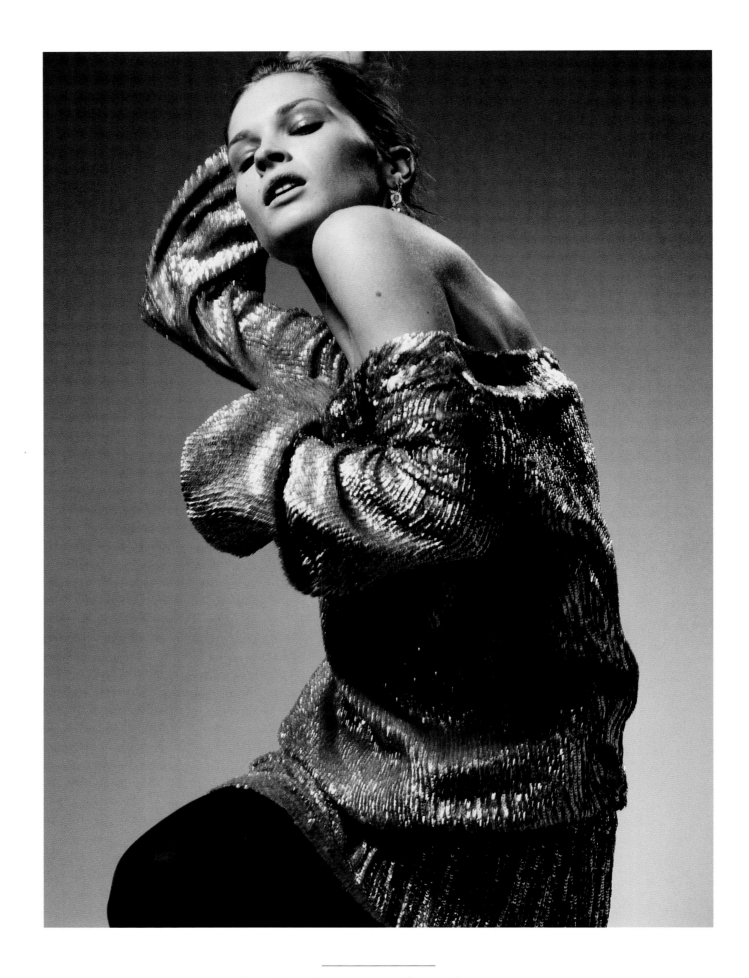

Above: I love the way this dress from 2003 shimmers.

Opposite: You can wear sequins any time, not just at night.
Mixed with this bomber jacket, the look is very modern, 2011.

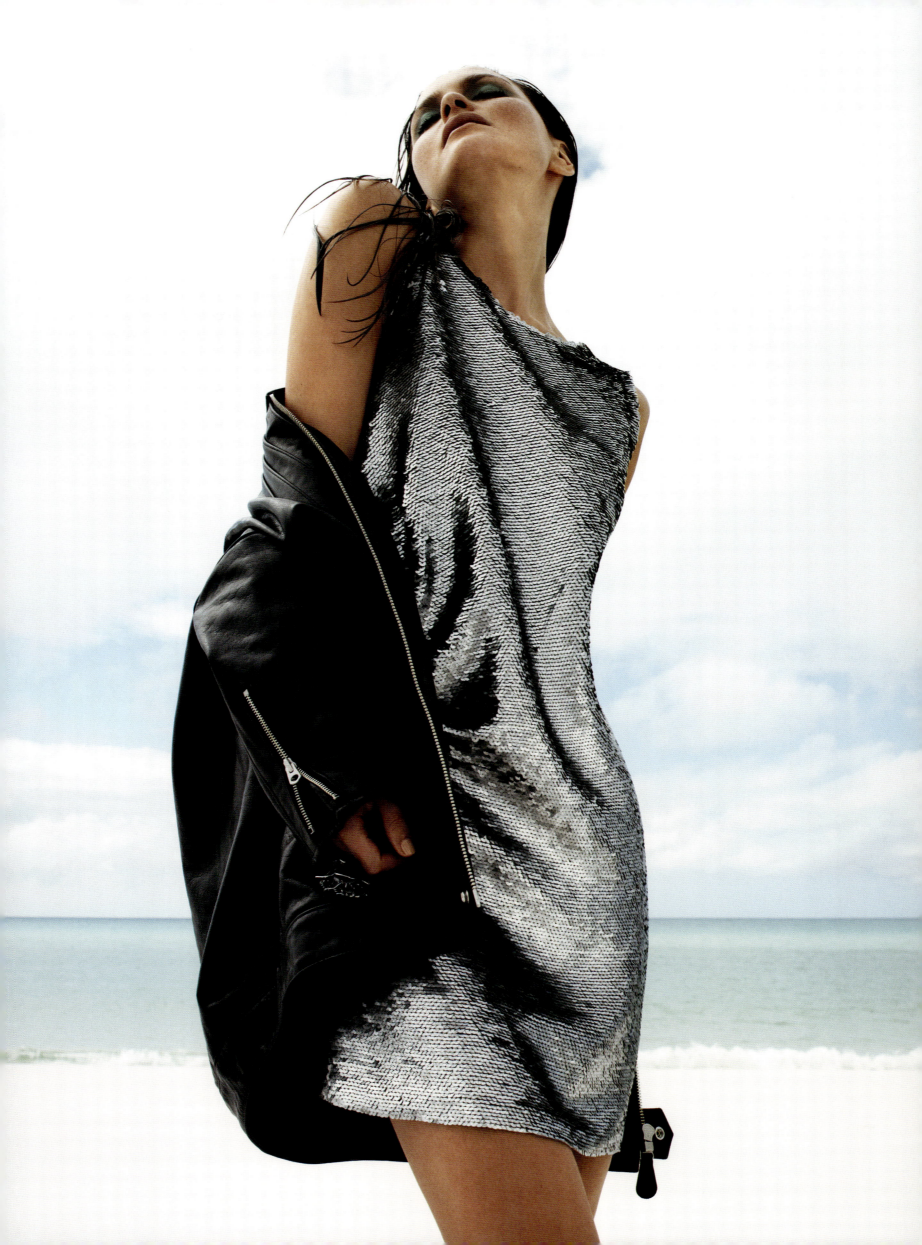

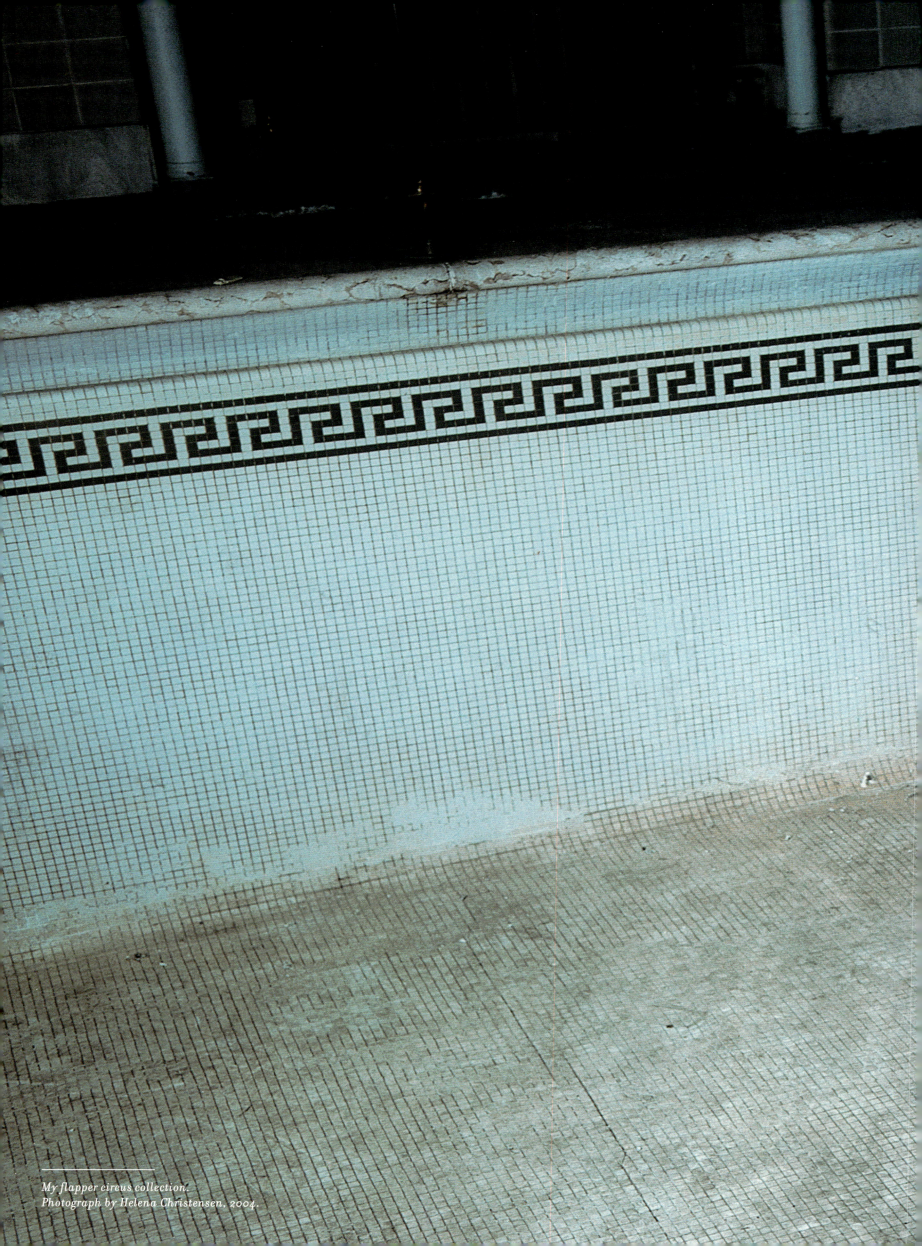

My flapper circus collection.
Photograph by Helena Christensen. 2004.

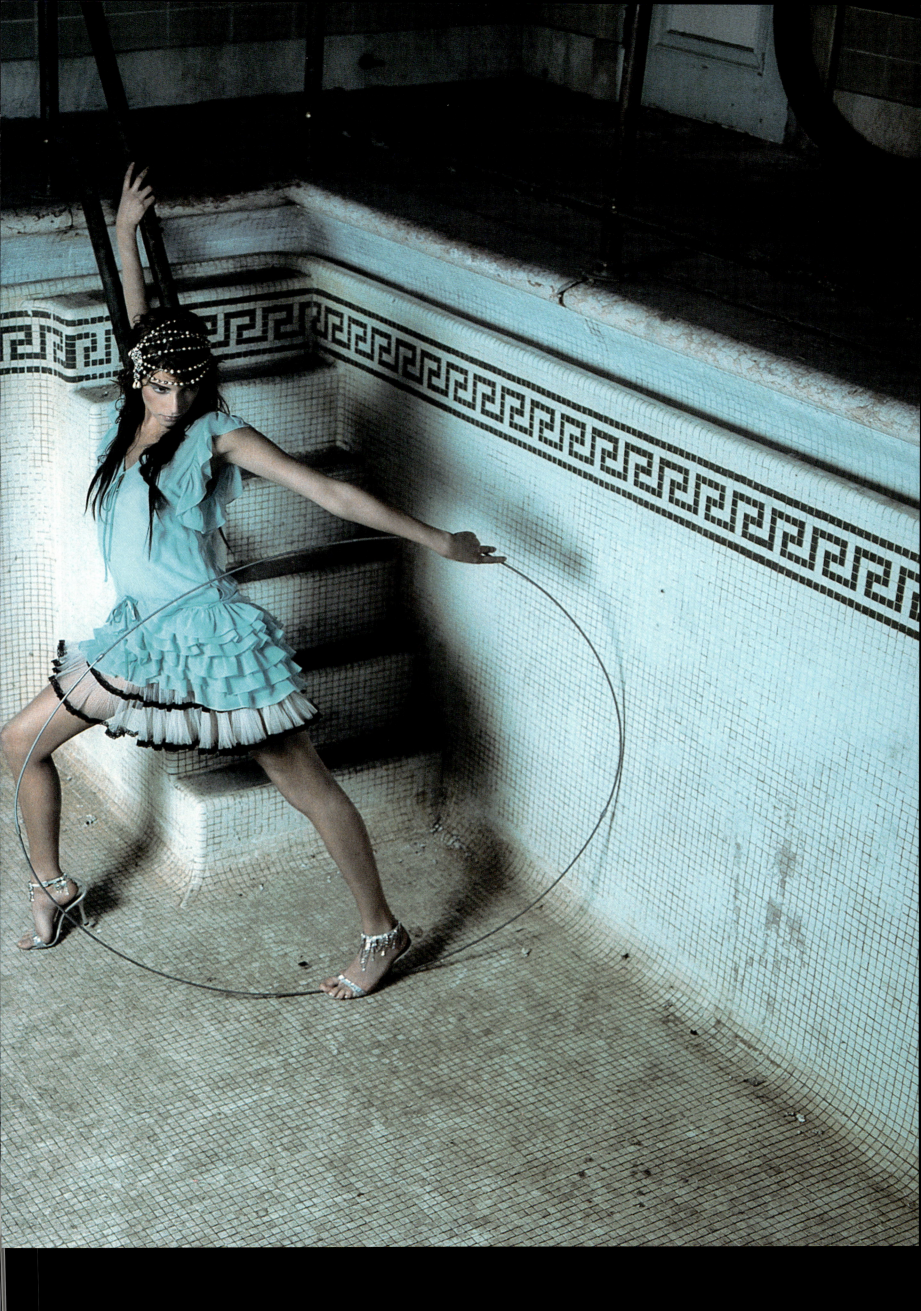

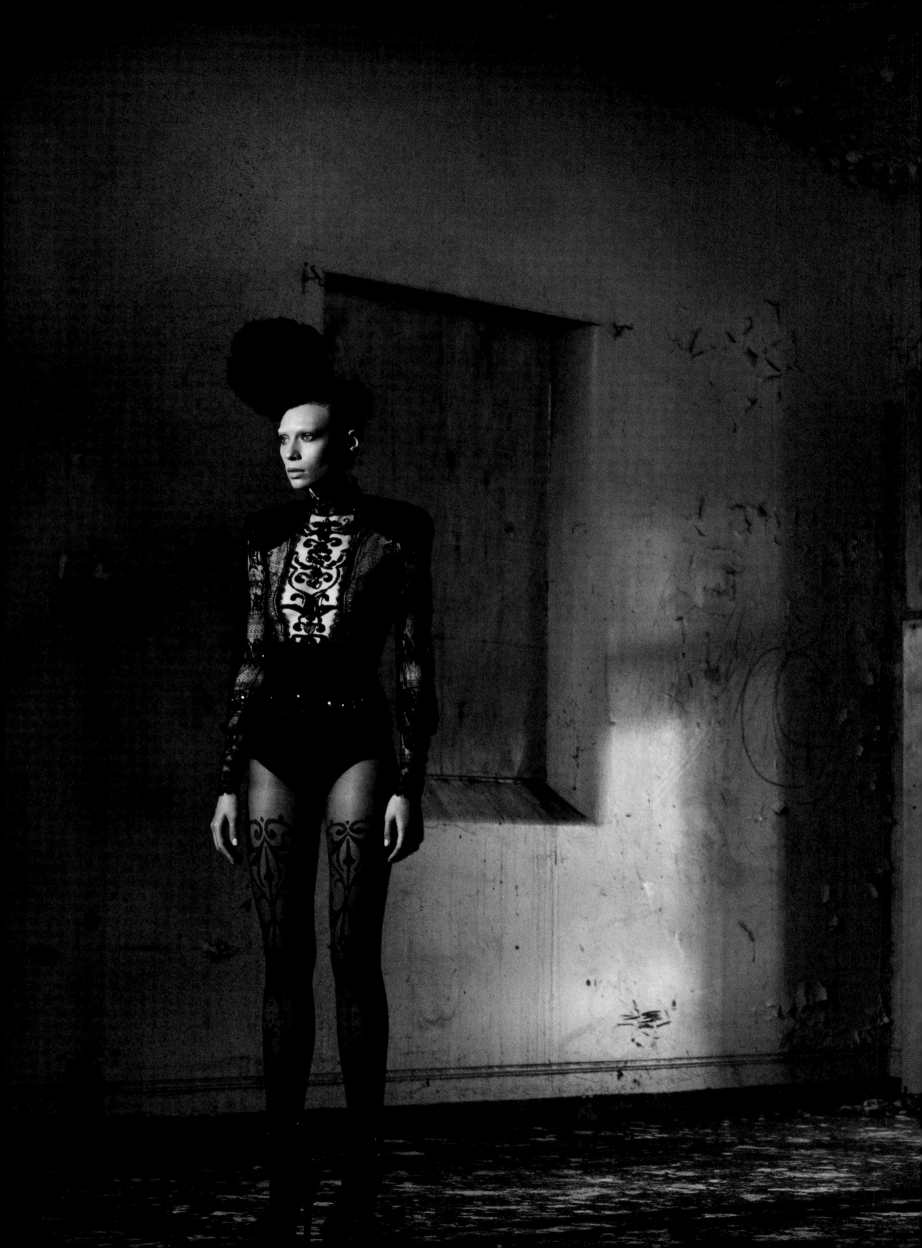

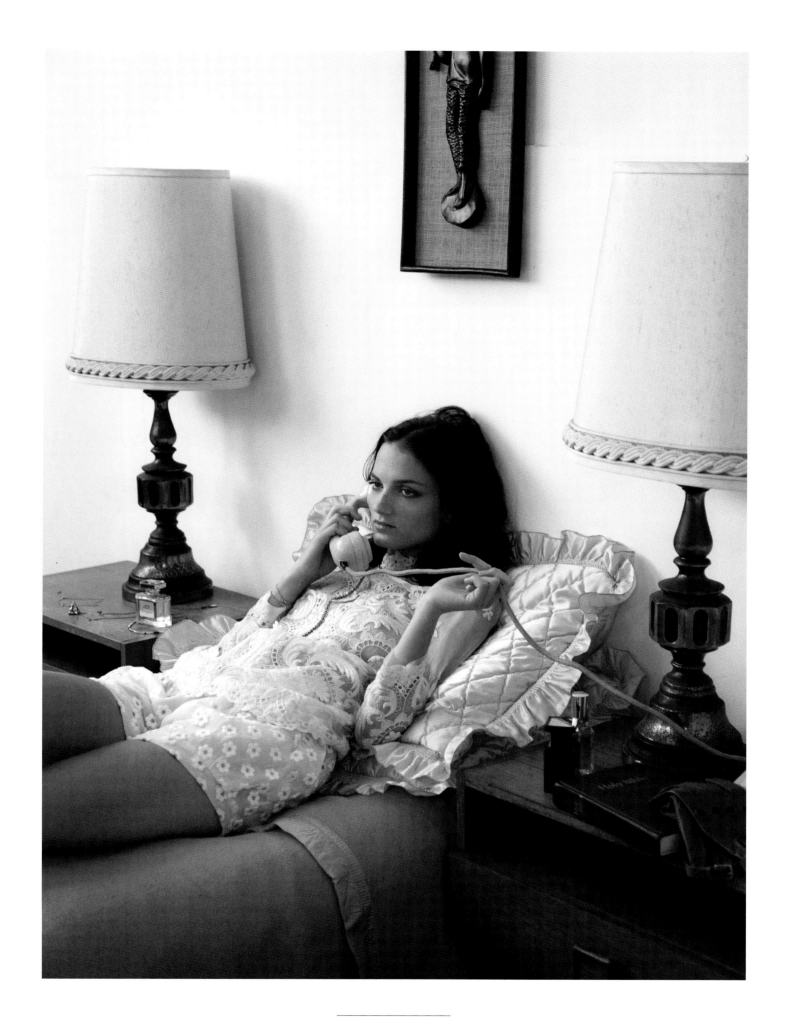

*Opposite: Android romance – a mix of the hard
with the soft, 2009.*

Above: 70s romance in 2012.

IF ONLY

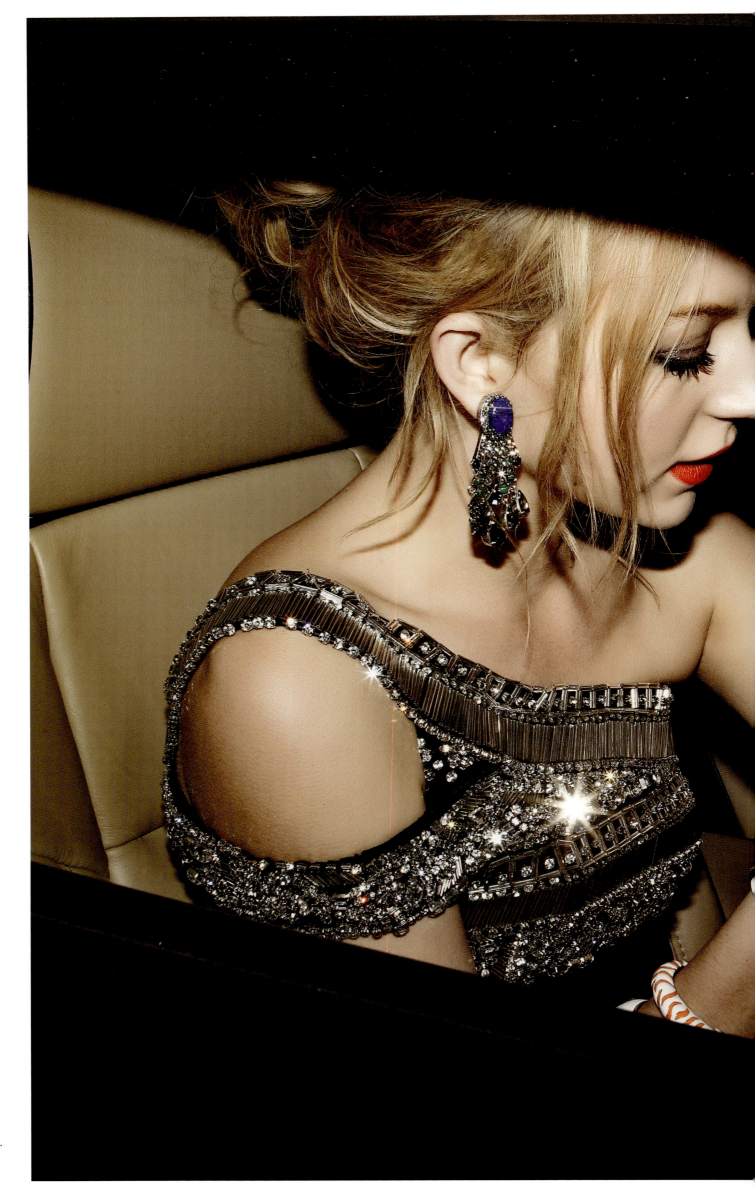

This shot epitomises rock-and-roll glamour in the contemporary world, 2006.

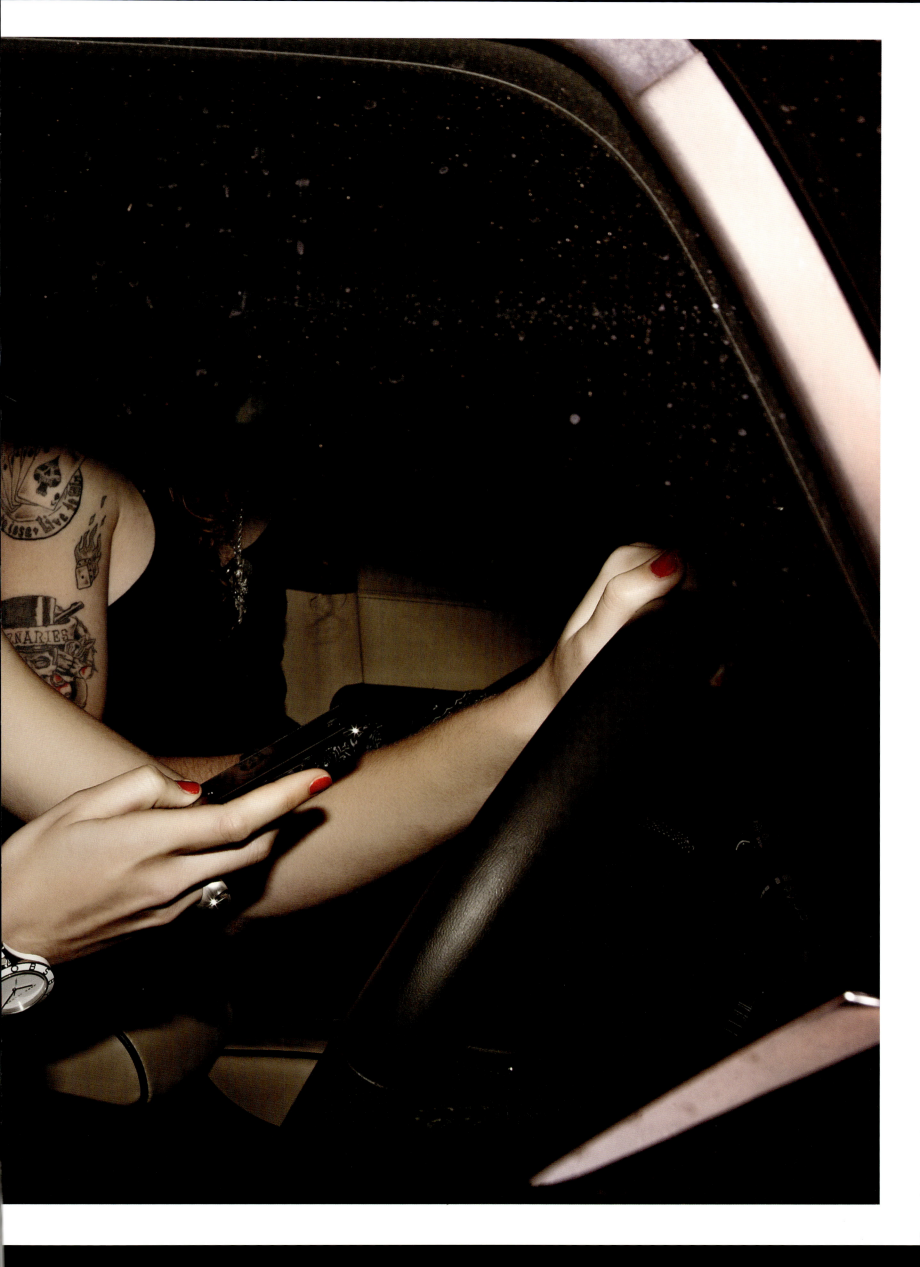

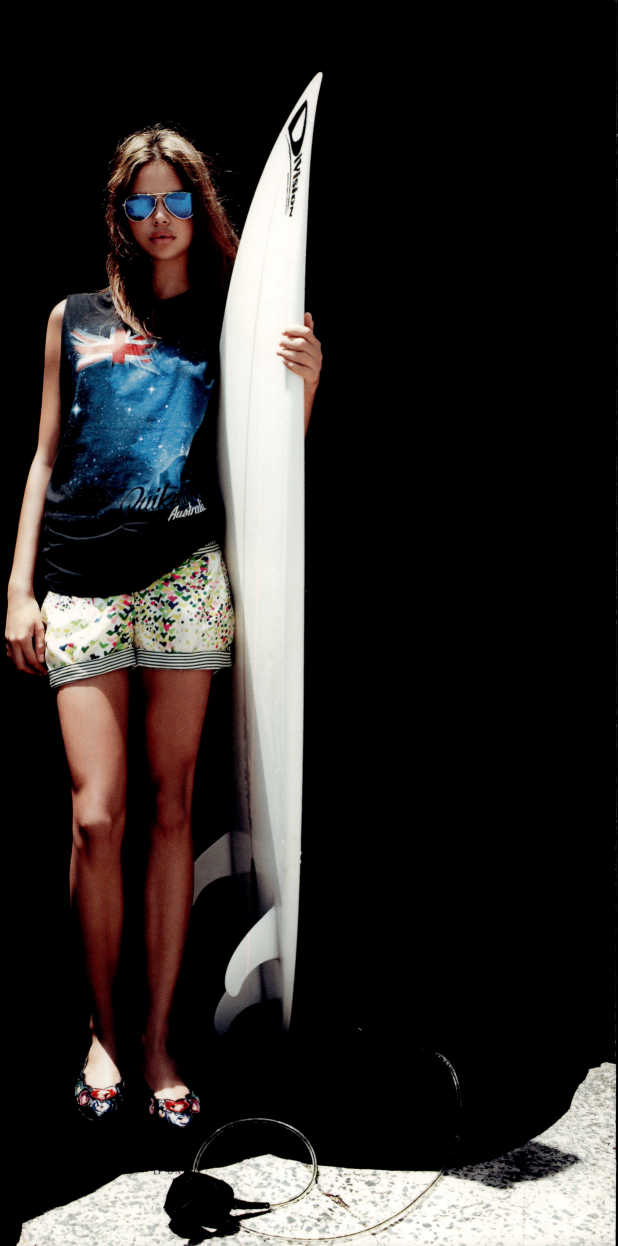

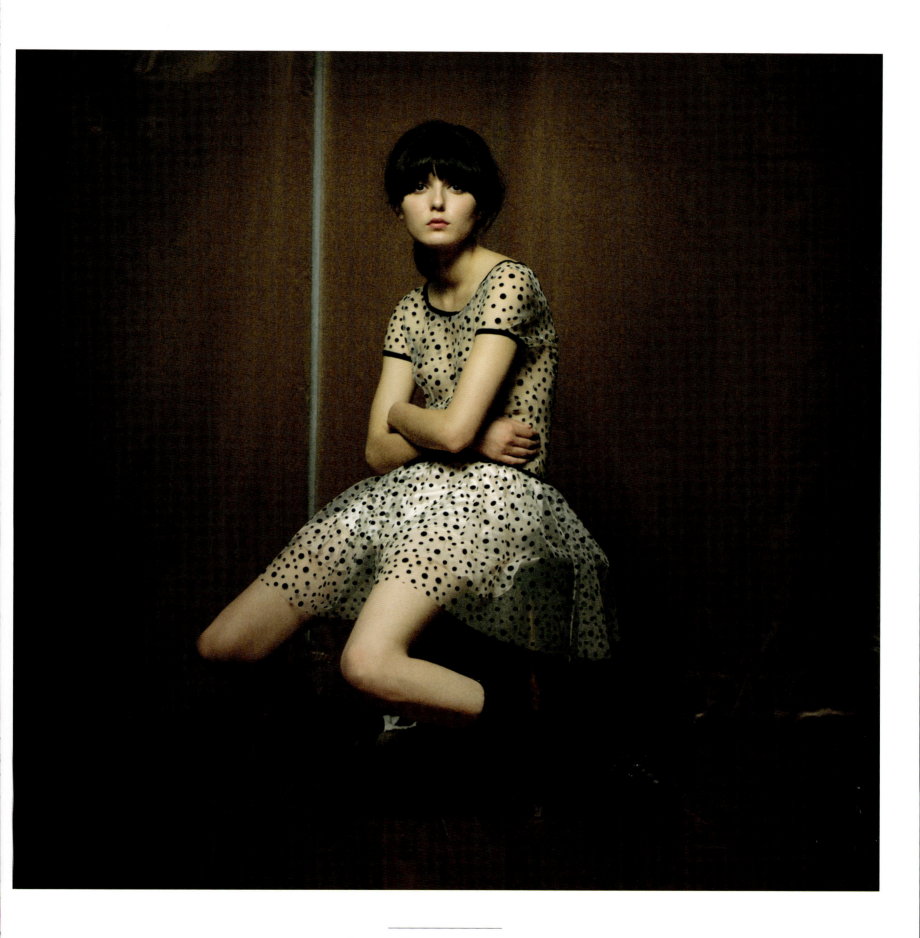

Opposite: *This shot is so Australian —*
it was taken at Bondi Beach in 2009.

Above: *The dark side of tulle, 2003.*

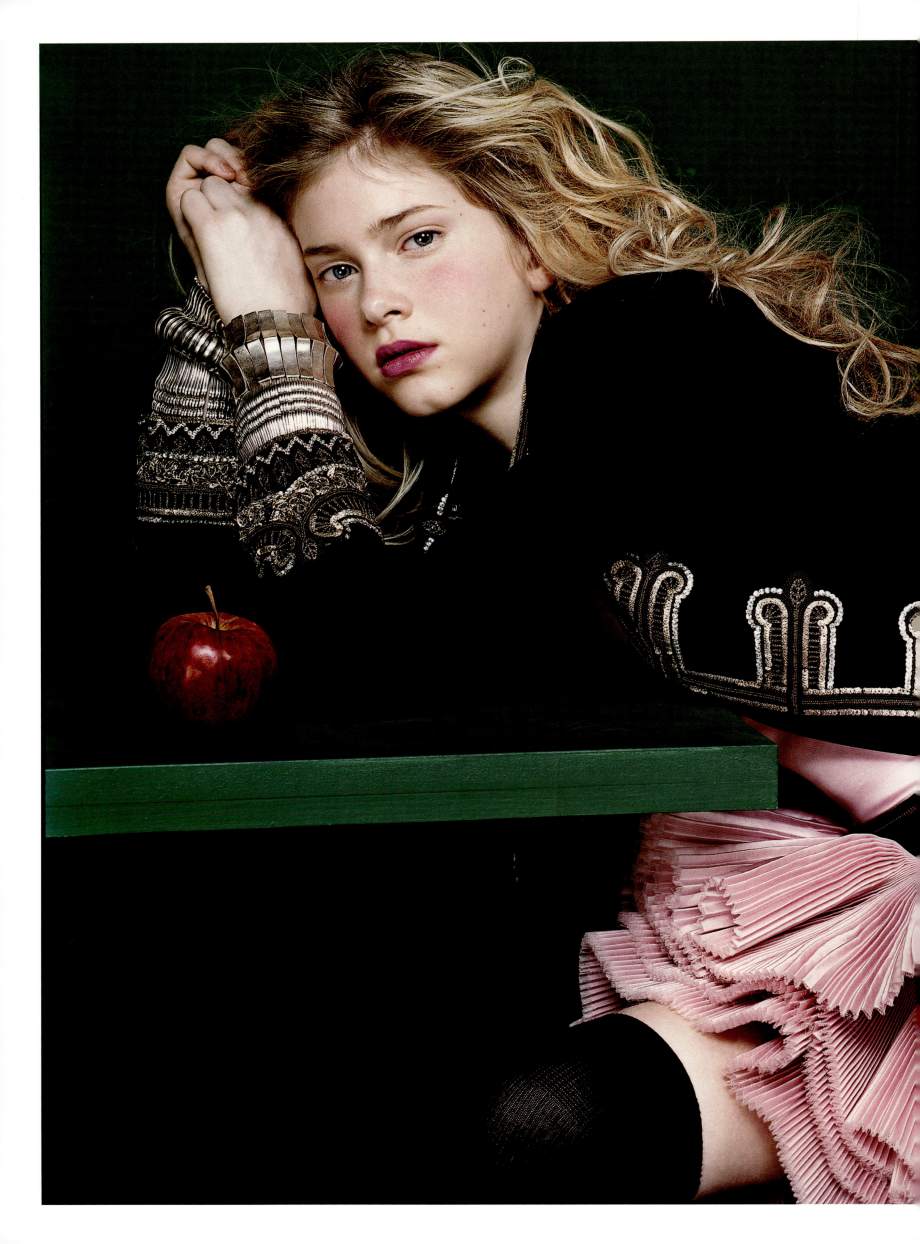

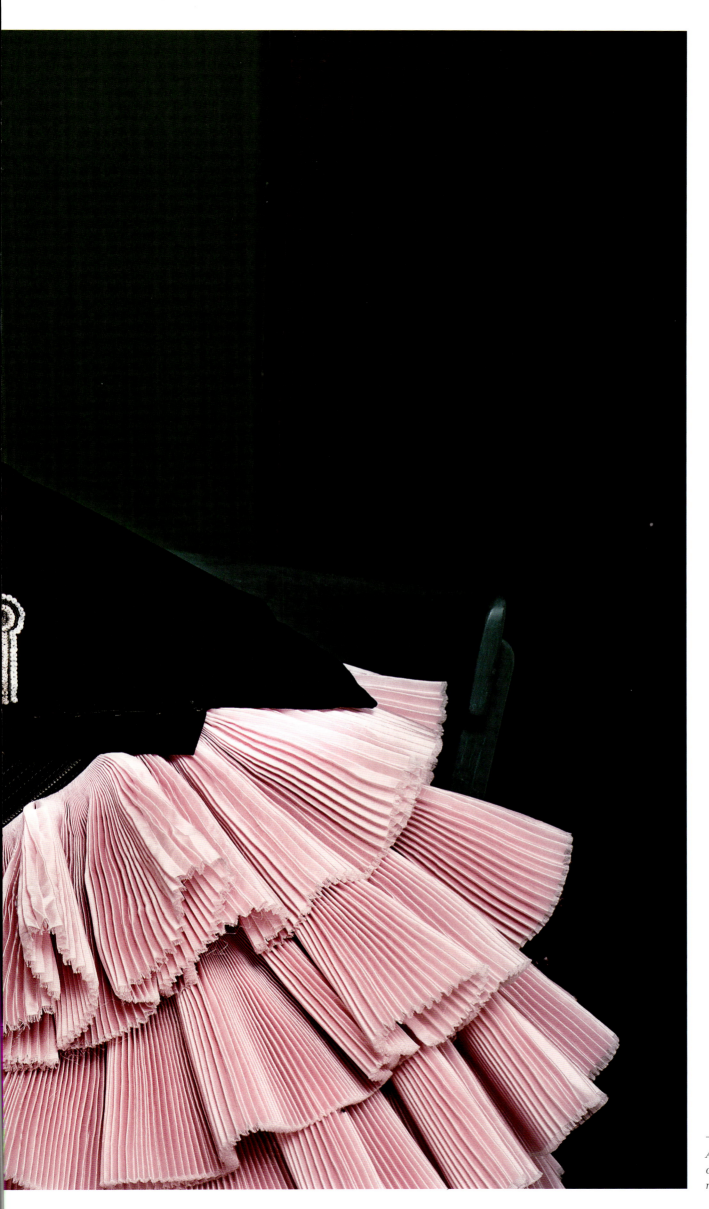

A hard-edged jacket is contrasted with a soft, romantic skirt, 2008.

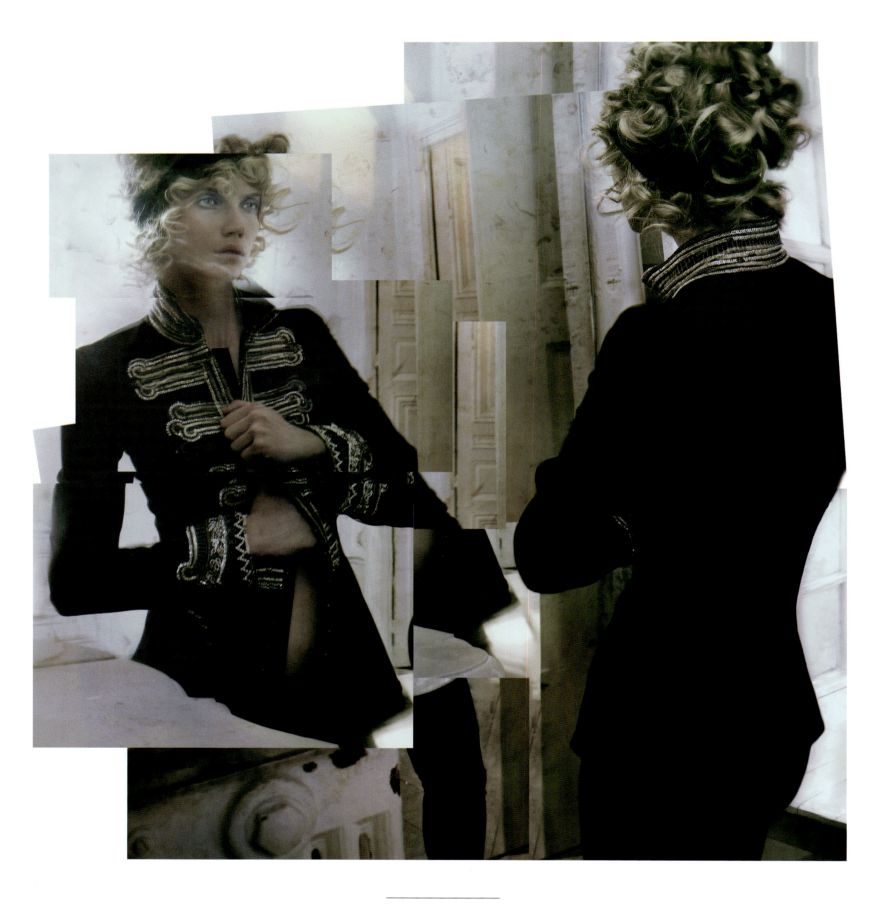

Above: A military moment, 2008.

Opposite: Miranda Kerr wears one of my favourite dresses,
made from a hand-painted, sequinned fabric, 2009.

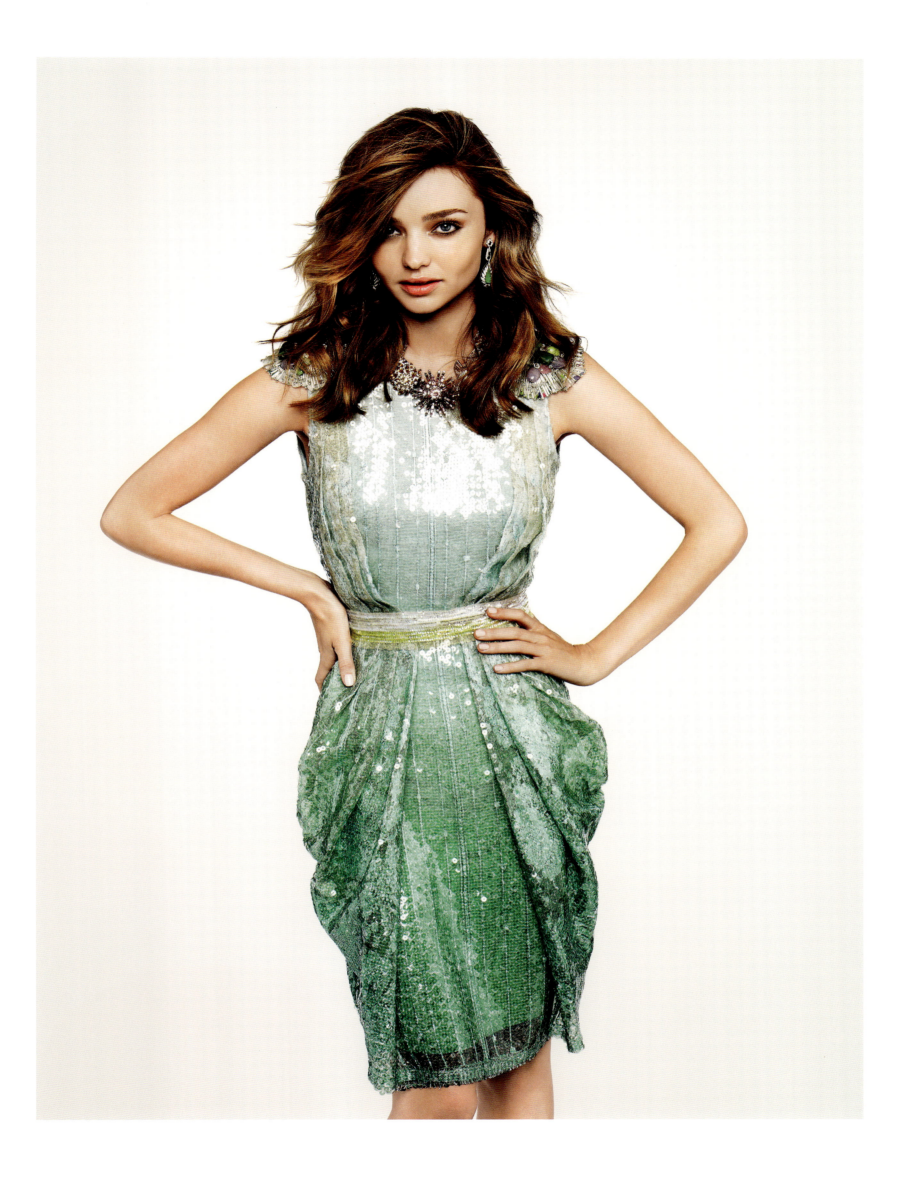

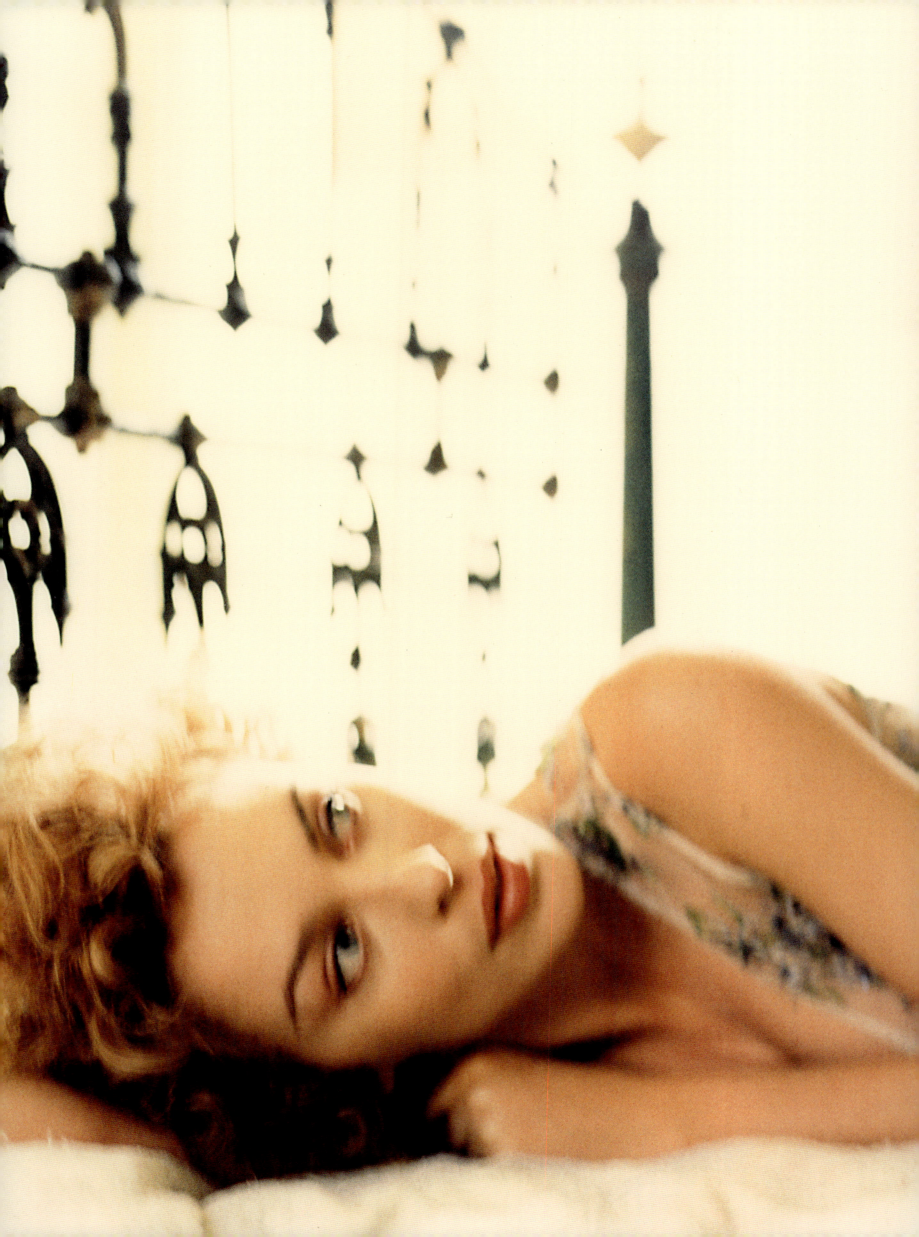

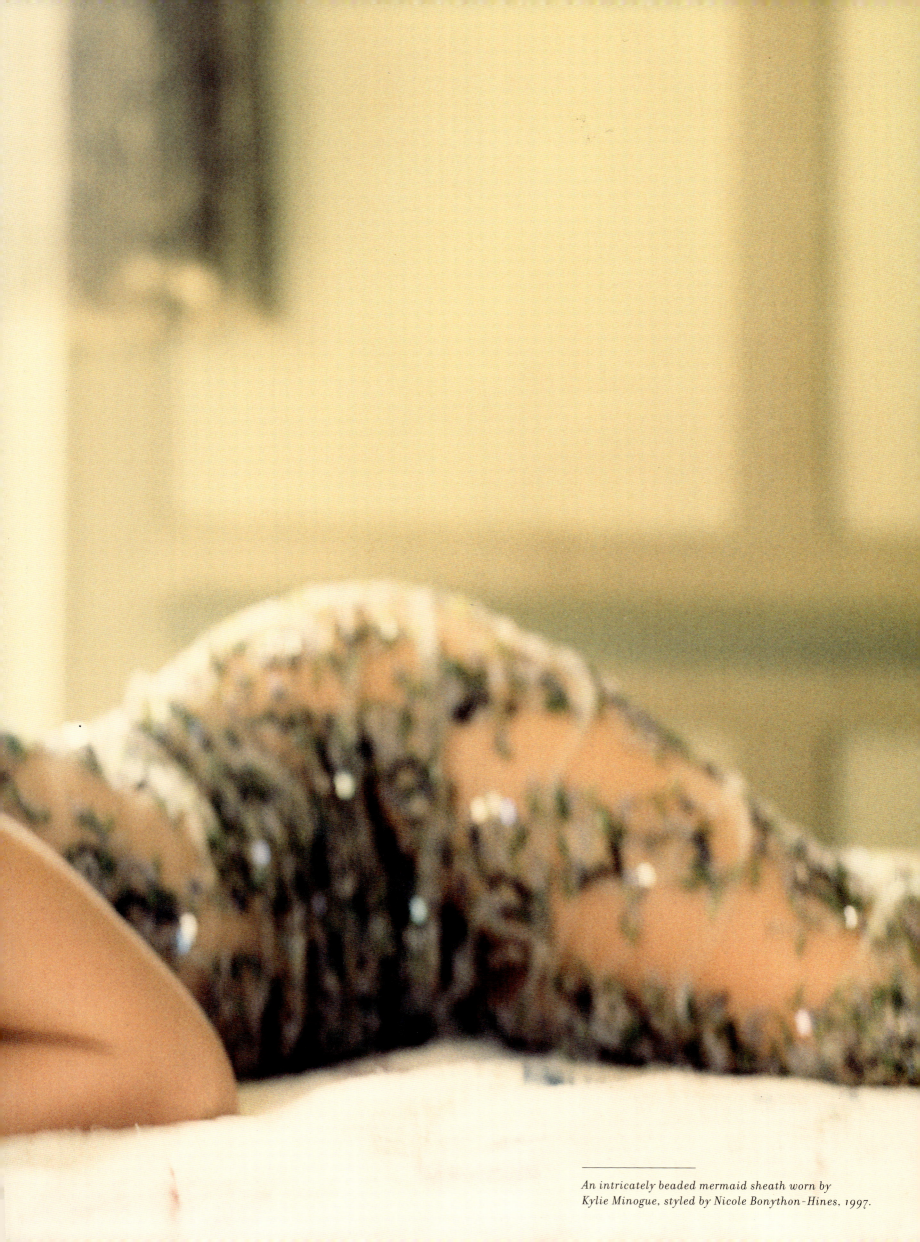

An intricately beaded mermaid sheath worn by
Kylie Minogue, styled by Nicole Bonython-Hines, 1997.

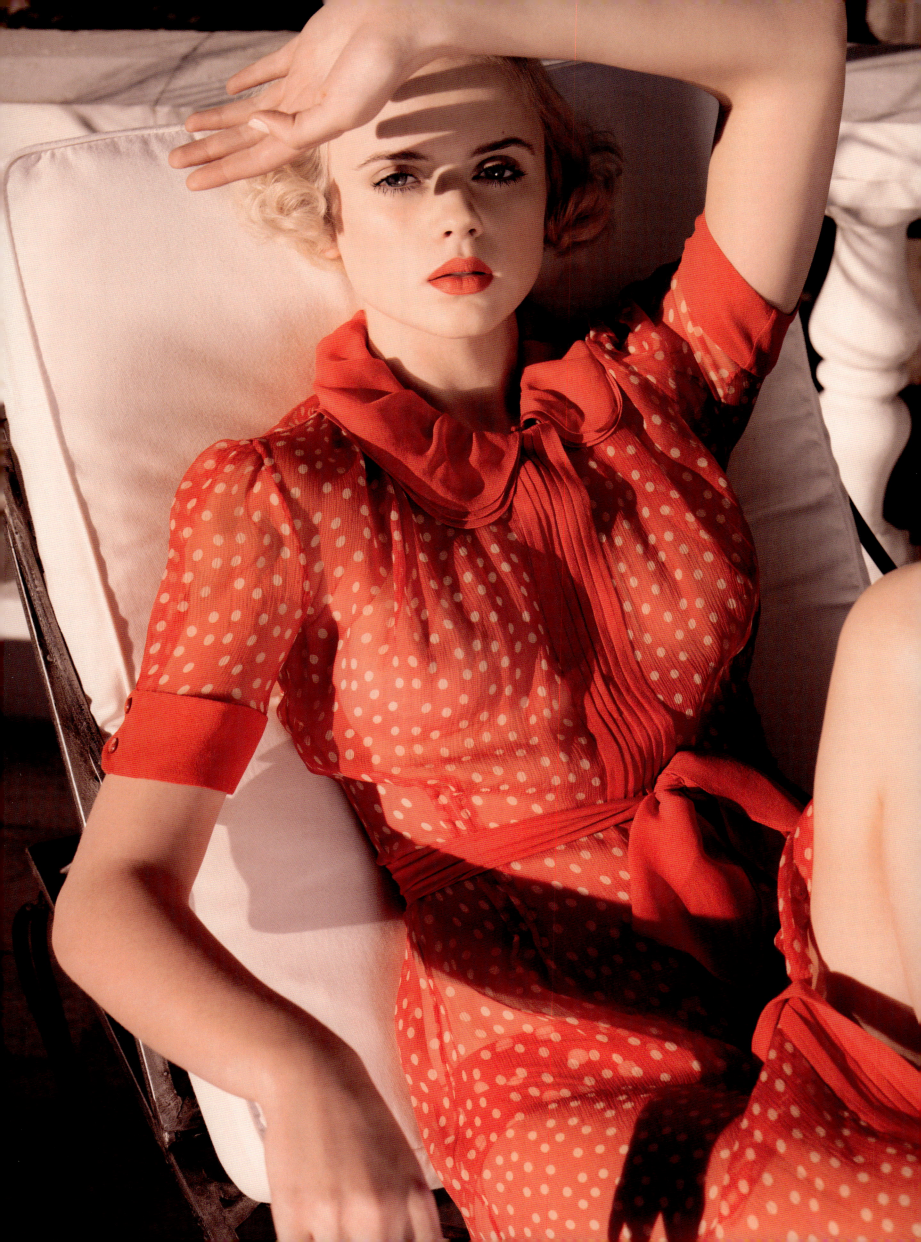

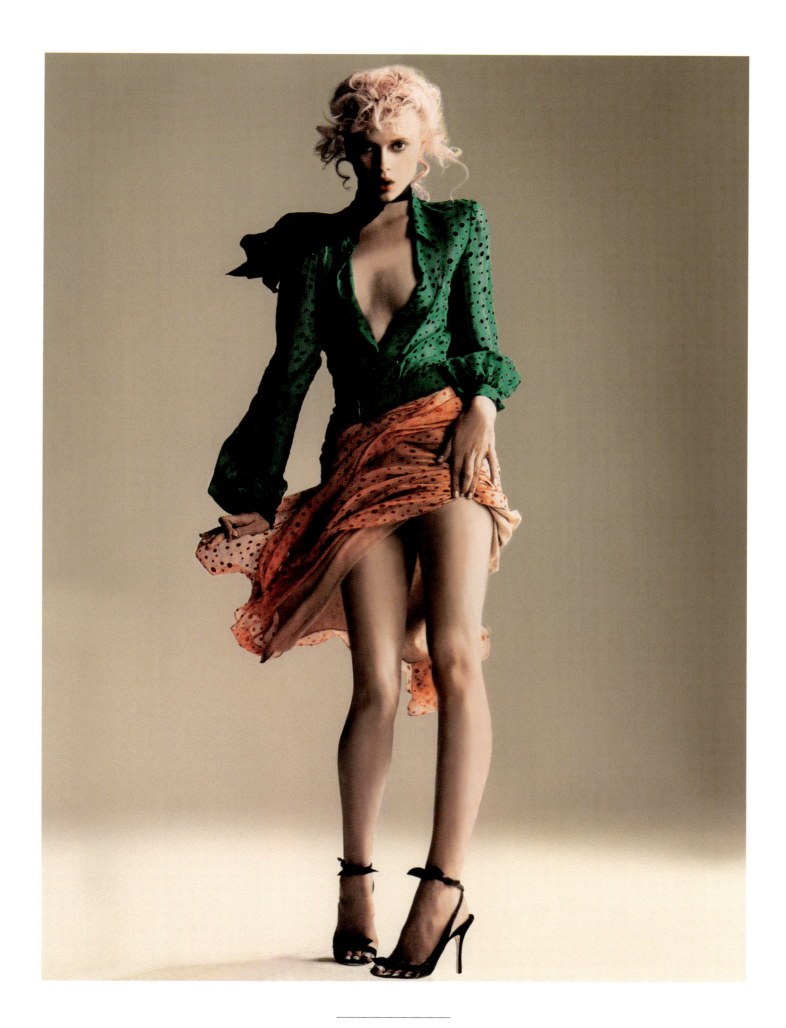

Opposite: My 50s-inspired collection.
Photograph by Richard Bailey, 2007.

This page: This shot is fun and fluid, 2005.

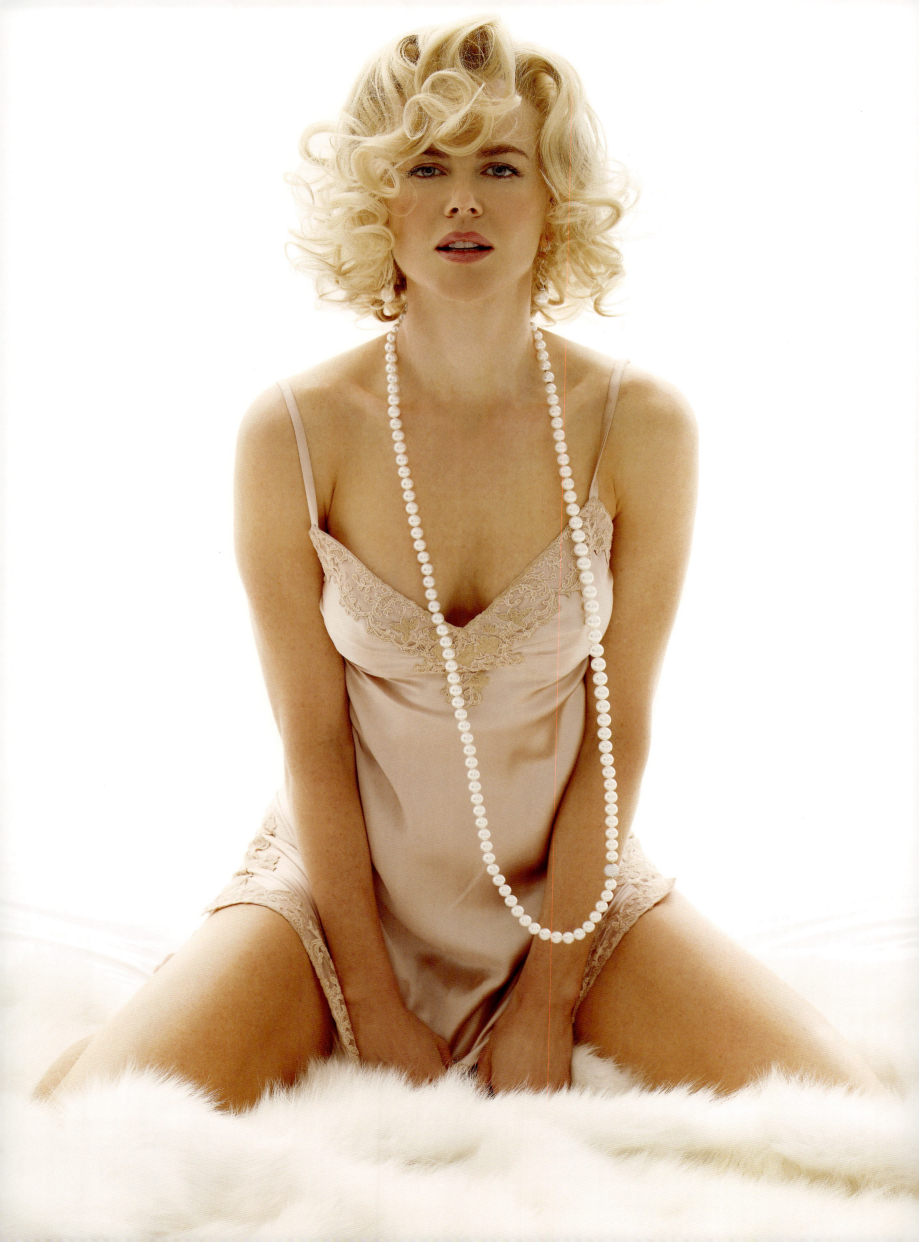

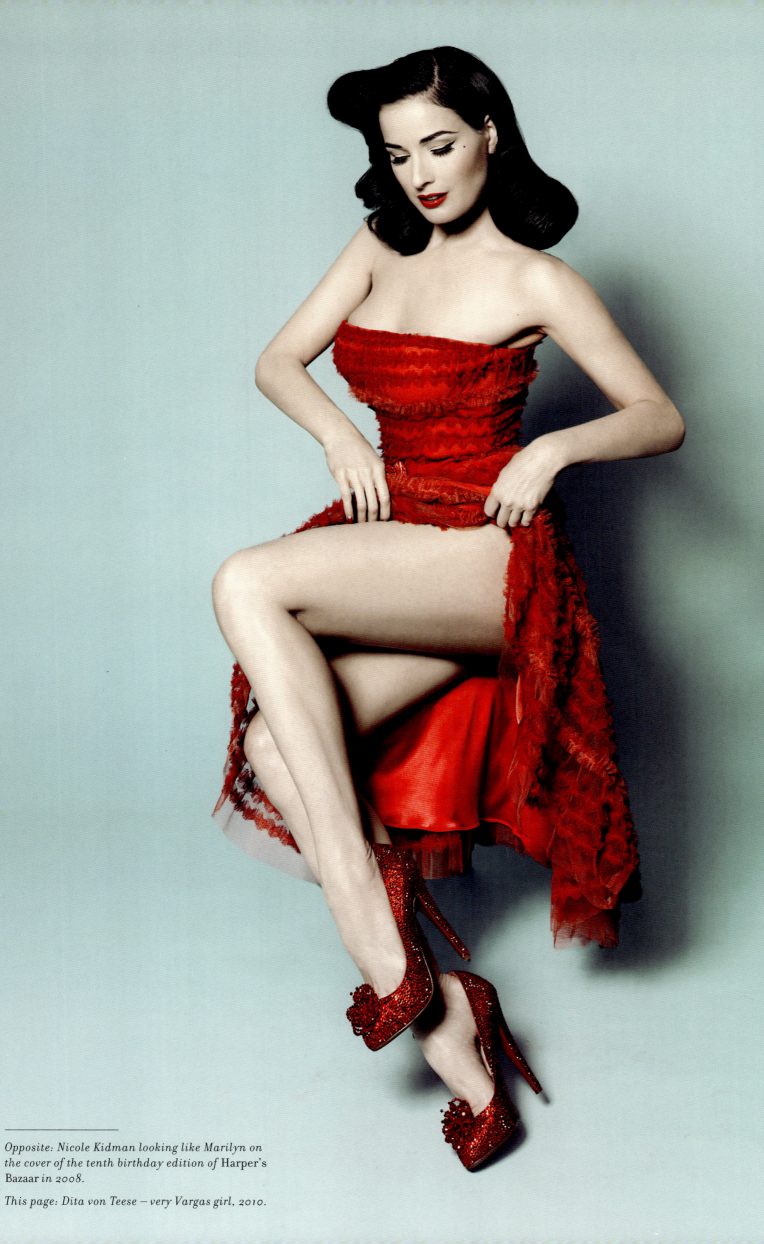

*Opposite: Nicole Kidman looking like Marilyn on
the cover of the tenth birthday edition of Harper's
Bazaar in 2008.*

This page: Dita von Teese – very Vargas girl, 2010.

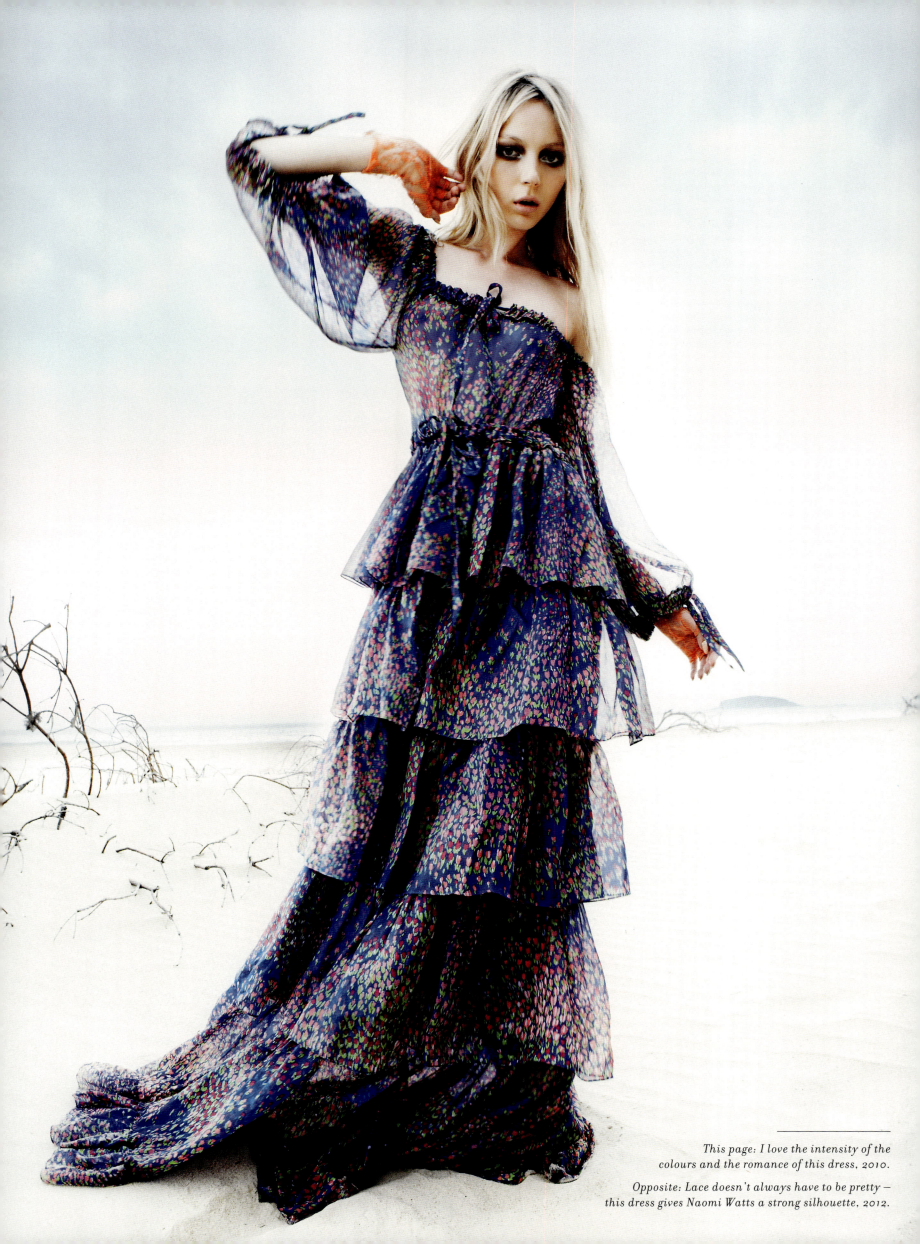

This page: I love the intensity of the
colours and the romance of this dress, 2010.

Opposite: Lace doesn't always have to be pretty –
this dress gives Naomi Watts a strong silhouette, 2012.

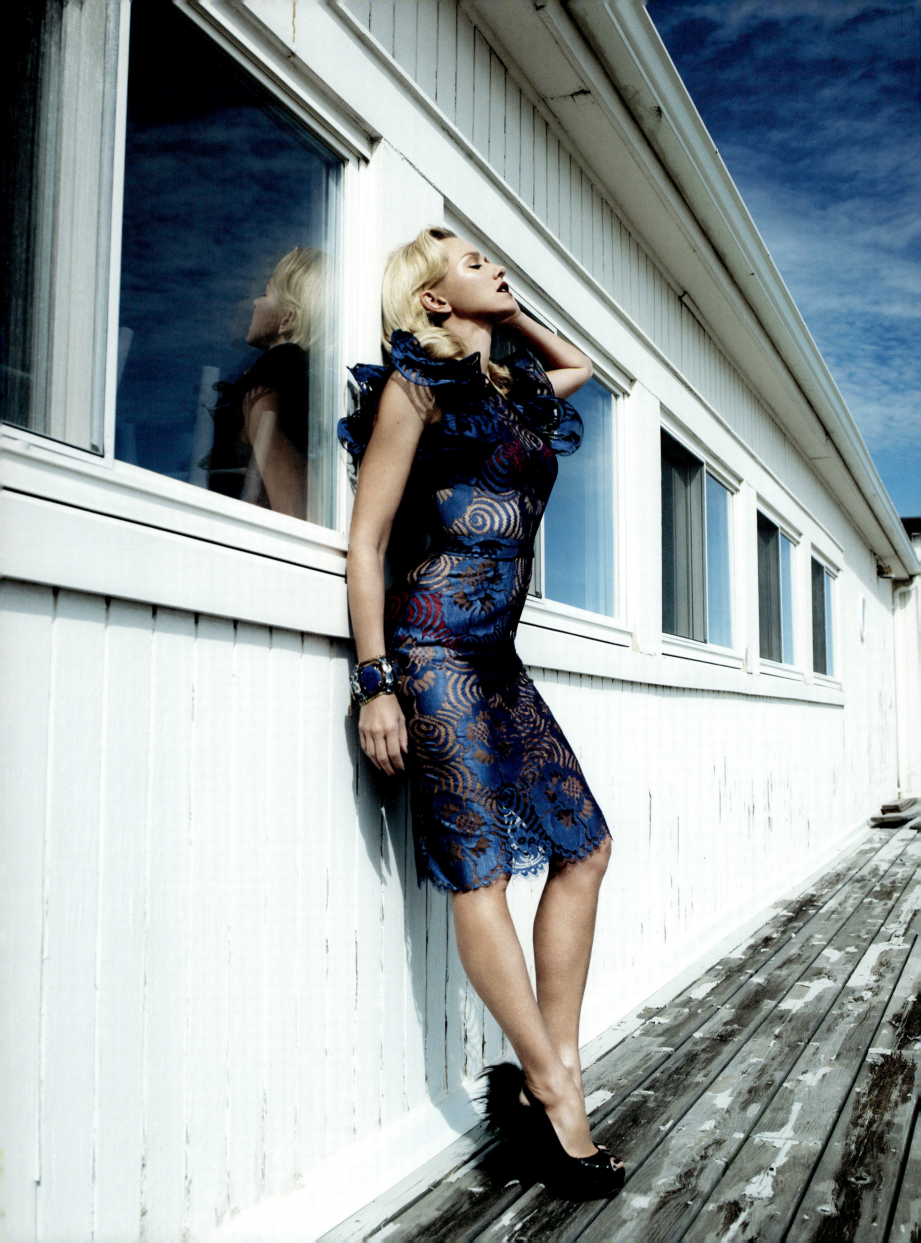

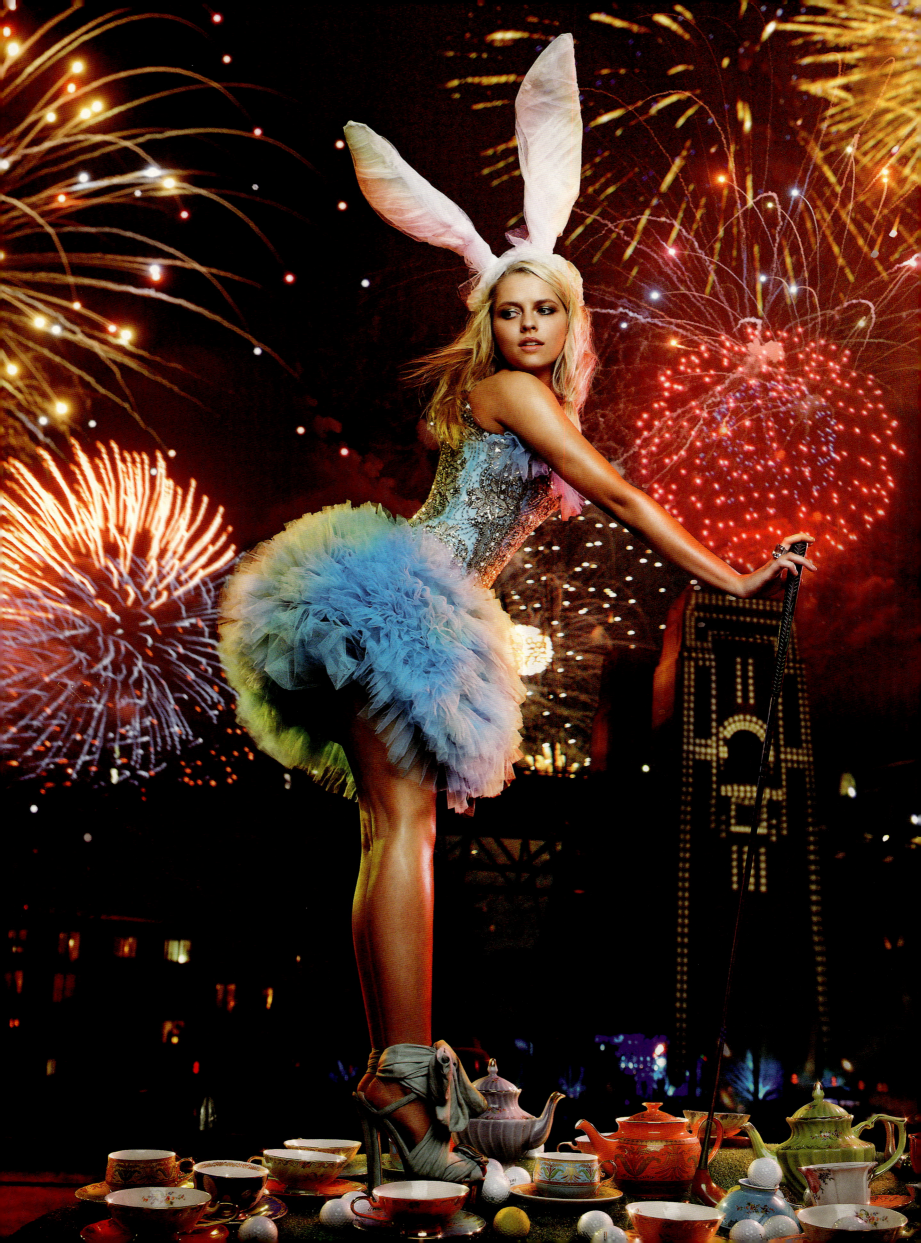

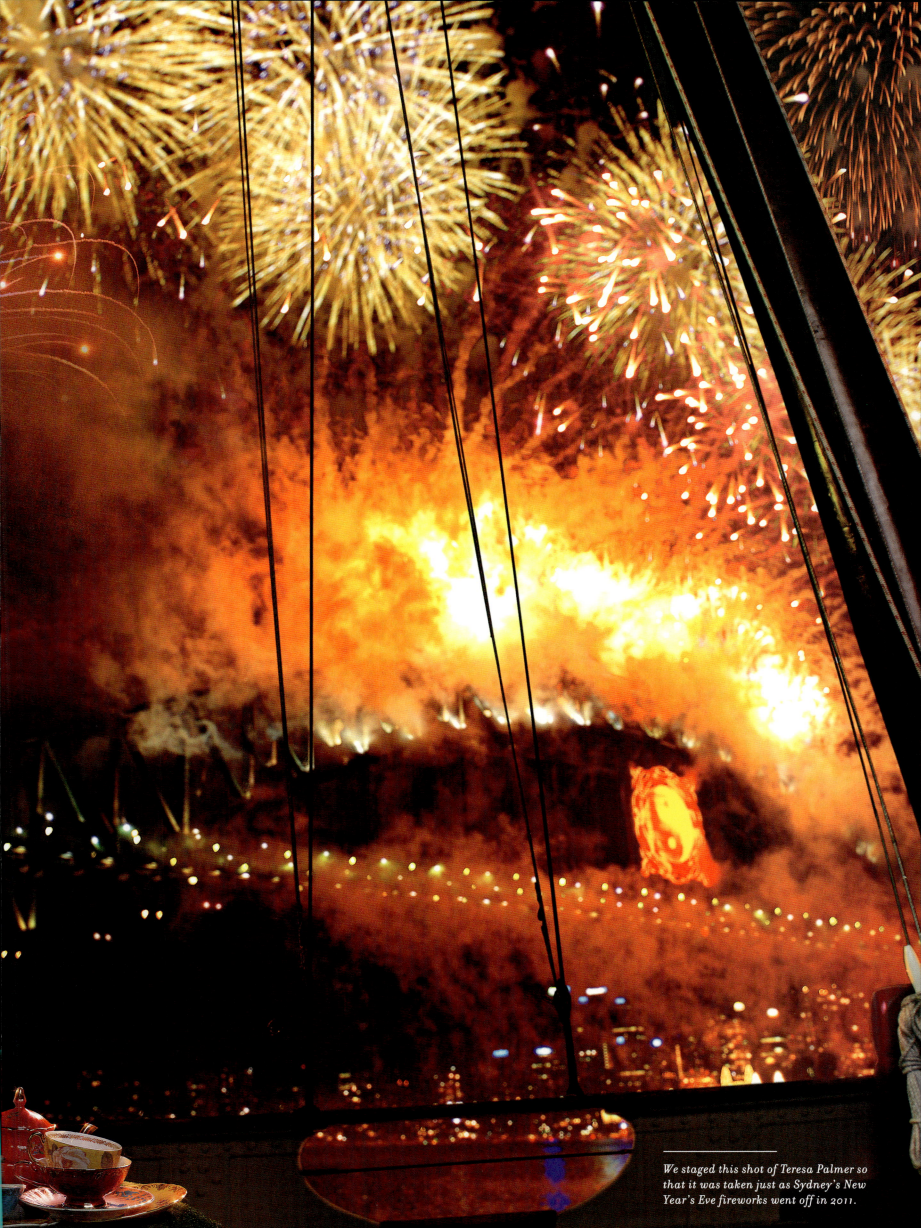

We staged this shot of Teresa Palmer so that it was taken just as Sydney's New Year's Eve fireworks went off in 2011.

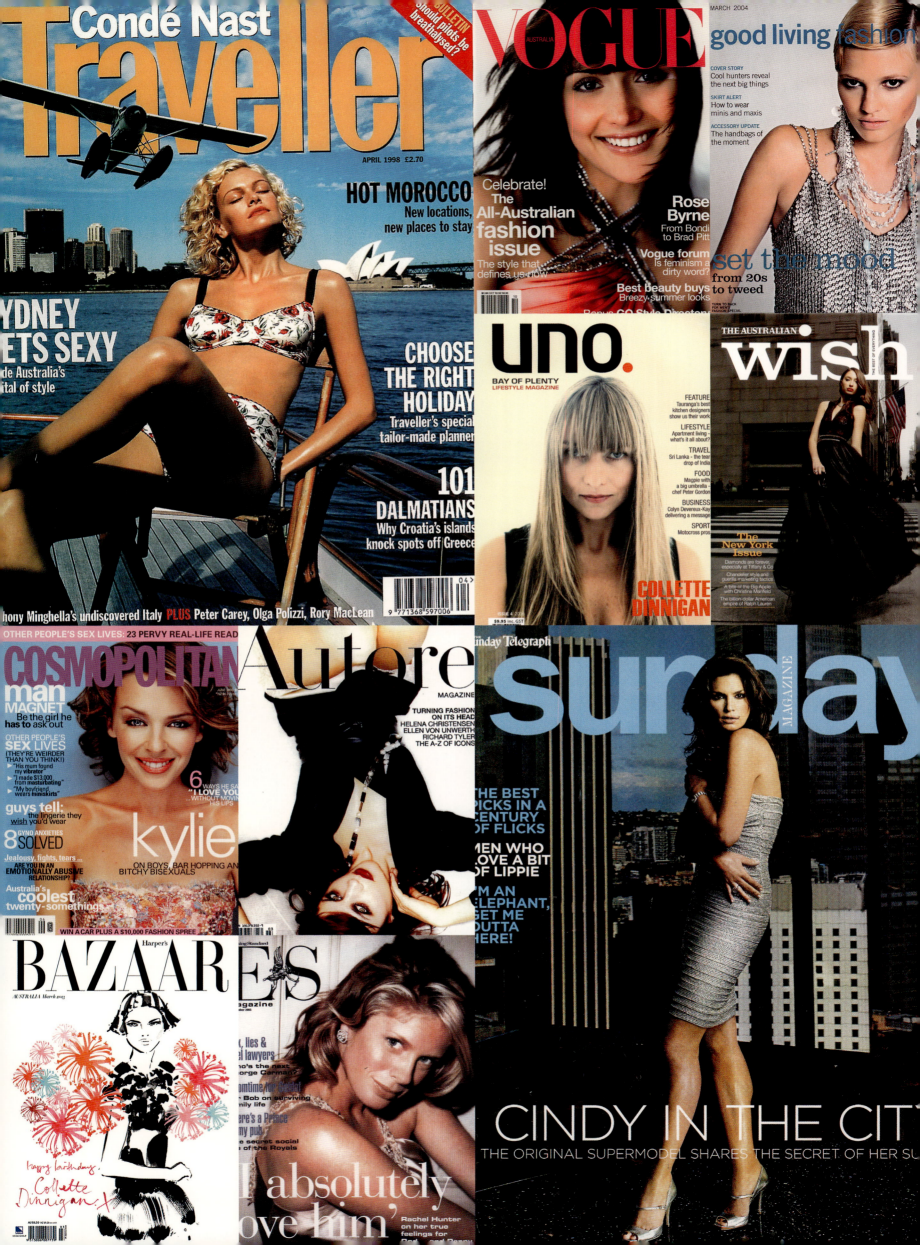

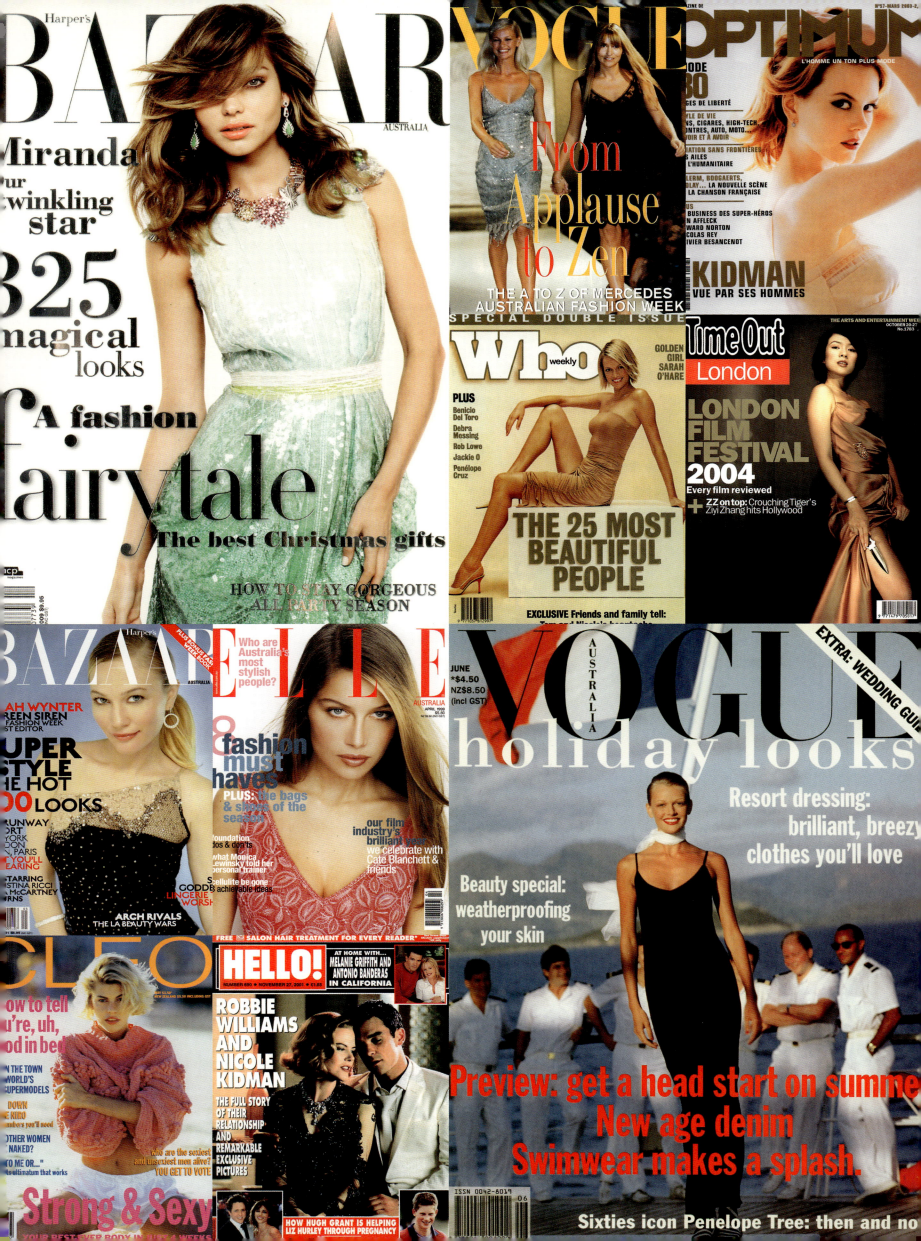

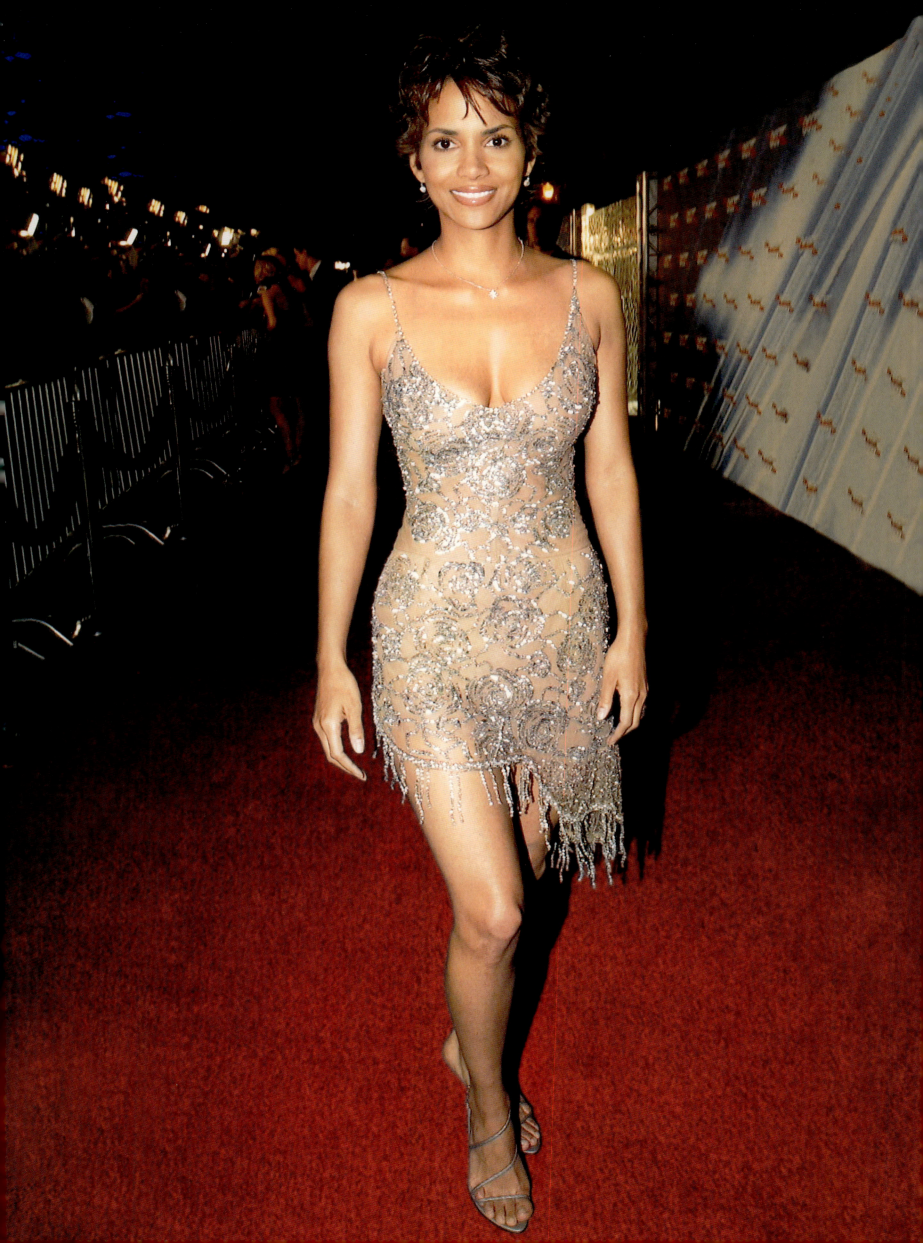

THE
JOURNEY
OF A
DRESS

From runway to

red carpet.

CHAPTER 7

ONCE IT LEAVES US,
EACH DRESS GOES
ON ITS OWN JOURNEY —

it might end up anywhere from

the red carpet to a palace.

THERE IS ALWAYS A GREAT

BUZZ IN THE STUDIO

WHEN SOMEONE INTERESTING

WEARS OUR CLOTHES.

It doesn't necessarily mean that we will

get a flood of requests for that particular dress,

but it certainly increases brand awareness.

THE RED CARPET

is a big part of my business —

THE WHOLE WORLD

WATCHES THOSE EVENTS,

and it's all about

WHO WEARS WHAT,

AND WHERE.

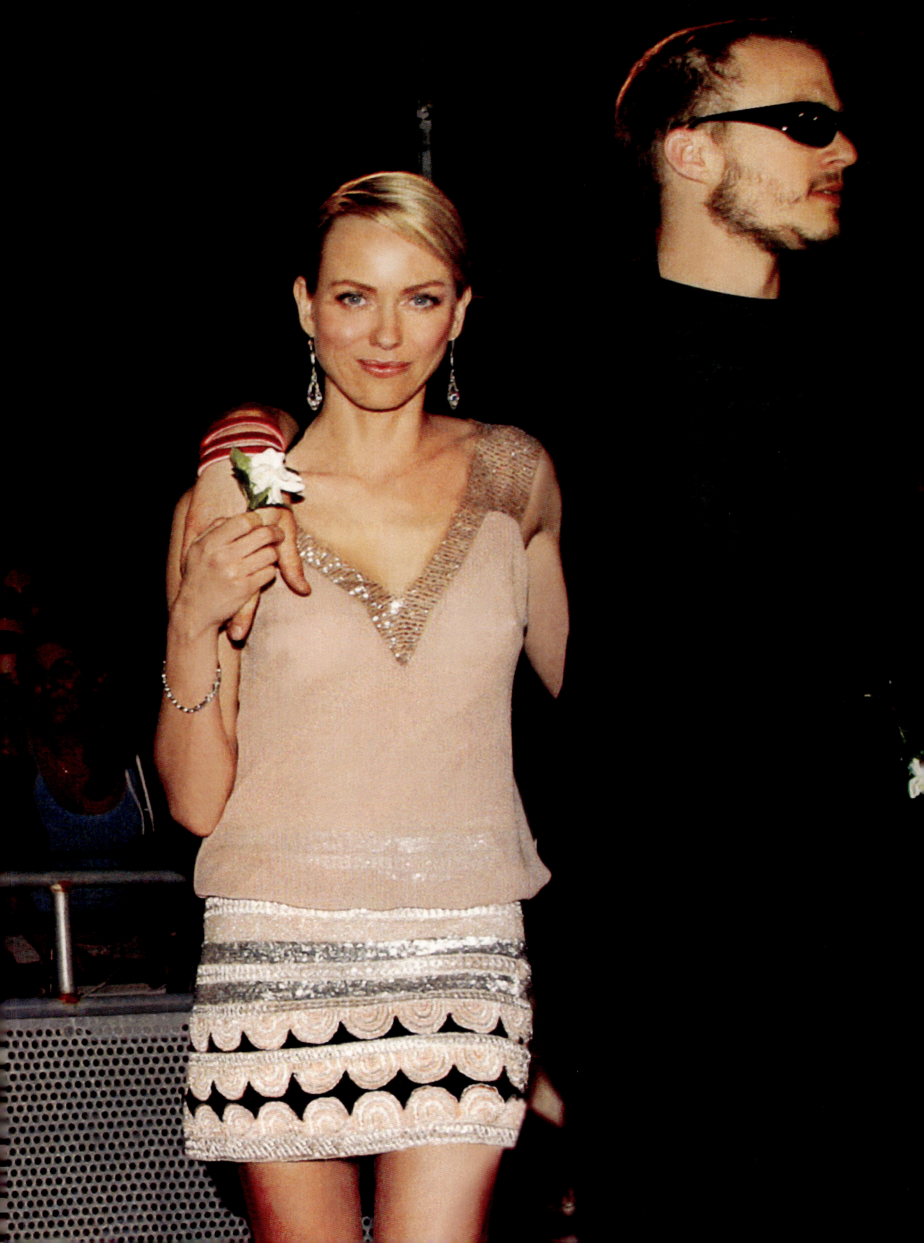

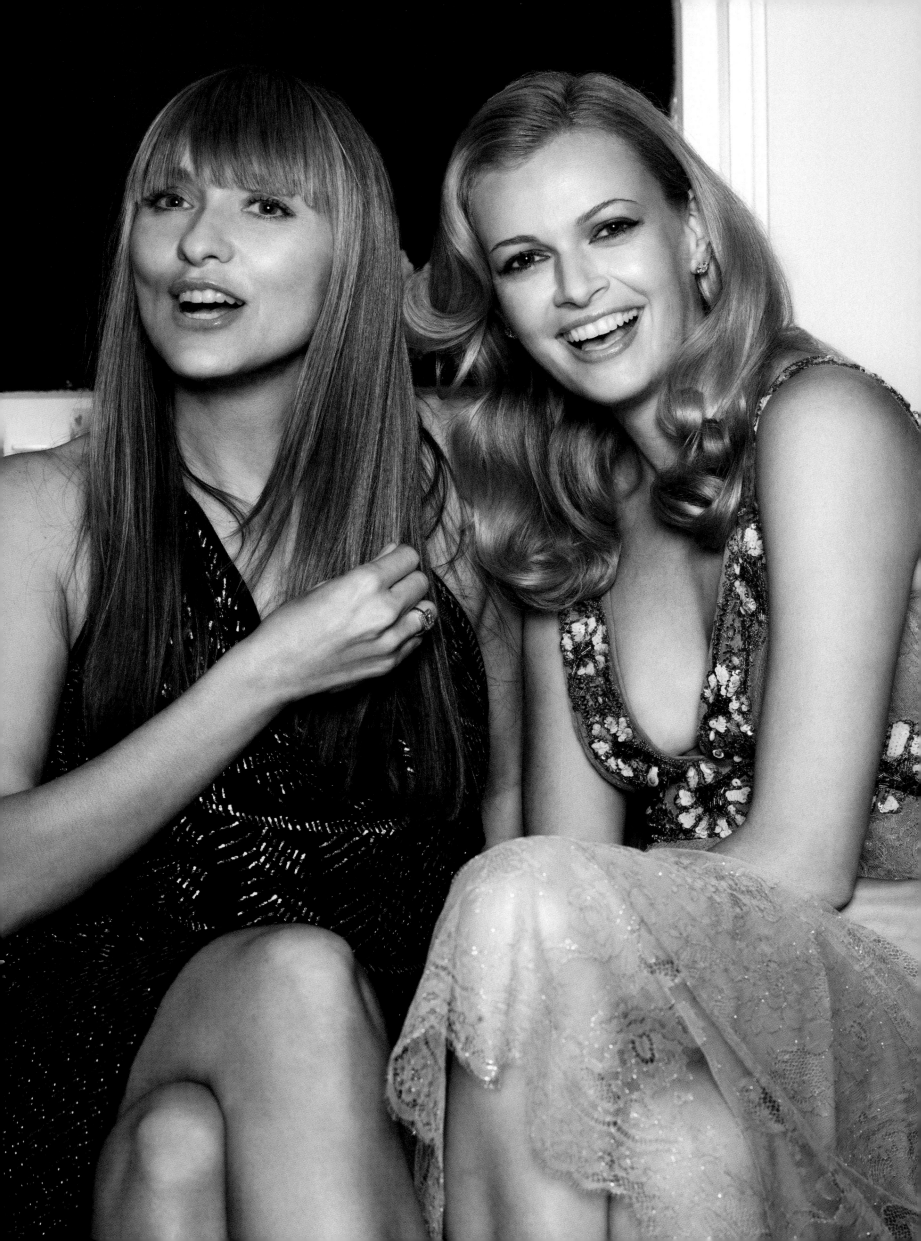

These days, I think most awards ceremonies are over-styled,

and a lot of actresses end up looking too conservative. Years ago,

before the stylist boom, awards ceremonies were more fun to watch.

∞

Today, if I am dressing an actress for an awards night, I have to deal with a whole entourage of people, all of whom have different opinions about how she should look. It is much harder than dealing with the actress one on one, as I used to do. There is so much pressure to get everything perfectly right, so that the actress feels comfortable all night – a lot of thought goes into it.

Some of my early Australian supporters were Cate Blanchett, Nicole Kidman, Naomi Watts, Kylie Minogue, Elle Macpherson and Sarah Murdoch. I would either make them a dress, or lend them one. All of them have since become great supporters and friends, who regularly wear my clothes. I love dressing each of them – they all look so fabulous in my clothes.

Even after all these years, I still feel flattered and proud when I see my dresses worn on the red carpet. Unlike some of the larger, more international design houses, I don't actively seek out that business. We don't have the budgets to compete, as we are a small bespoke design house, so we make very few of each dress. Some designers virtually set up ateliers in Los Angeles at Oscars time – I don't.

What usually happens is that a stylist who has been to one of our shows, or has seen our look book on style. com, will contact us and say, 'So-and-so loved the silver beaded dress with the short sleeves in your resort collection – could you please make it up for her?' They might ask for some variations, 'Could it be longer? Could it be shorter? Could it be made without the sleeves?' We always let them know when the dress will be in-store, so they

know that if it is worn after that date, it is already available for purchase. They send us the actress's measurements, and we make the dress up to fit her and send it over. We have a book of measurements with some very interesting information in it. I keep that under lock and key.

If the client is in Australia, I do the fittings myself if I am here. People ideally like to have somebody fit the dress who designed it. I have developed some close relationships with some of the women I dress regularly. Often the most high-profile people are the most private, and I respect that privacy. One thing I will say is that everyone is intimidated when they take off their clothes, no matter who they are. Unless they are models, not many women are totally comfortable with their bodies; there is always something they don't like, whether it is arms or bust, waist or hips. A fitting is very intimate and personal, so even the most beautiful woman can feel quite vulnerable. No one is perfect – and even film stars can have a bad underwear day!

I sometimes design a dress especially for a particular client, but more often I adapt an existing design that she or her stylist has seen. That said, the year Catherine Martin won two Academy Awards for *Moulin Rouge*, I did design her outfit especially for her. That was planned from the other side of the world, which was a bit frightening, as she has such an incredible eye for detail. As it happened, she just trusted me completely – if anything, it was her husband Baz Luhrmann who put the pressure on.

I was also really thrilled when Jacki Weaver asked me to design a dress for her to wear to the Academy Awards

---

Previous pages: Picture perfect. Halle Berry at the Die Another Day *premiere in Los Angeles, 2002 (page 108);*
Naomi Watts looking fabulous with Heath Ledger at the Ned Kelly *premiere at Fox Studios, Sydney, 2003 (page 111).*

Opposite: Sarah Murdoch and me at a dinner I hosted at my home in Paddington in 2005. Photograph by Richard Bailey.

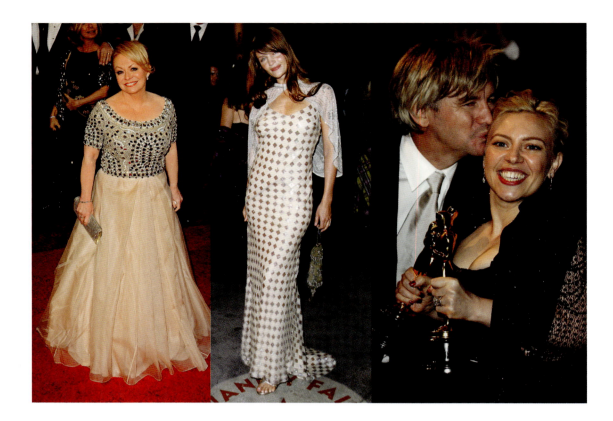

in 2011, when she was nominated for *Animal Kingdom*. She was delightful to work with – she gave me a few ideas, but then left it to me. I think she looked absolutely radiant in her dress.

Another dress that I designed especially was for my friend Kathy Lette's daughter, Georgina, who, in 2009, aged sixteen, was invited to participate in the famous Debutante Ball at the Hôtel de Crillon in Paris. Georgina was the first Australian to be invited to what is one of the most fashionable debutante balls in Europe. She would be rubbing shoulders with royalty and aristocrats from around the globe. The top European fashion houses were vying for the opportunity to dress her, but Georgina asked me to design her dress, which was a great honour. I was the first Australian designer to dress someone at that ball, and was thrilled to hear later that it had been voted the most beautiful dress there.

I have been fortunate to dress some of the most beautiful women in the world over the years. I will never forget when Halle Berry wore one of my dresses in 2002 to the Los Angeles premiere of the James Bond film she had just starred in, *Die Another Day*. The dress was from my latest Paris collection, which had an Indian theme, with lots of silver antique jewels on flesh-coloured silk.

I remember vividly that I was in the toilet paper aisle of the supermarket (of all places) when I received a call from Los Angeles from her stylist, Phillip Bloch, saying that Halle wanted to wear one of the dresses from that collection to the premiere. This was on a Friday, and the premiere was to be on the Monday, so we had to get it on a plane to her straightaway. I rang the office and arranged for someone to send over the dress in her size. The next day Phillip called to say he was sorry, but she had decided to wear another dress. I was a bit disappointed, but I understand that you can't make a final decision about a dress until you try it on.

Anyway, on Monday I started to receive calls from journalists wanting to interview me about the dress. I kept telling them that they had made a mistake, and Halle had not worn my dress. Then I saw Halle's photo in the paper when I got to work, and I realised that it was my dress after all. She looked amazing – the colour was perfect on her, and the dress fitted her like a glove. It caused quite a sensation in the press because it looked like Halle had nothing on underneath. All that any of the journalists wanted to know was whether she was wearing underwear. When I explained that the dress was fully lined with

Above: Dresses I have made for the Oscars –
Jacki Weaver, Helena Christensen and
Catherine Martin (with Baz Luhrmann).

Opposite: Halle Berry dazzles – I love
the antique beading on this dress.

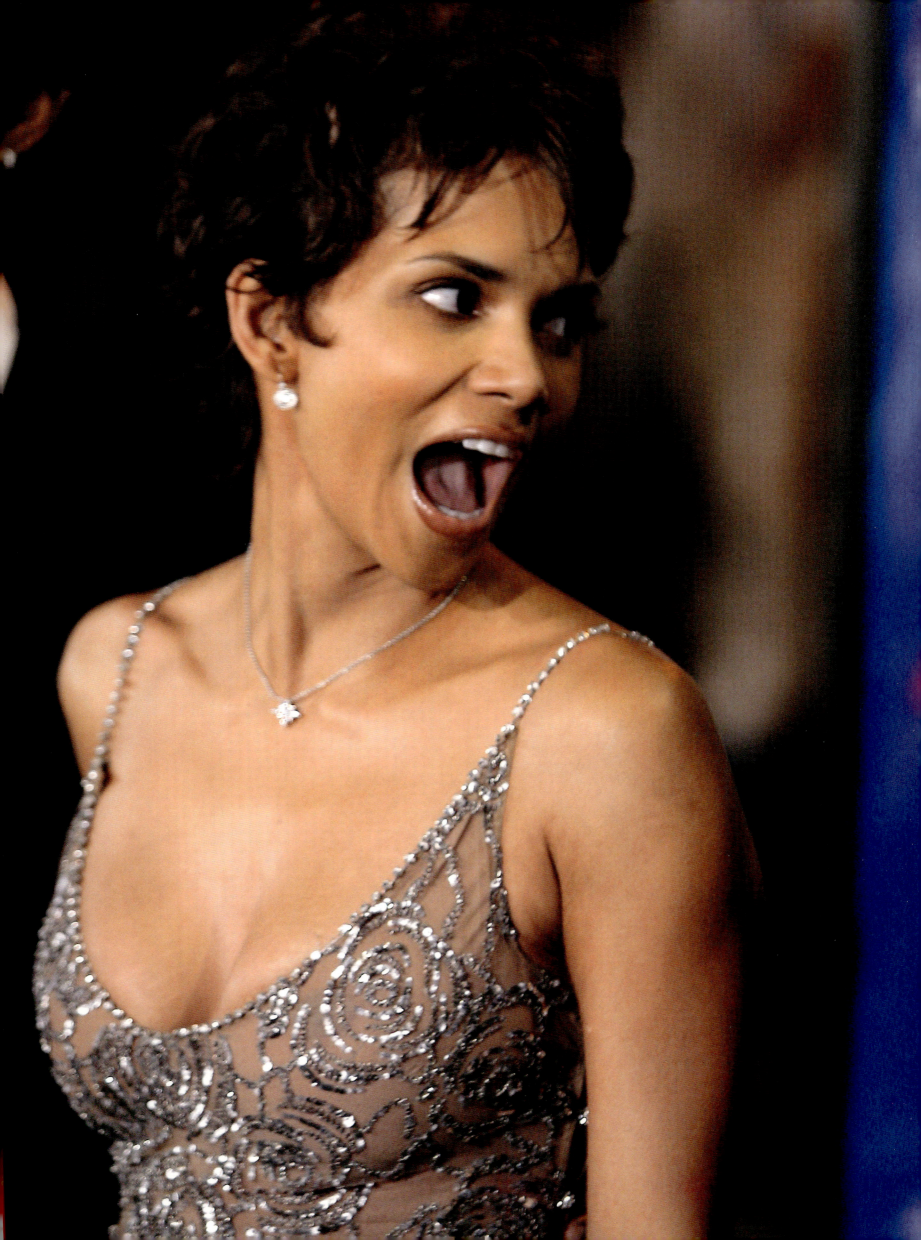

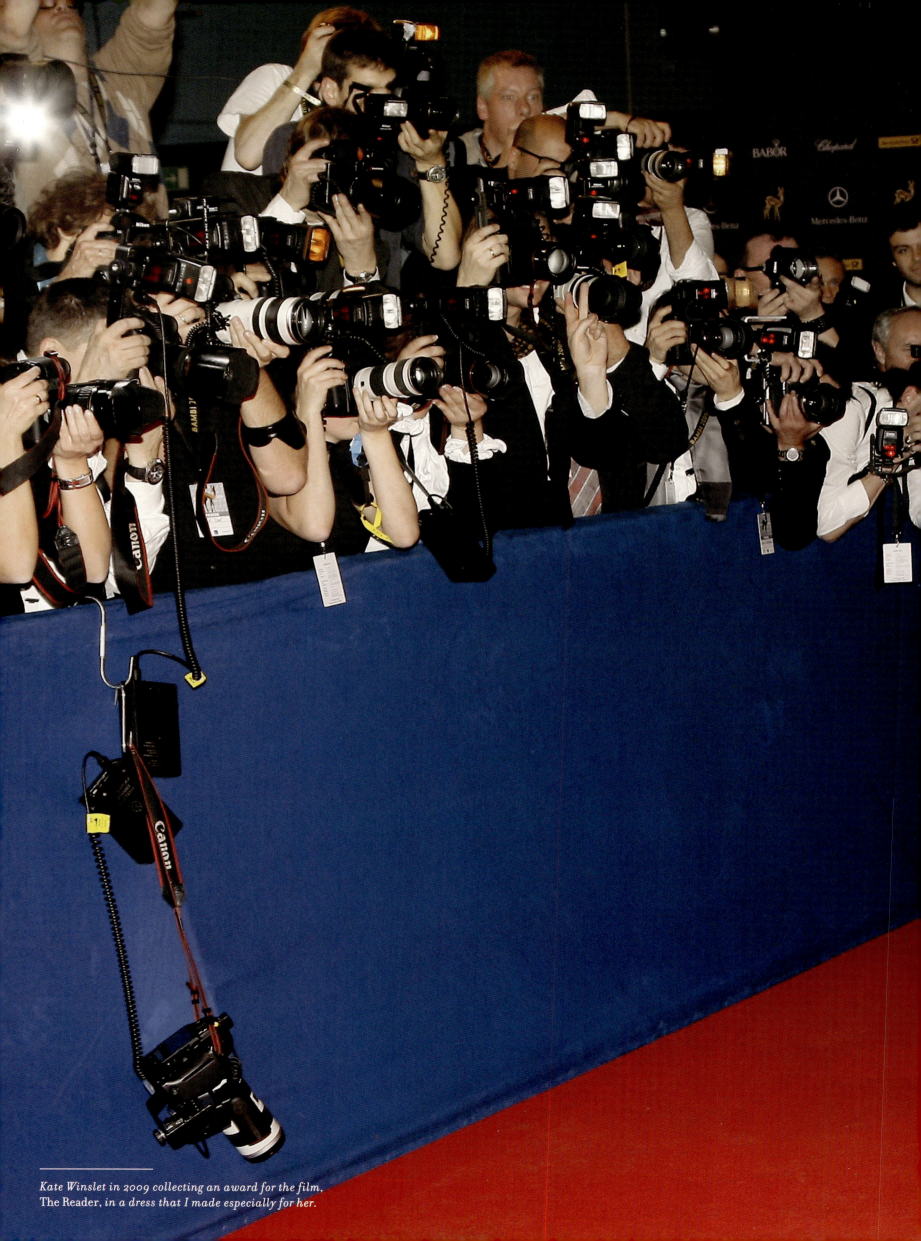

Kate Winslet in 2009 collecting an award for the film,
The Reader, in a dress that I made especially for her.

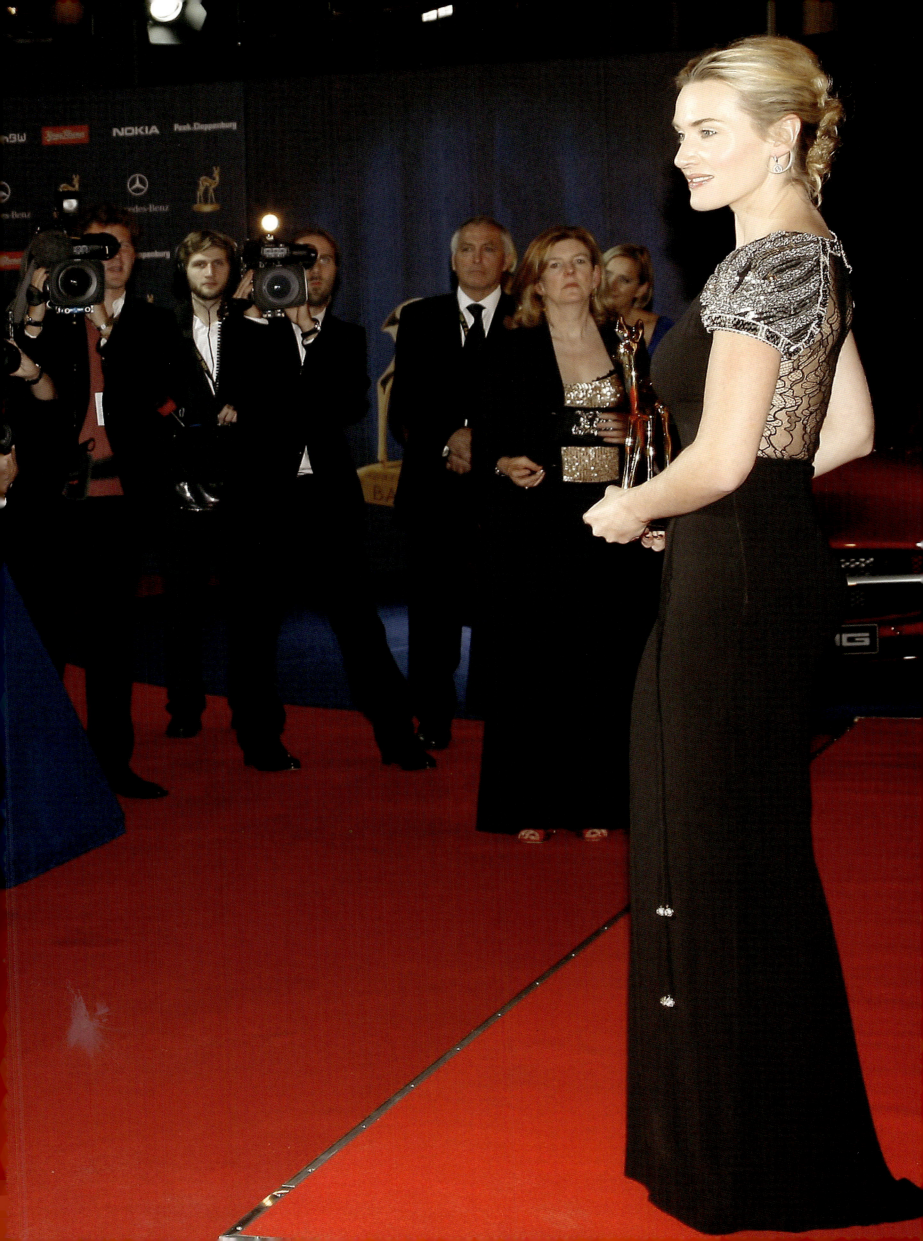

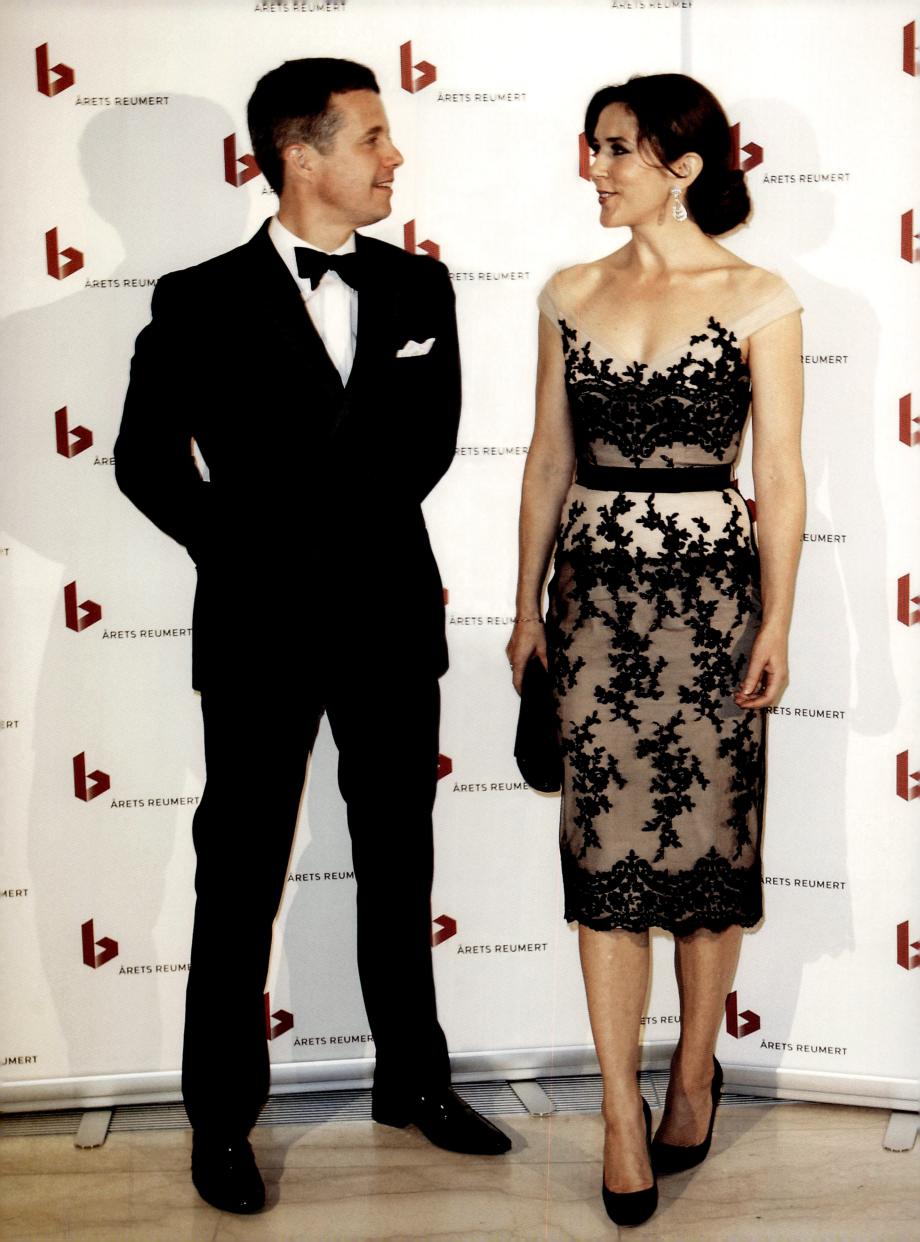

a flesh-coloured fabric, and that she certainly was wearing underwear, they lost interest in the story.

One dress that has been on quite a journey is the Mirabella dress, from my 2012 collection. I had decided to do a collection of limited edition pieces using sample lengths of black corded French lace. The idea was to create something very elegant and ladylike, and to do a small run only. It was quite challenging for my design team, as they couldn't just order a certain number of metres of lace, but had to use the pieces we had left, which were in all different shapes and sizes. Every piece had to be cut by hand and re-appliquéd. I was thrilled with the outcome. That dress is one of my all-time favourites – it was elegant, it had a beautiful neckline, it was sophisticated and also very feminine.

I loved the dress so much that I wore it to Buckingham Palace when I was invited to a function for prominent Australians in London. I remember opening the invitation from the Palace when I was in bed, and Estella was with me. She was so excited – she was six at the time, and mad about princesses and castles, and she insisted that I go. So I did, and it was quite the experience.

I arrived with my friend Marc Newson. I remember telling him I was worried because I didn't know how to curtsy, and he said, 'For God's sake, you're not going to meet the Queen. I've been to these things before, there'll be hundreds of people there'. Anyway, when

I presented my invitation at the door I was ushered away in the opposite direction to Marc and everyone else. I was quite rattled – I thought I must have done something wrong. When I asked the man who was escorting me what was happening, he said, 'Haven't you been briefed?

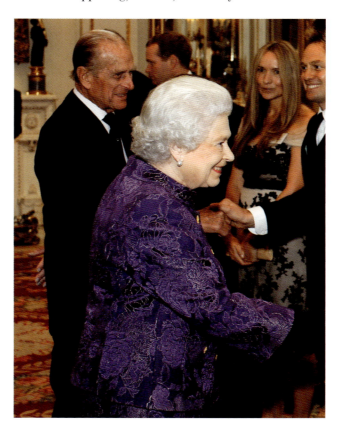

Opposite: Crown Prince Frederik of Denmark, with Crown Princess Mary in one of my all-time favourite dresses – the Mirabella – in 2012.

Above: I loved the Mirabella so much that I wore it myself when I was invited to Buckingham Palace to meet the Queen in 2011.

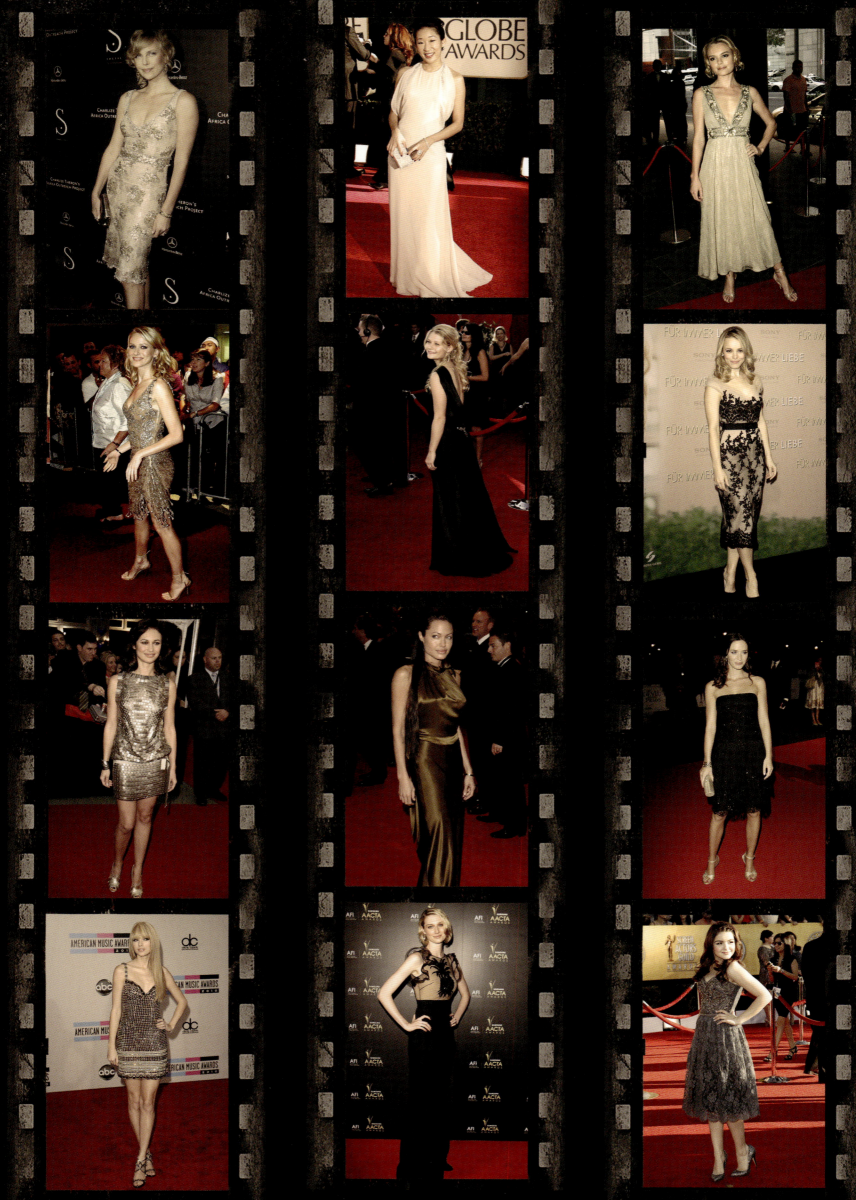

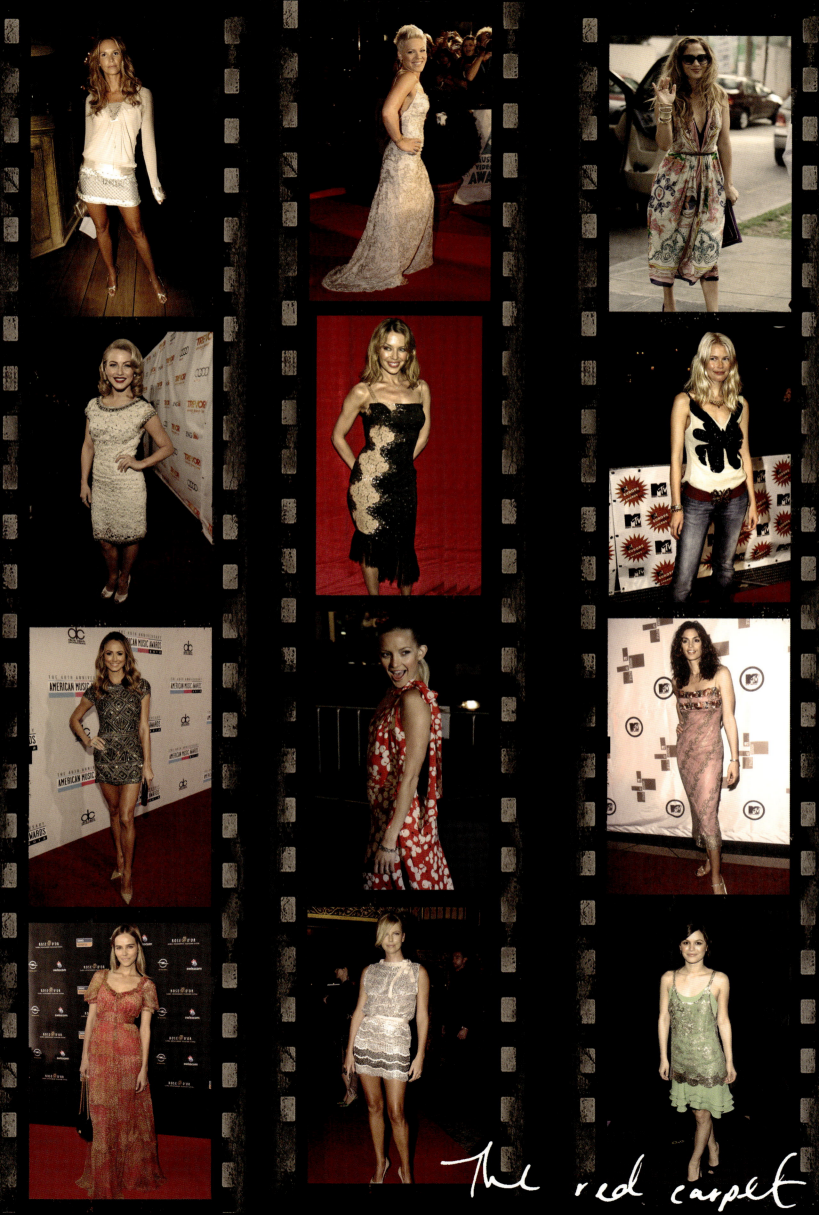

The red carpet

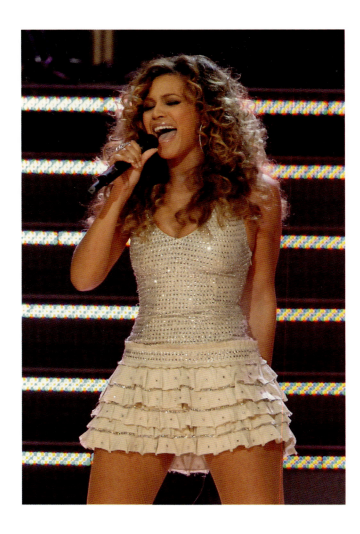

Above: Beyoncé on stage in Tokyo, 2006.

You're about to meet the Queen and Prince Philip.' That took me totally by surprise. Before I had time to panic, I was shown into a beautiful room, decorated in red (of course) where I saw Hugh Jackman, Elle Macpherson, Jason Donovan and the film-maker, Tom Hooper.

About fifteen minutes later, the Queen and Prince Philip arrived, with Prince Edward and his wife Sophie, the Countess of Wessex. They had obviously been briefed on each of us, and the Queen was very gracious. It was a very special experience, and I felt very honoured to be singled out like that. We chatted for about twenty minutes, and then the doors opened and we went into a large ball-room, where the rest of the guests were waiting – there were about three hundred people there. Later, a Palace official told me that they had had a bit of trouble research-ing me, as the Palace computer system kept blocking access to my website because of all the lingerie!

I feel incredibly proud when royalty, like Crown Princess Mary of Denmark, or Catherine, the Duchess of Cambridge, choose to wear my clothes, given that they have the choice of any of the designers in the world. Before she married Prince William, Kate Middleton was a regular customer of my London shop; she would often come in with her mother and try things on.

It is very different for her now that she is married – she obviously can't just come into the shop. She does still wear my clothes, though. Recently she wore a red lace outfit of mine to a wedding, and she got a lot of press, as she looked gorgeous. Of course, everyone then wanted that dress. It is a delight to dress her – she has such a great sense of style, and she dresses very appropriately. She seems to have the knack of crossing over from high street fashion to haute couture quite effortlessly.

Opposite: Helena Christensen at the Oscars, 1998.

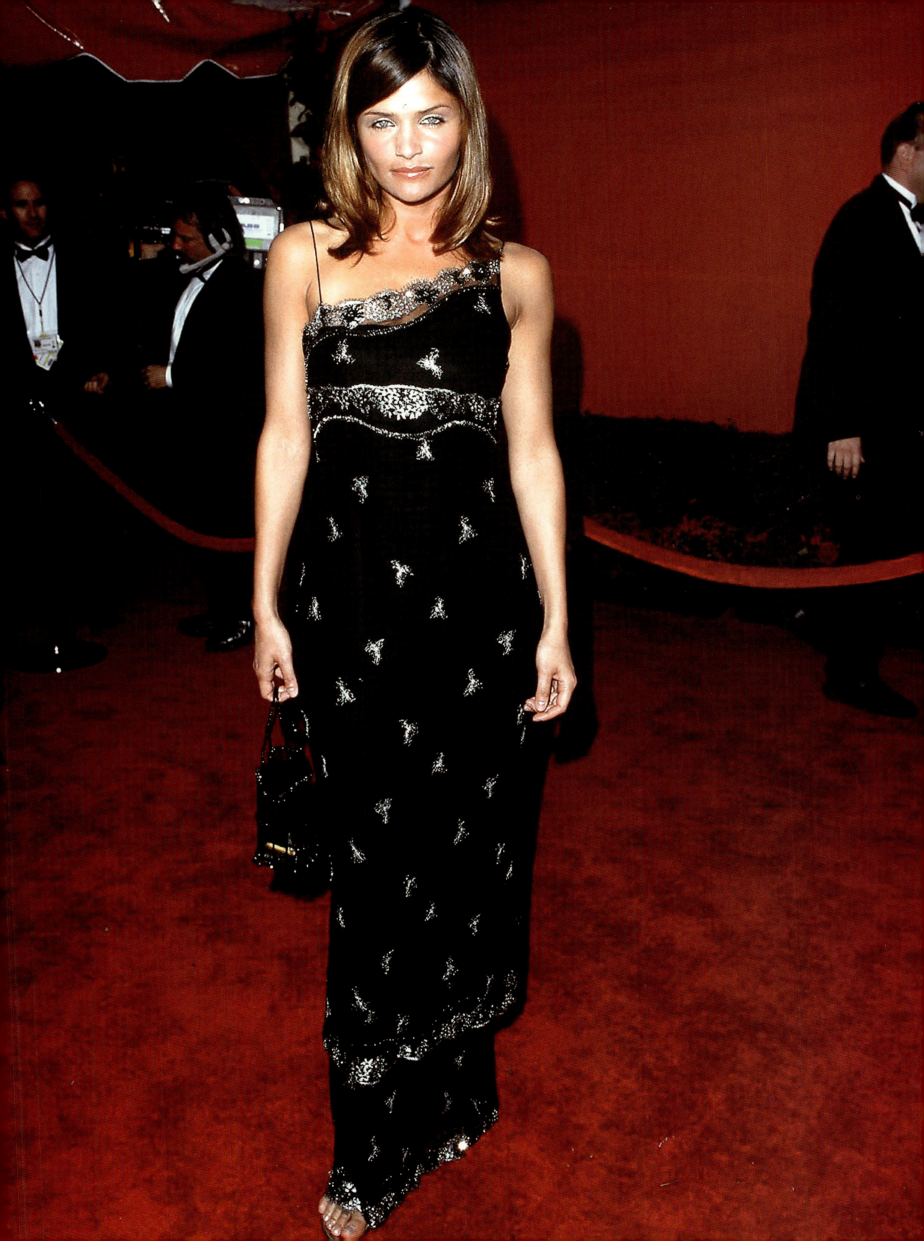

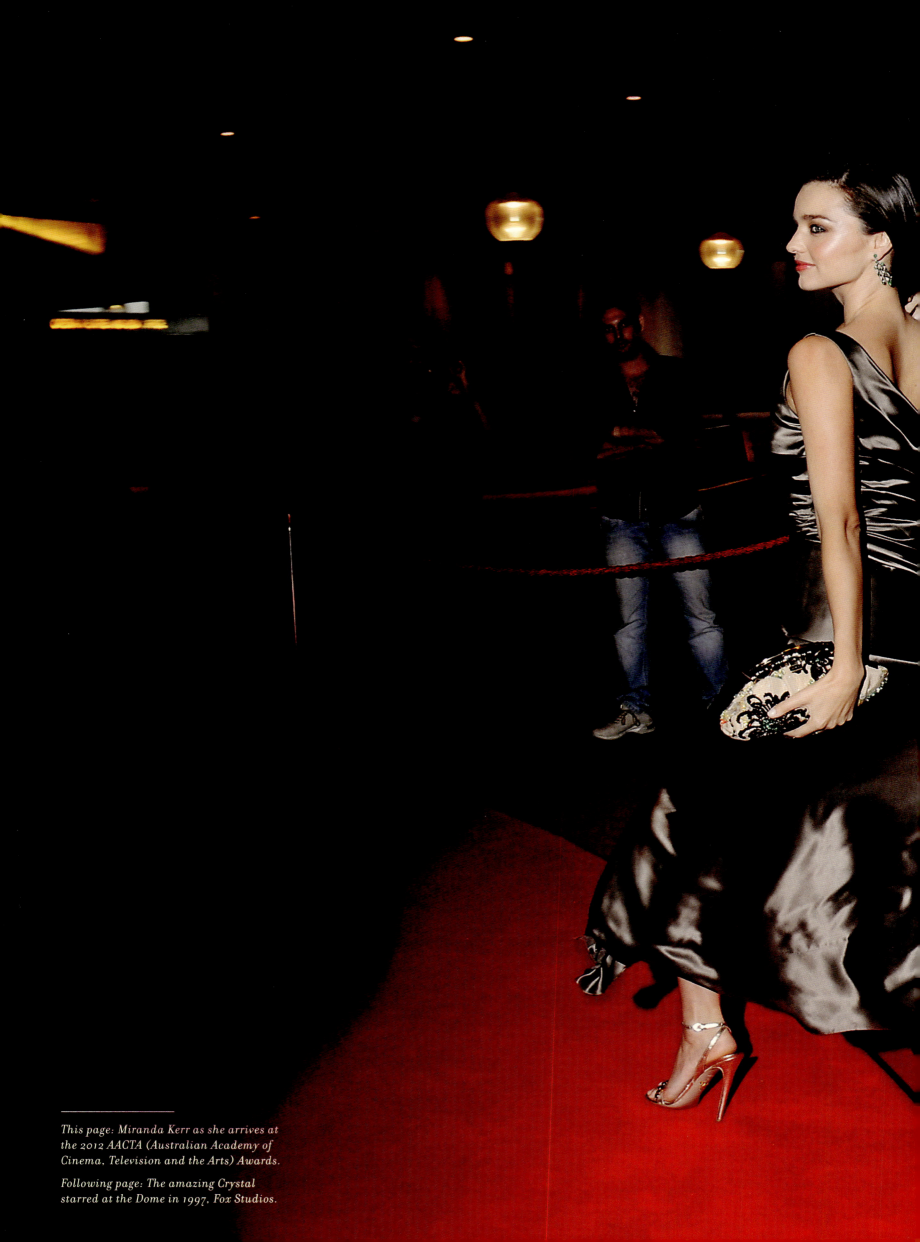

This page: Miranda Kerr as she arrives at the 2012 AACTA (Australian Academy of Cinema, Television and the Arts) Awards.

Following page: The amazing Crystal starred at the Dome in 1997, Fox Studios.

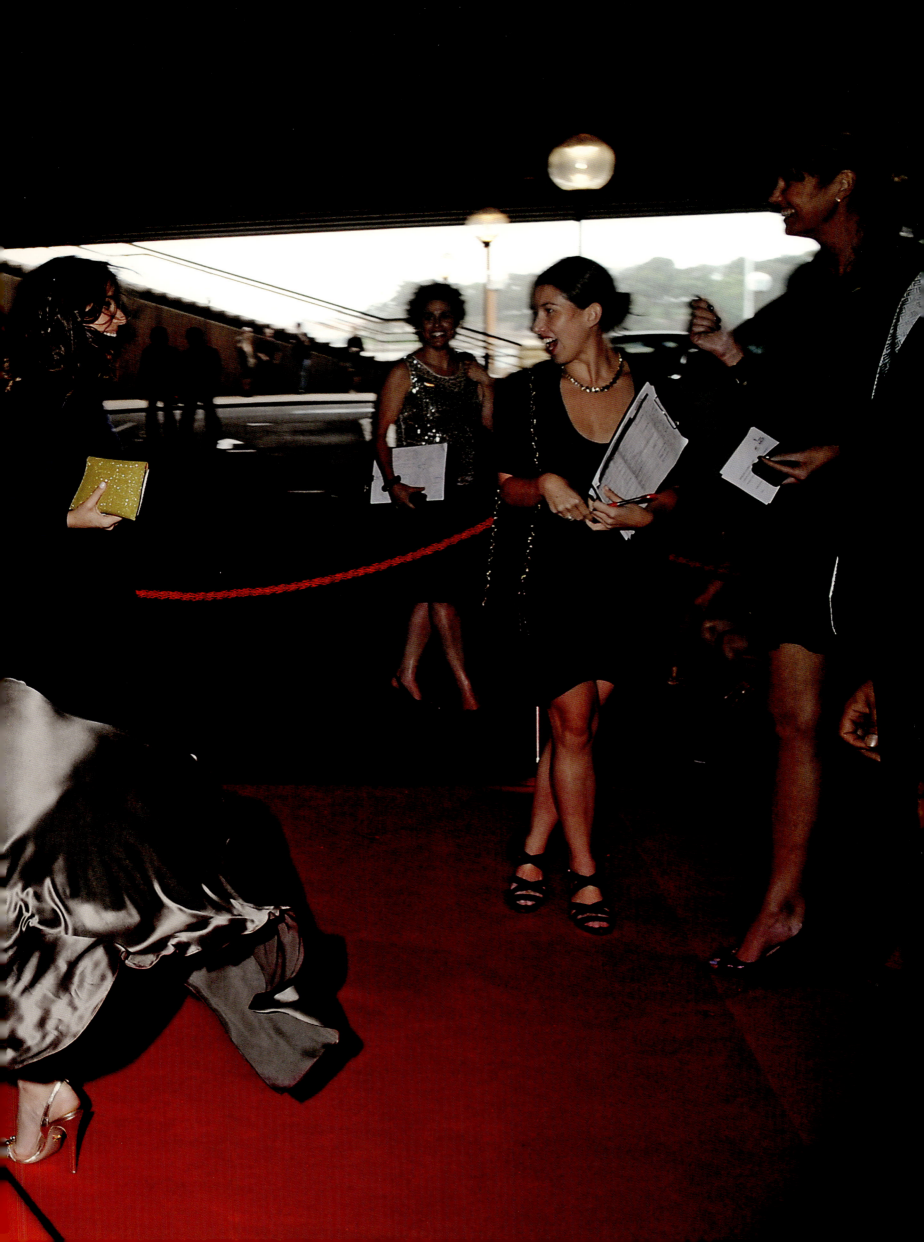

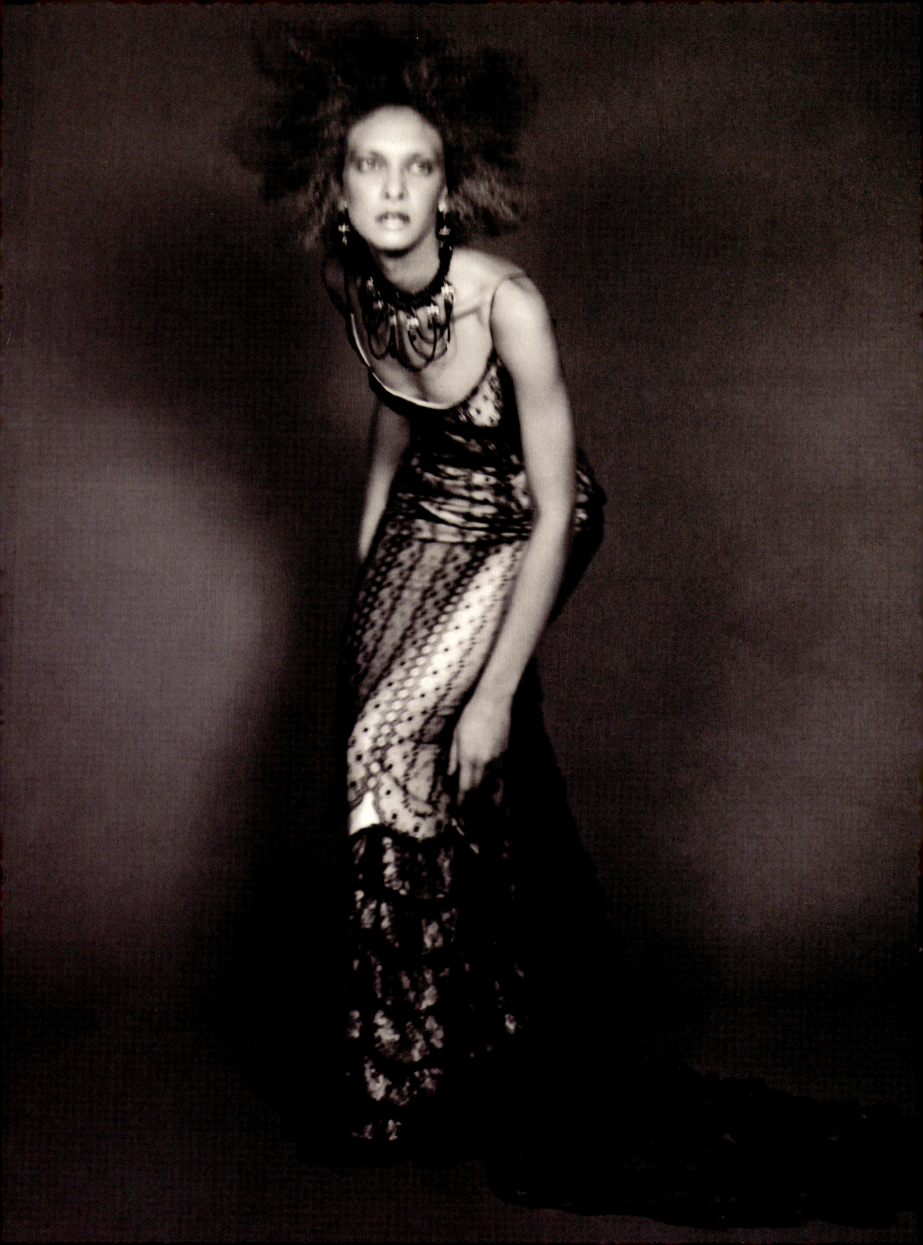

LIKE *attracts* LIKE

Baz Luhrmann and Catherine Martin,
Neil Perry, Marc Newson —
collaborations that count.

MY FELLOW

OBSESSIVES

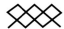

CHAPTER 8

I have been lucky to have worked with

some fantastic creative people over the years.

IT IS REALLY IMPORTANT

TO ME TO WORK WITH

PEOPLE LIKE MYSELF,

who are absolutely passionate

about what they do;

USUALLY IT IS AN

OBSESSION.

If you are creative,

EVERY EXPERIENCE

IN LIFE IS IMPORTANT,

whether it is what you wear,

what you eat or what you watch.

I am at my best professionally

when I work with people who are

AT THE TOP OF THEIR FIELDS,

AND WHOM I TRUST ABSOLUTELY.

It also helps if we enjoy each other's company,

AND HAVE FUN TOGETHER.

LIKE ATTRACTS LIKE

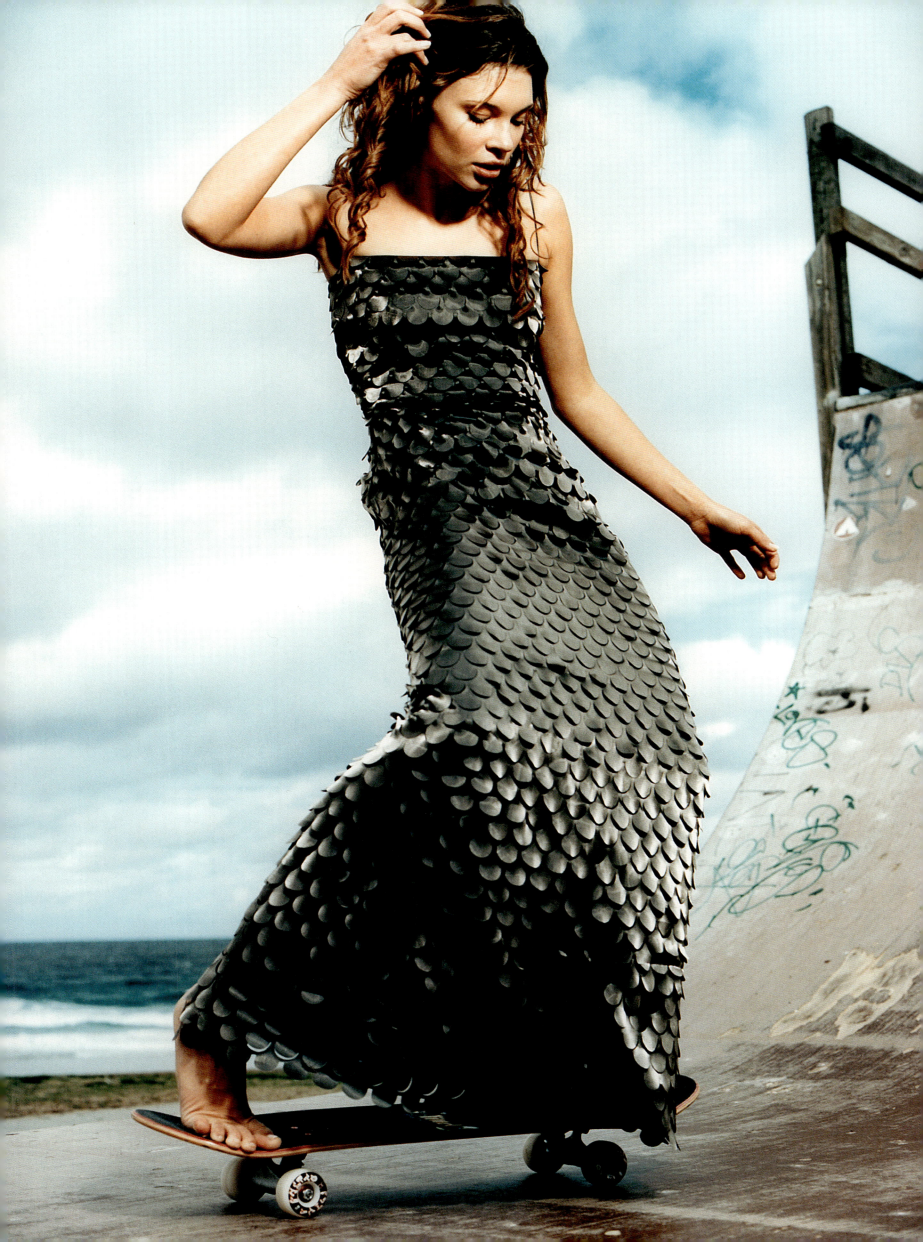

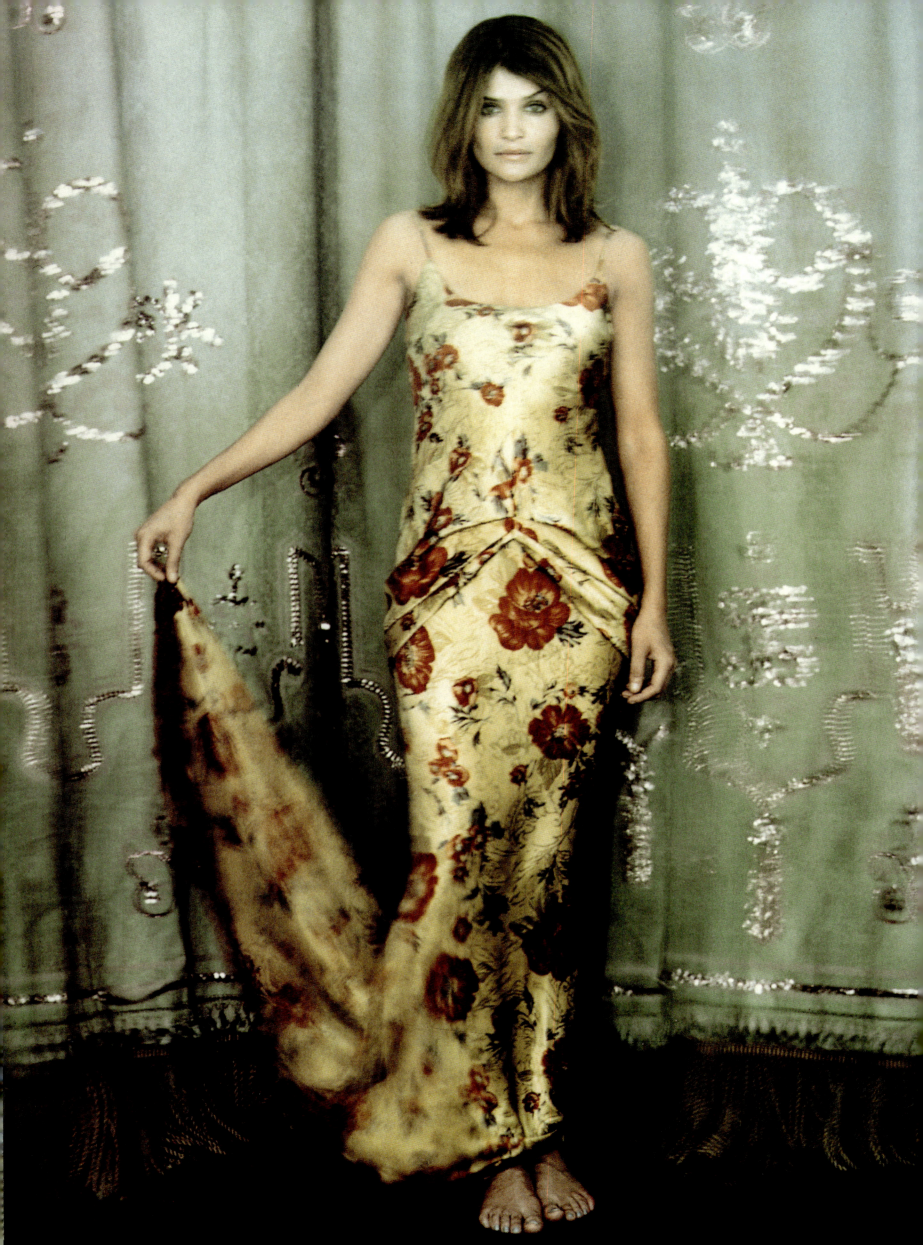

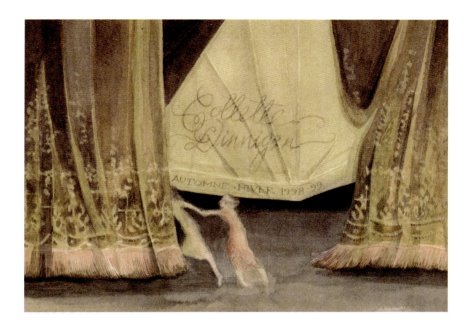

One of my most successful creative partnerships has been with Baz Luhrmann and Catherine Martin (CM). I first met them in 1994, when they were guest editors of Vogue Australia's *January edition, shortly after they had made* Strictly Ballroom.

The magazine was to include a calendar with photographs of celebrities, and they asked me to design the costumes. Baz and CM chose iconic Australian performers and we all had a great time working on that project. Baz was a fantastic director – he just had so much energy. It was all very intense – there was none of this: 'Oh it's six o'clock, we have to stop work and go home for dinner'. It just didn't matter. We worked until the middle of the night if we had to, and if we had to change something because it wasn't working, we would. I remember feeling a great sense of relief, to be working with like-minded people.

I became good friends with Baz and CM after that. None of us had children back then, so we saw a lot of each other. Just after they made *Romeo and Juliet*, I asked if they would be interested in directing my Autumn/Winter 1998 Paris show. Everyone was talking about them at the time, because of the success of *Romeo and Juliet*, so it was a real

coup for me when they said yes. I wanted to do something different from the usual Paris shows, something dramatic. Back then, other than John Galliano's shows for Dior, the shows weren't very theatrical at all. Baz said, 'You should just give this to CM, she's such a great creative and art director'. After that I worked mainly with CM, but it was great to have Baz as a sounding-board. When we started out we were going to rule the world, but we had to tone it down to stay within our budget.

CM designed the set, which featured fabulous, ornate curtains. It was great working with someone with such an eye for detail – it was amazing the way she directed and story-boarded the whole show. Usually I would have a fashion stylist style the show, but this time I wanted someone from outside the fashion world, who had a great clothes sensibility. We chose Lucy Ferry, who was married to Bryan Ferry, of Roxy Music. She had never styled a show

Previous page: My silver mermaid dress, styled by Nicole Bonython-Hines, 1999.

Opposite page: Helena Christensen in front of the theatrical curtains Catherine Martin designed for my Autumn/Winter 1998 show in Paris.

Above: James Gordon designed the invitation for the show Baz Luhrmann and Catherine Martin art-directed in Paris in 1998.

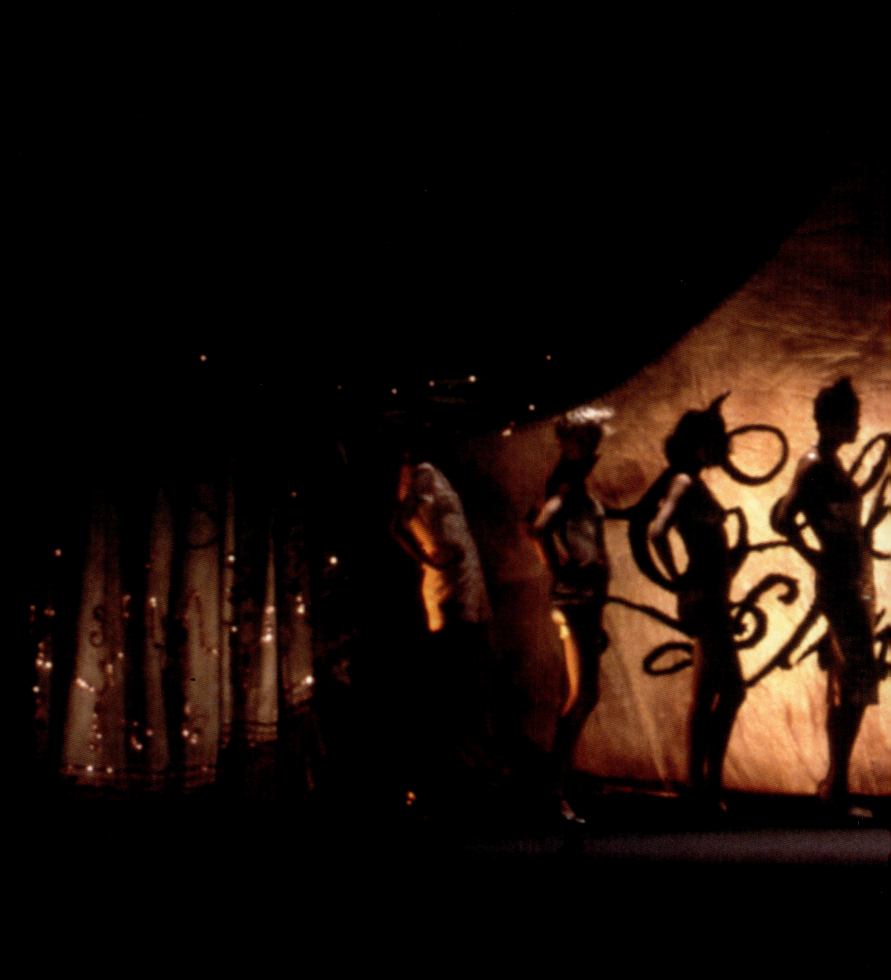

The dramatic opening of the curtains at the
Paris show art-directed by Baz and CM in 1998.

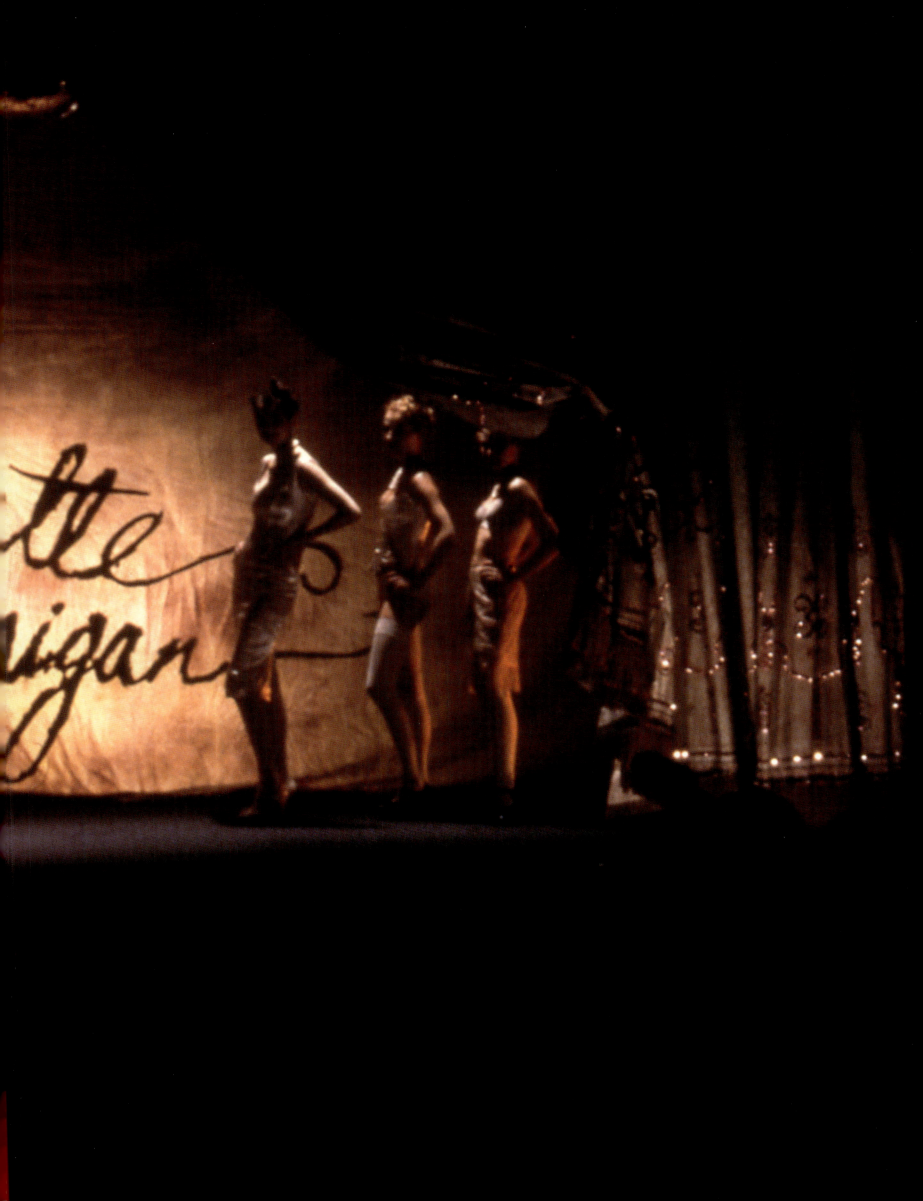

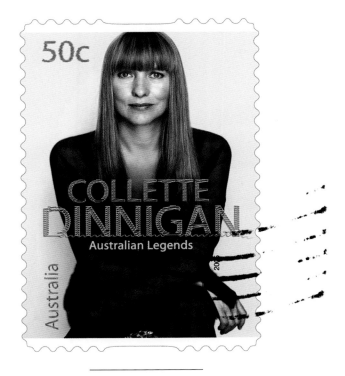

Above: In 2005, Australia Post put me on a stamp as part of their Australian Legends series, which honours people who have made a 'unique contribution' to Australia's way of life.

before, but she wore clothes well and had an incredible sense of style. So, while CM brought a film perspective to the show, Lucy added an English eccentricity. I asked the fabulous John O'Connell, known as Cha Cha, to choreograph the show. He had worked on *Romeo and Juliet* and *Moulin Rouge*.

We originally thought the show was going to be in an old mansion, but I was invited at the last minute to show in one of the specially built salons under the Louvre Pyramid. This was a real honour, because that was where Yves St Laurent and Christian Dior held their shows. It did mean a last-minute reshuffle, though – CM only had one week to prepare.

The show opened with a little girl tap-dancing, which was very unexpected; the audience didn't know what they were in for. There was a great sense of mystery about the curtains, and what was behind them. That mystique is very important to me with everything I do – it's all about the intrigue, what is left to the imagination, and how you

can be surprised and uplifted. Suddenly these big, beautiful, theatrical curtains opened, and the models came out wearing corsets and lingerie. The collection itself was very much about boudoir corsetry, with a bohemian twist, modelled by Helena Christensen and other top models of the day.

Another person I have had some great collaborations with is chef, Neil Perry. We've done shows together, and we've hosted dinners, and it's always so opulent and creative. I have absolute faith in him, because I know that he is as passionate about food as I am about clothes. He is a very positive person, with so much energy. Nothing is impossible with Neil. I trust him implicitly, as I know that we are on the same wavelength. Plus we have fun together.

I will never forget when he catered for an after-show party I put on at The Casbah, a nightclub in Paris. We took over the whole restaurant, and Neil planned to cook a wild boar, or *sanglier*, but it went missing in transit. We all became quite obsessed – I was getting daily briefings

Opposite: I met Baz and Catherine Martin when they asked me to collaborate on the design of the costumes for the calendar to accompany the January 1994 edition of Vogue Australia, *which they were guest-editing.*

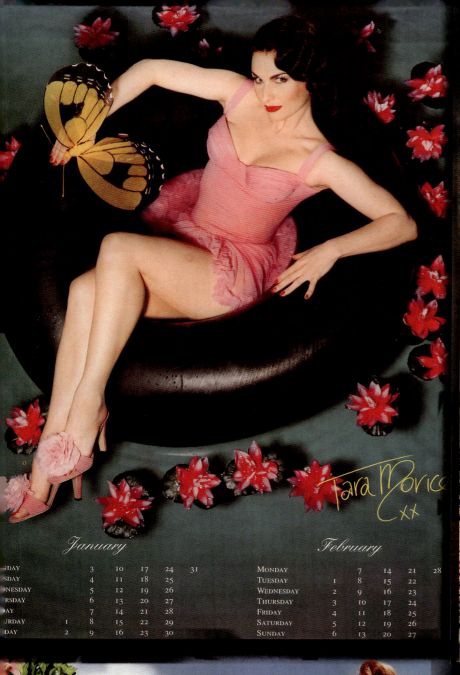

Tara Moñca
xx

January

~~DAY~~	3	10	17	24	31
~~SDAY~~	4	11	18	25	
~~NESDAY~~	5	12	19	26	
~~RSDAY~~	6	13	20	27	
~~AY~~	7	14	21	28	
~~RDAY~~	1	8	15	22	29
~~DAY~~	2	9	16	23	30

February

MONDAY		7	14	21	28
TUESDAY	1	8	15	22	
WEDNESDAY	2	9	16	23	
THURSDAY	3	10	17	24	
FRIDAY	4	11	18	25	
SATURDAY	5	12	19	26	
SUNDAY	6	13	20	27	

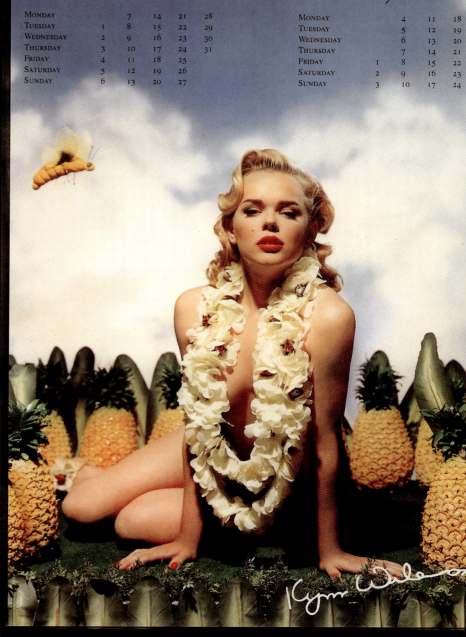

March

MONDAY		7	14	21	28
TUESDAY	1	8	15	22	29
WEDNESDAY	2	9	16	23	30
THURSDAY	3	10	17	24	31
FRIDAY	4	11	18	25	
SATURDAY	5	12	19	26	
SUNDAY	6	13	20	27	

April

MONDAY		4	11	18
TUESDAY		5	12	19
WEDNESDAY		6	13	20
THURSDAY		7	14	21
FRIDAY	1	8	15	22
SATURDAY	2	9	16	23
SUNDAY	3	10	17	24

Kym Wilso

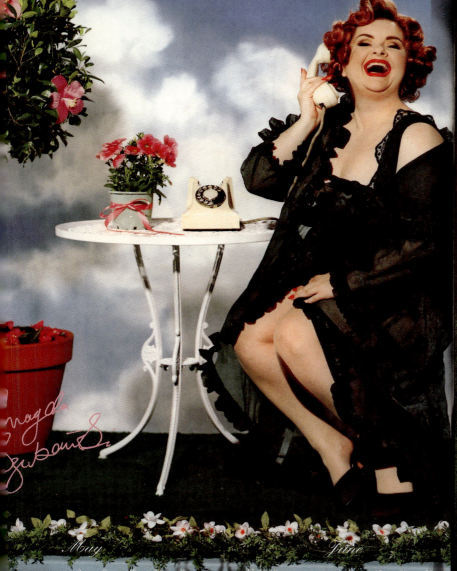

Magda
Subons

May

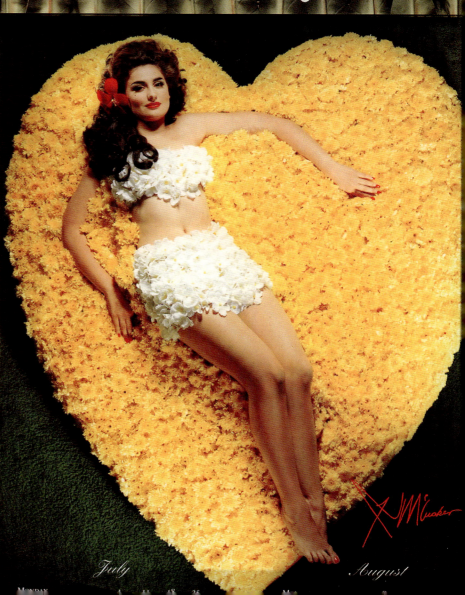

McEued

July

August

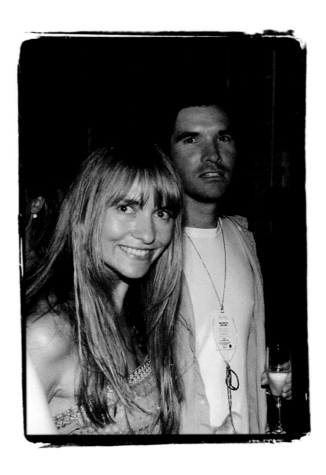

on where he was up to with his wild pig. I think he even ended up asking the Australian Embassy for help. It finally arrived just in time. He also had scallops coming from Tasmania, as it was meant to be an Australian feast, but they didn't turn up at all!

Cha Cha choreographed that show too, and we had Bulgarian tango dancers who tangoed right across the tabletops. It was a really lavish party, and people stayed and partied until three or four in the morning. It got lots of press and people were talking about it for a long time afterwards. Later, Neil told me that seeing such a beautiful show inspired him and his team to 'cook like angels'.

Neil, Cha Cha and I also worked together on a show I did in 1997 for Australian Fashion Week at the Dome at (what was then called) Fox Studios. I was just back from Paris and didn't want to do another catwalk show – I wanted something a bit different. So, we transformed the Dome into a Chinoiserie-style supper club, and the whole atmosphere was more like a soiree, than a fashion show. It was very dark, with lots of red velvet, and Neil had set

up dim sum trolleys everywhere, as well as a noodle bar. Guests sat around at small tables, and they all thought they had been invited for dinner. It was so authentic that no one suspected anything.

We had Todd McKenney, the actor, dressed as a waiter serving drinks. Later, talent agent Ann Churchill-Brown told me that when she saw Todd, she thought how sad it was that times were so tough that he had to wait tables. There were only about twelve models, and when they entered they just draped themselves against the pillars, so no one noticed them at first. All of a sudden, Todd dropped his tray of drinks, and the next minute he was up on the stage. Then everything started to happen; the music began, Todd performed the tango with a dancer in a red dress, the models walked onto the stage wearing beautiful long dresses, and it all felt like some sort of bordello. Cha Cha did the choreography. He worked his magic and, because he's so talented, the models performed like dancers – it was all quite fantastic. It was great to surprise people like that.

Above: With my number one collaborator –
my brother Seamus – at a millennium party
on New Year's Eve 1999.

Opposite: A night to remember, the Dome,
Fox Studios, 1997.

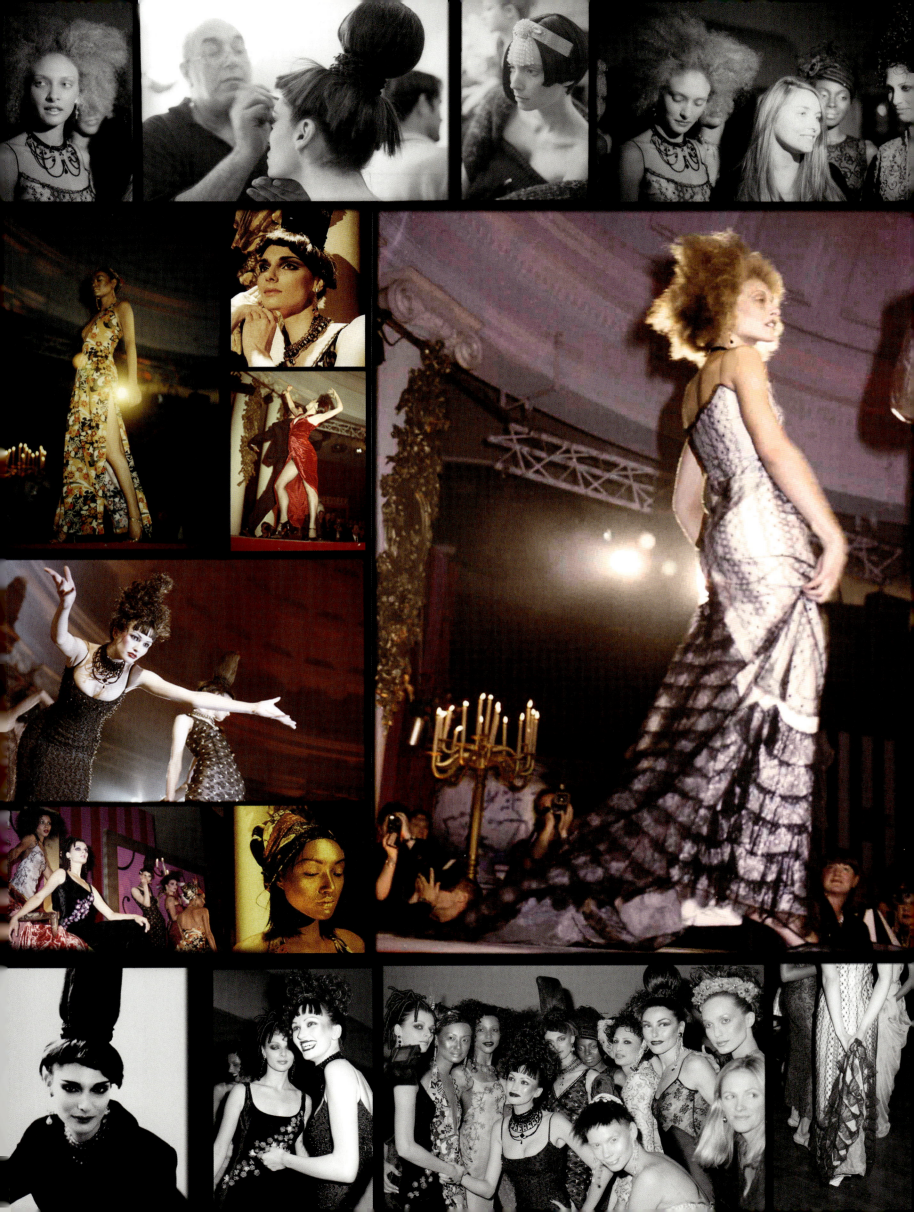

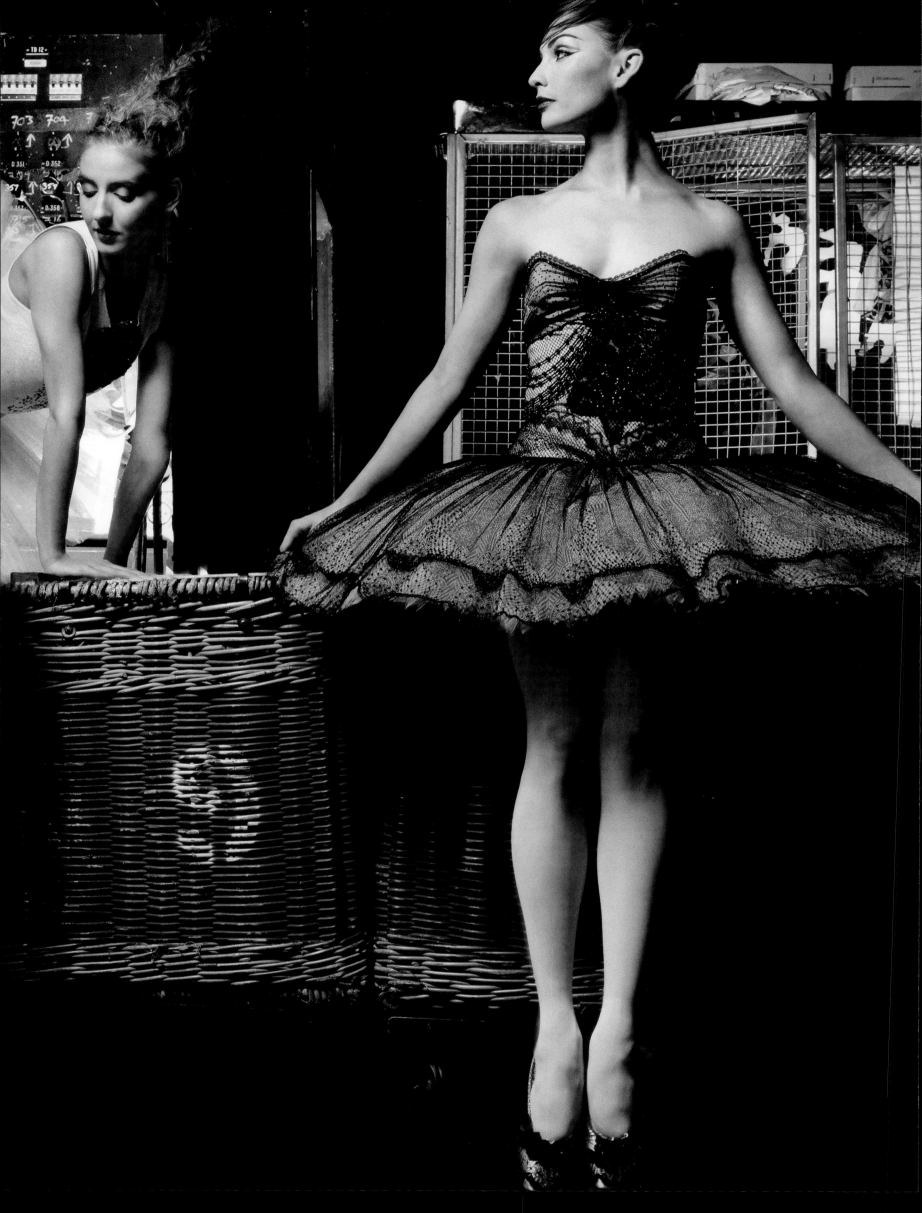

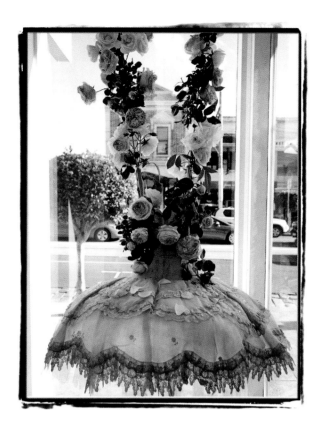

That was the night I met Marc Newson, because his girlfriend at the time, Crystal, had a leading role. Everyone was having such a good time that no one wanted to leave. Then it started to rain, torrentially, and suddenly the roof collapsed. Someone called the fire department because there were hairdryers floating around in the water. It was total chaos.

I got some amazing write-ups in the press the next day. Harry M. Miller, celebrity agent, whom I didn't know very well, sent me flowers and was quoted in the newspaper as saying: 'I don't know how she did it, but she really shocked the whole Sydney social set last night – she just blew them away. We all want to go back to that club she created!'

Neil also cooked for a show I did in 1999 for my resort collection at Boomerang, a magnificent old home in Elizabeth Bay, Sydney. The theme was French Riviera, and everything was blue and white stripes, and crisp linens. I designed it all – the awnings, the cushions, the chairs.

Neil served a fabulous three-course meal, with beautiful wines. The surprise element there was that the dining table turned into a stage after people had eaten – Kate Ceberano just danced down the middle of the table, singing. It was more than just a fashion show – it was entertainment. Events like that are a lot of fun to work on, even though they are hard work, because I was not just designing a collection, but designing everything else as well, right down to the menu covers. It is about way more than just the clothes.

Another event that Neil and I worked on together was the Mission Australia 'Best of the Best Dinner', held in 2002. Mission Australia at that time was holding annual fundraising events, aiming to raise a million dollars each time. They asked if I could help former Prime Minister Bob Hawke and television presenter Gina Boon organise the dinner, and I agreed. I suggested the 'Best of the Best' theme – that instead of just doing the usual cocktail party,

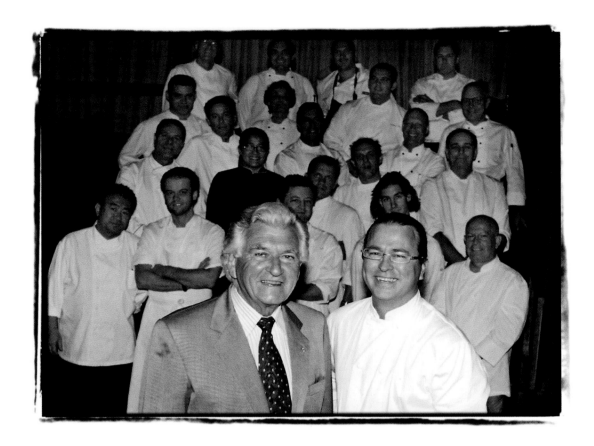

Above: Neil Perry has been a great collaborator at countless events.
Here he is with former Prime Minister Bob Hawke and a group of the top
chefs in Australia at that time. They cooked up a storm at the Mission
Australia 'Best of the Best' dinner I helped organise in 2002.

they get the best chefs, the best entertainment, and the best of everything. We needed surprises and personalities. We invited people like Ian Thorpe, Elle Macpherson, Sarah Murdoch, Rachel Ward and Bryan Brown.

I basically designed and styled the whole dinner – from the invitations through to the furnishings and the seating plan. We held it in the old White Bay Power Station building in Rozelle, where everything was falling apart. Baz and CM helped to organise the entertainment – we had a band of marching girls on stage, and a tango dancer I had met through Jean Marc Loubier from Paris. I brought Neil on board as head chef, and he helped round up some of Sydney's best chefs of the day, including Guillaume Brahimi, Kylie Kwong, Matt Moran, Damien Pignolet and Tetsuya Wakuda. We asked all the chefs to sign the plates, and people could take them home.

The chefs each cooked different meals, so no one knew what they were getting – it was all a big surprise. We had one long table, and the guests were seated in an

unconventional manner. It was quite the exercise working out who was to sit where – a brain surgeon might be sitting next to a sports star. It was all a great success – everyone had a great time, and danced the night away.

Another kindred spirit is Marc Newson. He is more of a friend than a collaborator, and just as obsessive as me. He always says he doesn't know anyone else he can complain to in quite the same way; he knows I understand the sheer frustration of getting it just right. He designed the First Class Lounge for Qantas, and invited me to do a show there for its opening in 2007. I think Qantas was expecting something more corporate, but we wanted the launch to be fun, and touched with the true glamour of how First Class travel used to be.

It was much more than just a fashion show – it was all about capturing an experience, creating a sense of something amazing. The lounge was perfect, because it was a bit like a catwalk. My resort collection is all about the glamour and luxury of travel, and the fantasy that when it

Opposite: The Dom Pérignon Lounge I designed
in 2009 for Dom Pérignon in The Establishment in
Sydney. I was the third designer – after Marc Newson
and Karl Lagerfeld – to be asked to create one.

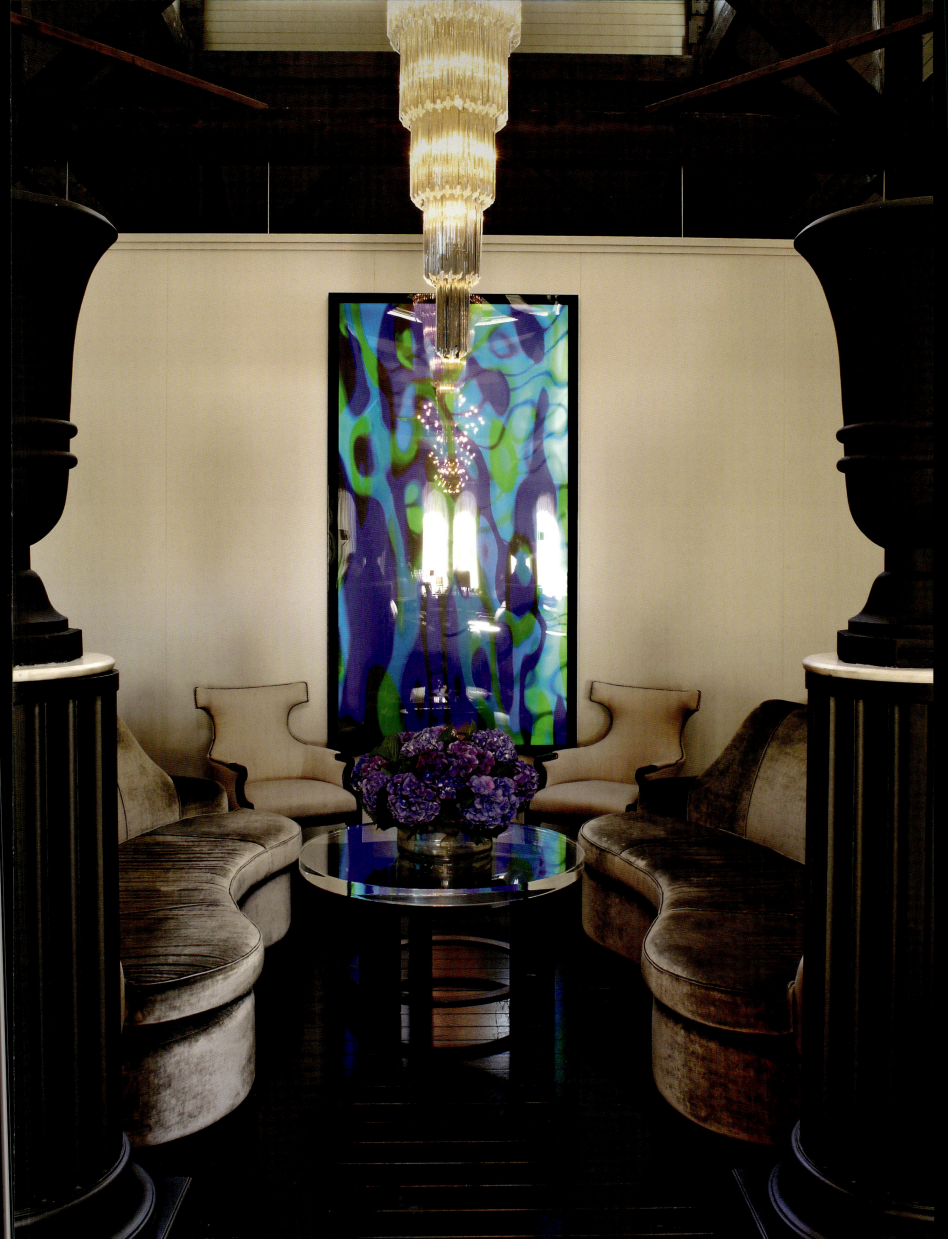

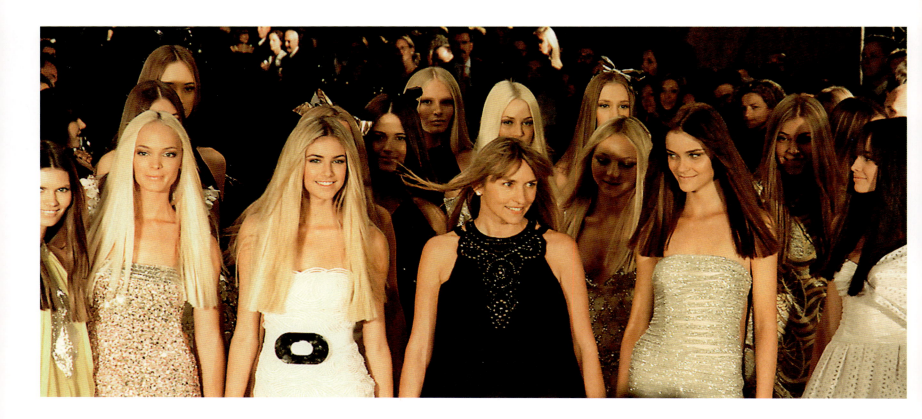

Above: A show I did in 2007 for the opening of the
Qantas First Class Lounge, designed by Marc Newson.

Opposite: Sarah Murdoch and me at a show I did in 1999
at Boomerang, a grand historic house on the water
in Sydney's Elizabeth Bay. Sarah is not only a close
friend, but one of Australia's best ever models.

is winter here, you can escape to summer in the Turks and Caicos Islands, or the French Riviera, or wherever. I loved working with Marc and his wife, Charlotte Stockdale, a stylist and fashion editor in London. It worked out well for Qantas too; instead of just having a corporate crowd, they had a whole different group of people – designers, fashion people, journalists, all interested to see what would happen next.

I've had so many wonderful collaborations, with photographers, artists, stylists and others I have worked with over the years. Many of them have become close friends, like Tory Collison and Nicole Bonython-Hines. I remember a shoot Nicole did once at Bondi Beach. She got a fabulous shot of Chloë Maxwell, barefoot on a skateboard, wearing my silver mermaid dress. I loved it so much that we used it on the invitation to an exhibition of my clothes at the Victoria and Albert Museum in London in 2000. They featured me in their *Fashion in Motion* series, in which they showcased the works of particular designers for a month at a time. I was the only Australian designer included – other designers featured were Alexander McQueen, Vivienne Westwood and Roland Mouret.

Throughout the years my biggest collaborator and confidante has been my brother, Seamus. He has an incredible eye for detail, a great sense of humour (most of the time), and I know I can always rely on him one hundred per cent to get the job done.

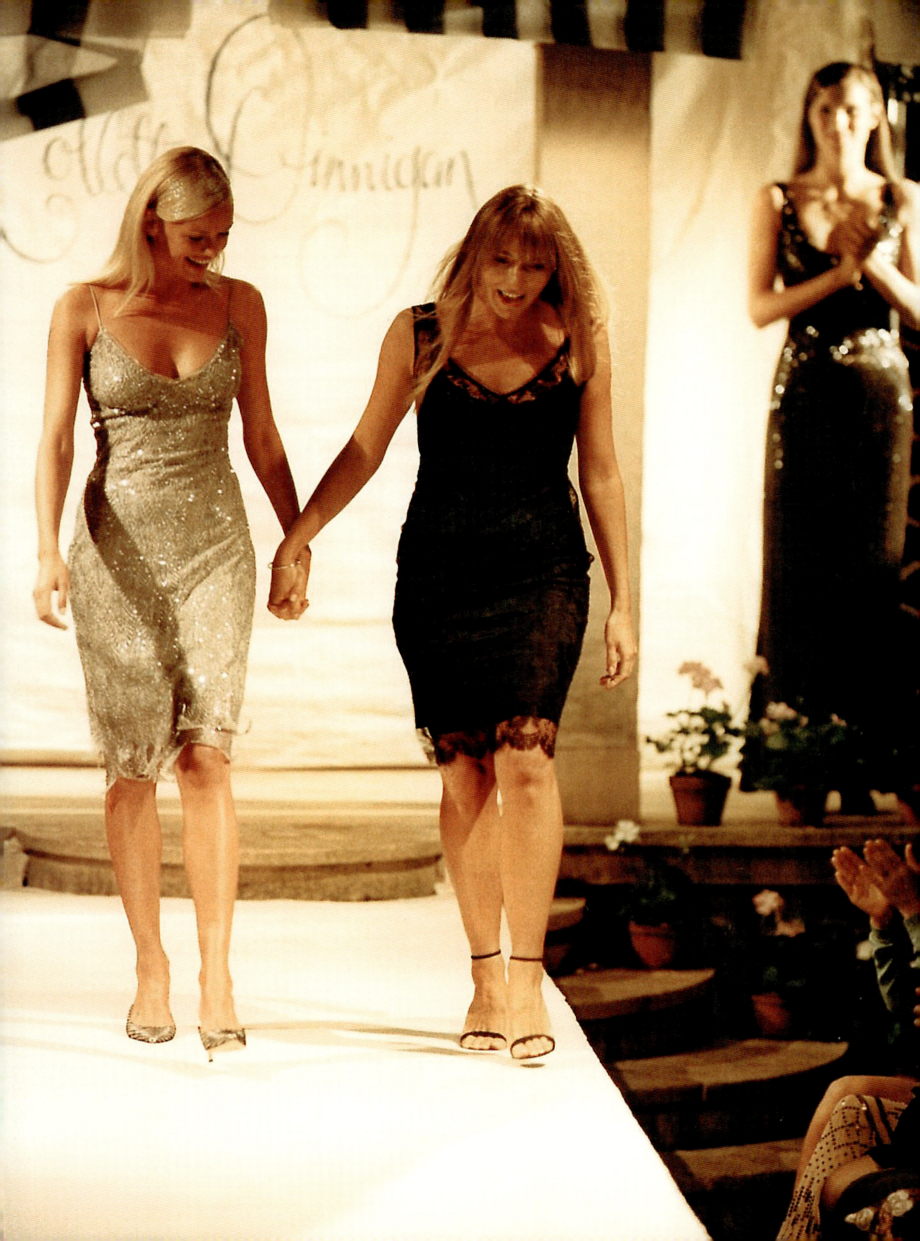

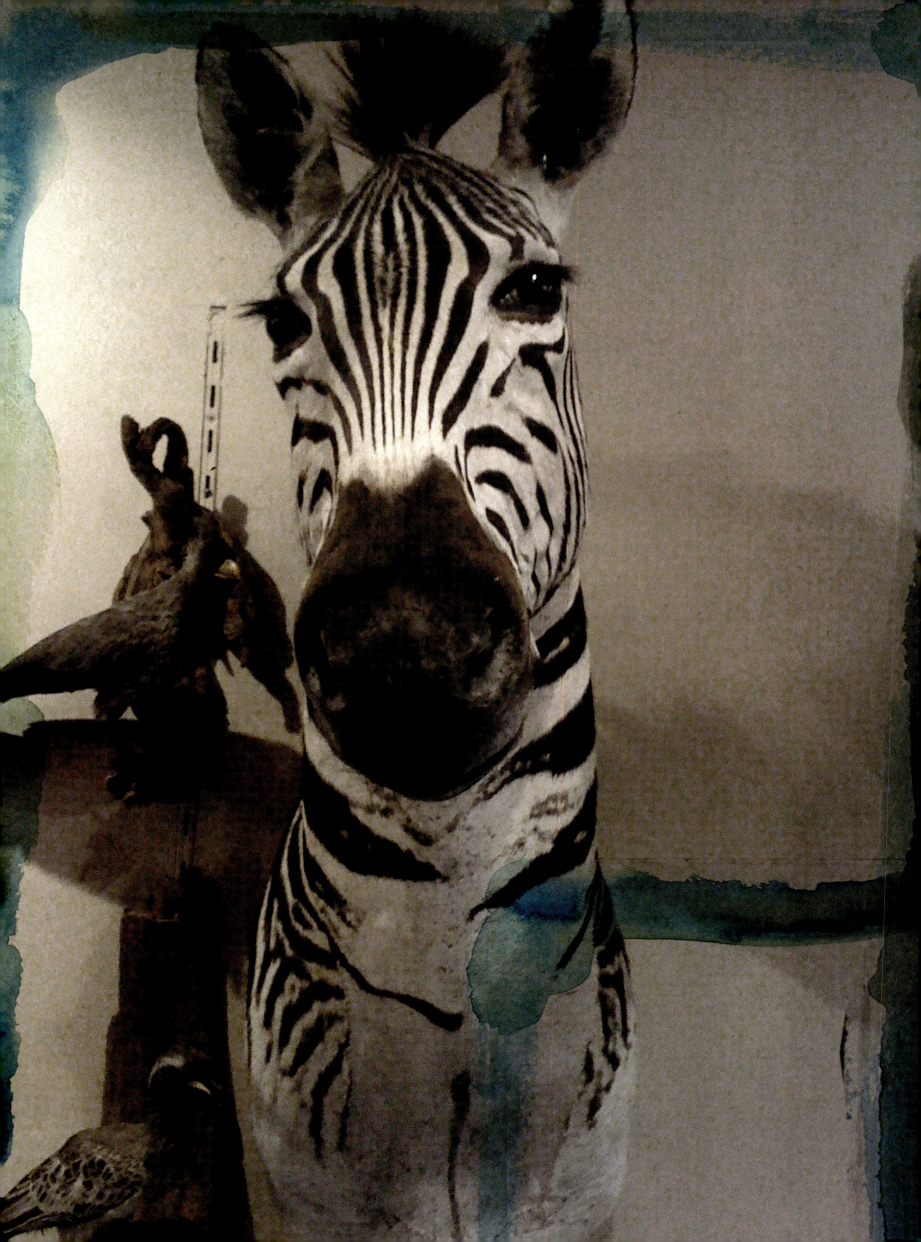

WE ALL HAVE AN EYE

*Things flotsam, whimsical;
fields of flowers, random acts
of nature inspire me.*

ME AND MY CAMERA

CHAPTER 9

I HAVE HAD AN INTEREST
IN PHOTOGRAPHY SINCE I WAS
IN MY LATE TEENS.
I started using an old Kodak camera of Dad's,
but as I got older I remember wanting
something that looked a bit less seventies
than the old Kodachrome film.
MY PARENTS GAVE ME
A KONIKA CAMERA, AND WHILE
I WAS AT FASHION SCHOOL
I DID A PHOTOGRAPHY COURSE.
I shared a darkroom in Wellington
where I did all my own developing,
AND I'D SPEND A LOT OF
MY SPARE TIME TAKING
PICTURES OF FRIENDS,
AND JUST EXPERIMENTING.
I love the texture of old photographic paper,
and the excitement of the whole developing process.
I USED TO WANT TO BE A PHOTOGRAPHER —
A PART OF ME STILL WANTS THAT.

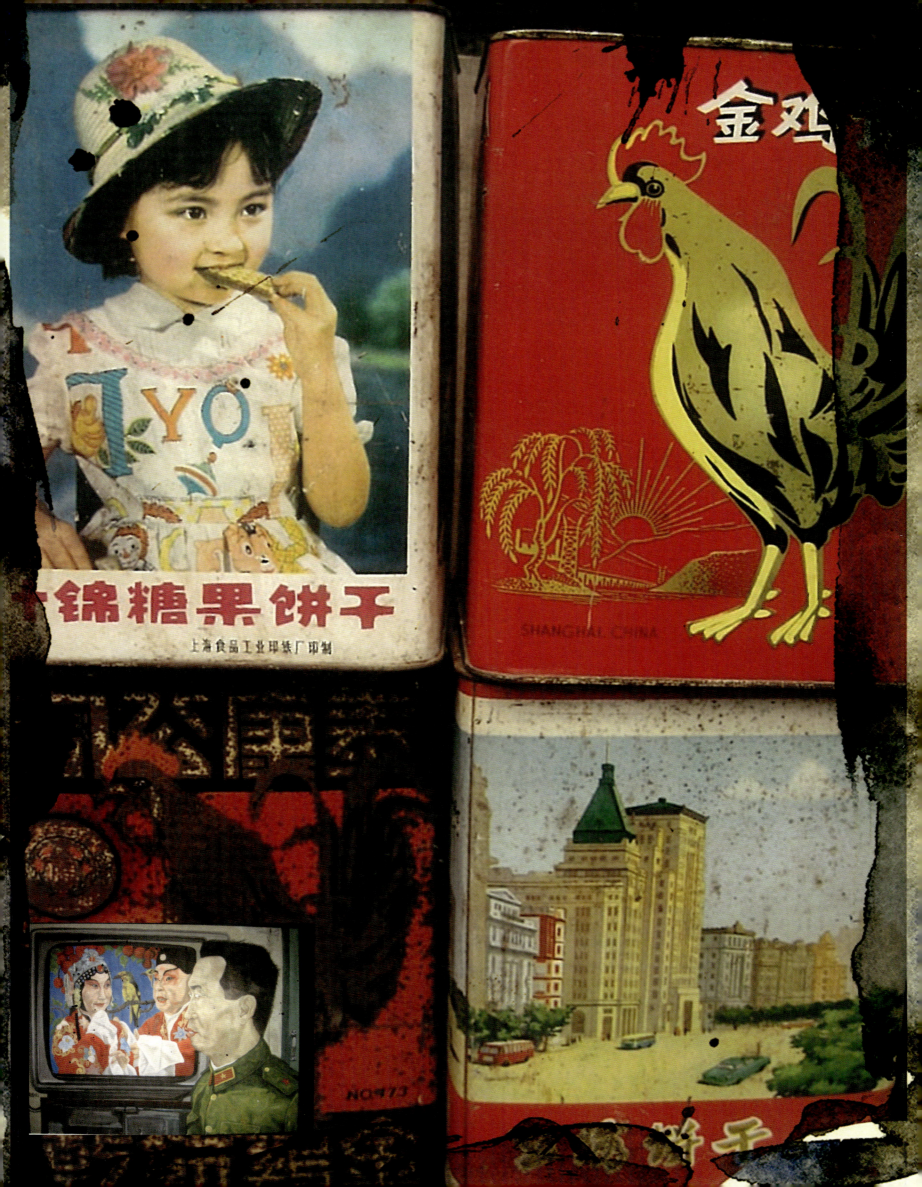

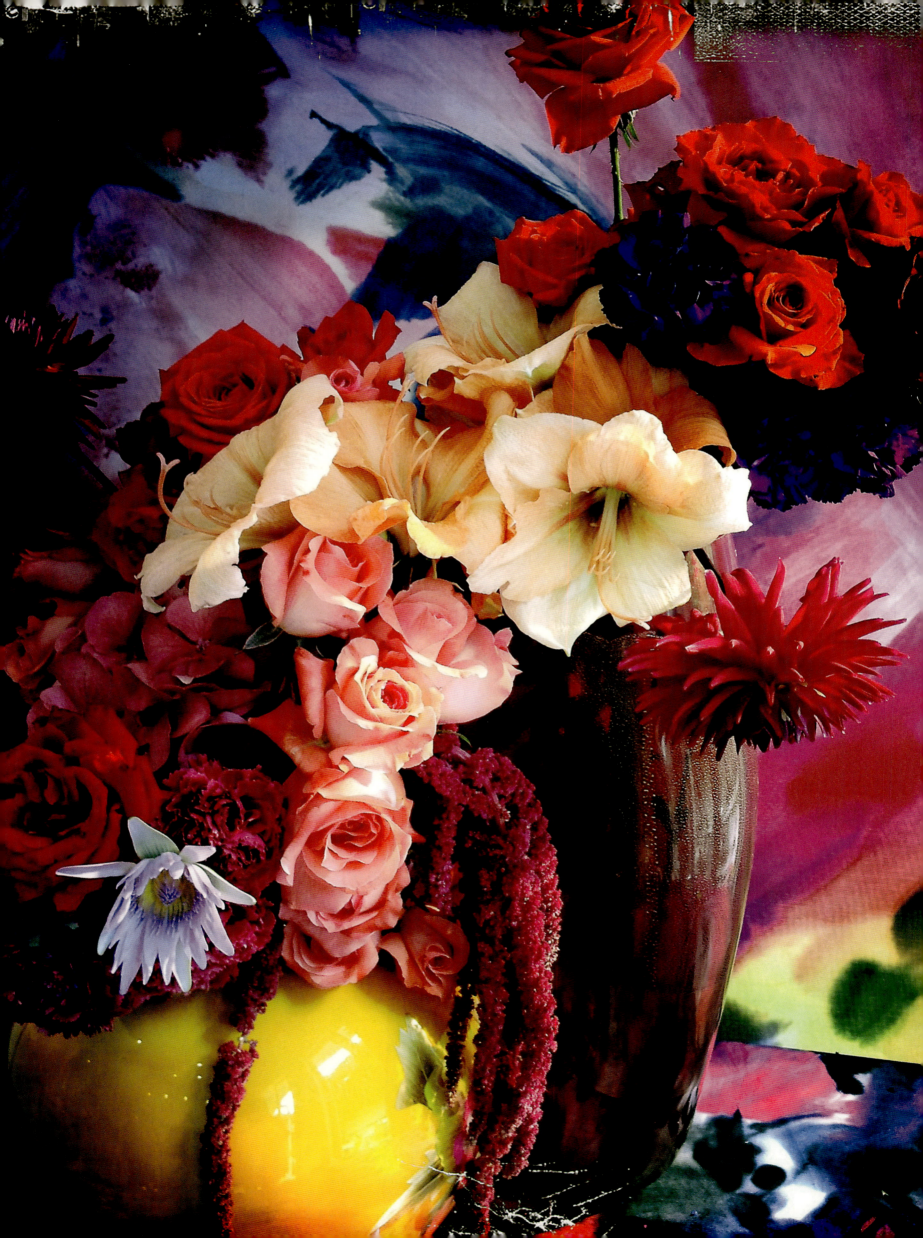

When I take photos for myself I feel self-indulgent —

it is not about pleasing other people, it's about the things I love.

I just wish I had more time to edit and frame them all.

What interests me most is the composition of a photograph. The picture is very much in the eye of the beholder – I love catching people off guard, or capturing a building or landscape in a particular light. Having an eye is all about seeing something that no one has seen before – you must look all around, not just straight ahead, because if you don't look, you won't see. When I am travelling, I especially love to photograph people, and I like each photo to tell a story – where they've come from, their history, their costume. I love the intrigue of the lives they've led. I like to surprise people with my photographs – it's the hardest thing to do, and when you can deliver, it makes people stop and think.

I love vivid colour, which is why I take so many photos when I'm in India. Everything there is just so visually powerful. I love the tiles, the art and architecture, and the bright colours the women wear, especially in Rajasthan, where you see every shade of pink. Everything doesn't have to be beautiful; beauty can be quite ugly, and I love that. Everything can be so ordered, in a chaotic way. It is a place of contrasts. You might see the most peaceful, gentle person, sitting calmly next to a freeway, not showing any stress.

When we are doing photo shoots I look at the shots to see their composition, whether they're too light or too dark, and what personality is coming through. I'm less worried about the detail of the clothing – the most important thing is the mood of the photo, how provocative it is, and what sort of emotional connection it conjures up.

I have worked with some fabulous photographers over the years – a highlight was working with Ellen von Unwerth and Helena Christensen. Ellen's energy and her sense of style come through so clearly in those photos, which are provocative and also quite moody. Hugh Stewart is another photographer I love to work with. He captures a personality, an atmosphere, a nonchalance.

I collect photographs; there are so many photographers whose work I admire – Mario Testino, Helmut Newton, Paolo Roversi. They all have very particular styles, which make them who they are. I think Sarah Moon is wonderful, and I also love Peter Beard, and the way he integrates his life experience and travels into his work. Miroslav Tichý is a Czech photographer I admire immensely. He made a camera from tin cans, cardboard and rubber bands and took photographs mainly of women (usually unsuspecting) around his home town of Kyjov.

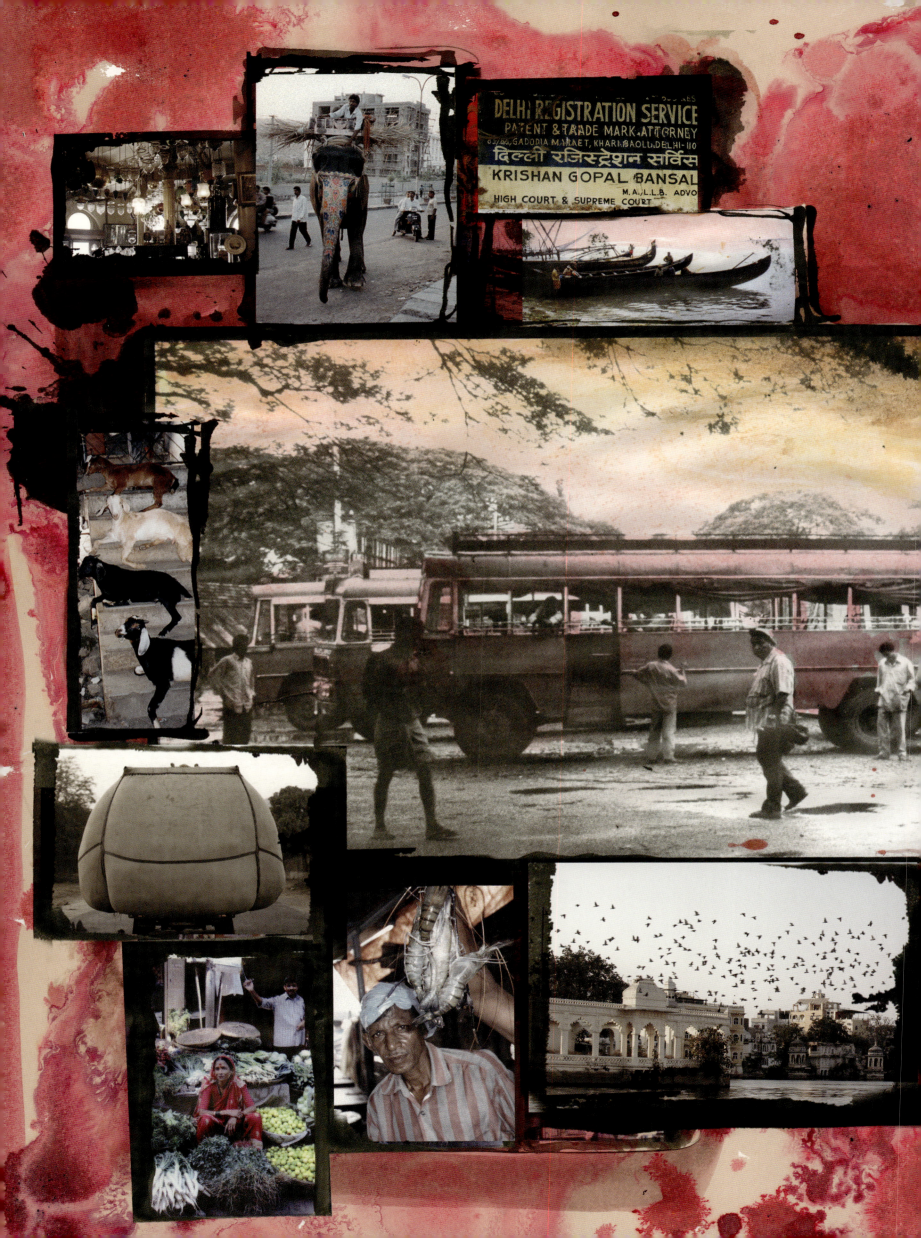

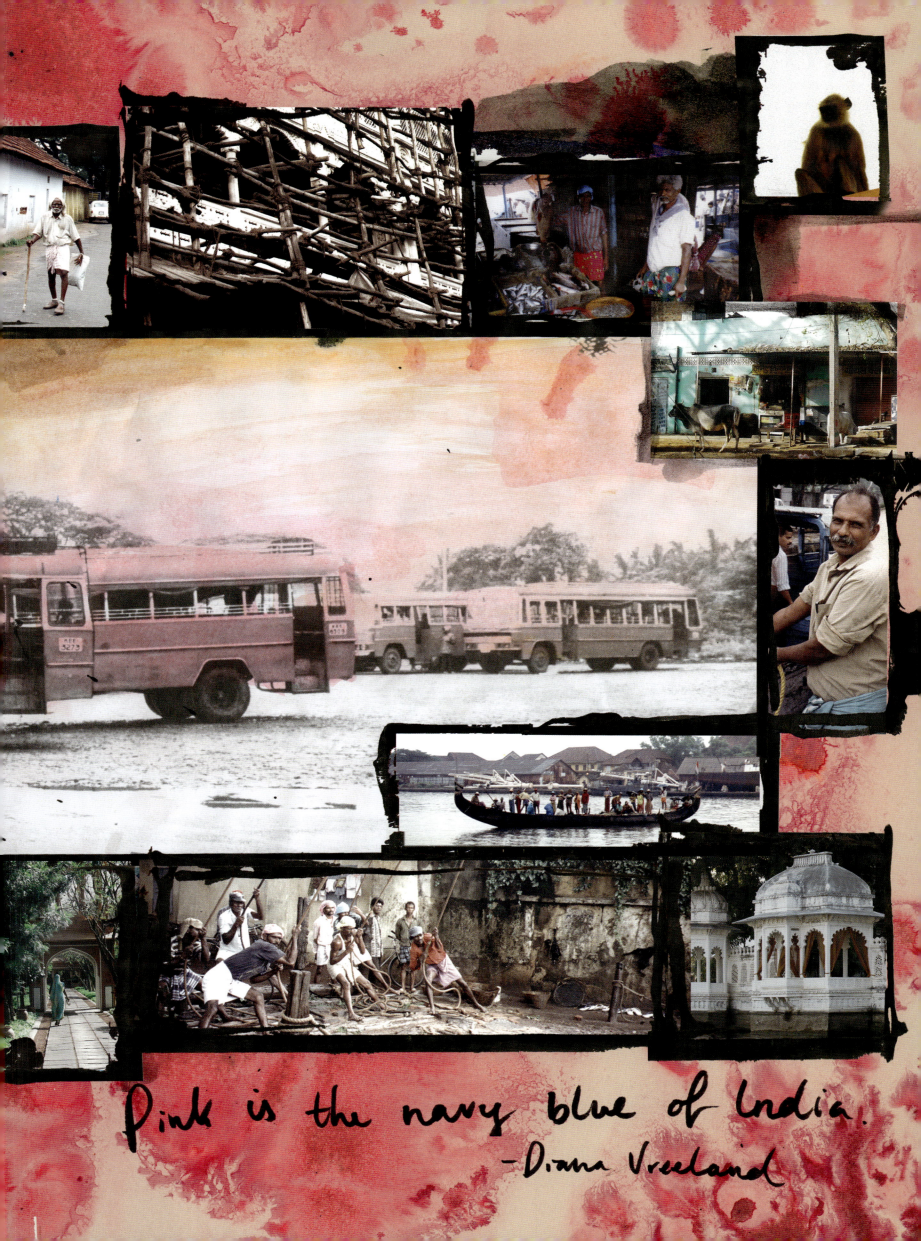

Pink is the navy blue of India.
— Diana Vreeland

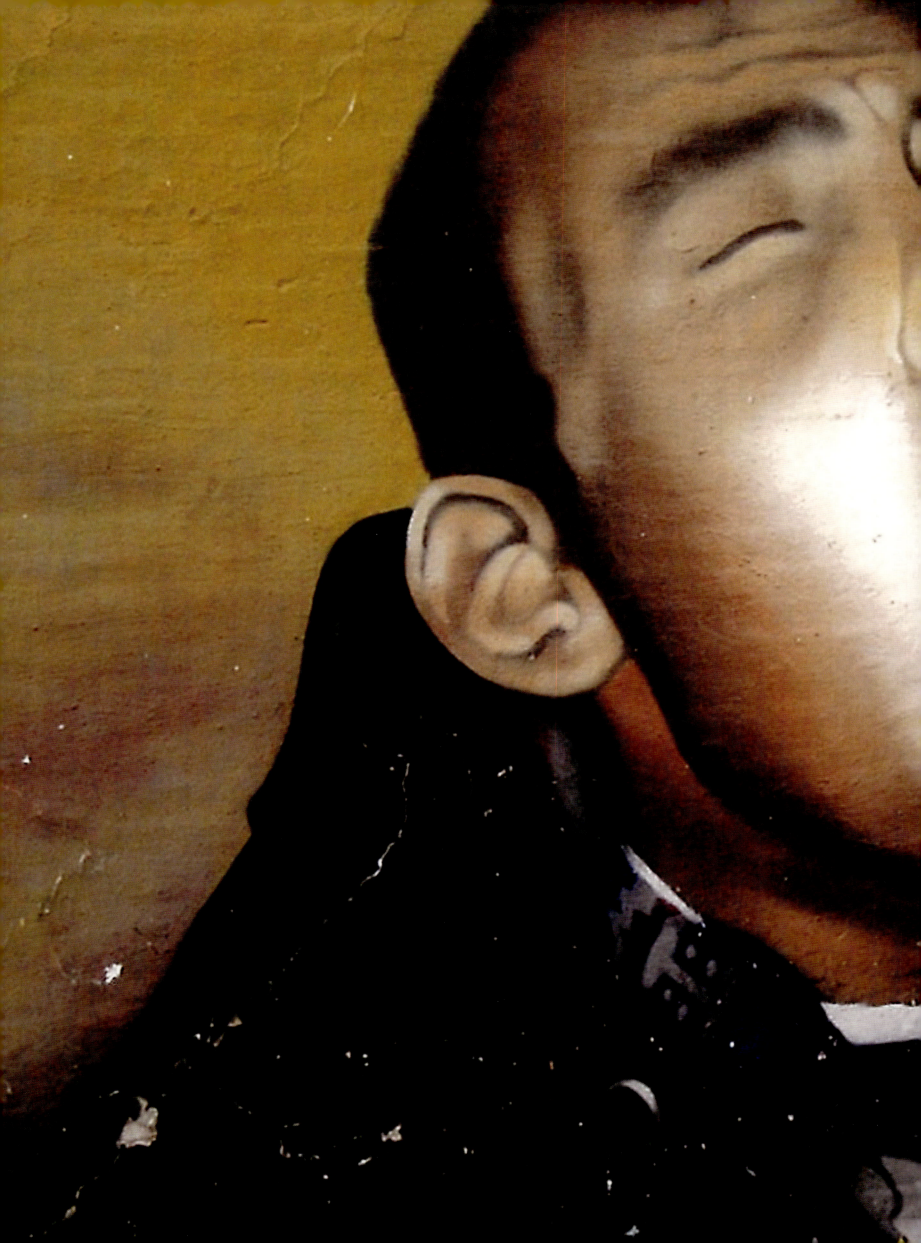

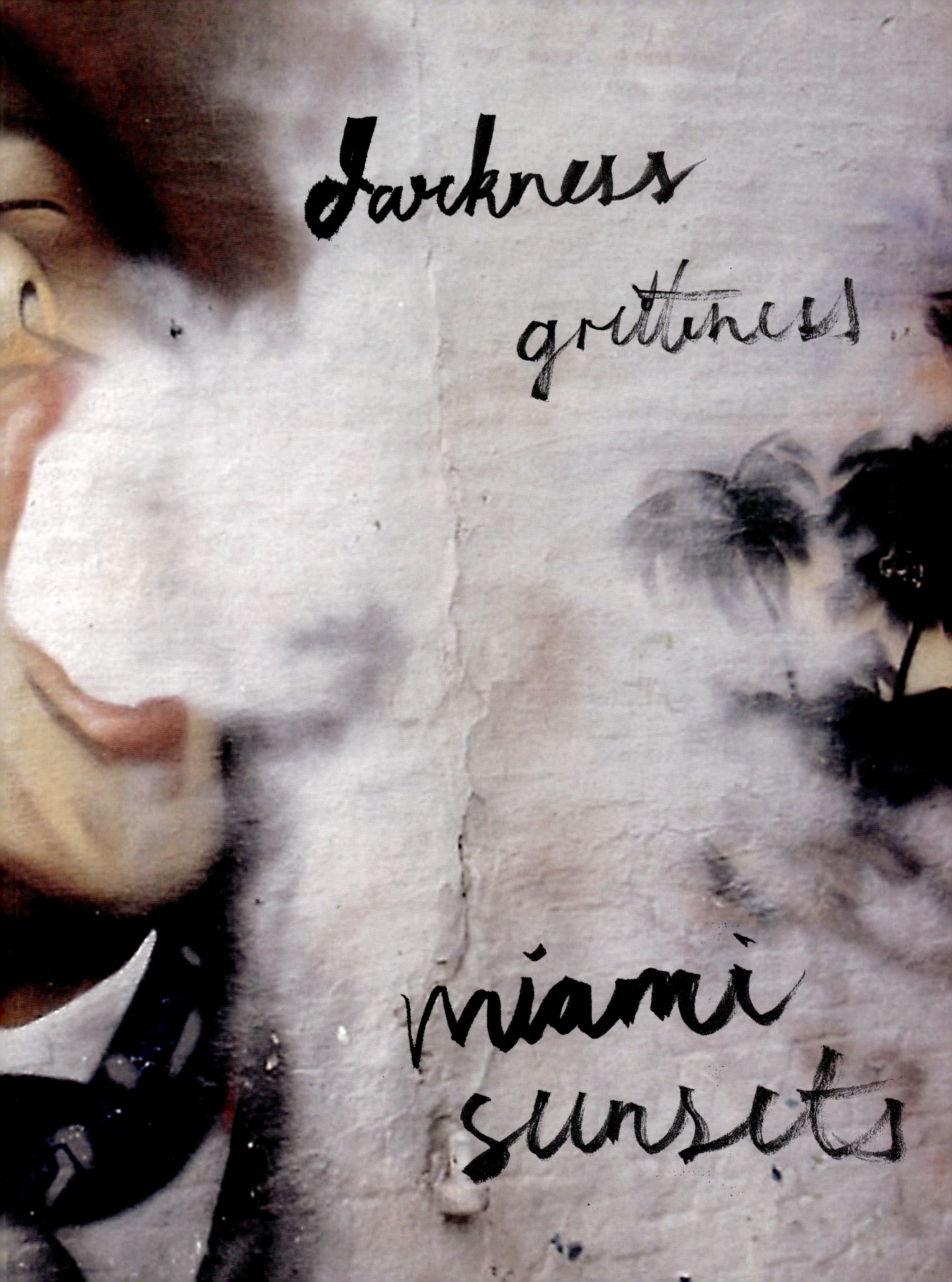

darkness
grittiness

miami
sunsets

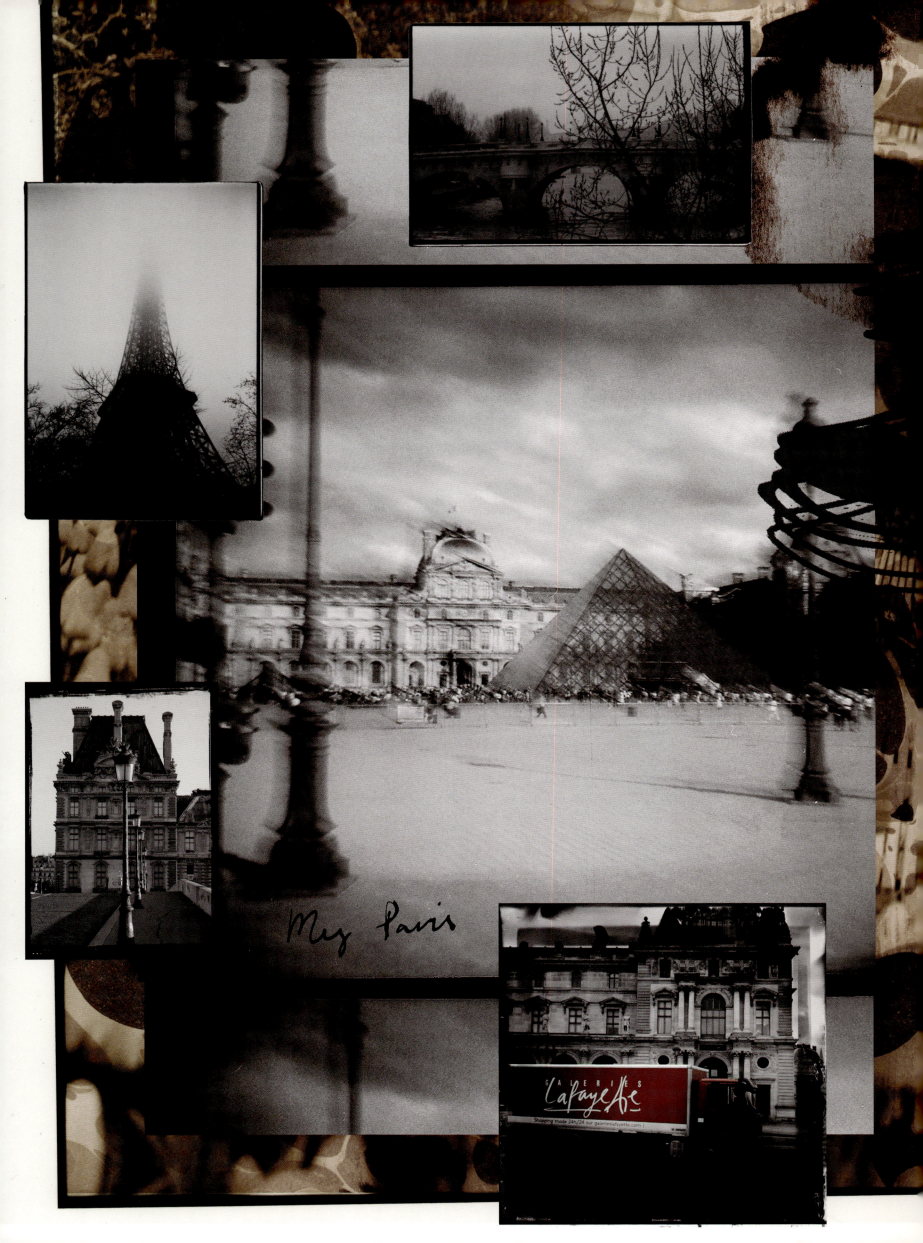

My Paris

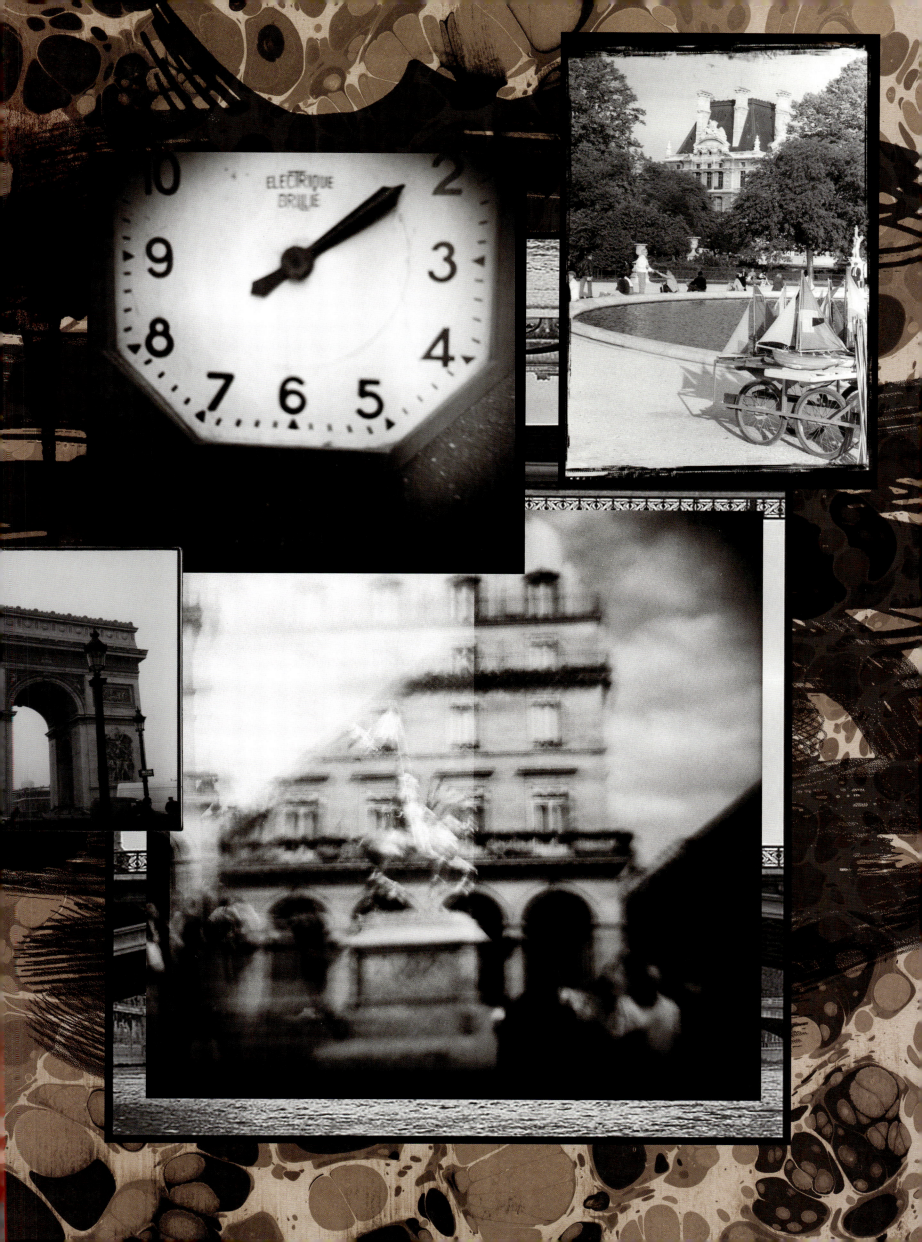

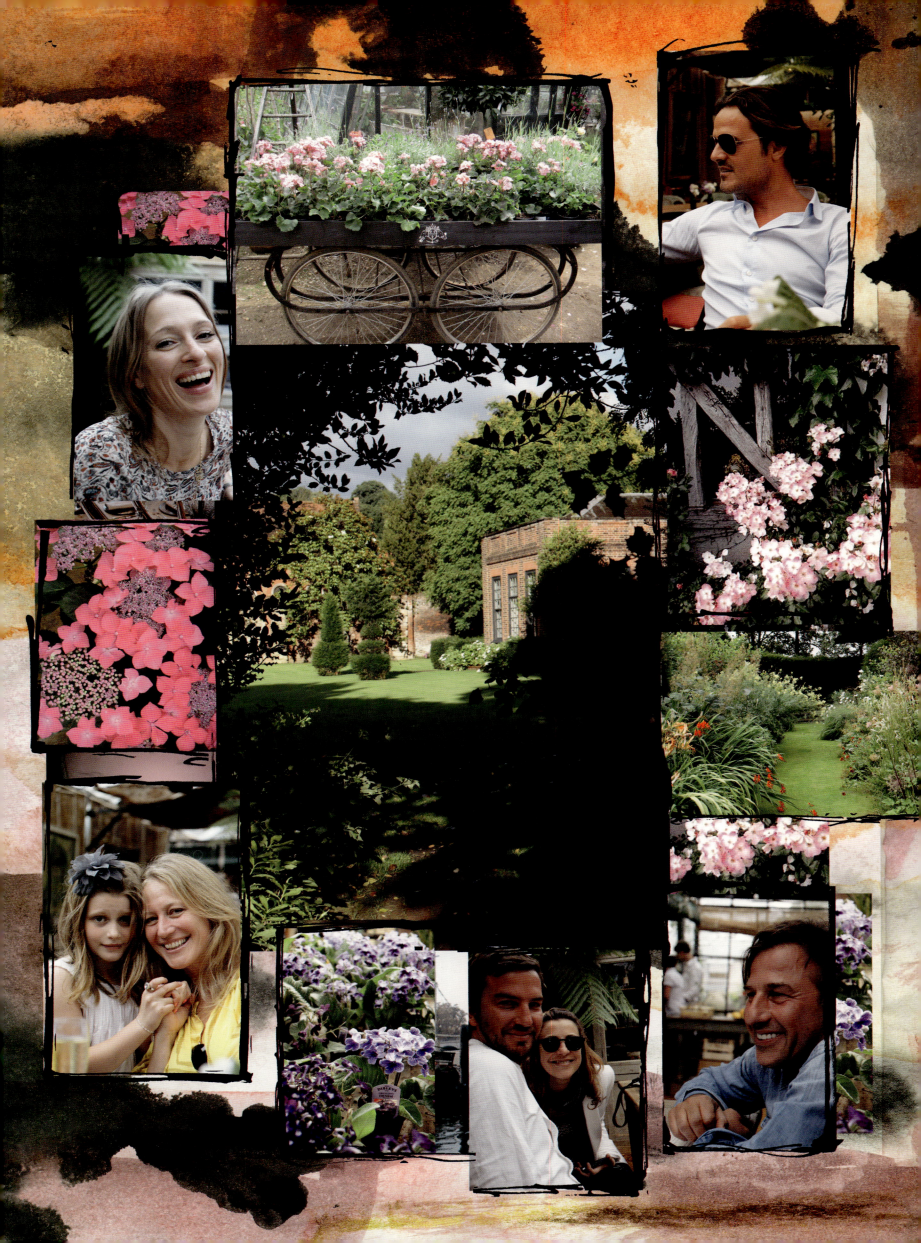

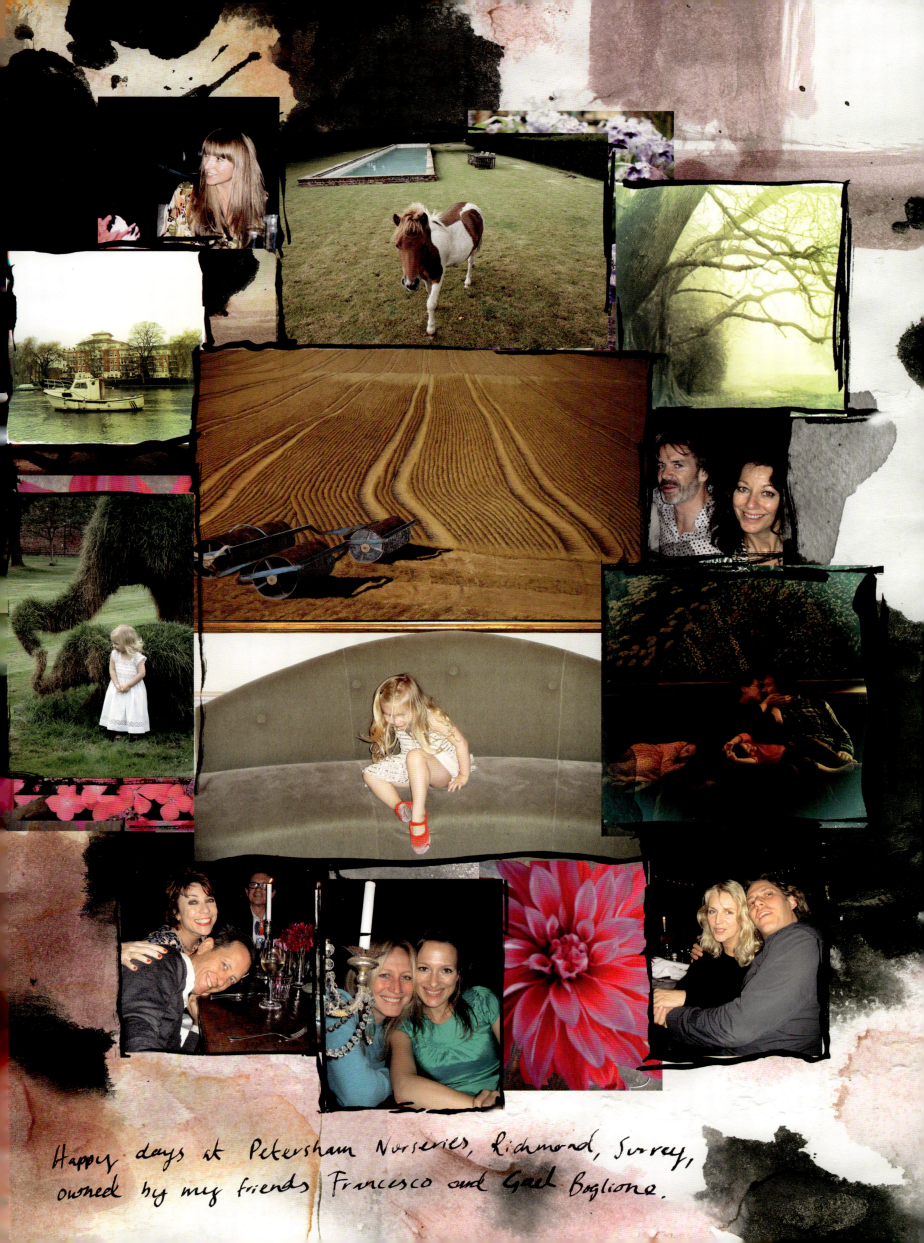

Happy days at Petersham Nurseries, Richmond, Surrey, owned by my friends Francesco and Gael Boglione.

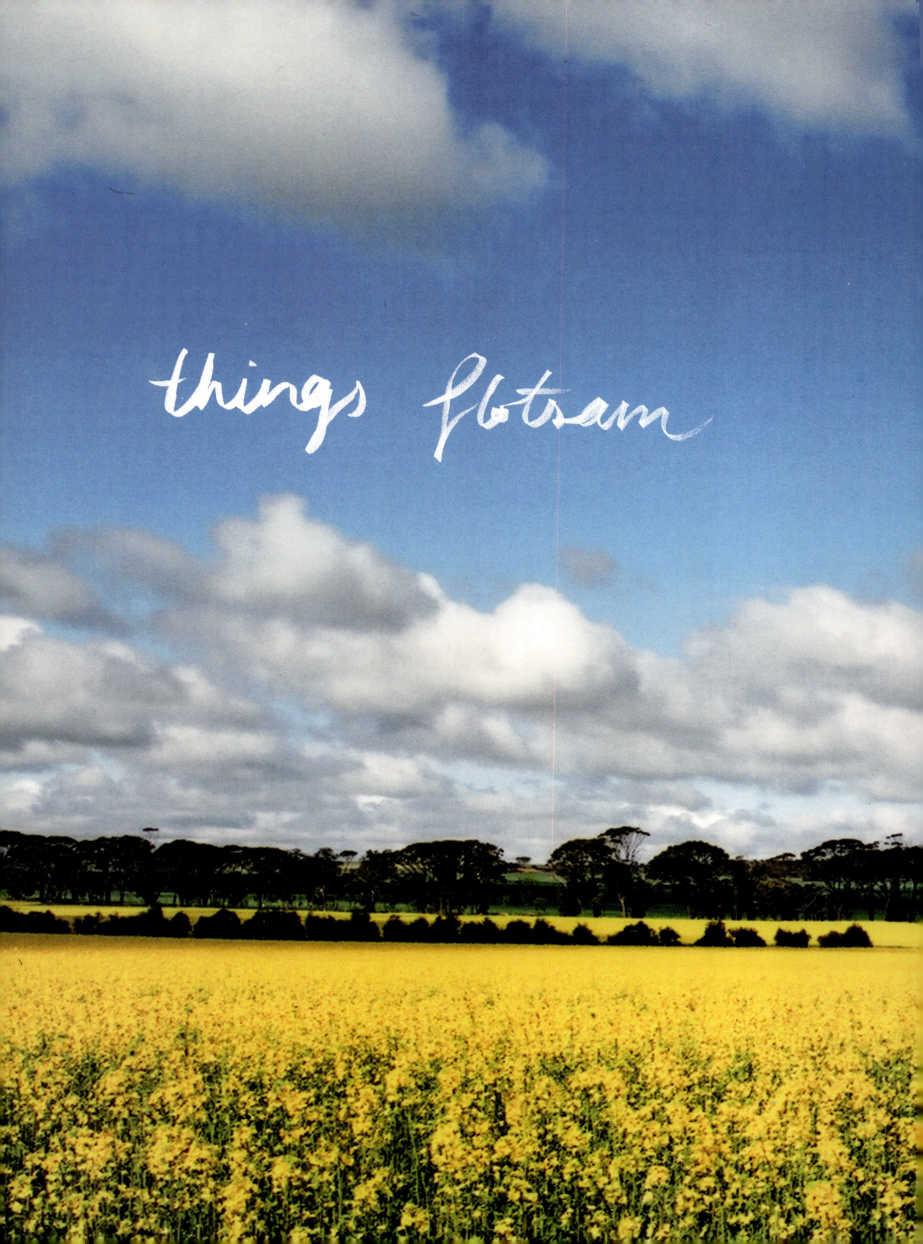

things flotsam

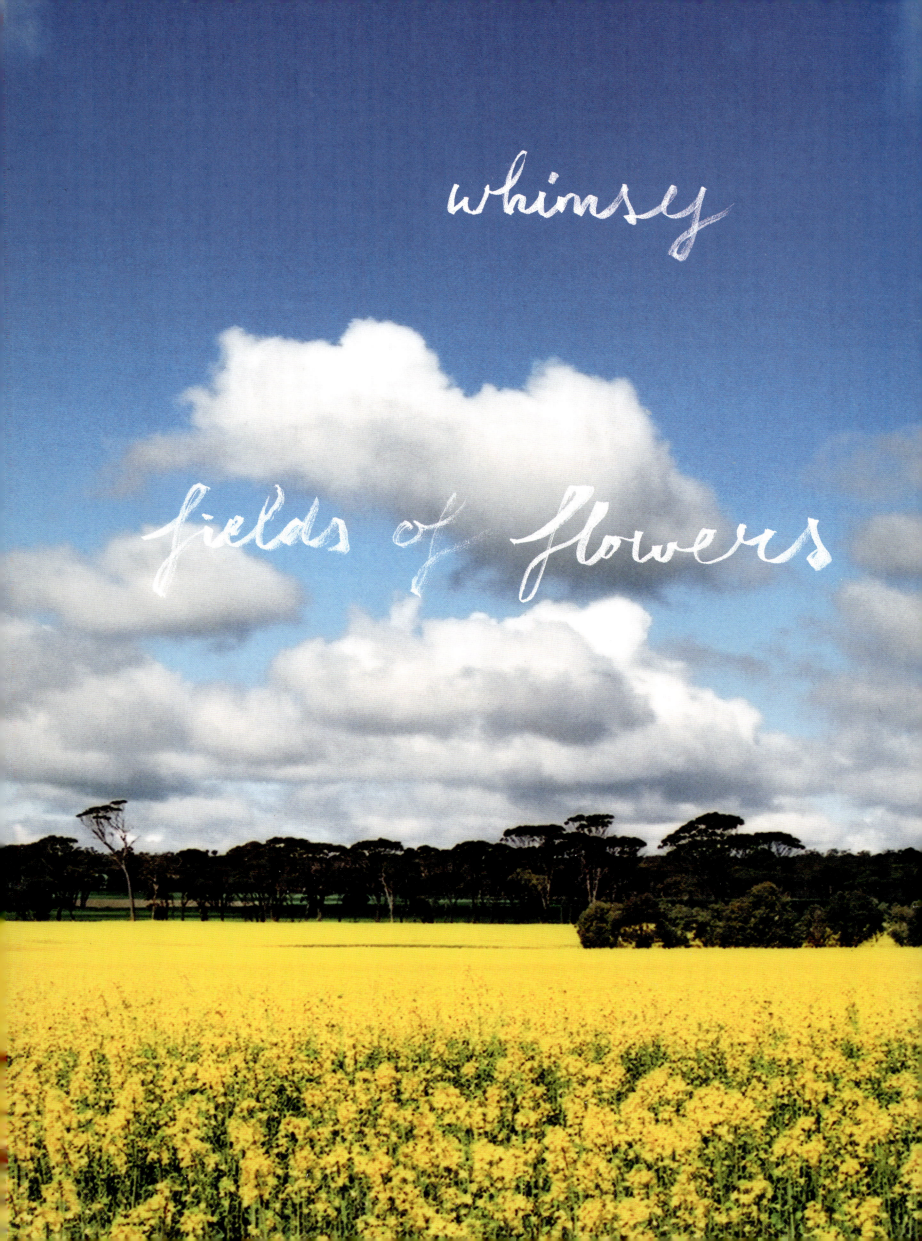

whimsy

fields of flowers

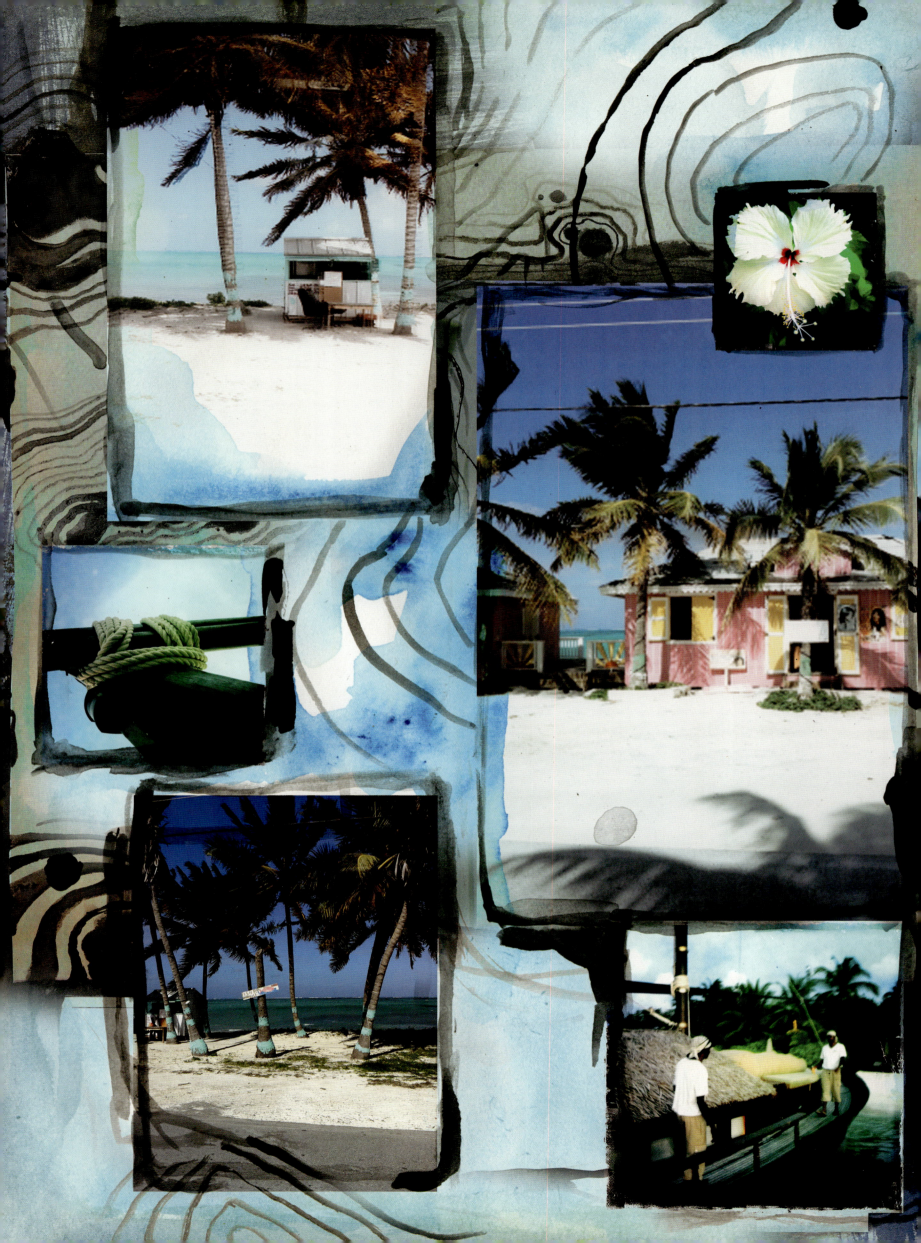

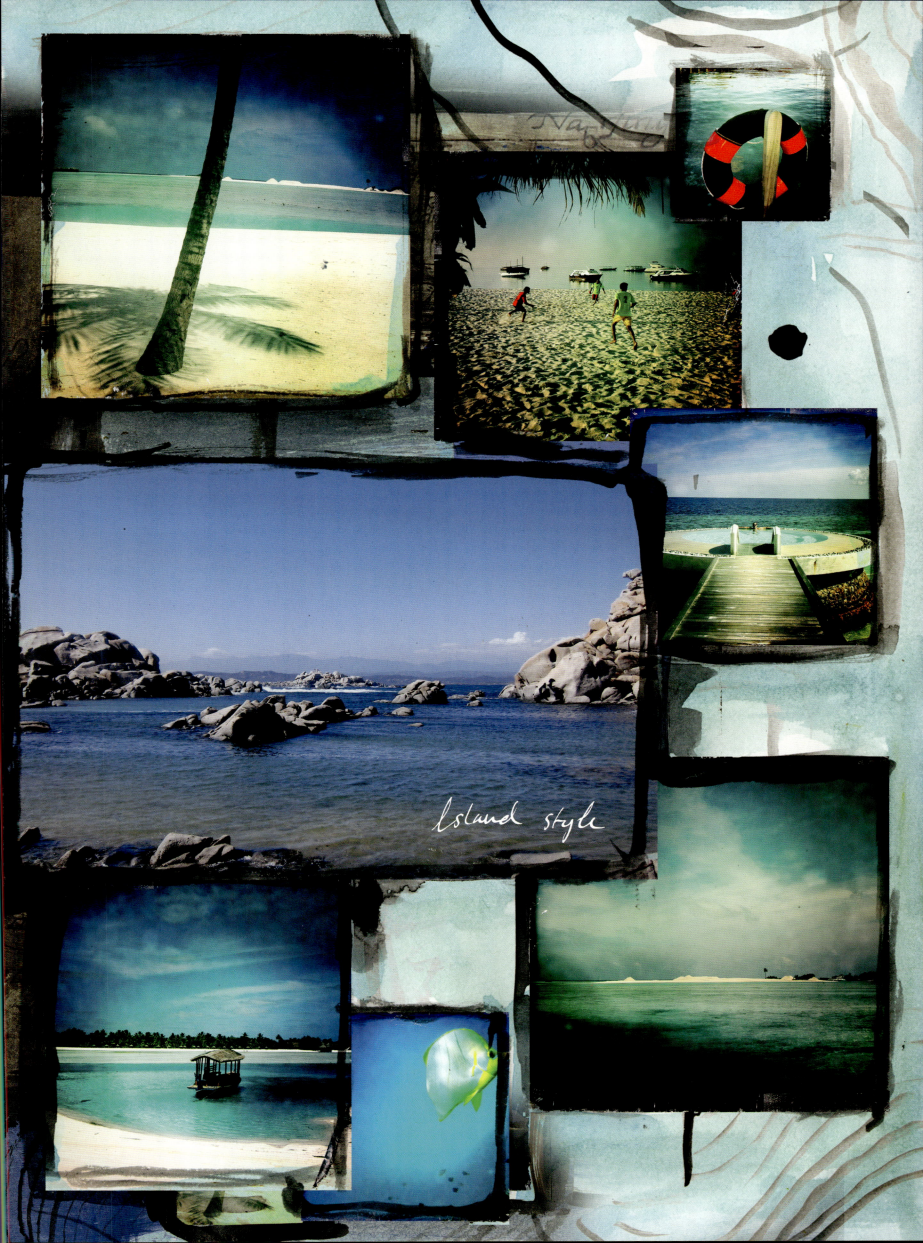

Island style

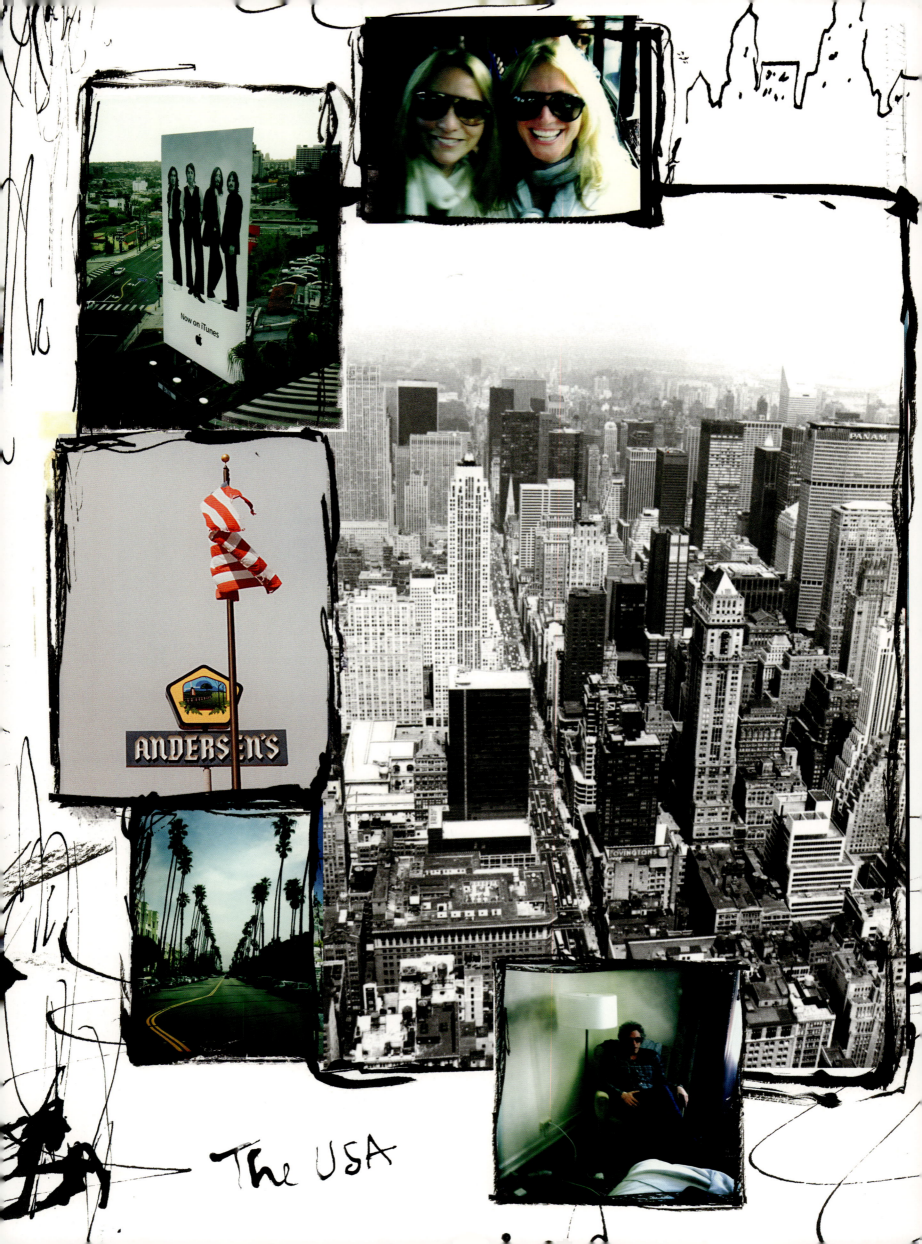

The USA

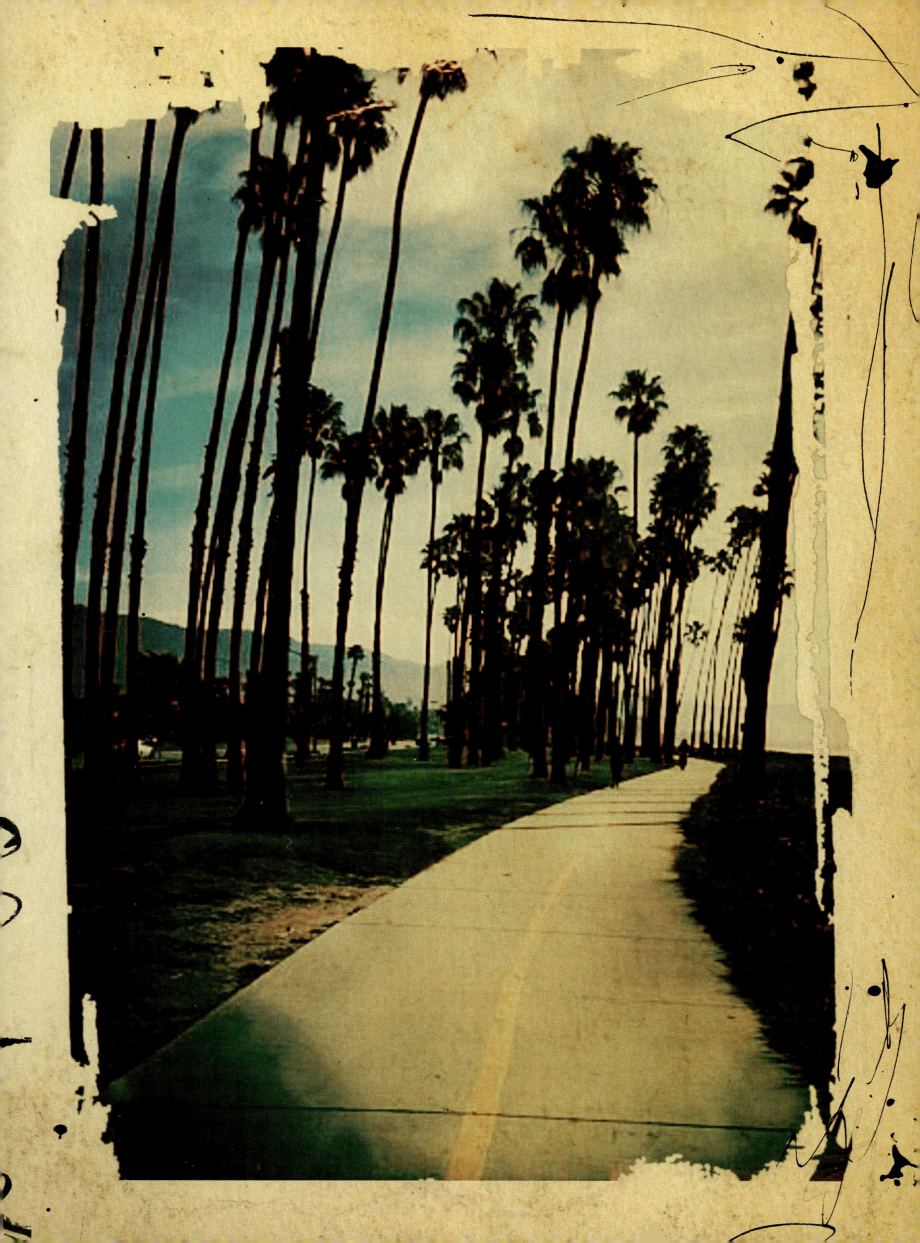

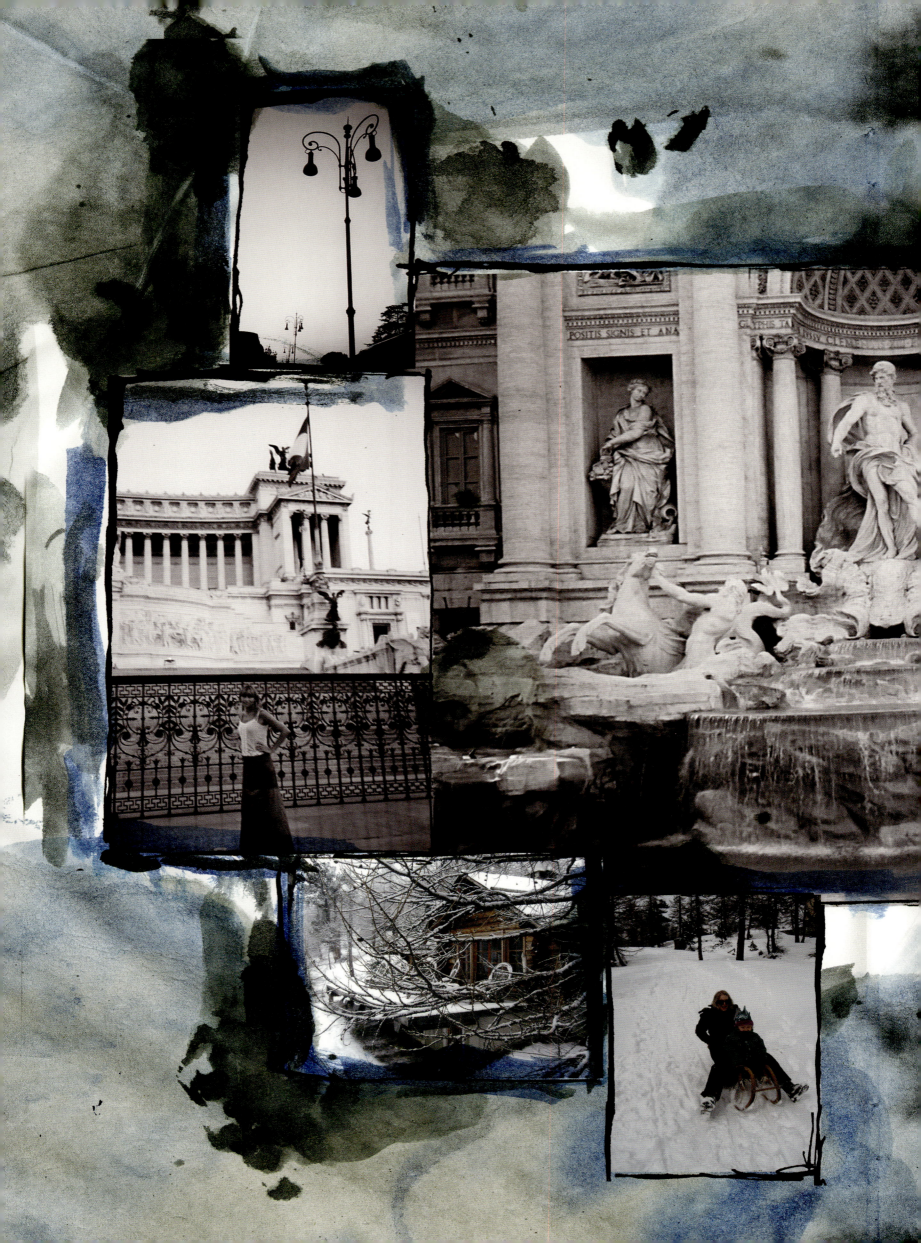

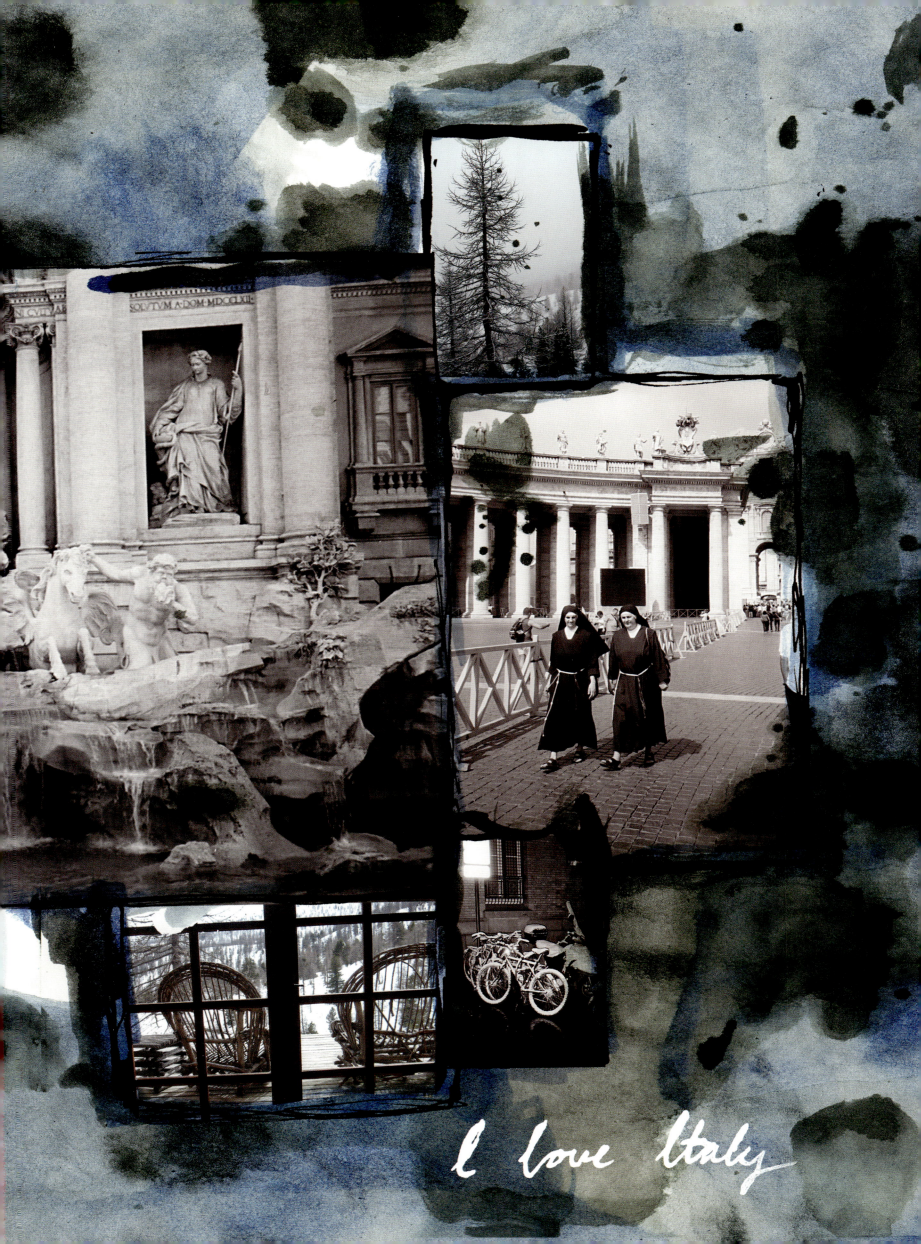

I love Italy

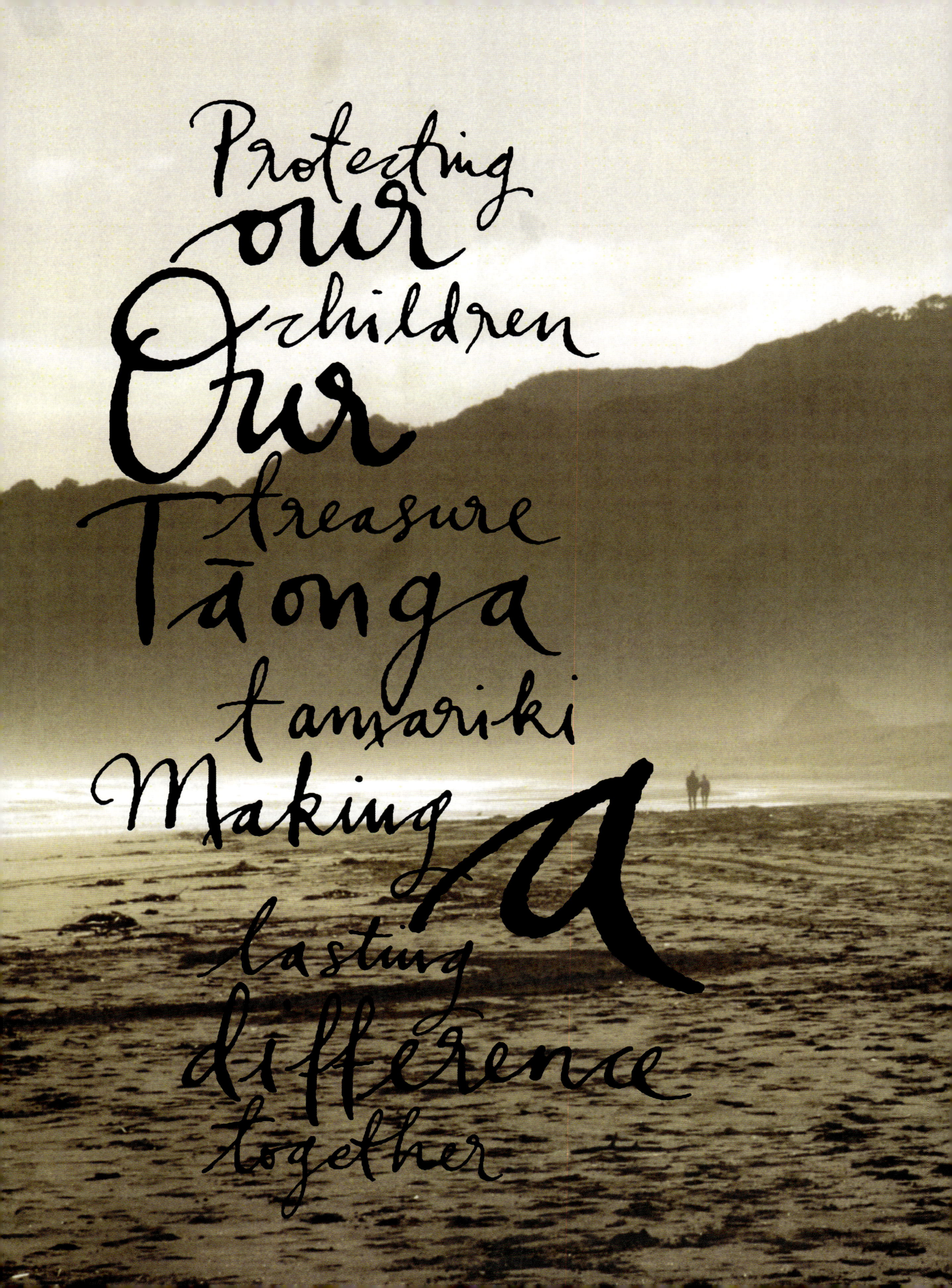

Protecting our children

Our treasure

Tāonga

tamariki

Making a

lasting

difference

together

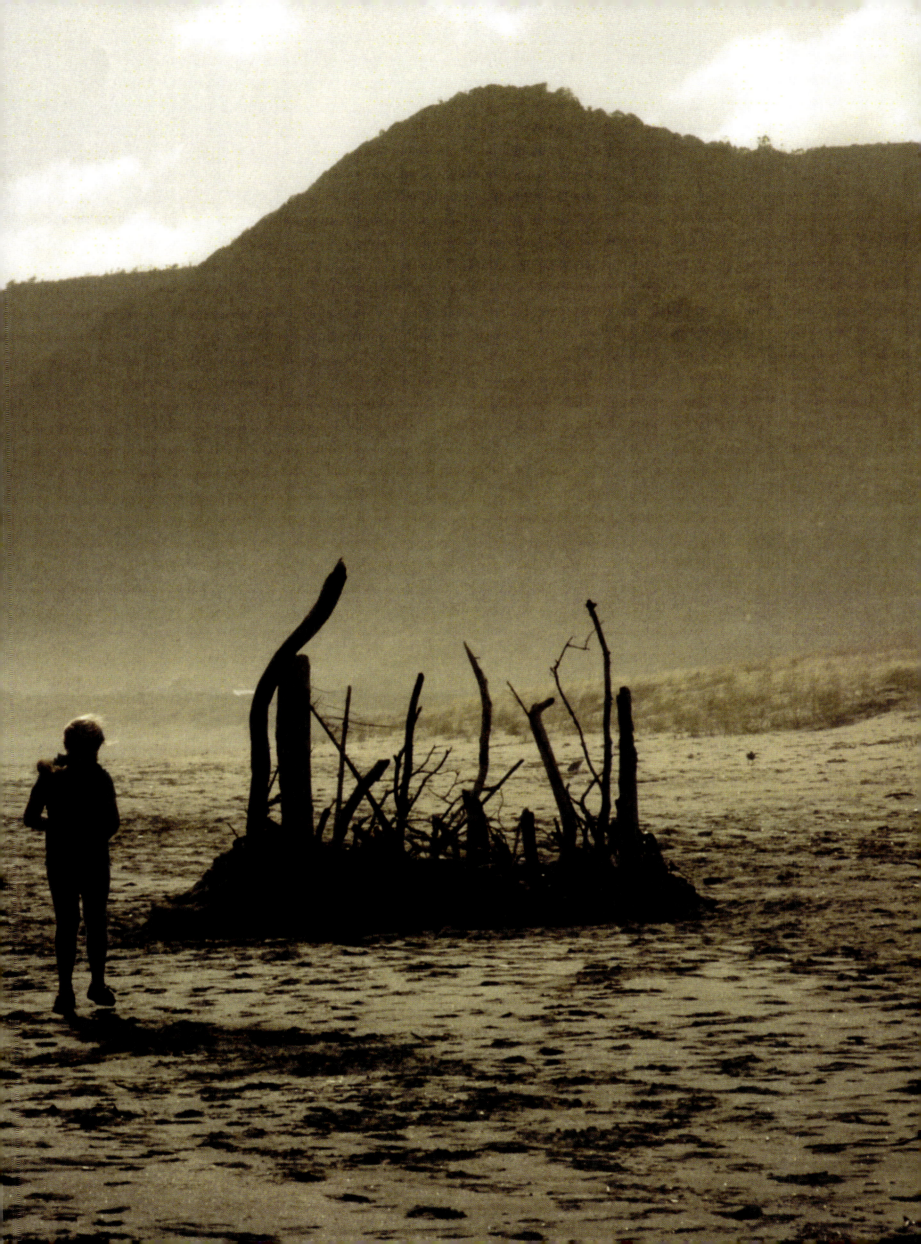

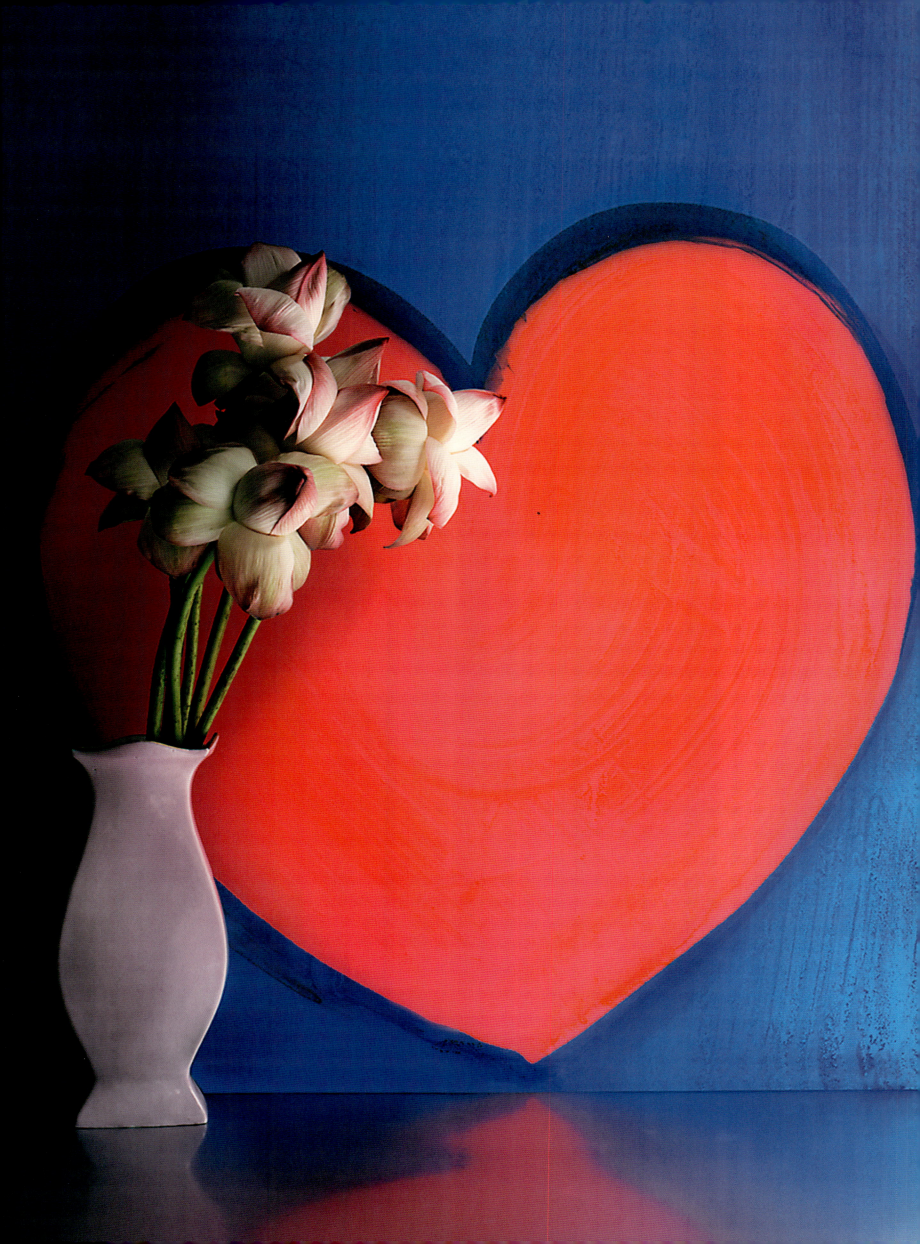

HOME IS WHERE THE *heart* IS

Downtime at Milton;
entertaining at home;
interior design — mixing the
old with the new.

CHAPTER 10

I FIND IT HARD TO RELAX
AT HOME IN SYDNEY –

there is always something that needs to be done.

BRADLEY SAYS THAT THE ONLY TIME
HE HAS EVER SEEN ME RELAX

was when we were on our honeymoon.

I had just found out I was pregnant,

and I had terrible morning sickness,

so all I could do was lie in bed,

OR SIT UNDER A PALM TREE
AND TRY TO READ A BOOK.

I was forced to do nothing,

but that's not my idea of relaxing.

I'D RATHER BE DISCOVERING
A NEW MARKET, *shopping for fabric,*

jewellery, old photos or even furniture,

OR COOKING A MEAL
FOR FRIENDS.

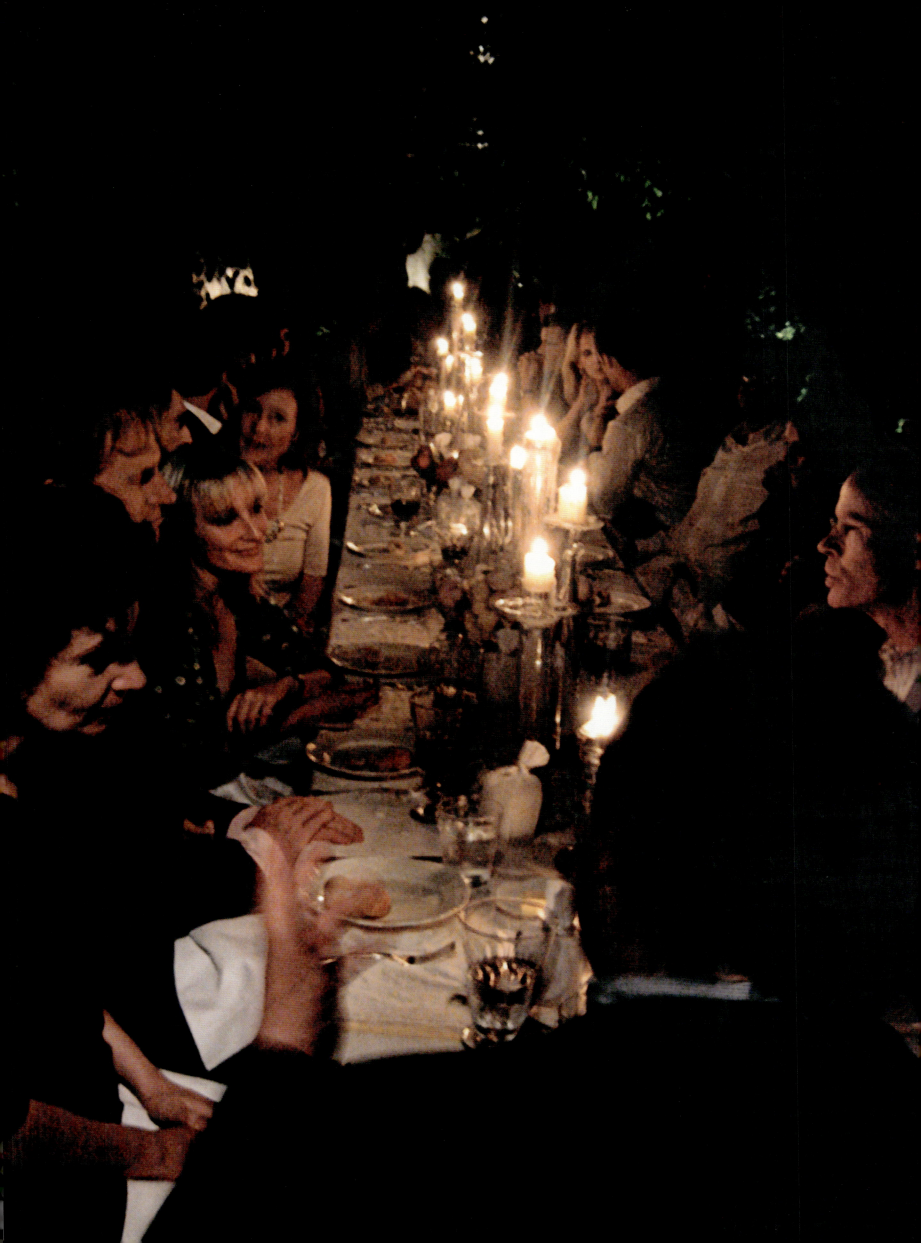

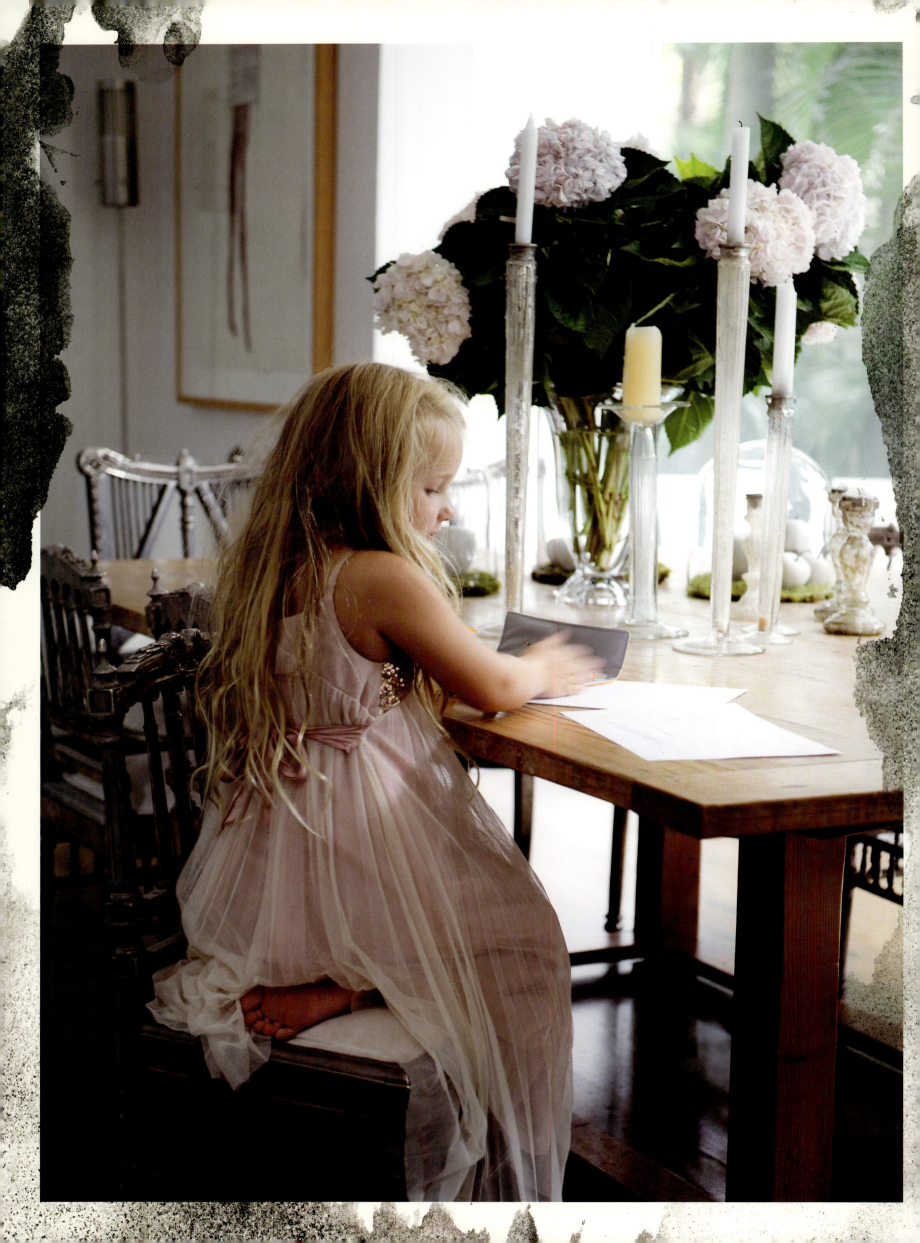

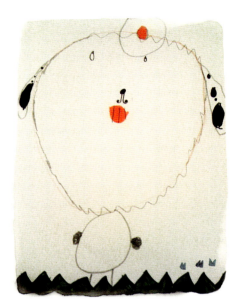

*My life is pretty hectic, especially now that I have Hunter. I work a
six-day week, most of the time. On weekdays I drop Estella at school
after making her breakfast and lunch, then I head to the office.*

Each day is different, depending upon where we're up to in the calendar – there might be design room fittings, production fittings, designing fabrics and colour schemes, sales meetings, designing invitations, meeting people who are in town – it's never the same. I am usually in the office for eight or nine hours a day, then I will spend some time at home on email. I used to run and exercise quite regularly, but there are days now when I just can't find the time. I try to walk to work every day, as a minimum, but sometimes I can't fit that extra twenty minutes into my day. I need to find the time and the discipline.

The place where I do unwind is at Milton, on New South Wales' South Coast, where I have a lovely old farmhouse which I bought about seven years ago. It was quite funny the way it happened – I had always wanted a place by the beach, and was just about to sign the contract for a house in Coalcliff, right on the water, when my friend, Peter Weiss called me and said: 'I know this property at Milton, with the most beautiful garden – it's magical. You have to go and have a look.' I had just returned from the Gold Coast, and I headed straight down to see it. It's an old dairy farmer's house, about one hundred and eighty years old, with the most stunning garden. It's about a four-minute drive from the beach, and I just fell in love with it and bought it straightaway.

The garden is quite English in style, with large magnolia trees and an orchard of sorts, with oranges, lemons, plums and other stone fruit. There are also the most beautiful wisteria and roses. I started a vegetable garden, where I spend a lot of my time when we're there. I love pottering around – Bradley's always telling me to come and relax, but that is my way of relaxing. I just think it's so amazing to plant something and then come back and see how much it has grown. I also love the idea of us eating seasonal produce – there's nothing better than going to the beach and catching fresh fish, then serving it with potatoes and salad from your own garden.

I think everyone should have a garden to relax in, no matter how small. I remember when my friend Joy Smithers had just had her first baby (Sasha, my god-daughter)

HOME IS WHERE THE HEART IS

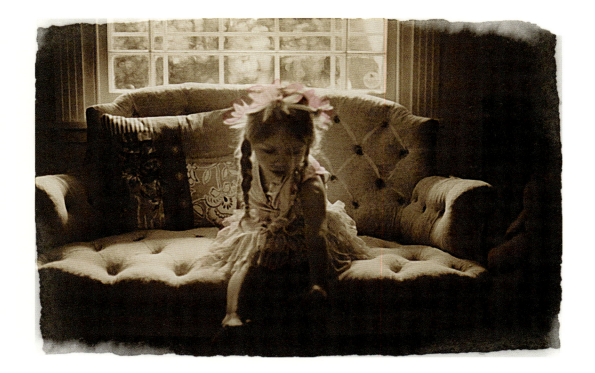

Above: Estella, at home.

*Opposite: I found these fabric petals in a market
in Paris. They used to be used as colour swatches.*

and I went to visit them in her small rented home. I was appalled to see that all she had for a garden was a patch of cement. As my gift to her and Sasha, I turned it into a garden so that they had somewhere sunny to sit together.

We try to get to Milton as often as we can, because we love being there – it is so peaceful. We spend summer holidays and Easter there, and usually one other school holiday as well. It takes three hours to get there (it took seven hours the first time we attempted it when Hunter was a newborn!) so we don't tend to go just for a weekend. Milton itself is quite special – it's not one of those sleepy little towns, it has a really vibrant, productive community. It is lovely to be so close to the beach, too. We spend most of our time in the garden or on the beach, just relaxing. The South Coast beaches are so stunning – there are lots of gum trees and native bush where the land meets the sea, and there aren't many houses right on the beach. I love going for long walks along the beach. In Milton it's all about the simple things in life.

We have a lot of great family time at Milton, but we also end up doing a bit of entertaining there, especially over summer, when many of our friends from overseas are home visiting families in the area. It is all very relaxed and low-key, simpler somehow than it is in Sydney, quite European. We sit outside on the veranda, and everyone pitches in and helps with whatever we're doing – shelling prawns, shucking oysters, or cooking on the barbecue. We have a long, lazy lunch, followed by an afternoon sleep (a real luxury) then we'll all go down to the beach for a swim.

I have always loved entertaining – I get that from Mum. She was always having friends round, and, like all children, we would sit at the top of the stairs and listen secretly to the adults partying the night away. Our home was always filled with music and laughter. Estella is just like I was – she loves to be involved, she wants a tray, she wants to serve people. It is never a chore for me to cook and entertain – it is wonderful to bring people together,

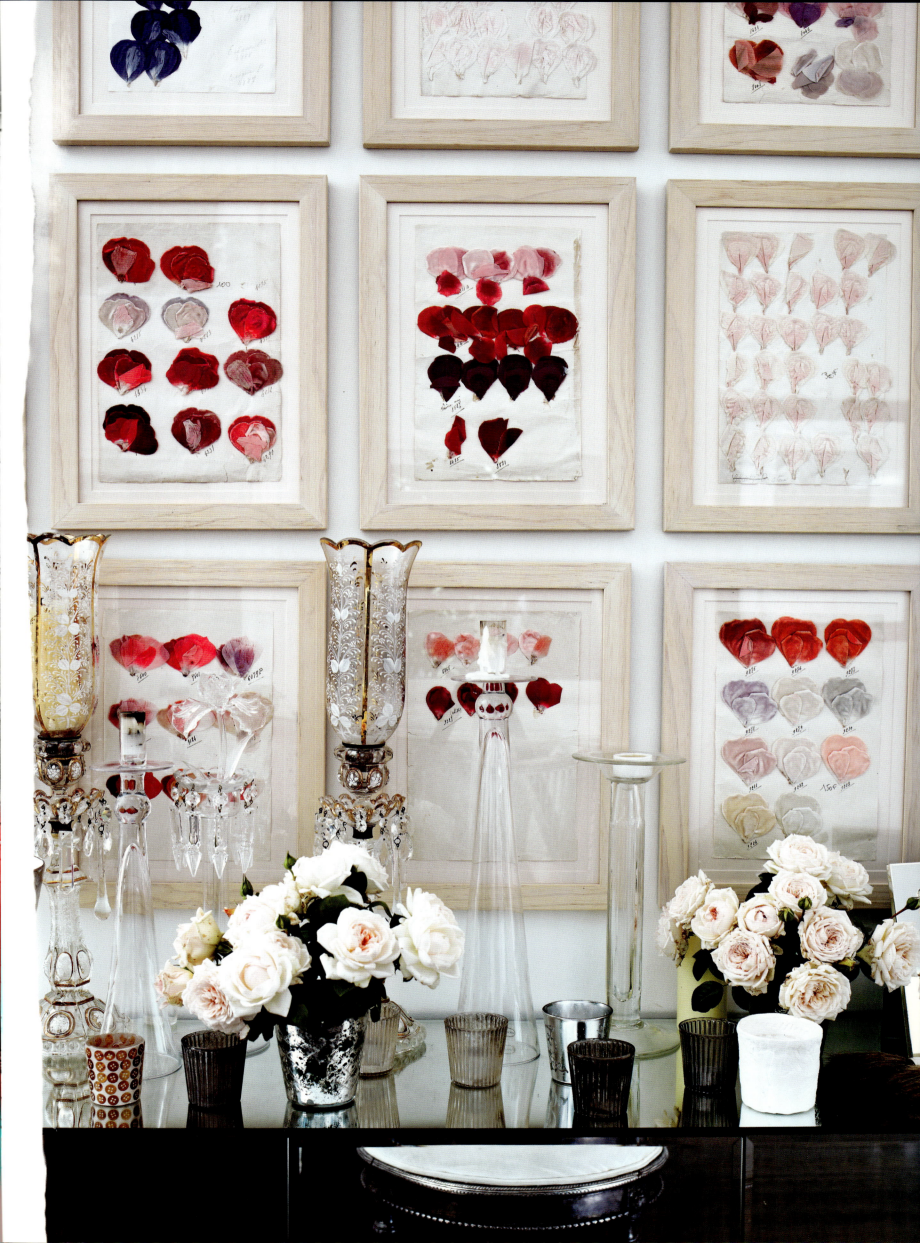

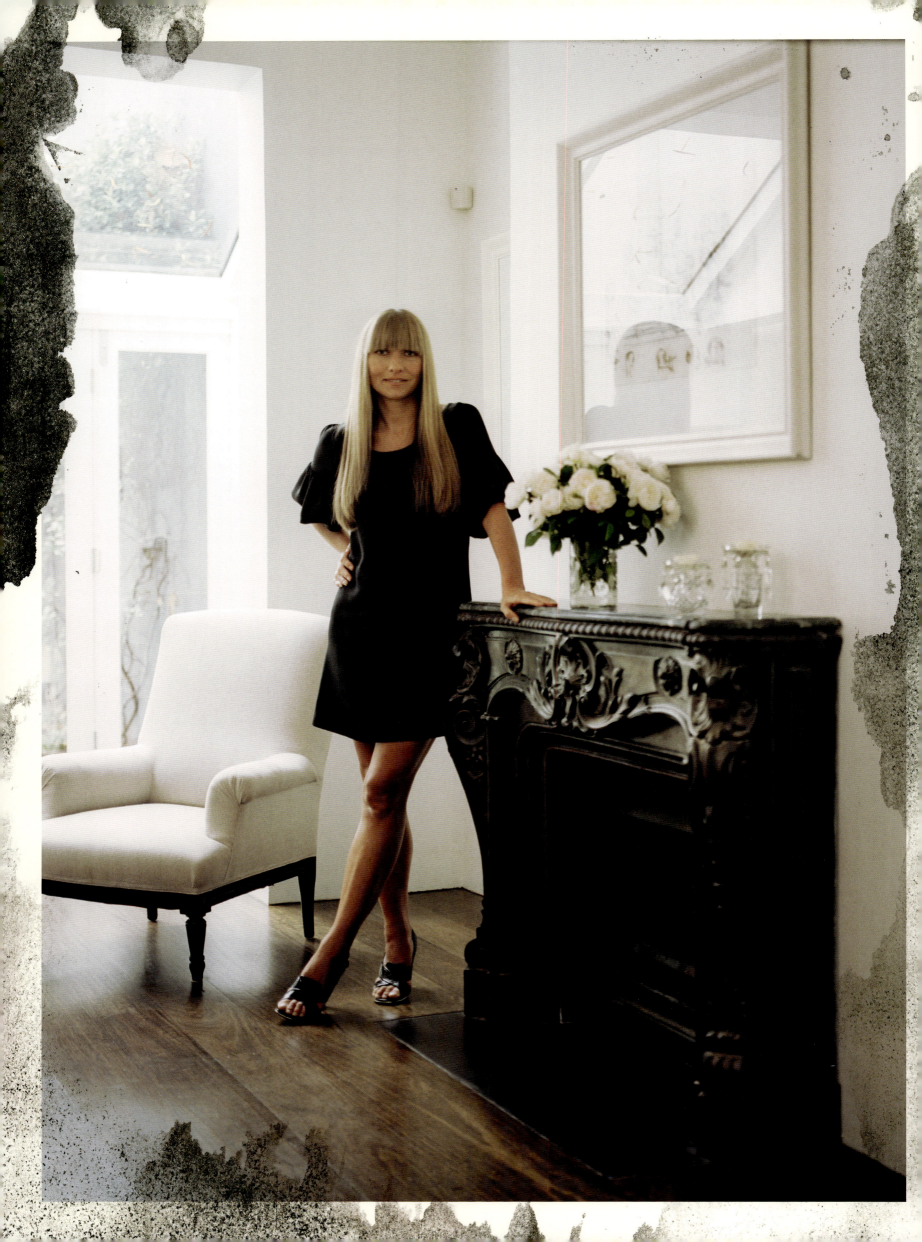

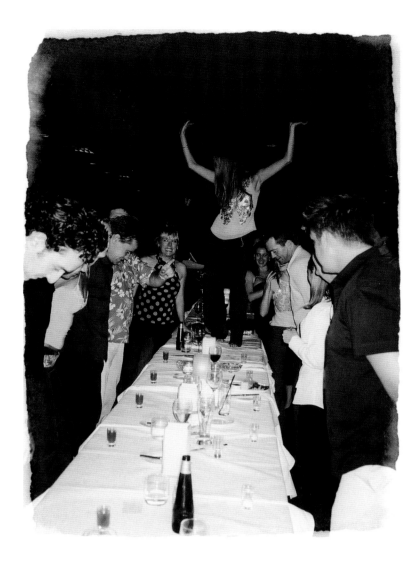

and it is nice to know that I have helped to create some lasting friendships.

When we entertain in Sydney it is all pretty laid-back and informal. Good wine is essential, and we eat in the dining room, which is lit by a beautiful old chandelier filled with candles – there are no electric lights. I think carefully about who to invite, because at the end of the day, it is always about the people, no matter how good the food and wine are. Much as I love cooking, people don't come for the culinary experience. Like us, our friends are creative or they have high-pressure jobs, and they just want to have a few glasses of wine, let go, share some laughs and not be scrutinised. They usually don't want to talk about work, but if they do, this is a safe environment for them.

I have had a lot of fun over the years renovating the homes we have lived in – putting my own stamp on them. I am a bit obsessive about interiors – so much so that when I walk into a new space, I can't help redesigning it in my head. I have a strong sense of colour, and proportion,

and I find it so frustrating to see a room or building with character, where the layout or the colours are all wrong. I think that in Sydney there's often a lack of respect for beautiful, old buildings – I can't understand how councils allow some things. My eye for detail can be the bane of my life though – I will walk into a room and say, 'Oh God, why did they paint it that colour?' I can't just relax, or switch off – and it drives Bradley mad. We will walk in somewhere and he will look at me and say, 'Don't you even think about it.'

For my own homes, what I like most is to mix the old with the new – the modern with the more traditional. I love warm finishes, with timbers and stone and other natural elements, and I like to work with tactile things. I love marble in the bathrooms. Proportions are very important – at home, everything is all about a feeling, a sense of space and balance. I love high ceilings and lots of natural light, and there must be a good airflow – a place which has those things always has potential.

*Opposite: In the drawing room
at my old home in Paddington
in 2007.*

Above: We all love to have fun!

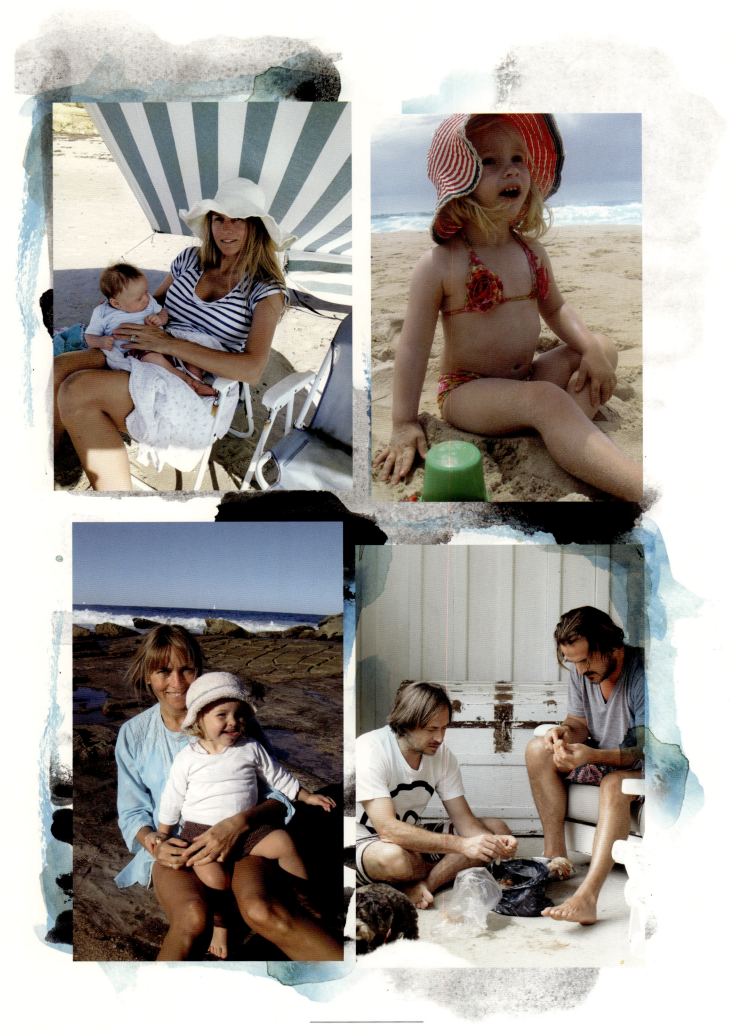

Above: Life at the beach.

Opposite: At my beach house at Palm Beach in 2011.
I love the painting behind me by Paul Haggith.

HOME IS WHERE THE HEART IS

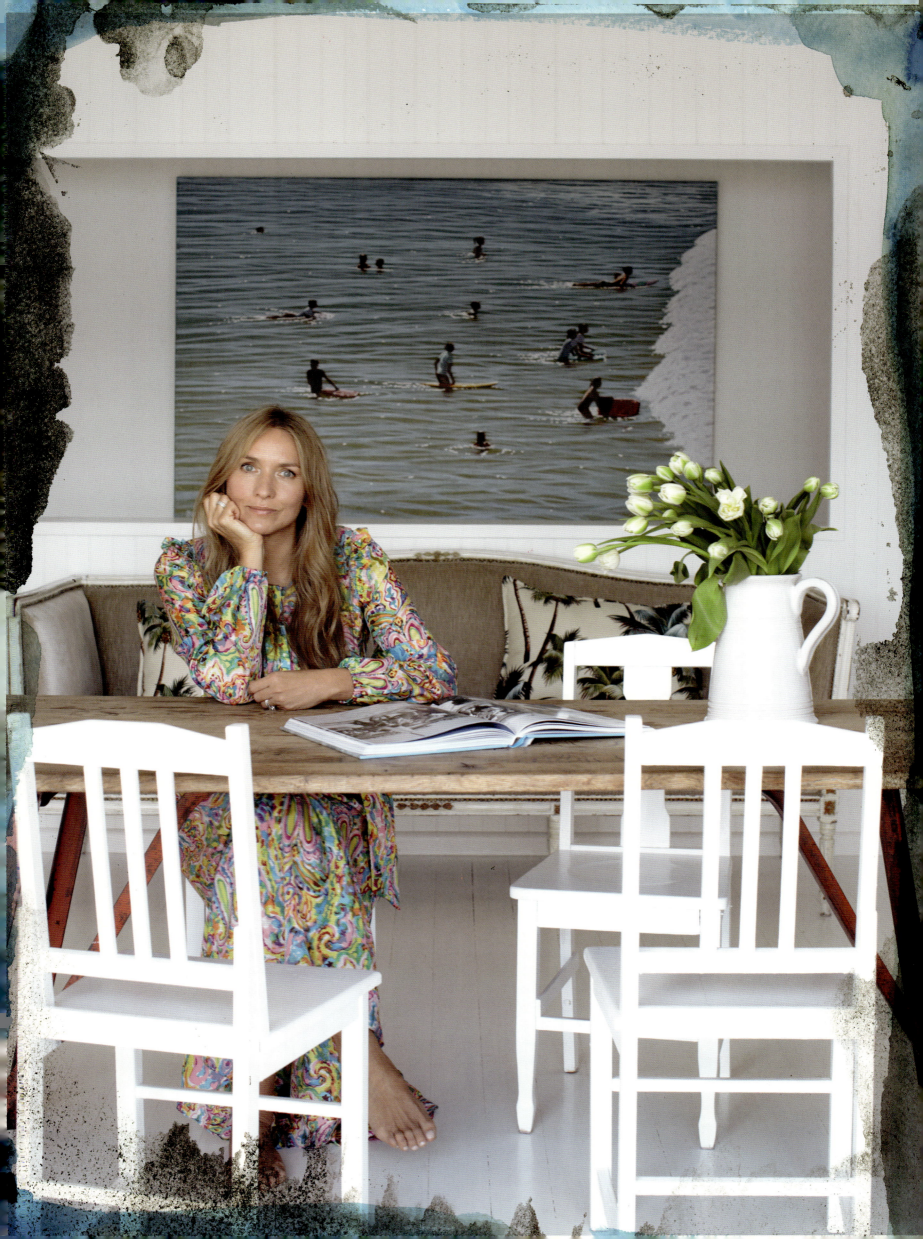

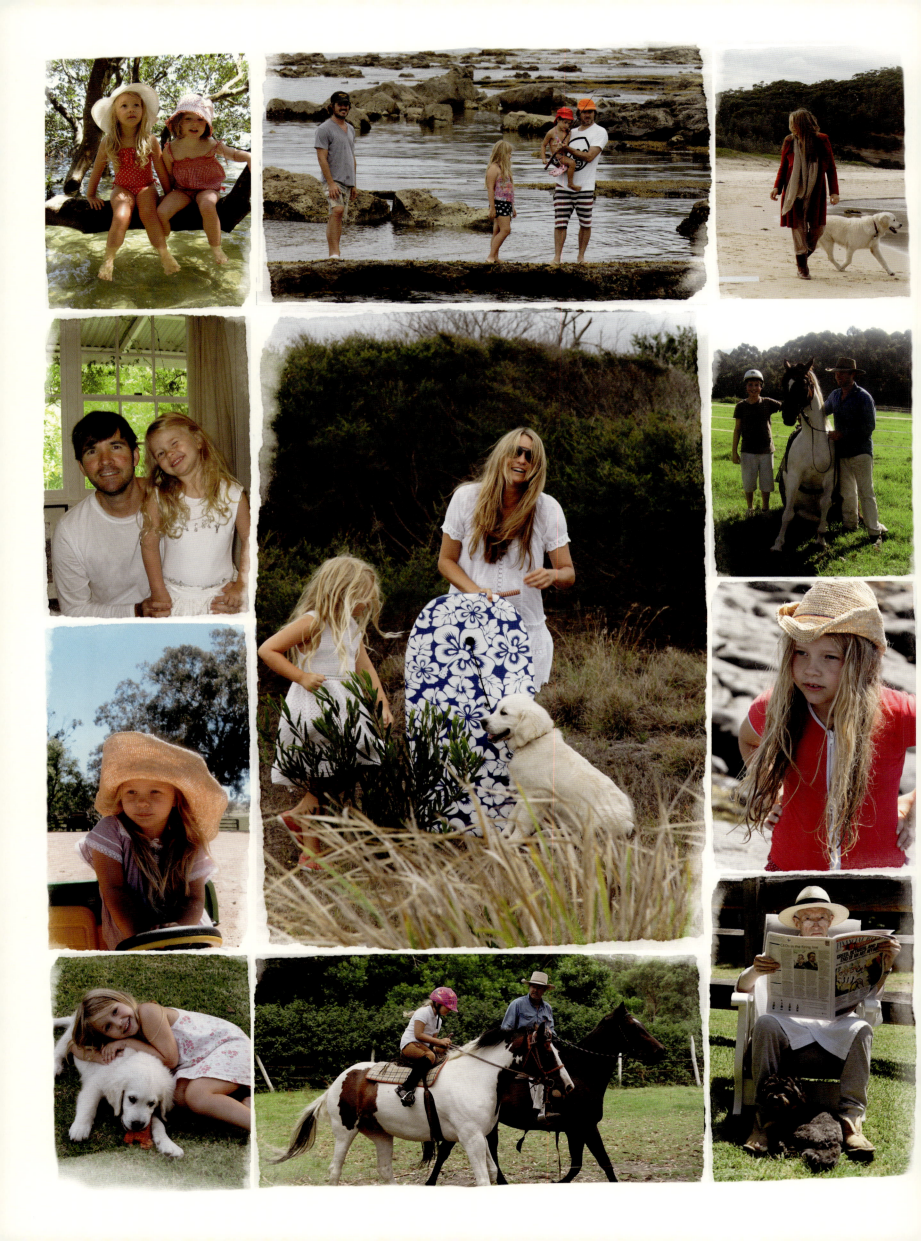

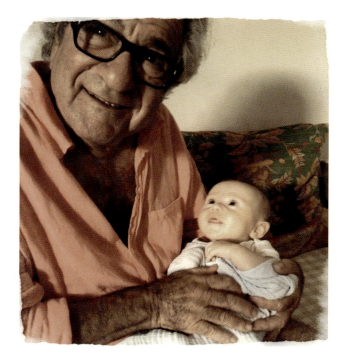

Above: Hunter, three weeks old, with
Papa Peter (Peter Weiss), his godfather.

I like my home to feel peaceful, because my work studio is so full of energy. Although I try to keep home calm and less messy, it's not easy, with dogs, babies, children and friends – there's always chaos somewhere in the house. It's never quiet – but it's a good noise, not an annoying noise. I believe the most important thing is that a home feels lived in – and mine certainly does.

There are lots of things I love – and some things I can't stand. I love stand-up lamps and I loathe down lighting; it's so unflattering. I like a sense of breeziness, so I much prefer curtains to blinds. I love Carrera marble, and old timber floors, in greys and whites – I don't like using red tones at home. I'm very resourceful, I like to recycle, especially old furniture. With fabrics, I love linens, silks and cottons printed with unexpected designs. I really like botanicals and tend to use them in unusual ways, like printing them on fabrics for sofas. My favourite room at home is our bedroom – it is simple and charming, with exposed beams, a lovely outlook over some trees, and a beautiful old stone fireplace. Plus, it's always cool and breezy.

I have renovated every home I have ever lived in – I can just walk into a space and imagine how it would be if I lived there. Sometimes even I have to admit that I take this to extremes. In my 'nesting' period just before Estella was born, I decided that I couldn't bear the floorboards in my home any longer, so I set about ripping them out, digging up the flooring underneath, laying new floorboards, then staining, sanding and sealing them. Estella was born two weeks later.

It took nearly two years to renovate our home in Paddington. We changed the layout of the rooms, opening them up and putting in lots more doors and windows. I took out the new floor and replaced it with old floorboards from a woolshed in Perth. It was a big project. Next time, I think I would live in a house for a little while before renovating.

Ironically, when we last moved it was to downsize, but now, with Estella growing up and Hunter's arrival,

Opposite: Precious family time at Milton. Clockwise
from far top left: Estella and Daisy; Bradley, Estella, Marc
and Imogen; with Louis; Luke, who takes Estella riding,
with Christian; Estella; Dad; Estella and Luke; Estella
with Louis; Estella on a tractor; Estella with Seamus.

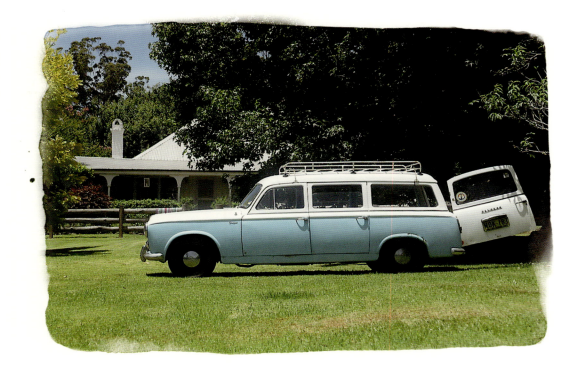

Above: A friend's old Peugeot at Milton.

Opposite: Estella and Louis.

we are thinking that maybe we need more space. In a few years' time, when she's a teenager and he's an active little boy, she may want a music room, he will probably want a backyard – I need to be quite mindful about where we go next, rather than impulsive. As far as Bradley's concerned though, I am not allowed to fall in love with some derelict old mansion. He says: 'Leave it to someone else, I will divorce you if you take on another house.'

I can't say I blame him – I do love to redecorate, to make a home my own. I made minimal changes when I bought my farmhouse in Milton, though. It was more redecorating than renovating. It is such a comfortable home, and it has a great spirit. It is all on one level, which

I love, so everything is smaller and more intimate. It is all quite informal there, in the country – people just drop in, without phoning first, and you never know what's going to happen. We have a lovely old fireplace, and everyone just sits around and chats. There's a lot of outdoor space, with beautiful gardens as well as my vegetable gardens. In summer, it's very much about living outside.

When we bought the house at Palm Beach, the idea was to keep it simple, perhaps just repaint, but as it turned out we did quite a lot of work to it. We put in a new balcony, new bedroom and new bathroom. Pretty much the whole house was redone. That's why Bradley says he knows me too well now – it will never be just a coat of fresh paint.

Following page: Our wedding, at the Town Hall in Positano, Italy in 2011. Behind me is a bougainvillea-covered arch. It was our dream wedding.

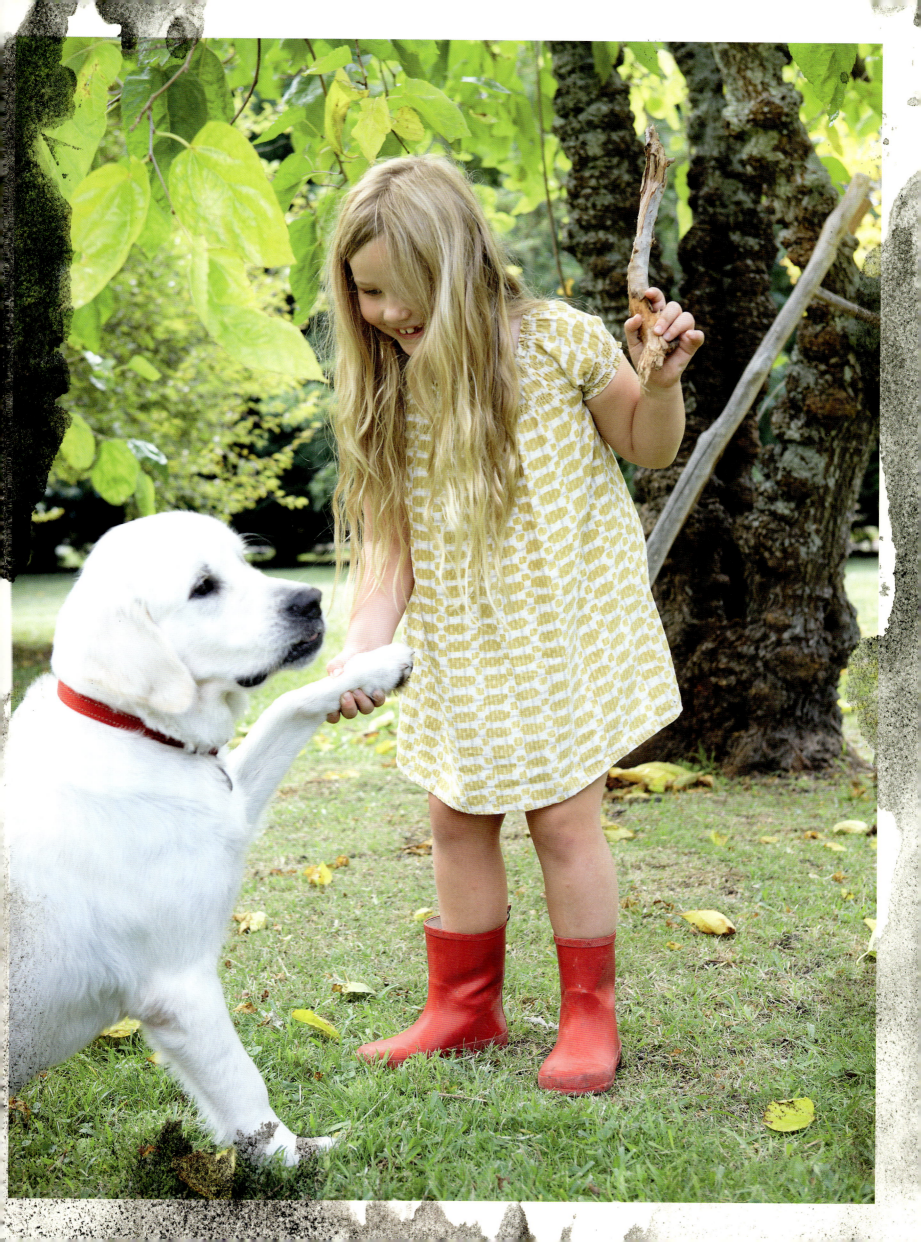

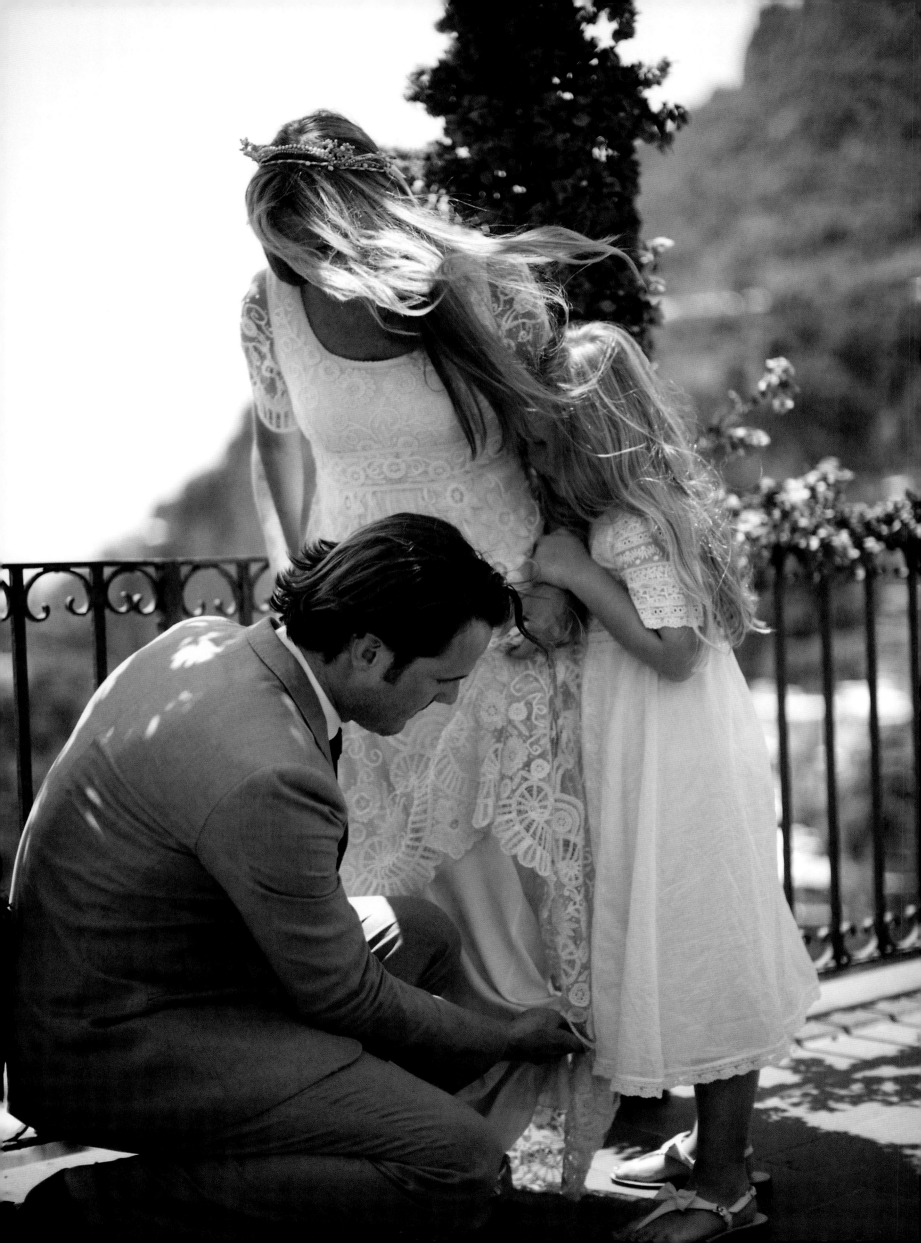

THAT'S AMORE

Wedding bells in Positano;
Dom Pérignon and Fanta on the water;
designing a bridal collection.

LOVE AND NUPTIALS

CHAPTER 11

FOR A WHILE,

WHEN I WAS IN MY THIRTIES,

I really discounted the whole idea of

ROMANCE AND WEDDINGS,

but in my forties I have come to

see how important it all is,

PERHAPS BECAUSE I HAVE

FOUND HAPPINESS MYSELF.

When Bernie and I separated

I was in my thirties.

My other significant relationship

was with Richard, Estella's father.

WE HAD MANY MEMORABLE

MOMENTS, BUT IT WAS

NOT MEANT TO BE.

I never gave up hope that

I would find the right person —

I AM A DREAMER, AND I LOVE

BEING IN A RELATIONSHIP,

so I kept on hoping for the best.

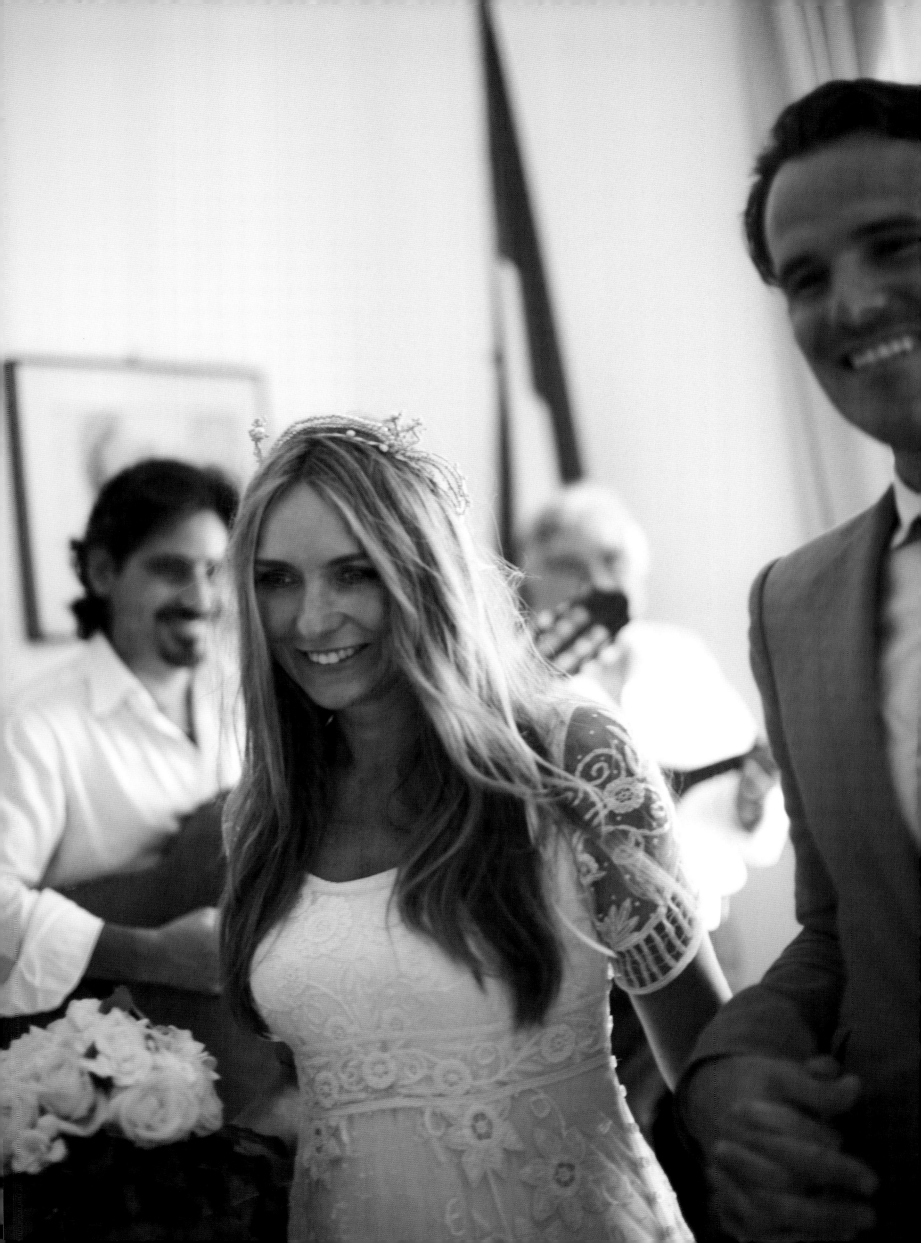

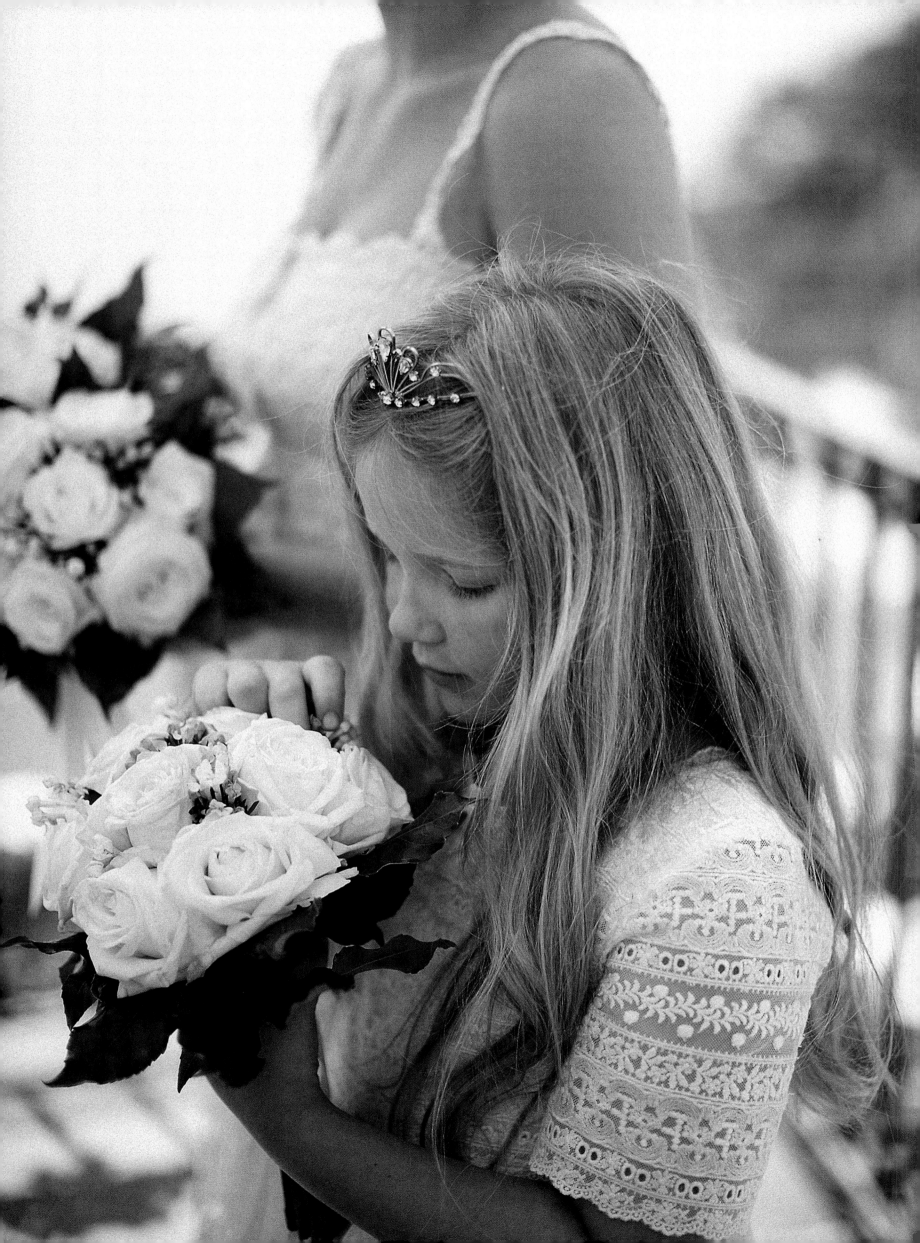

*I met Bradley Cocks in 2007 at a party I wasn't even
planning to go to. My friend Nikki Andrews introduced us.
We started chatting, then suddenly I realised I had been
talking to this man for an hour and a half.*

I remember being very attracted to him, and sensing that it was mutual. The next night I was hosting a dinner at home to celebrate *Vogue Living*'s fortieth birthday – they had done a profile on me and my home. I had invited about fifty people, a mixture of friends, fashion people and architects, a very creative group. As someone had just pulled out, Nikki suggested I invite Bradley. So I asked him that night, and, being Bradley, his response was, 'Only if I can sit next to you.' He's very charming. I said, 'Of course' – what else was I going to say?

He fitted in perfectly. The next day everyone was interrogating me – the usual questions were asked . . . We started to meet quite regularly for coffee and lunch. There were also a lot of phone conversations. After about six months, we both happened to be in India staying at the Taj Hotel, at the same time. As far as I know, that was just by chance. I don't think he's the kind of man who would have changed his plans so he could see me – if he did, he's never told me.

That was that. He moved in the first week we were back in Sydney. I was trying so hard to take it slowly and he was cautious, too – so much so that he moved in, moved out then moved back in again. He realised he couldn't just jump into a relationship with someone who had a child, and a public profile – but it's hard to take it slowly when you have strong feelings for each other. It didn't take long for me to think that he might be 'the one'. As you get older, I think you focus on what is most important for you.

Bradley had a very genuine relationship with Estella, right from the start. That was crucial – I needed to know that he was the right person for her as well as for me; I didn't want him to play a big part in her life and then just disappear. Estella took to him from the word go, I think because he's quite childlike, like a lot of boys, who never really grow up. He teaches her all sorts of things that I can't – like how to bake. I don't bake at all, but it is something they love to do together. She adores him and he adores her – when she's upset about something, she'll often say 'Where's Bradley? I want Bradley'. We all just have a really good time together.

Bradley has very similar values to me, and I think that's essential in a relationship. He's genuine, he respects people, he has good manners, he cares for his family, and we have the same priorities. He also has a great sense of humour. This relationship has just been so easy, despite our age difference. I think age is irrelevant – he is very

Previous page: Man and wife.

*Opposite: Estella wore a dress from my Enfant
range, and she and I both wore tiaras I had found
at the flea markets in Paris, years before.*

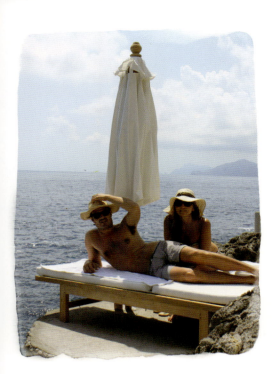
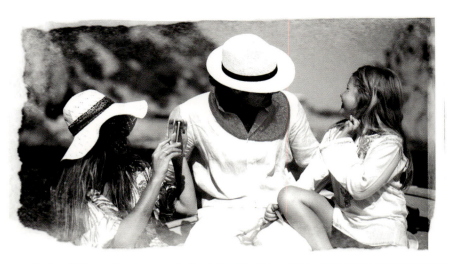
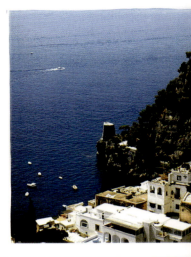
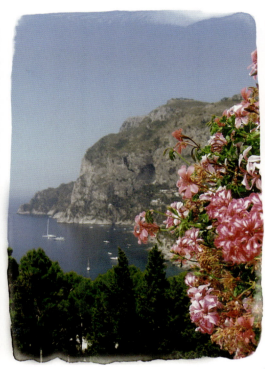
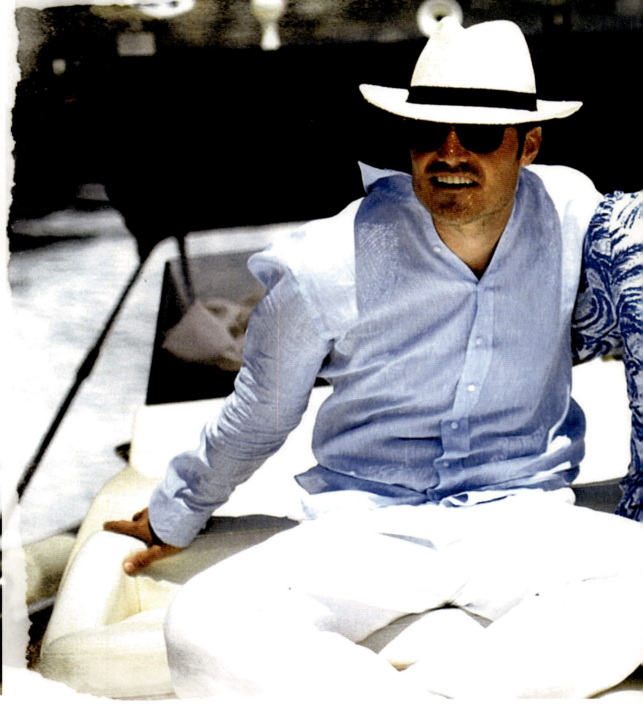
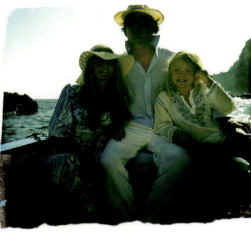
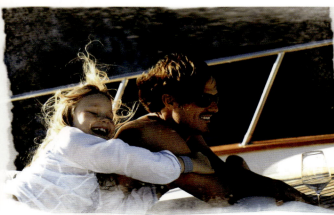
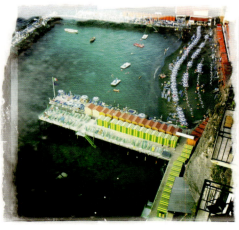
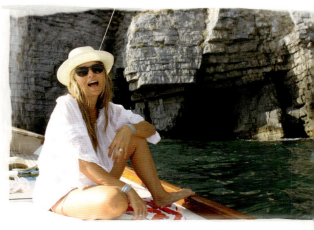

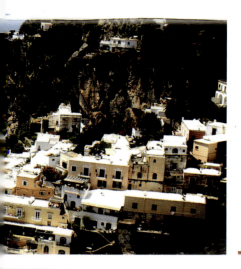
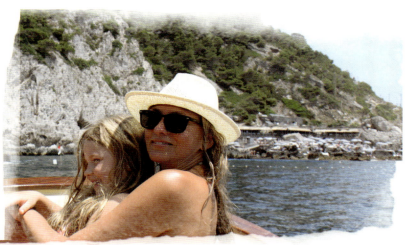
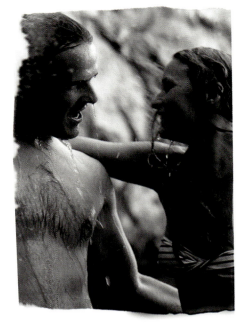
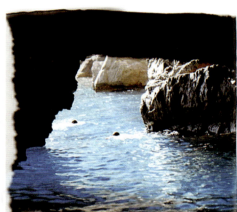
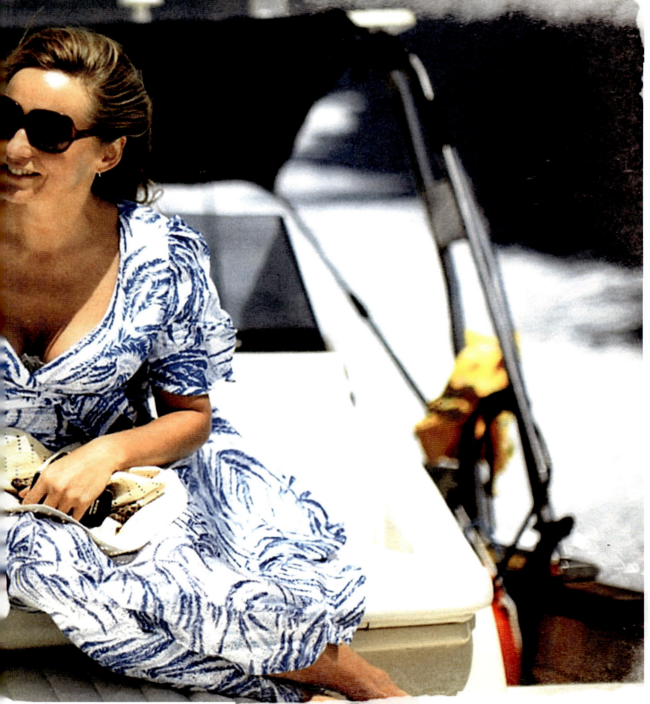
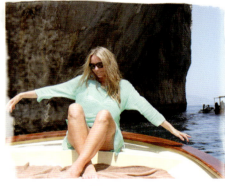
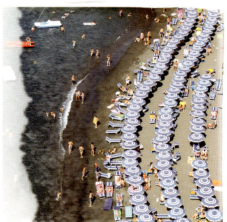
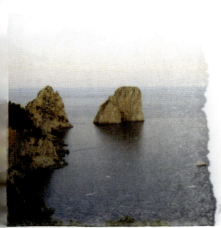
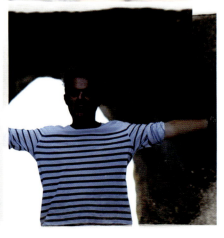
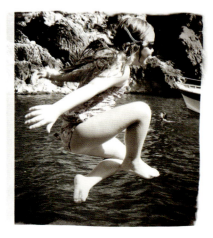
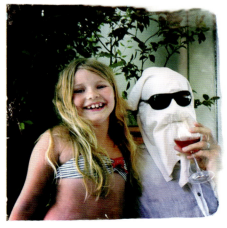

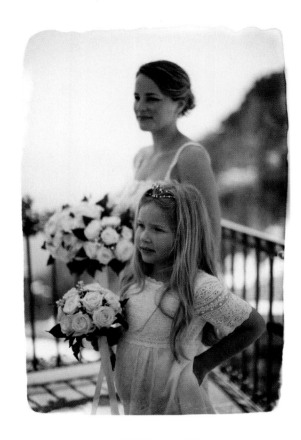

Previous pages: After the ceremony, we hired a boat and cruised around Positano and Capri for the afternoon. It was idyllic – all that I could have hoped for.

Above: The only people at our wedding apart from Estella were David Loftus, who doubled as photographer and best man, and Alice Goozee, a family friend who came along to help with Estella. This is Alice with Estella during the ceremony.

mature, and I am quite mischievous, and young at heart. I love his honesty, his humour, his integrity and his thoughts.

Bradley had always said that he couldn't understand why people got married, and that he wasn't the marrying kind. I was the one with the old-fashioned values – I probably dreamed of getting married, though I thought he wasn't up for it. It didn't really bother me, as I always felt that we would be together. So when he did propose – on New Year's Eve, after a bottle of Dom Pérignon – I knew he was genuine. The next day we woke up and it was still true. It was our secret, because we both really wanted a small wedding, which is hard when you have so many good friends.

Six months later he proposed more formally, on his birthday, on bended knee in front of the fireplace at Milton – it was so romantic, and I was not expecting that at all. He presented me with a ring that he had designed himself. Then we told people we were engaged – they didn't realise that we had already planned our whole wedding and were eloping to Positano two weeks later.

I didn't even have a wedding dress to start with – I was just planning to wear a white linen dress from my diffusion collection, to keep it casual. Anyway, the week before the wedding I was in India working with Chetan, and when I confided in him that I was getting married he said, 'You must have a dress'. So we spent a day looking for laces and trims, draping and designing, creating my dress. We sent the embroidered fabric back to Sydney to be made up secretly in my studio. Bradley brought the dress over to Italy with him (without looking at it!) and I tried it on for the first time two days before our wedding.

We chose Positano because we had been there for the first time together a few years before, and we both loved it. I am so glad that we eloped there, as everything was just so easy and stress-free – the opposite of my work life. Alice Goozee, a family friend, came with us to help with Estella. I ordered simple posies of roses and gardenias from a local florist for Estella, Alice and me. The one thing I did ask for was bougainvillea – and we ended up with an arch covered

Opposite: That's amore.

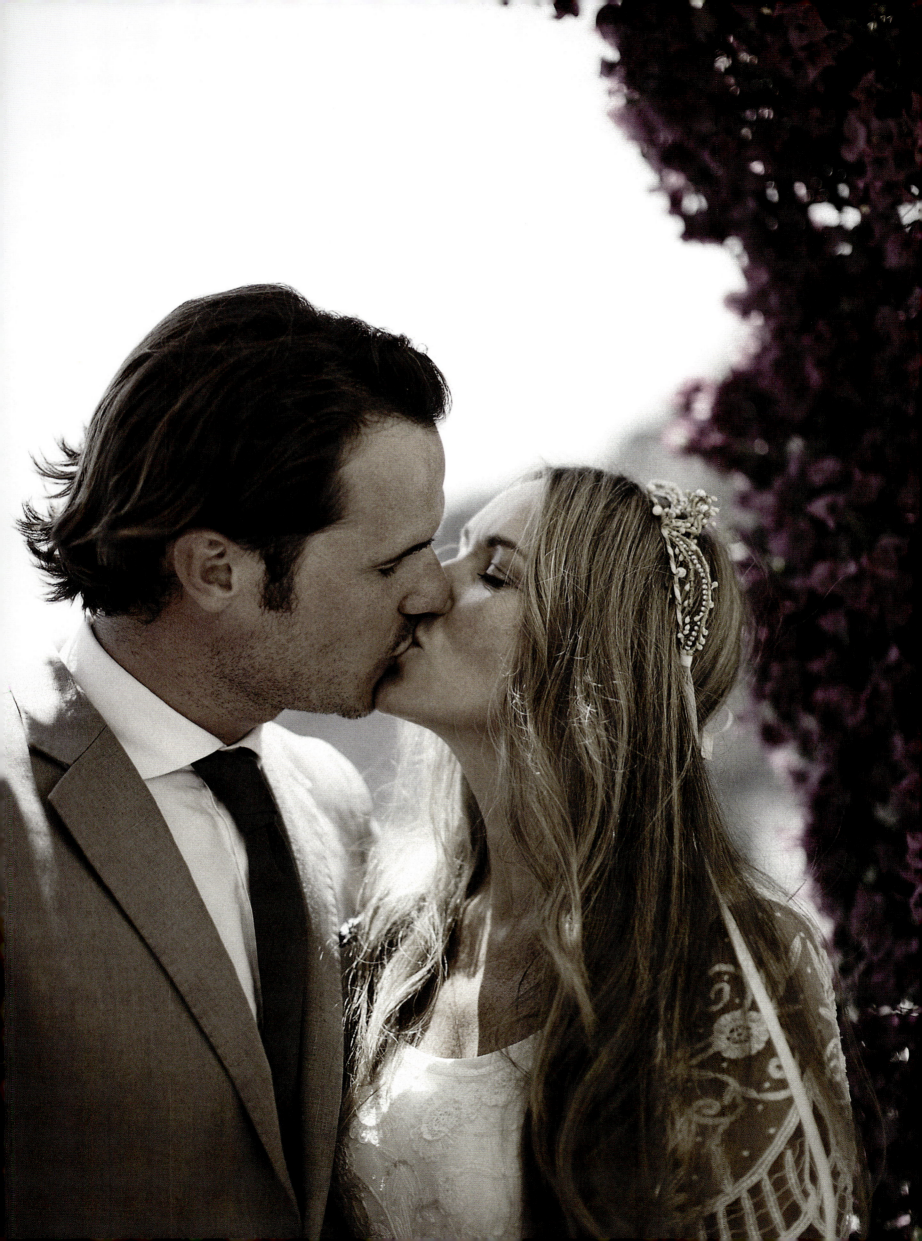

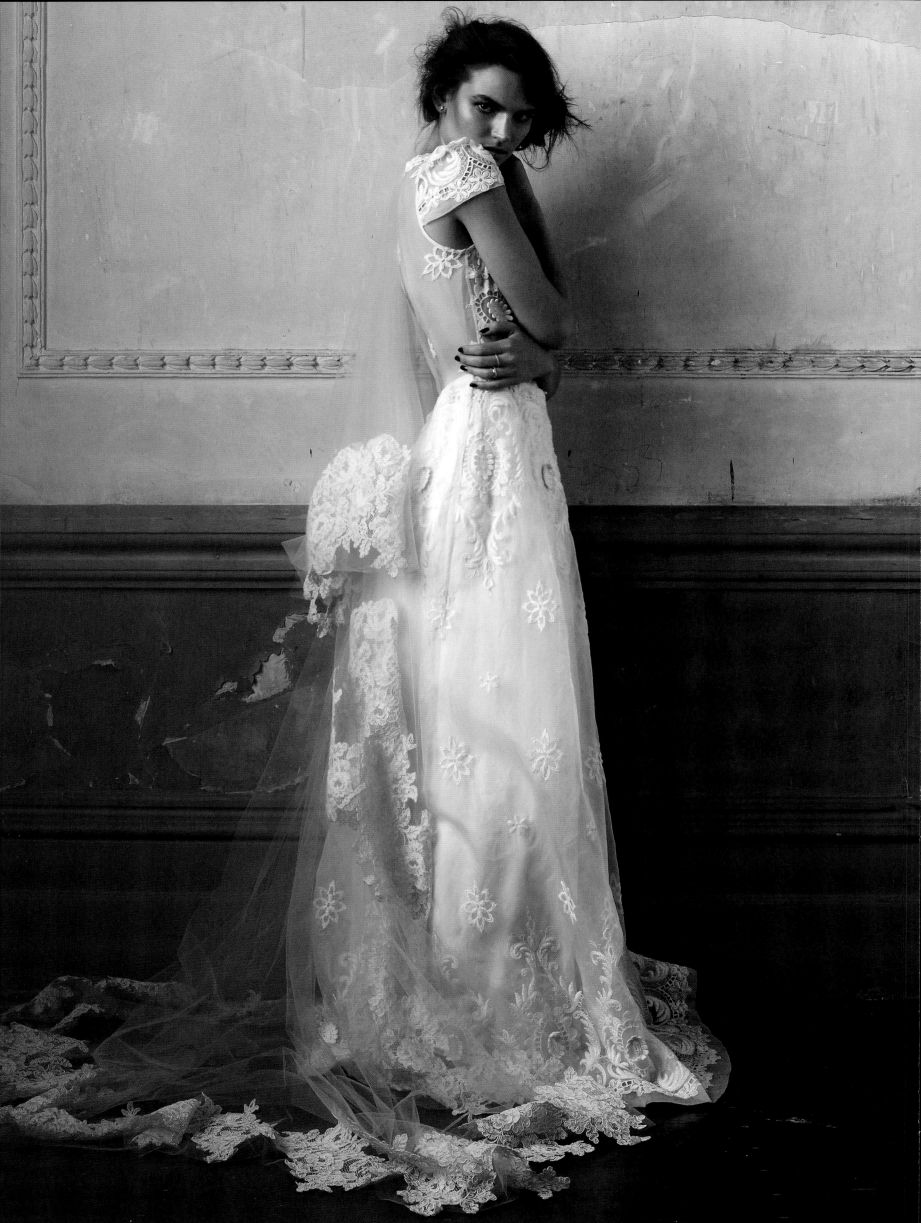

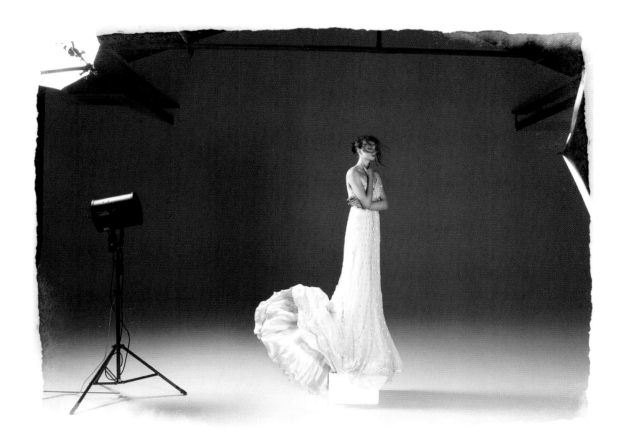

Above: Spotted silk tulle wedding dress, 2007.

in it, which was very typical of Positano. Estella chose the cake – a hazelnut and Nutella creation. I asked David Loftus, who lives in London and had done photographic profiles on me, to take some photos. He ended up as best man as well; Bradley met him half an hour before the ceremony. There were no other attendants (or guests) apart from Alice.

We were married by the mayor at the town hall, which is up on the hill and has a stunning view out over Positano. It was an incredibly hot day, but everything went perfectly. The ceremony was in Italian, which they translated for us. Bradley was very surprised at one part, which said something like '. . . and the husband shall help his wife in the house, with the cleaning, cooking and the raising of the children'. Who knew the Italians were so modern?

Bradley read me a poem by Somerset Maugham, and I read Estella *The Owl and the Pussycat*. It was relaxed and magical, and Estella was adorable – it was as much her dream wedding as it was mine. She wore a dress from my children's range, and we both wore tiaras that I had bought from the Paris flea markets years before.

After the ceremony we changed into swimsuits and casual clothes, then walked down to the water, where we had arranged for a private boat to take us to our favourite restaurant, La Fontelina, on Capri. We collected our wedding cake on the way, and, as a treat, bought Estella some Fanta and lemonade, which she drank on the boat while we shared a bottle of champagne. We had a lovely lunch of spaghetti alle vongole and spent the afternoon cruising around the island, and swimming. It was all just so carefree – everything you could possibly want. When we returned to our apartment we sat there and watched the sunset, then emailed some photos to friends, telling them we were married. I think people were quite shocked.

The idea of doing a bridal collection evolved over the years, as people started asking if we could make up particular evening dresses in ivory so they could wear them as wedding gowns. That kept happening, and eventually I realised that I needed to do a bridal collection, that we

Opposite: One of my favourite bridal gowns,
the rococo dress, 2011.

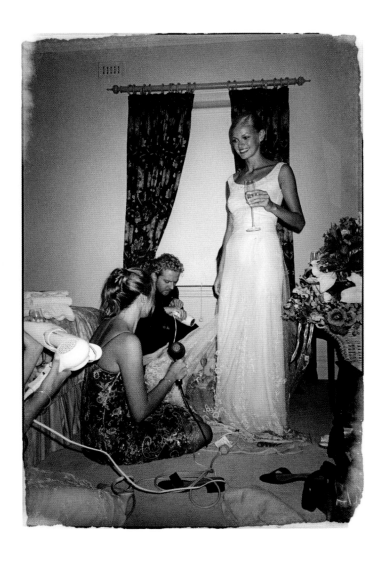

*Above: It was pouring with rain at Sarah O'Hare's wedding to
Lachlan Murdoch in 1999. Here Shane Paish and I are drying Sarah's dress
and train between the ceremony and the reception. Sarah was totally unfazed.*

could show and sell in the stores as a separate range. Collette Dinnigan Bridal was officially launched in 2007.

When I started I did two collections a year, one summer and one winter, but now I only do one, which is basically summer, because there isn't a market for winter wedding dresses. I have really enjoyed the creative freedom of designing dresses especially for brides, rather than converting dresses worn on the Paris catwalk into wedding dresses. My wedding dresses are quite ornate. While many of them are dreamy and traditional, with a vintage feel, I also do modern dresses; as well as the long, romantic dresses, I have designed Jackie O-inspired, tailored, knee-length dresses. Some have a trousseau-like feel to them, while others are more casual.

Every wedding has its own dramas, and I will never forget Sarah O'Hare's wedding to Lachlan Murdoch. They had built a special chapel on the Murdoch country estate, and on the day it was pouring with rain. Everyone was walking about with umbrellas, and after the ceremony, as Sarah was making her way to the marquee, her dress and train got soaked. We had to whisk her away to wash it out, and I remember a group of us surrounding her, with hairdryers, drying the back of her dress, as she was laughing and drinking a glass of champagne. She was such a relaxed and happy bride – some brides would have been hysterical, but she just thought it was funny. Nothing was going to spoil her day.

*Opposite: Sarah and Lachlan. I introduced them – Sarah
and I were doing a shoot on an old boat on Sydney Harbour
for* Condé Nast Traveller *(see cover shot of Sarah on page 106),
and I decided to keep it for the evening and invite some friends,
including Lachlan, to join us on board for drinks. That was it.*

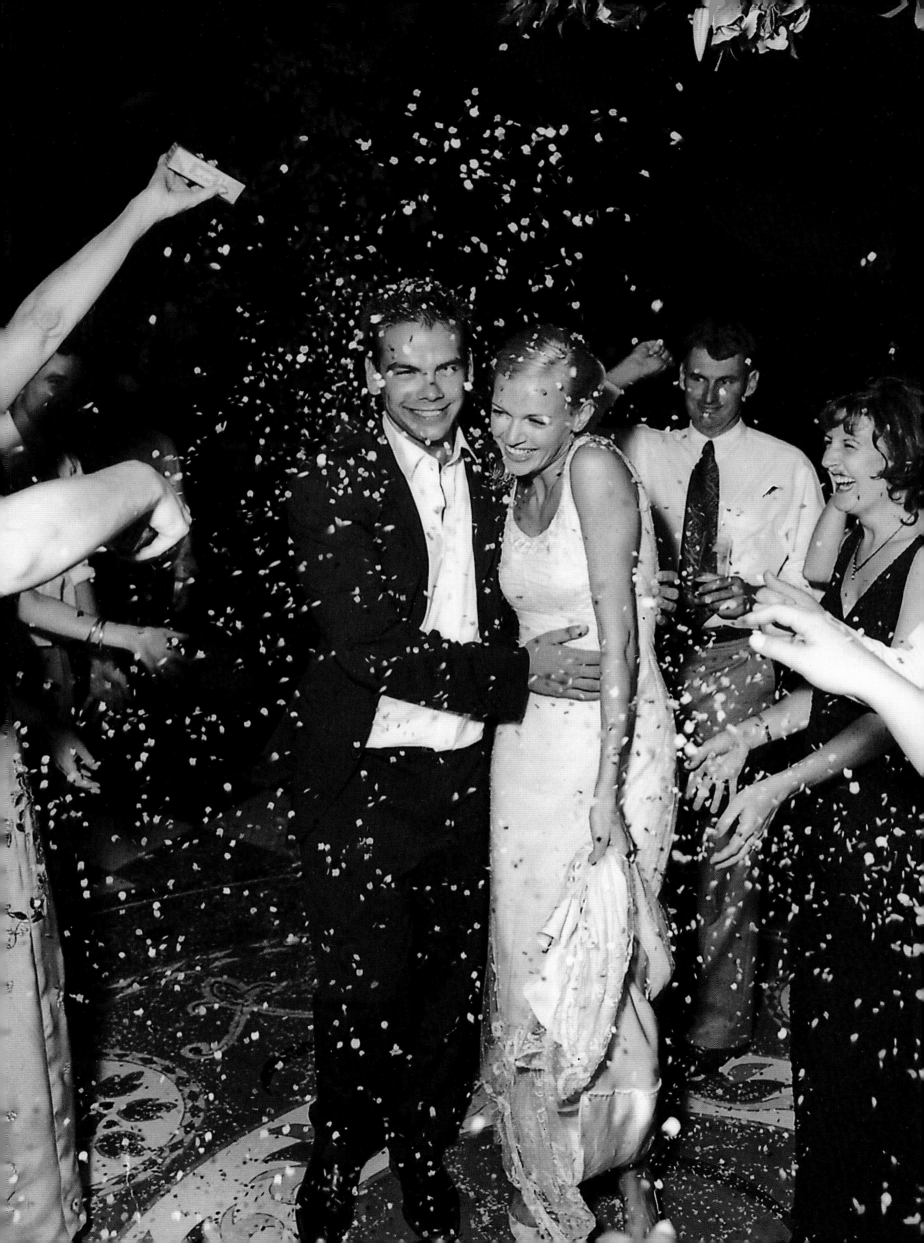

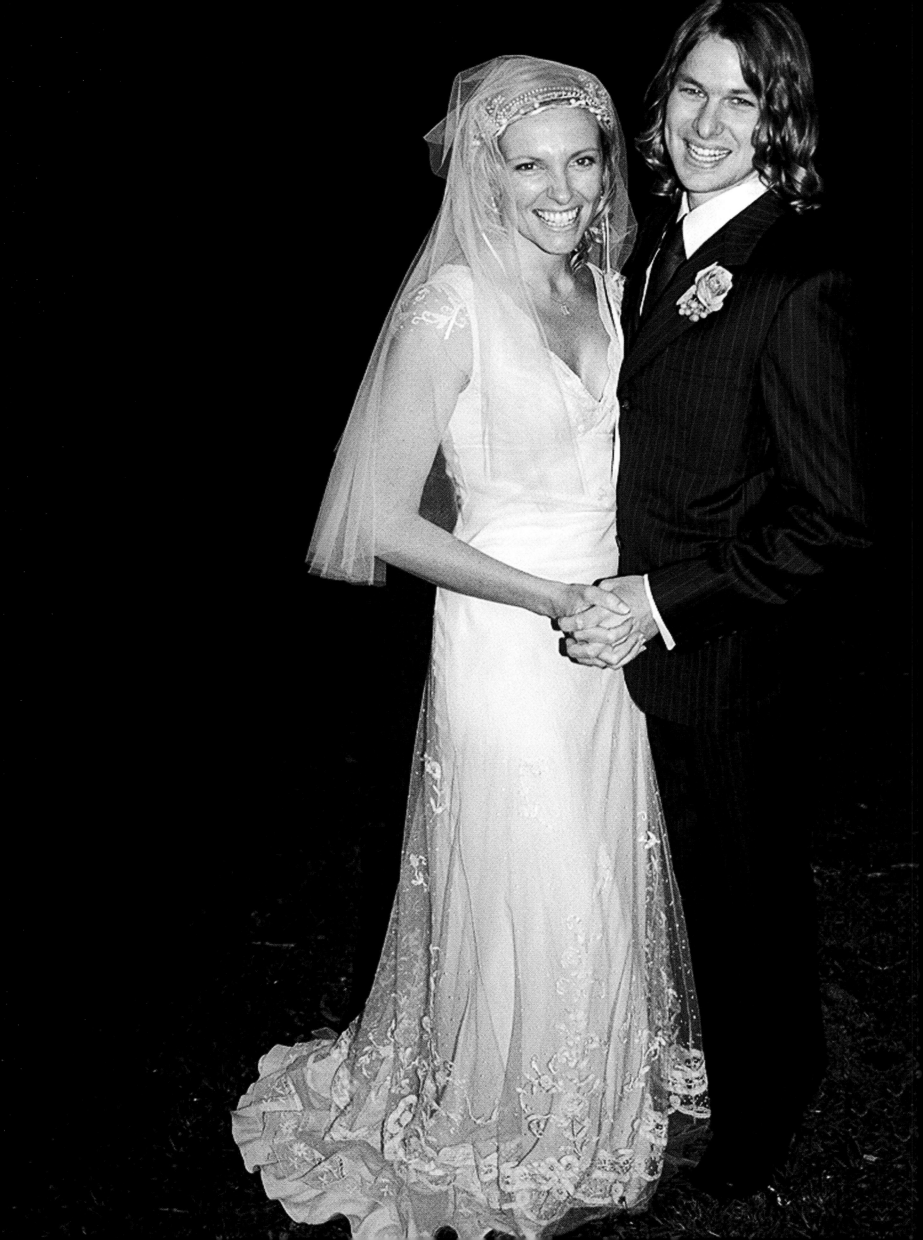

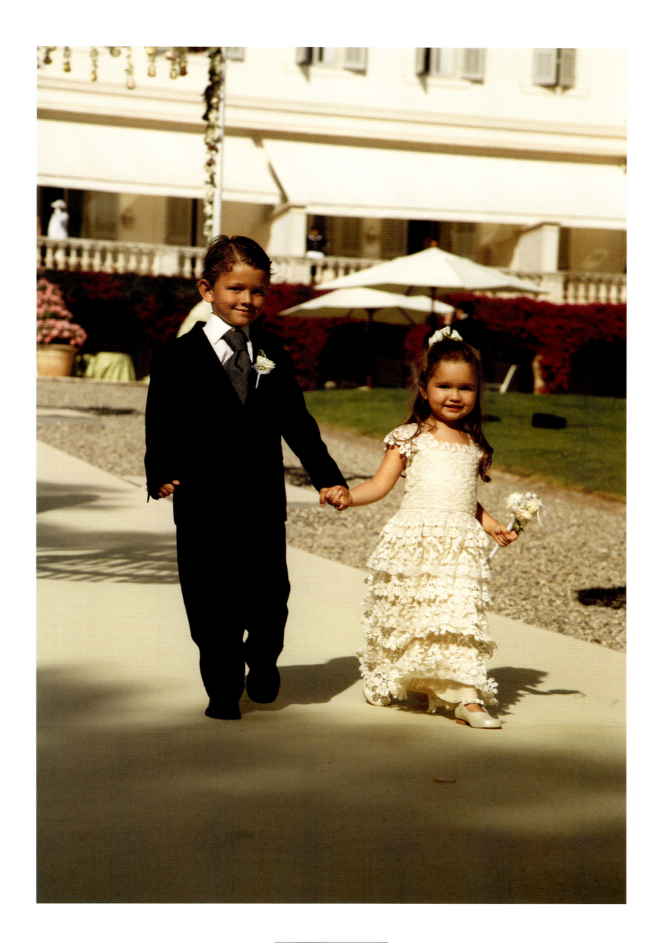

Opposite: Toni Collette weds musician Dave Galafassi
in 2003 in a dress I designed for her.

Above: Pageboy and flower girl at James Packer's wedding to Erica Baxter
in Antibes in 2007. I dressed the bridesmaids and the flower girls.

THAT'S AMORE

199

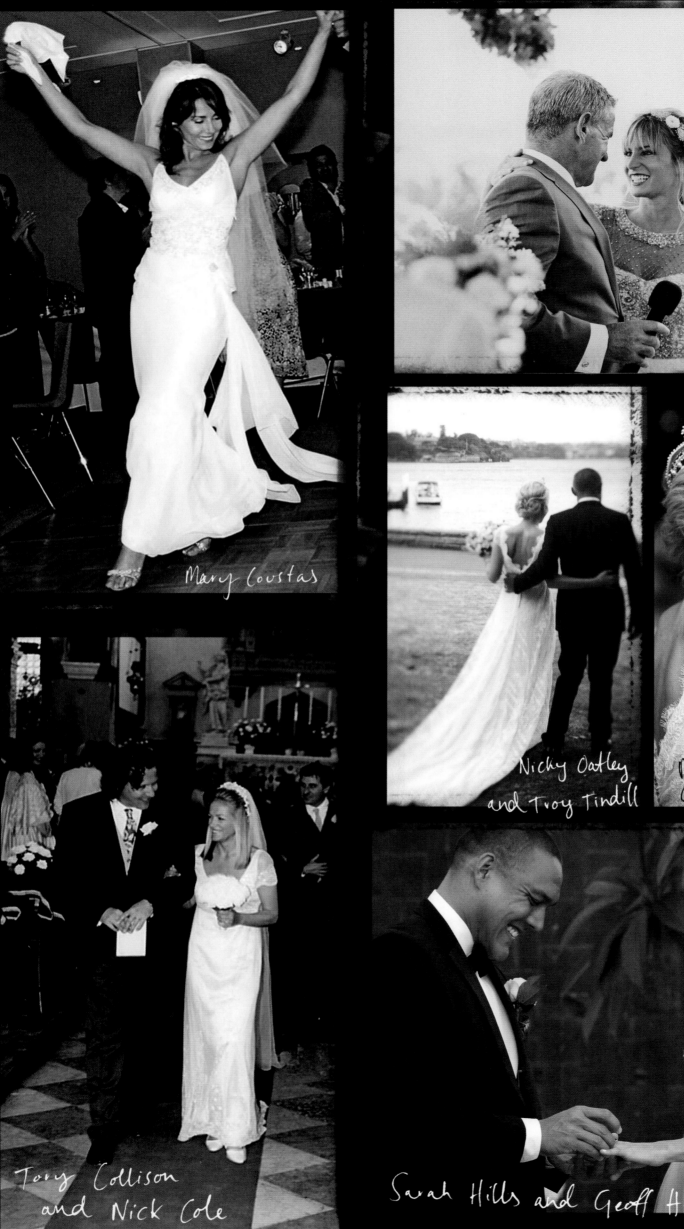

Mary Coustas

Tony Collison
and Nick Cole

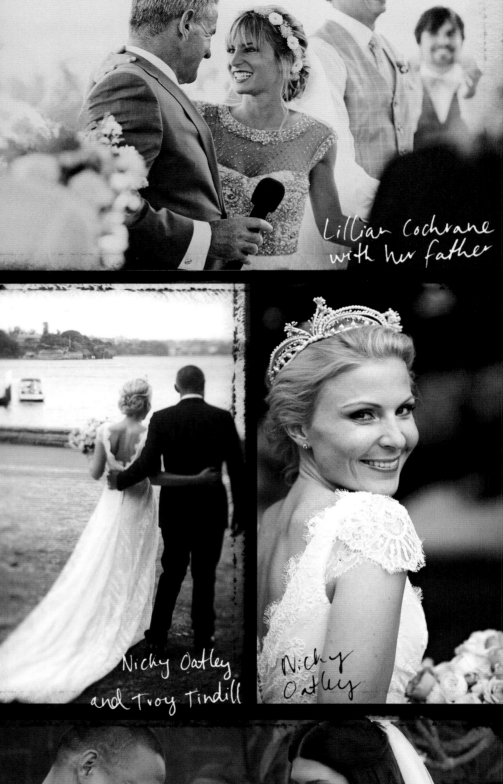

Lillian Cochrane
with her father

Nicky Oatley
and Troy Tindill

Nicky
Oatley

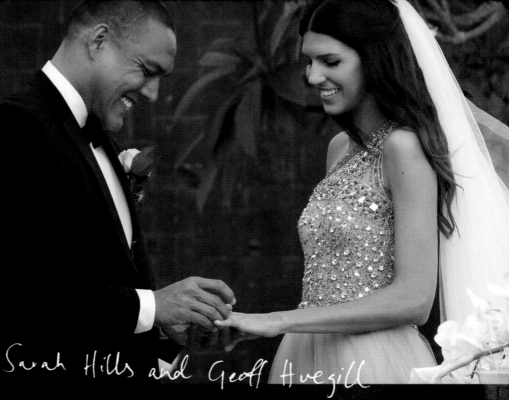

Sarah Hills and Geoff Huegill

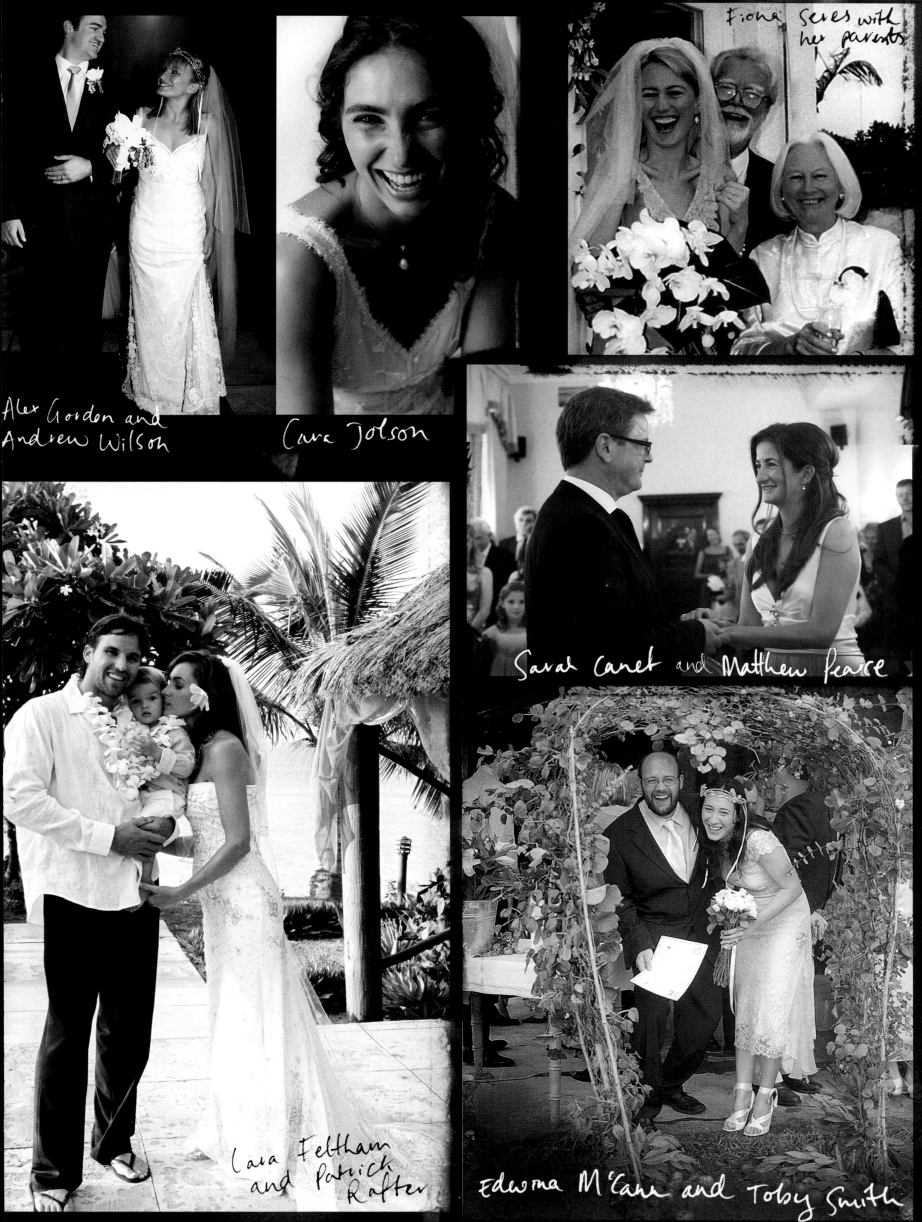

Fiona seves with her parents

Alex Gordon and Andrew Wilson

Cara Jolson

Sarah Canet and Matthew Pearse

Cara Feltham and Patrick Rafter

Edwina M'Cann and Toby Smith

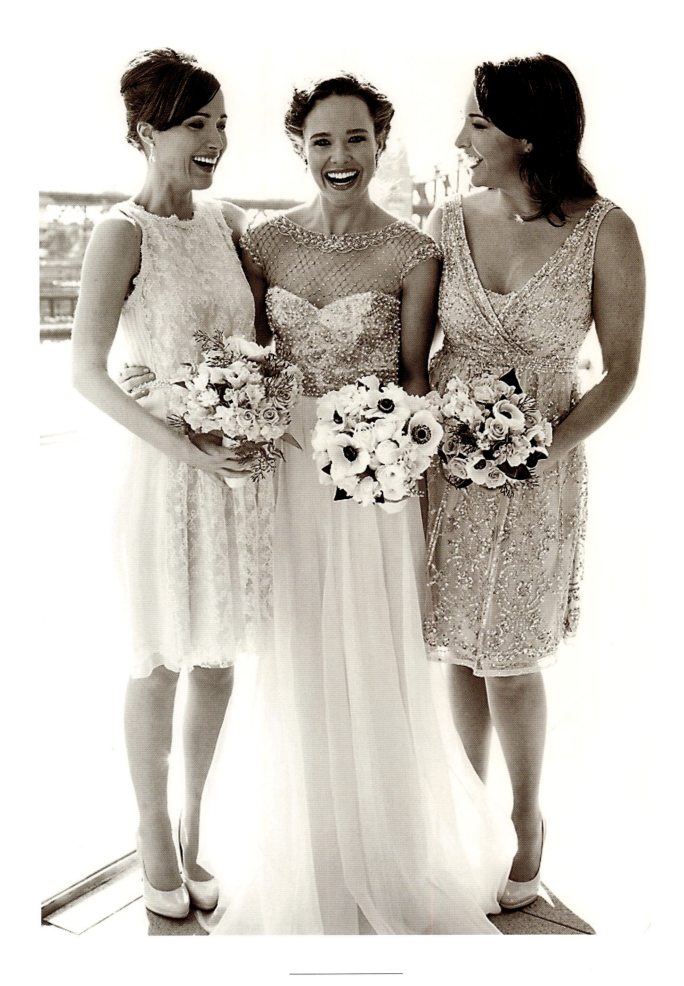

*Above: Krew Boylan at her wedding to Andrew Baud in 2012,
with bridesmaids Rose Byrne and Krew's sister Jodi.
I designed all of their dresses.*

Opposite: Jessica Rowe sparkles at her wedding to Peter Overton in 2004.

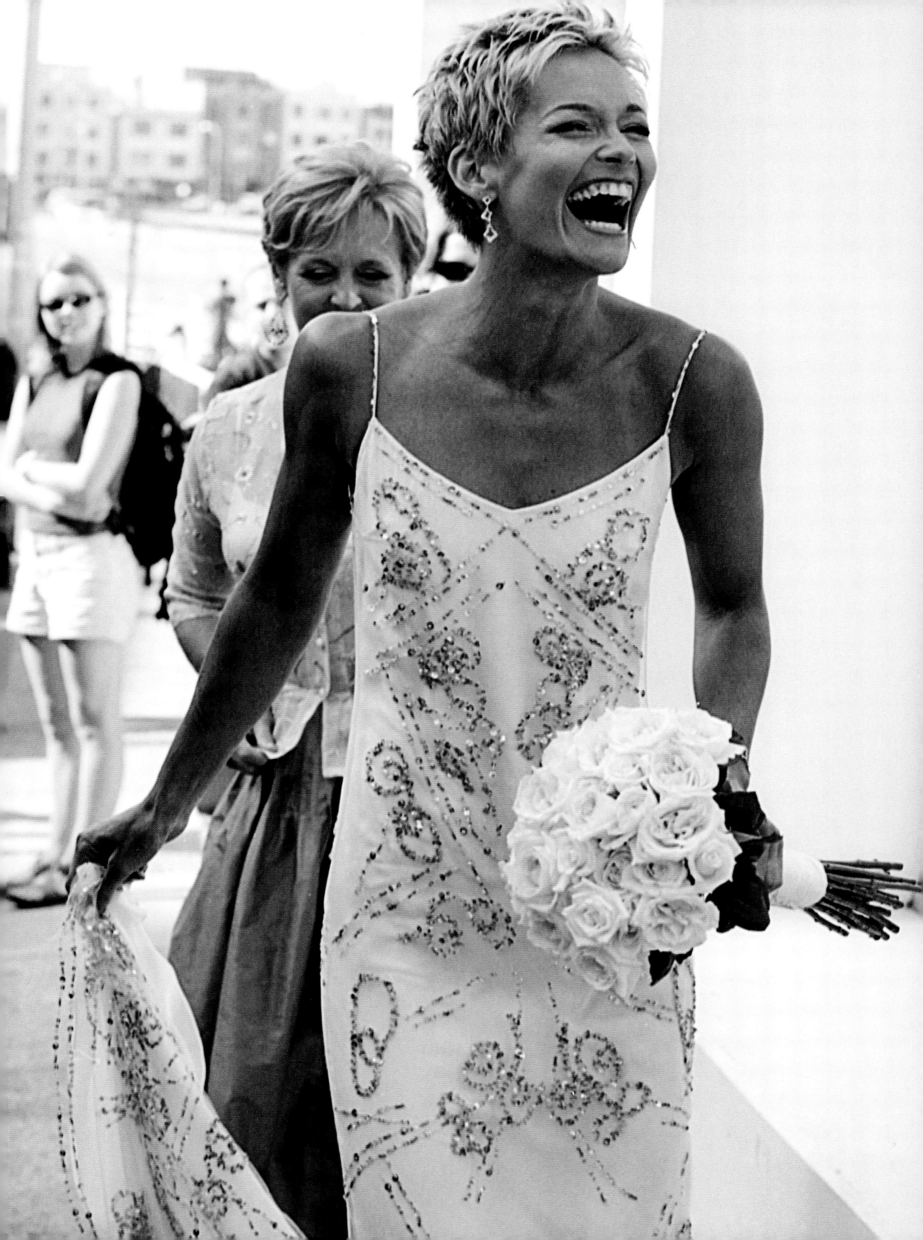

front row

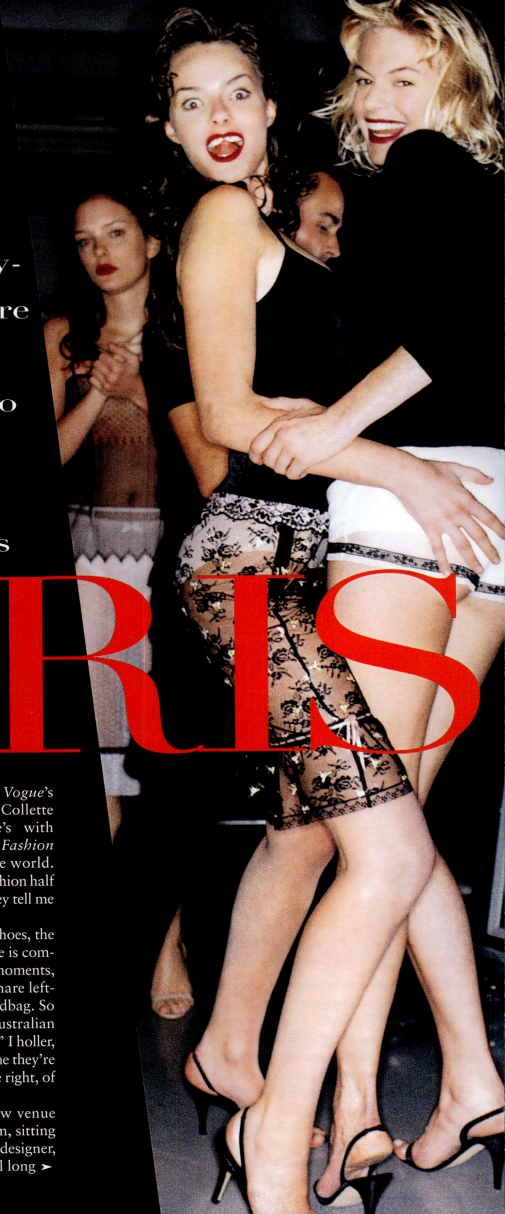

Onwards to the ready-to-wear in Paris, where Collette Dinnigan dazzles, John Galliano transports us to wonderland, and Rei Kawakubo confounds

PARIS

At **1.25pm** I spot American *Vogue*'s Kate Betts *walking away* from Collette Dinnigan's venue. Panic. She's with Jeanne Beker, host of Canada's *Fashion TV*, which is beamed all over the world. Double panic. Australia's finest fashion half hour is about to take place and they tell me they are off to get lunch.

While the fashion pack spend Milan shopping for shoes, the number-one priority in Paris is where the next baguette is coming from. There is never enough time to eat. In bleak moments, fashion doyenne, Suzy Menkes, has been known to share left-over breakfast toast fished from the depths of her handbag. So two of the women who can help make or break an Australian designer's career are heading off to chow down. "Wait!" I holler, as I charge along the pavement behind them. They tell me they're starving and that the show won't start for ages (they are right, of course), and with a click of high heels they're away.

I'm stressed, despite the fact that inside the show venue Paula Yates and Michael Hutchence appear quite calm, sitting as they are in a rosy bower created by the Sydney set designer, Jamie Gordon. Of course, the show doesn't start until long ➤

HOW TO STAGE A SHOW (OR 33) IN PARIS

Angelina Tearoom;
Chambre Syndicale;
backstage; the parties.

A

CHAPTER 12

I WILL NEVER FORGET MY
FIRST SHOW IN PARIS.
It was in 1995 and came about at
the suggestion of Mary Gallagher, from
Harvey Nichols in London, who had been
selling my clothes for a few years.
IN THOSE EARLY DAYS
I USED TO GO TRAIPSING
AROUND THE WORLD
with a suitcase of samples to show buyers
IN LOS ANGELES, NEW YORK,
HONG KONG AND LONDON.
One day Mary said to me
'WHY ARE YOU DOING
ALL THAT TRAVELLING?
WHY DON'T YOU JUST
GO TO PARIS
AND DO A SHOW?
People don't really understand how
to wear your clothes, with all the different layers,
SO YOU NEED TO SHOW THEM.'

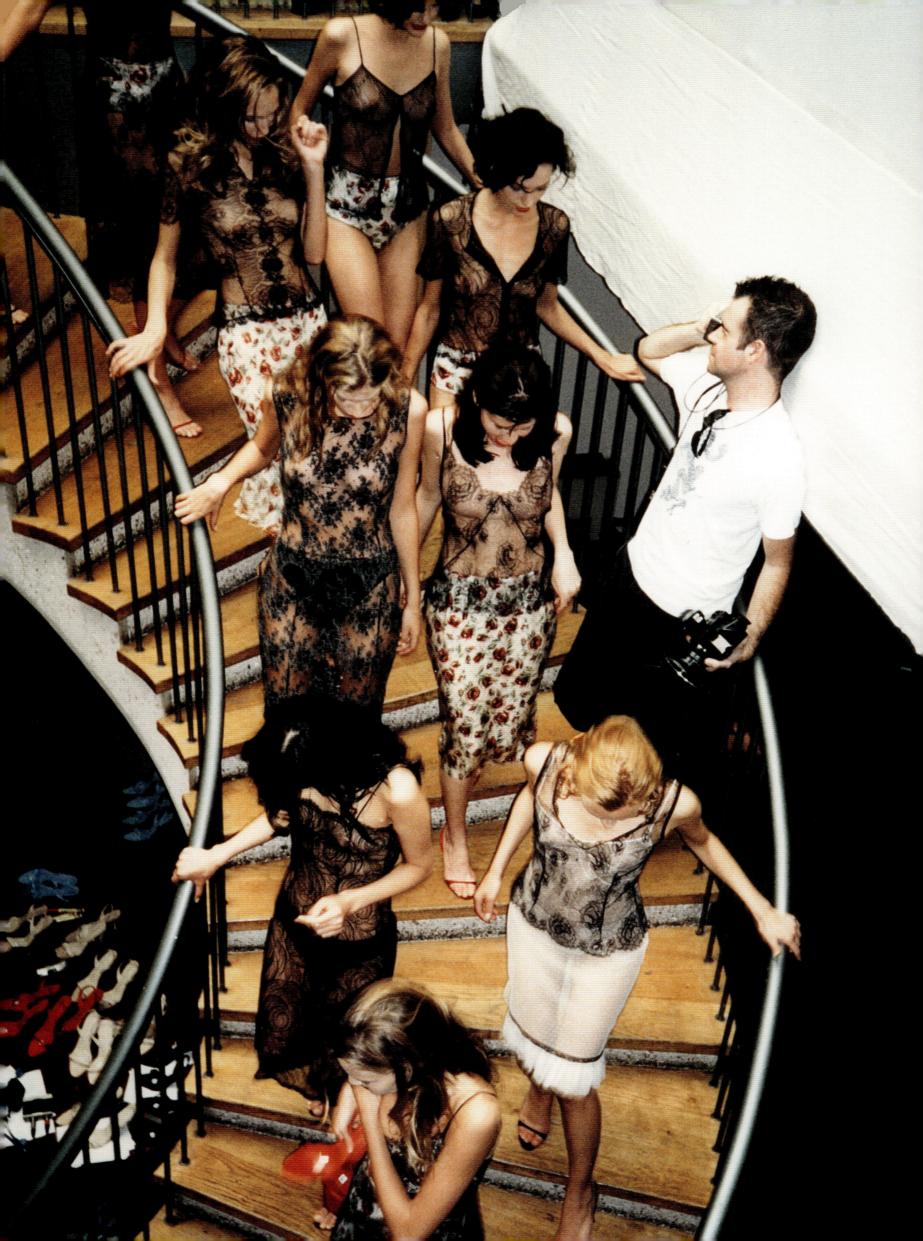

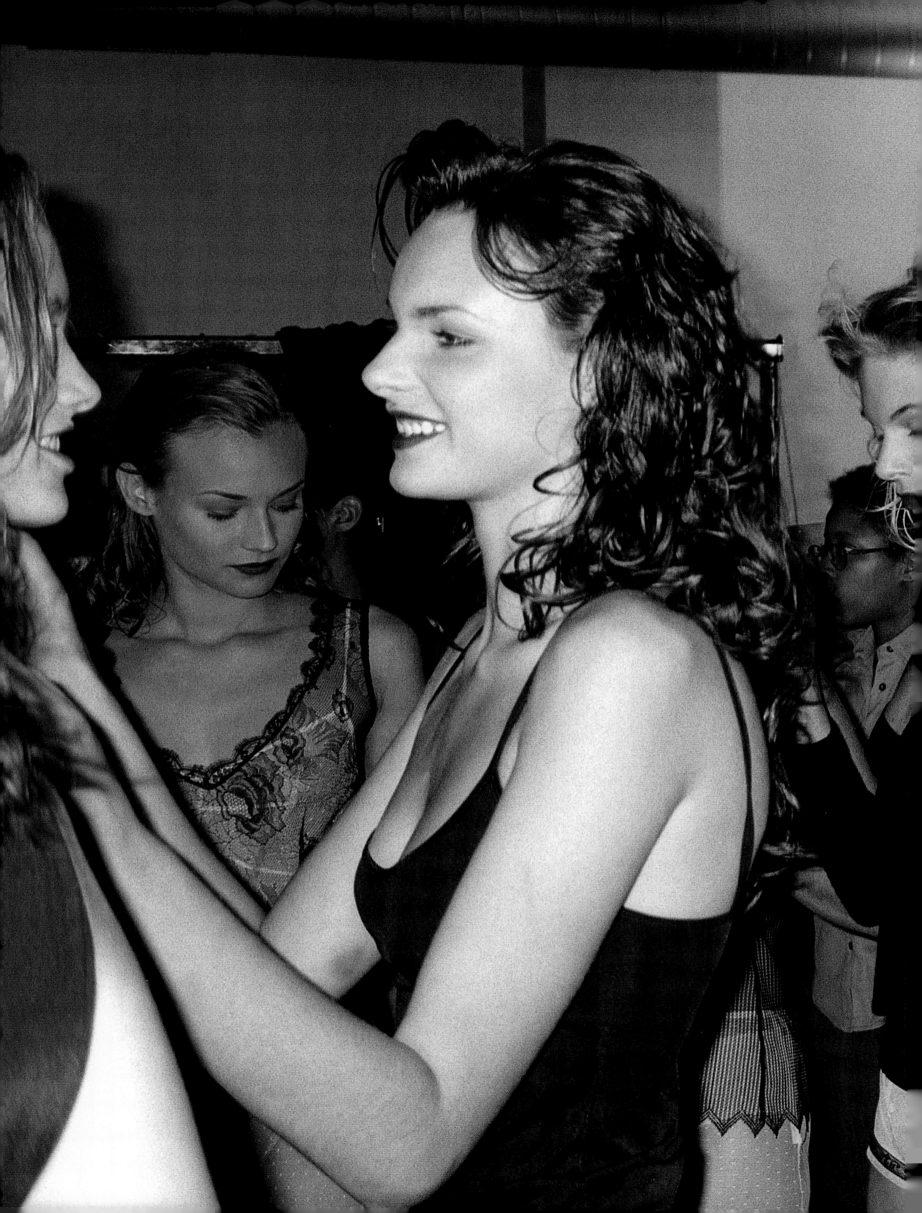

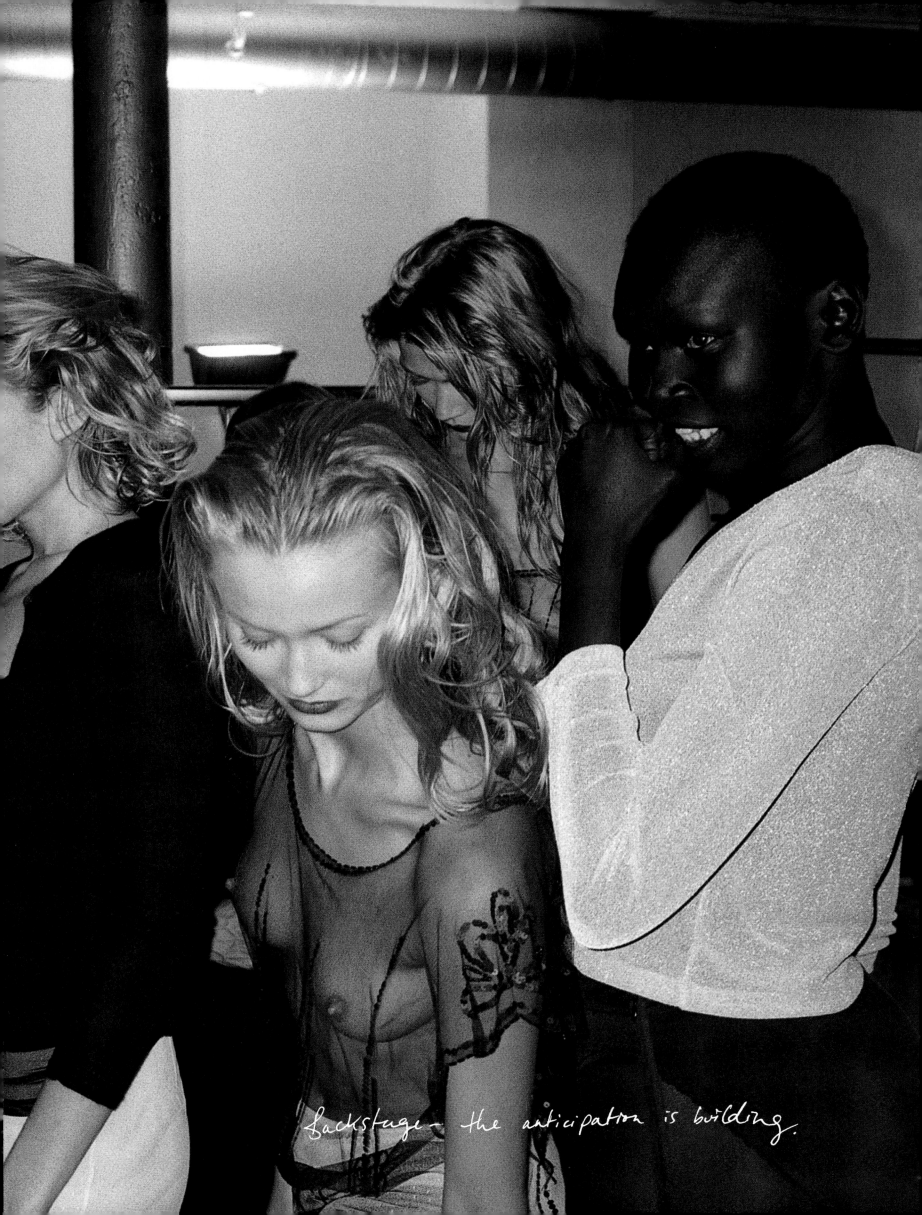

backstage - the anticipation is building.

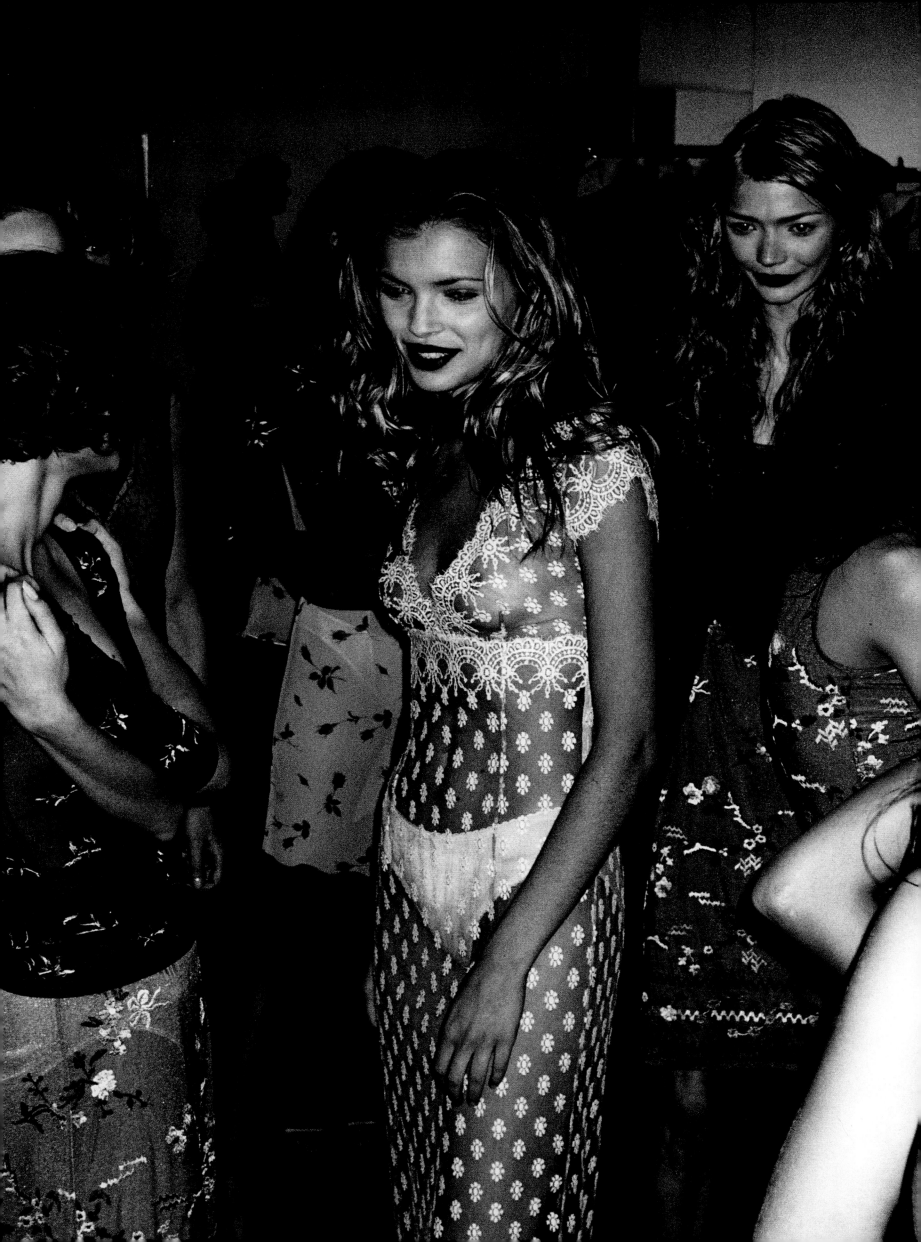

These days, people take photos with their iPhones and tweet them and put them up on their blogs almost immediately, so many fashion editors don't come to the shows anymore. This has taken away some of the magic and the anticipation, I think, which is a shame. Nothing compares to actually being at a show.

A

The only contact I had in Paris was Stephen Todd, a friend of Seamus's who wrote for *The Australian* newspaper, and he offered to help. He suggested I do the show at the Angelina Tearoom on the Rue de Rivoli, next to Le Meurice, and together we put together the show. I still don't know how we did it – I was just running on adrenaline. Stephen was an amazing support. My show was 'off schedule' as I hadn't been accredited by the Chambre Syndicale (the French body that runs the show schedule). I decided to show against Comme des Garçons, because Rei Kawakubo has a very different sensibility from mine, and I didn't think we would compete as much for press. I sent out invitations to the press and buyers, and a friend of Stephen's lent us her wardrobe of shoes, and off we went.

I showed a collection of my corsets, layered skirts and lace overdresses, and we got some really good press. People knew that we were already selling to Barneys and Harvey Nicholls and I think they were quite intrigued – they are always looking to discover someone new. I did another show later that year, and again had a good response from the press, and other designers on the official list started to complain that I was taking key press away from their shows.

After a year or so the Chambre Syndicale approached me about giving me an official timeslot. I was thrilled – only a small number of designers show on the calendar, and I was the first Australian designer to be asked. For the first five years they gave me the timeslot just before Christian Dior, which was great in terms of attracting press,

but a nightmare for casting models. In 2007 the Chambre Syndicale asked me to join their committee, which was a great honour, although, sadly, I can't make the meetings, which are held in Paris.

Much as I love doing them, organising two Paris shows a year from Sydney is a real challenge; it's not like you have your office just down the road. Back in the day I used to take a big team of ten or fifteen people with me, including public relations people, seamstresses and models. Now I take a much smaller team, and hire people over there, as it is simpler, logistically. I have the invitations made in Sydney, but post them from Paris. We aim to do thirty-six looks in a show, so we'll take about one hundred and fifty pieces and edit it down; we never show the whole collection to the press.

Ideally, I would like to arrive in Paris a week before the show, but these days I usually only make it there two or three

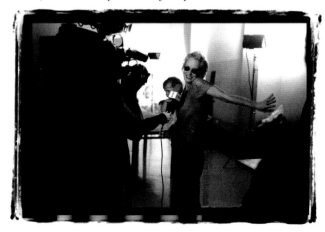

Page 207: Seamus snapped this shot of models passing Gavin Bond on the stairs. This was my Spring/Summer 1999 collection.

Opposite: Spanish model Esther Cañadas, backstage at my Spring/Summer 1998 show.

Above: Paula Yates, backstage with her daughter Tiger Lily, 1998. Photograph by Philip Castle.

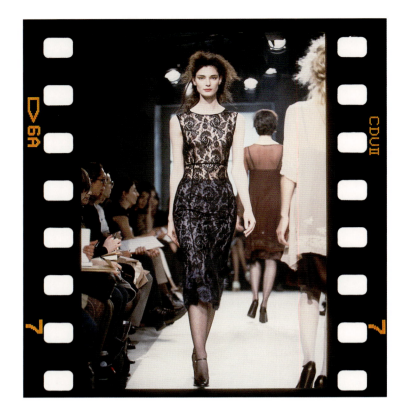

Above: Australia's Anneliese Seubert.

days before. After a production meeting, we start with styling and casting, which I do with the assistance of a casting director. We see about one hundred or more models, and choose twenty or so. They come from all over the world, many these days from Poland, Russia and the Ukraine, and they are all incredibly beautiful. Often they speak little English, but they know enough to be able to try on clothes and do the walk, and they are all very professional. Once we have chosen the models, there are rounds of fittings and rehearsals, and then I work with a stylist. I don't get involved in the production details of the show, but I am very hands-on in terms of anything creative.

On the day of the show, it is organised chaos backstage. The lighting and production crews get there about twenty-four hours in advance to do the installation, which I will have signed off on in Sydney. Three to four hours before the show the hair and makeup teams arrive, each with up to ten people, and then there are the stylists, the assistants, the dressers – there can be up to one hundred people backstage.

Shows run from nine thirty in the morning until nine thirty at night, for seven days, so it is a gruelling schedule. Each show takes about twelve minutes. The buyers and the press are very choosy about which shows they attend these days, and in fact many buyers don't come to the shows at all now. They just come to the appointments, which run from eight in the morning, twelve hours a day. It's a shame, because I don't think you get the real feel of a collection unless you are actually there at the show.

In the early days I had more freedom with my choice of venues – I chose romantic places that were a bit edgy: small art galleries, beautiful old buildings filled with character, and places in the red light district or Montmartre. There was an intrigue to taking people out of their comfort zones; it was exciting and a real experience. These days the venues are more conservative – it's important to be central, in the First Arrondissement, and you must have internet coverage. I have done several shows at The Louvre, in the rooms underneath, where all the main designers, such as Dior and Valentino, show. Obviously that is a wonderful venue, but I do feel it lacks the soul of some of my early off-site venues. More recently, my shows have been at Le Meurice, where I stay and have my showroom.

I have been lucky to have had some of the world's top models walk in my shows. It's hard to single anyone out,

Opposite: Audrey Marnay at
Espace Carole de Bona, 1997.

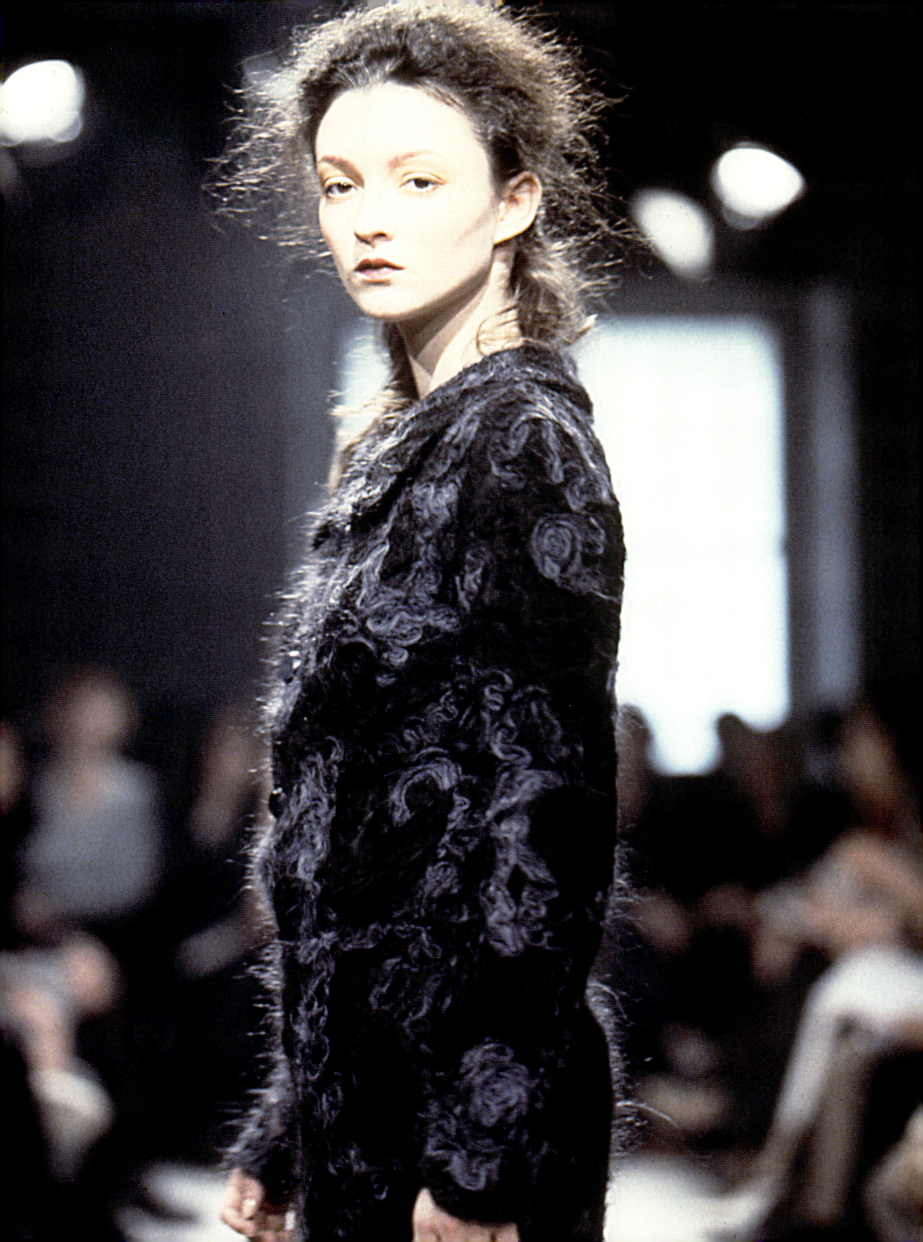

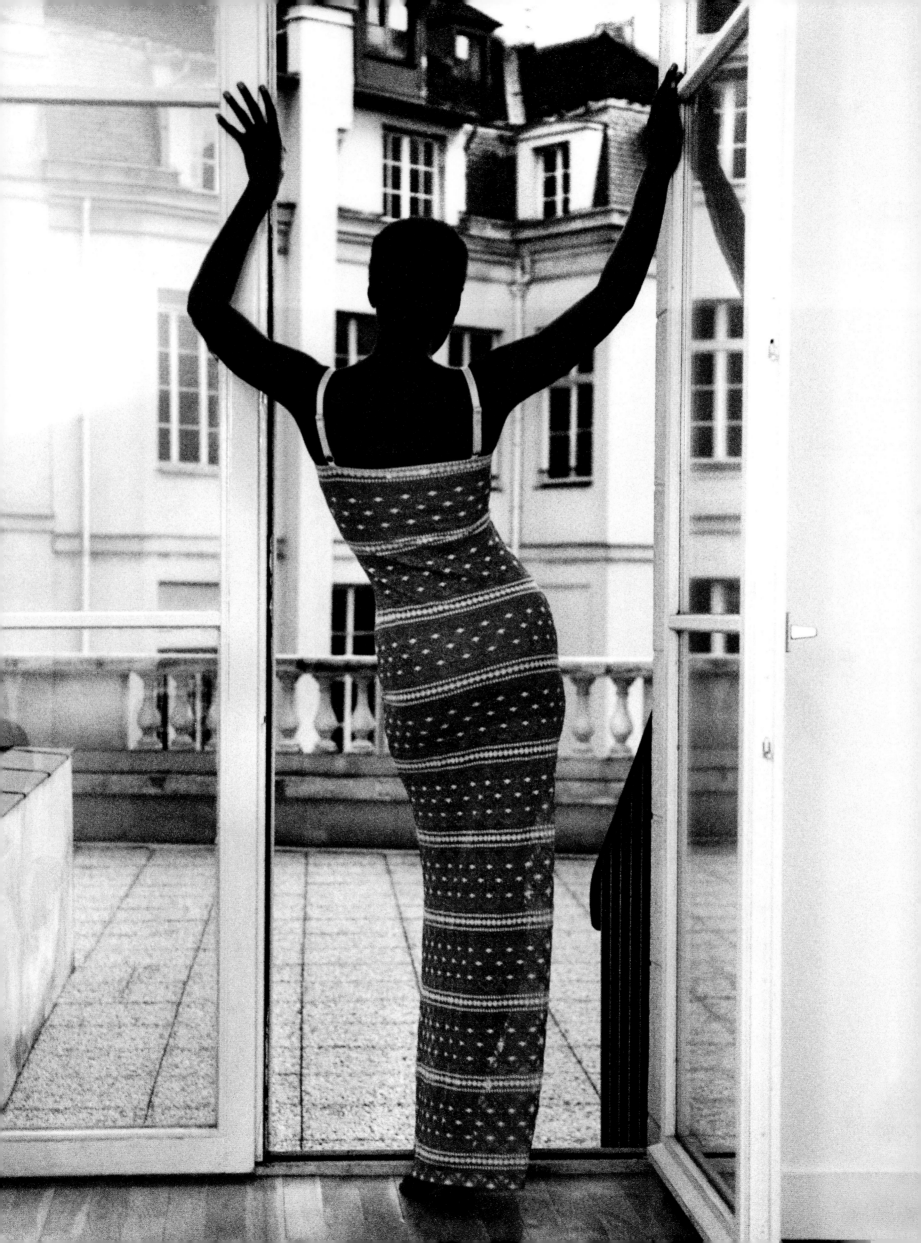

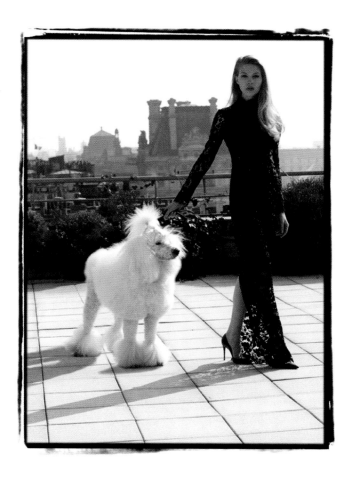

*Above: Model on the roof of Le Meurice
before my Autumn/Winter 2013 show.*

but Helena Christensen, who did three or four of my shows, does stand out. She was one of the true supermodels of the nineties – unbelievably professional, beautiful and alluring. Some of the other names who spring to mind are Esther Cañadas, Audrey Marnay, Alek Wek, Laetitia Casta, Jasmine Guinness, Honor Fraser and Rosie Huntington-Whiteley. Many of them have gone on to become big names.

Probably my favourite Paris show was the Autumn/ Winter 2004 show I did at The Louvre. It was dark, with a rock and roll edge to it, and the models had wild hair and dark eyes. There was a sense of cheekiness in that collection that I liked – it made you think of the rock-and-roll era back in the sixties and seventies. My winter collections are always a bit edgier than my summer collections; there is more tailoring, and construction; they are darker and more urban. My summer collections have a nonchalance to them – I think there is much more of an Australian influence, the light and colour, especially.

Every show has a story – we work so hard to make the whole production look seamless, but there are sometimes dramas behind the scenes. One show I will never forget. I was working with Tory Collison from *Vogue Australia*, who was styling the show, and at the last minute we realised we didn't have enough shoes – the ones we'd ordered hadn't all arrived. We ended up madly swapping shoes between models as they were going out for their walks, and one poor girl was sent out wearing two left shoes. The tyranny of distance – had we been based in Paris, we would have received the shoes weeks in advance, and could have sorted it out, but to get anything from Sydney to Paris via a human courier takes a minimum of forty-eight hours because of the time difference.

Paris has been an important part of my life in my thirties and forties. It is like a wonderful playground where I meet such interesting people; it is constantly entertaining, and so visually stimulating. I feel totally at home as

*Opposite: Alek Wek at a fittings and castings
session. Photograph by Philip Castle, 1997.*

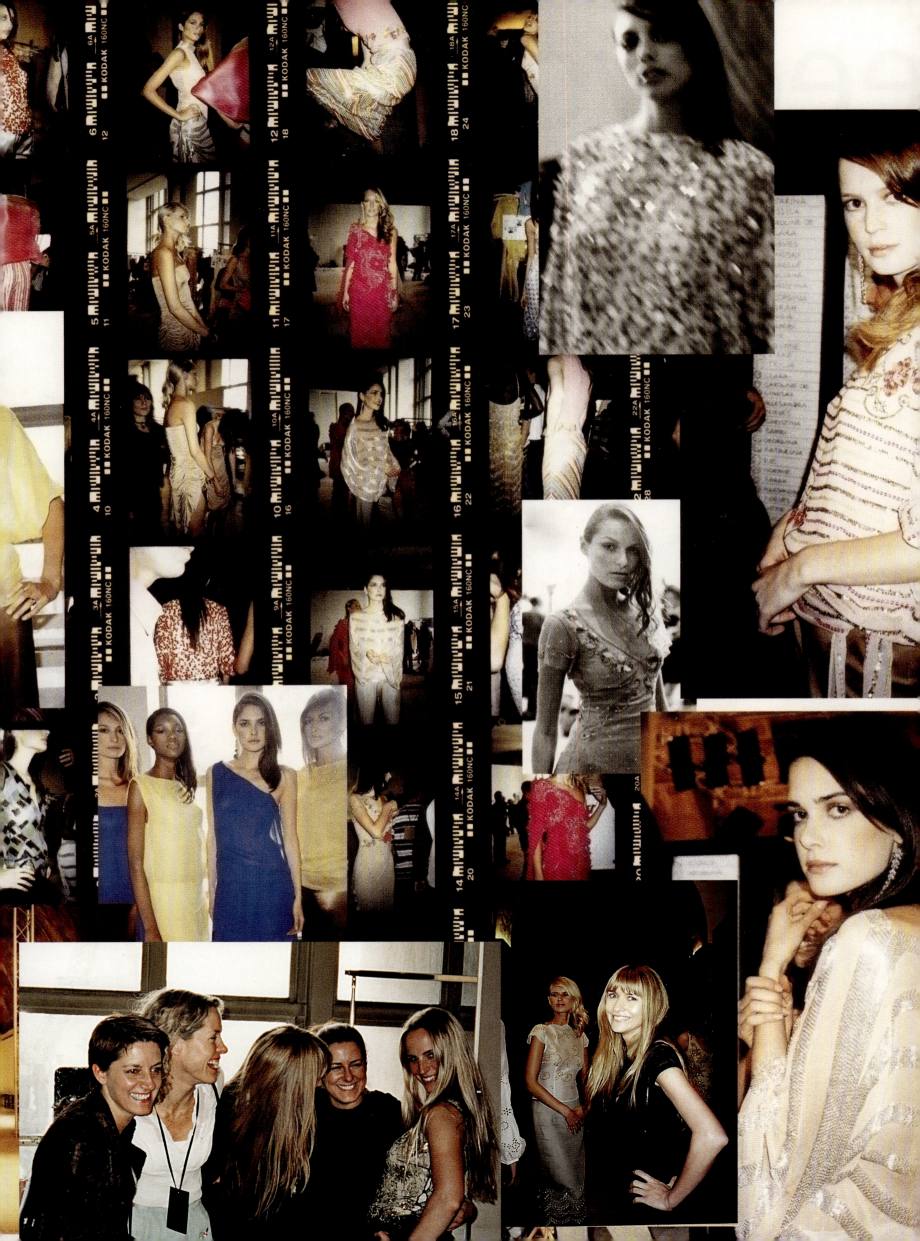

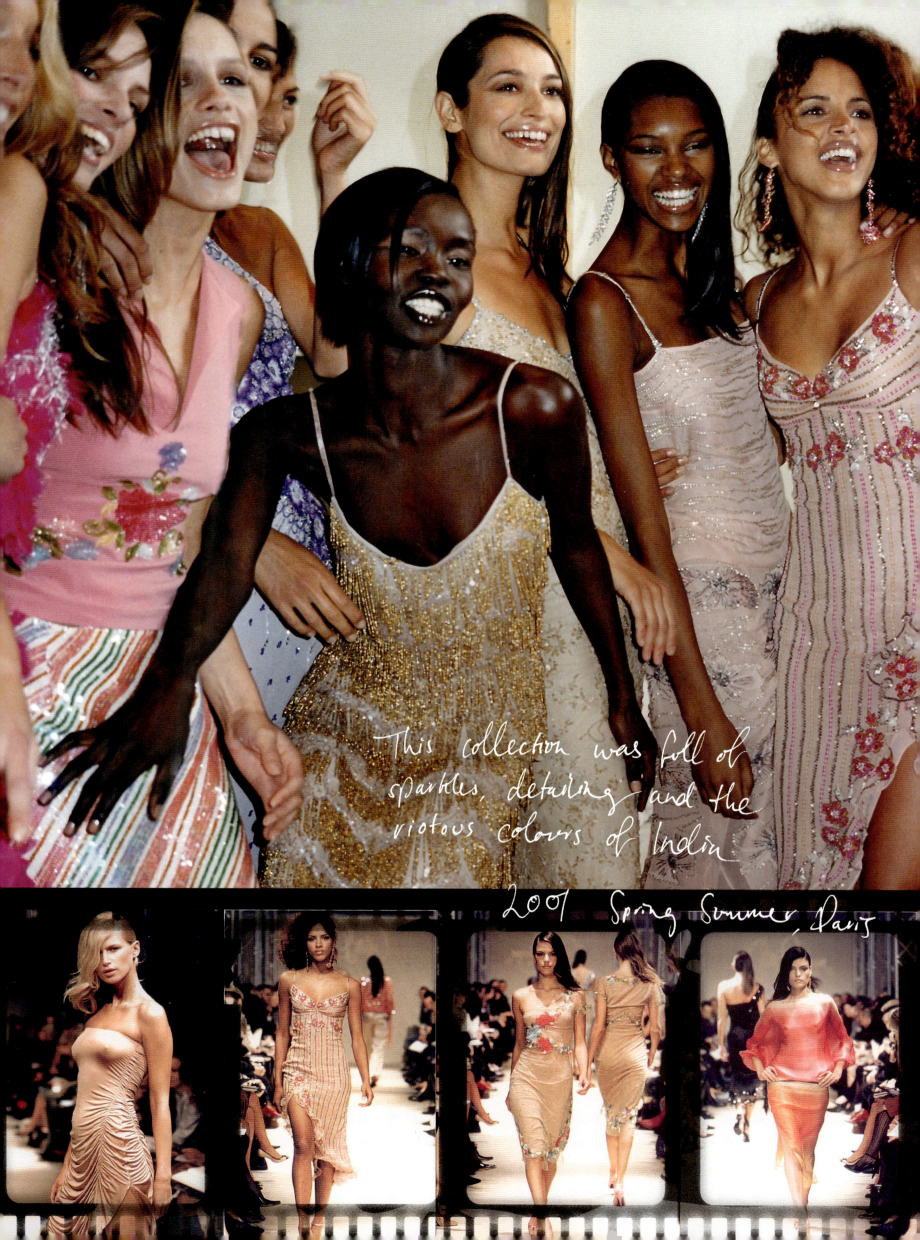

This collection was full of sparkles, detailing and the riotous colours of India

2001 Spring Summer, Paris

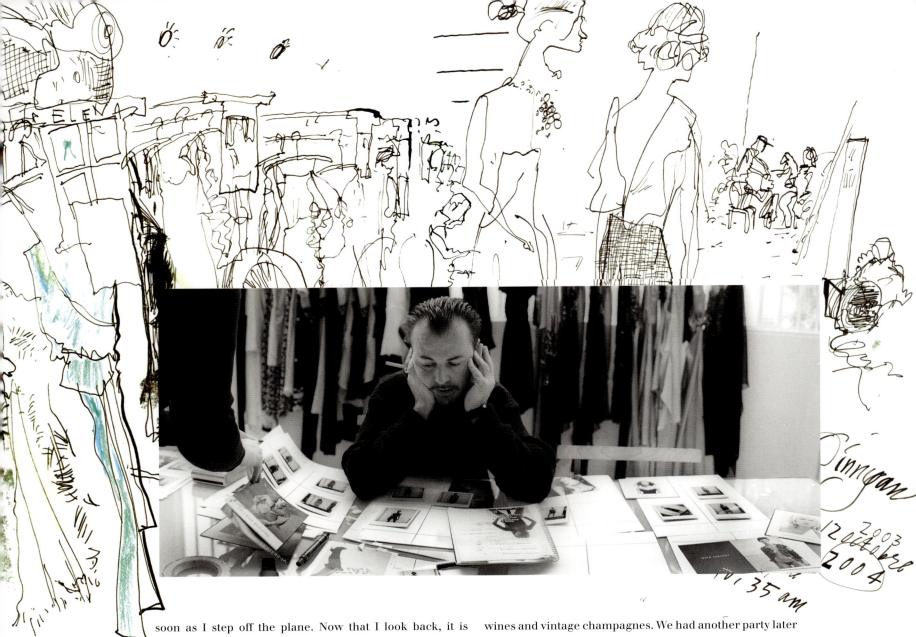

soon as I step off the plane. Now that I look back, it is amazing how quickly I integrated. I used to throw lavish after-show parties (everyone did, in those days), and invite loyal customers, key Australian and international journalists, as well as celebrities and friends of the brand. There'd always be fabulous French champagne flowing – word got out about what great parties they were.

I think the Australian and the French just blended really well – Australians know how to let their hair down, and the French have such an appreciation of good food and wine. Now it's a different story – with everything going digital, journalists are expected to file their reports half an hour after the show has finished. In the old days, if your show was on a Wednesday, you'd hope to make the papers by Friday, if you were lucky.

The last big party I hosted in Paris was in 2005, to celebrate ten years of showing there. I held a lunch at the Hôtel de Crillon for about one hundred and fifty people. We had the Salon Marie-Antoinette and Salon des Aigles with a wonderful balcony overlooking the Place de la Concorde. There was lobster and caviar, and exceptional Australian

wines and vintage champagnes. We had another party later that night at a little Moroccan bar called Andy Wahloo, and by midnight I was speechless with exhaustion. Apart from anything else, I was still breastfeeding Estella, who was six months old at the time.

Much as I love Paris, one thing that drives me mad is how hard it is to get a taxi, which makes life stressful as you are always running late. Once I was so desperate to get somewhere that I stopped a pizza delivery bike and asked the rider to take me where I needed to go. I would never do something like that in Sydney – it wouldn't seem right to hail a Dominos Pizza or Pizza Hut boy and hitch a ride. Somehow it is different in Paris.

Another time John Spender, then the Australian Ambassador to France, and his then wife, fashion designer Carla Zampatti, were hosting a cocktail party at the Australian Embassy to celebrate my show. The taxi I had booked didn't turn up, and as I was running through the streets desperately trying to find one I saw a policeman. He didn't speak a word of English, so I asked him in my best French to take me to the Australian Embassy. I was so relieved

Above: Philippe le Poder,
our casting director in Paris.
Photograph by Philip Castle.
Illustration by Stewart Walton.

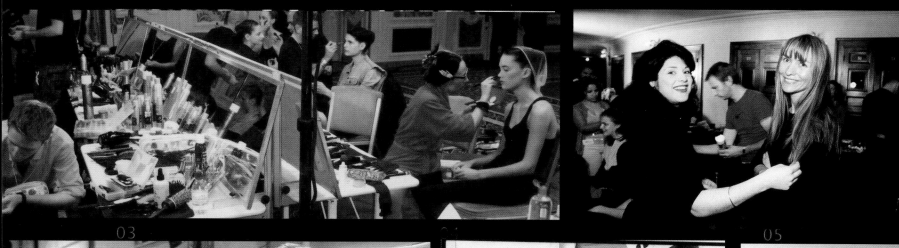

03   01   05

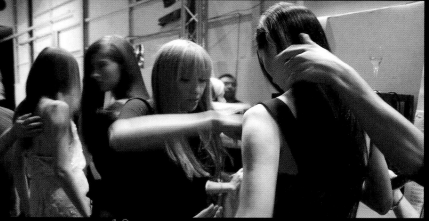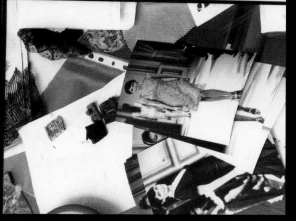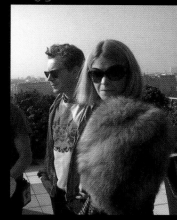

10   11   12

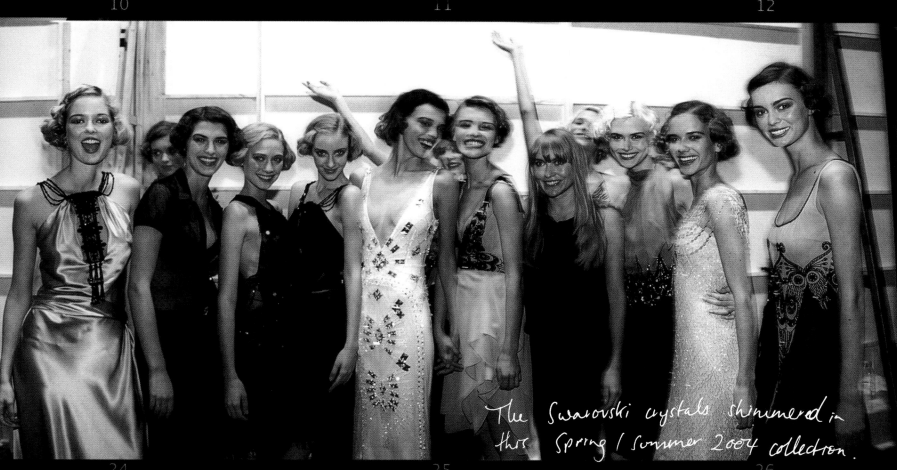

The Swarovski crystals shimmered in this Spring / Summer 2004 collection.

24   25   26

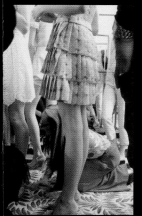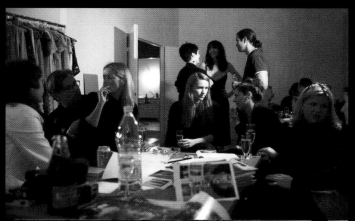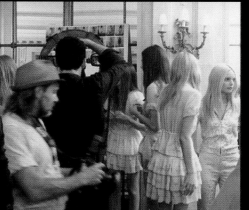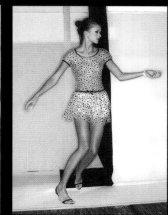

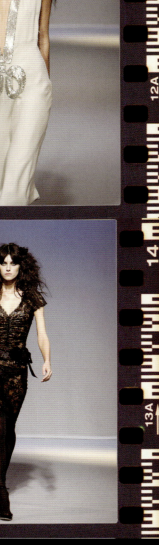
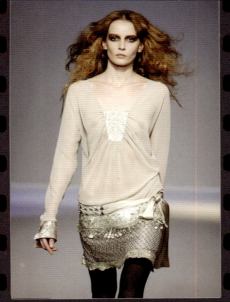
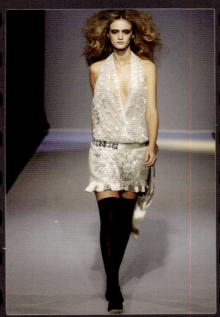
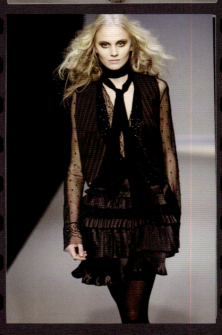
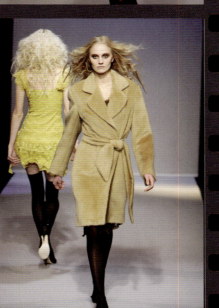
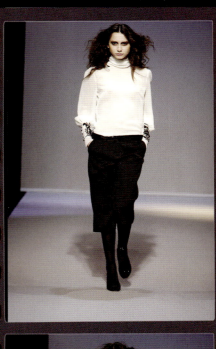
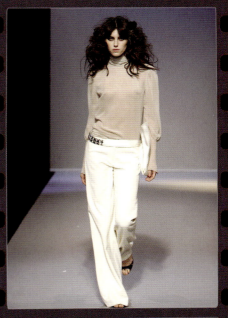

2004 Autumn/Winter, Paris

One of my favourite shows, staged at the Louvre, Paris. It was dark, with a rock-and-roll edge to it.

Collette Dinnigan

Automne-Hiver 2004

Dimanche 7 mars 12h30 salle Gabriel Carrousel du Louvre 75001 Paris

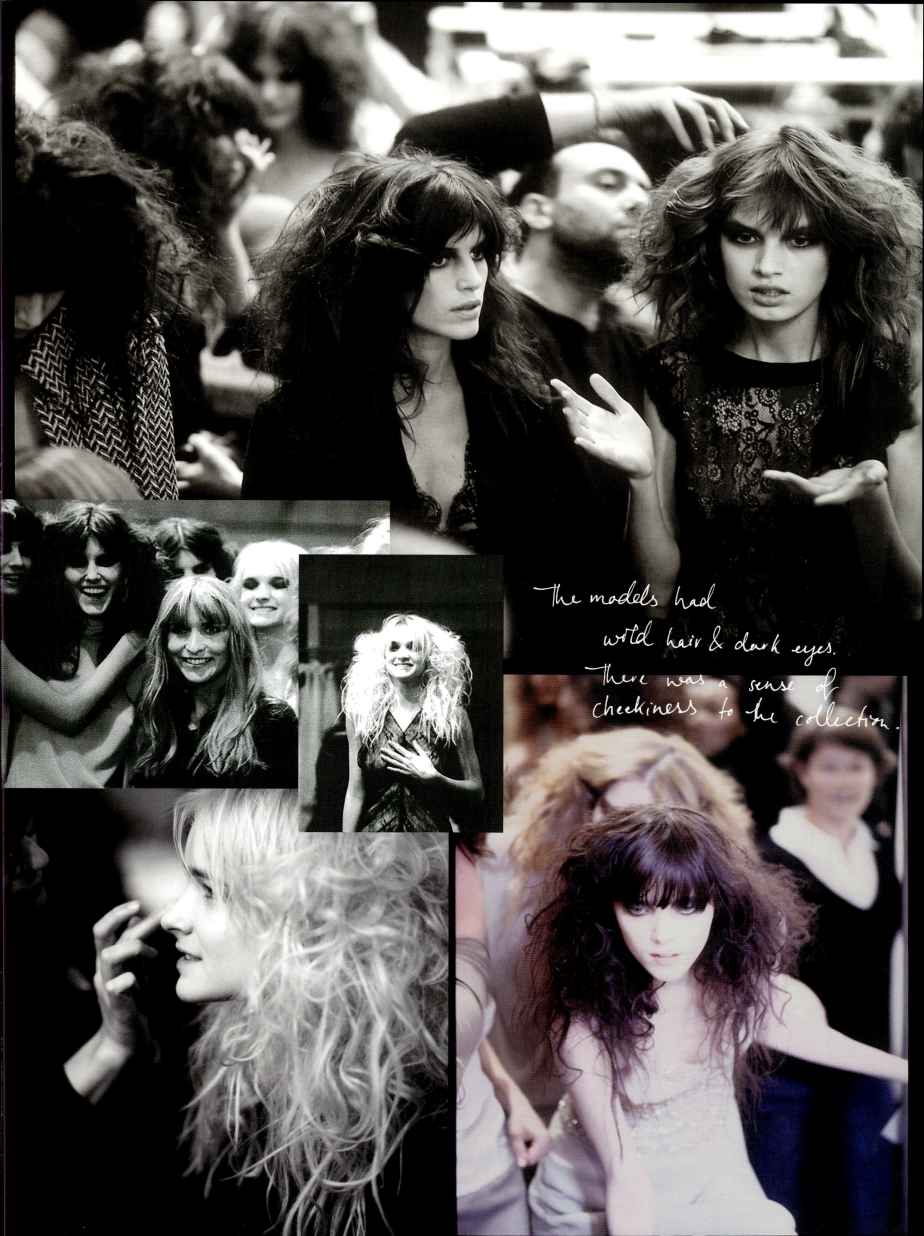

The models had
wild hair & dark eyes.
There was a sense of
cheekiness to the collection.

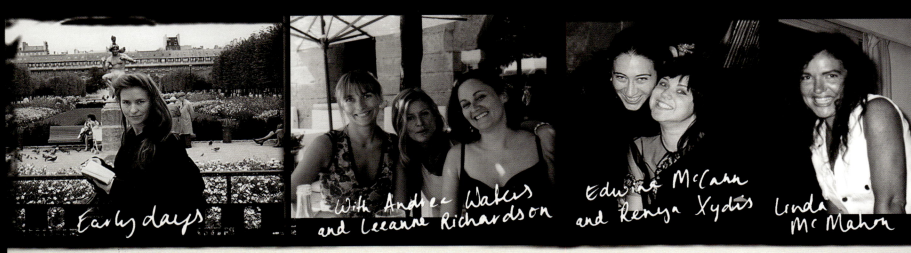

Early days

With Andrea Waters
and Leeanne Richardson

Edwina McCann
and Renya Xydis

Linda McMahon

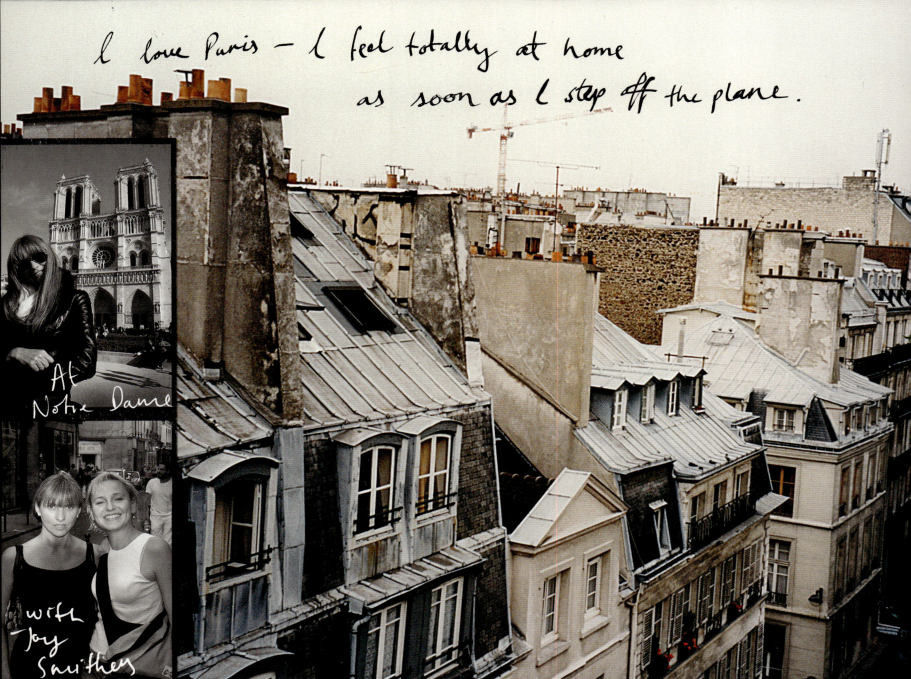

I love Paris — I feel totally at home
as soon as I step off the plane.

At Notre Dame

With Joy Smithers

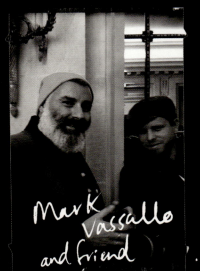

Mark Vassallo and friend

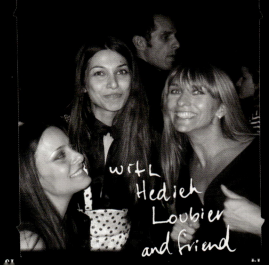

with Hedieh Loubier and friend

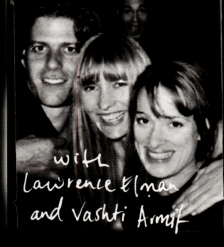

with Lawrence Elman and Vashti Armit

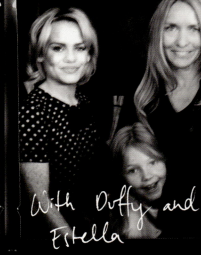

With Duffy and Estella

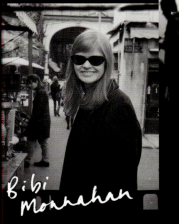

Bibi
Monnahan

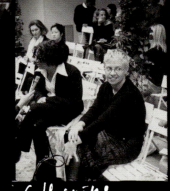

Michael Hutchence
and Paula Yates

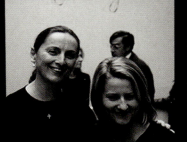

Catherine
Martin

Jane de Teliga
and Maggie Alderson

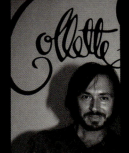

Marc
Newson

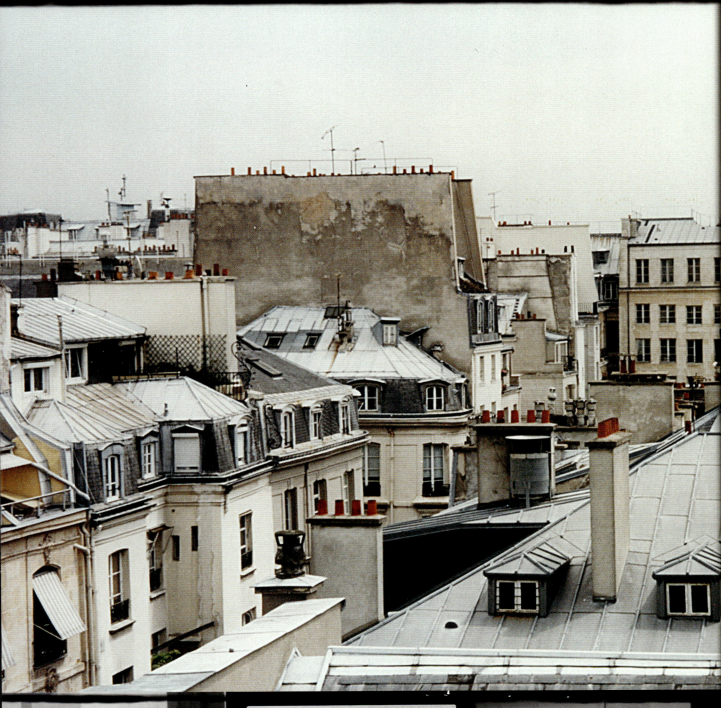

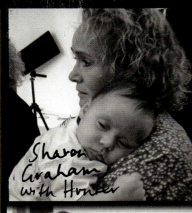

Sharon
Graham
with Hunter

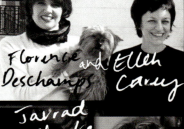

Florence and Ellen
Deschamps Carey

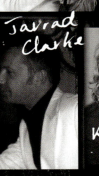

Jarrad
Clarke

Karl
Plewka

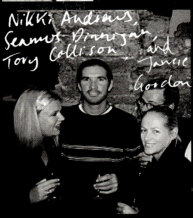

Nikki Andrews,
Seamus Dinnigan,
Tory Collison and
Jamie
Gordon

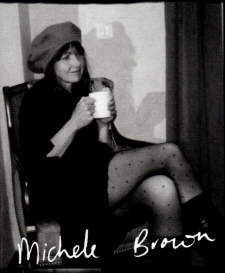

Michele Brown

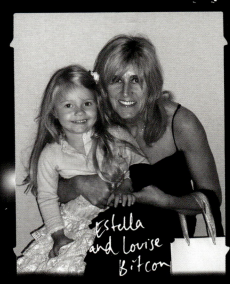

Estella and Louise
Bitcon

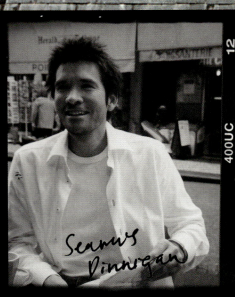

Seamus
Dinnigan

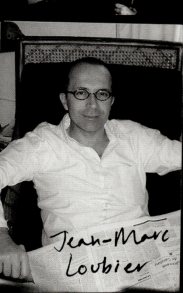

Jean-Marc
Loubier

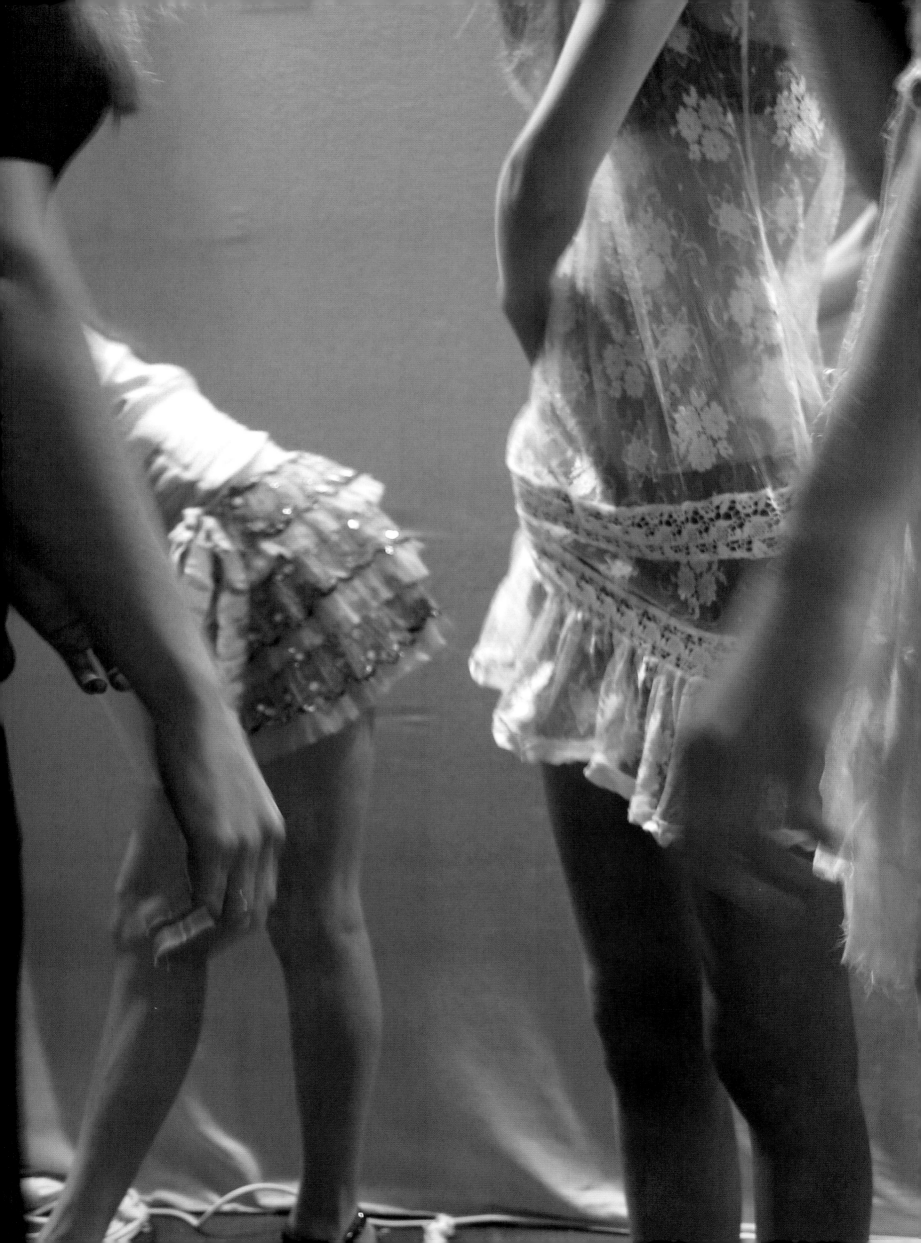

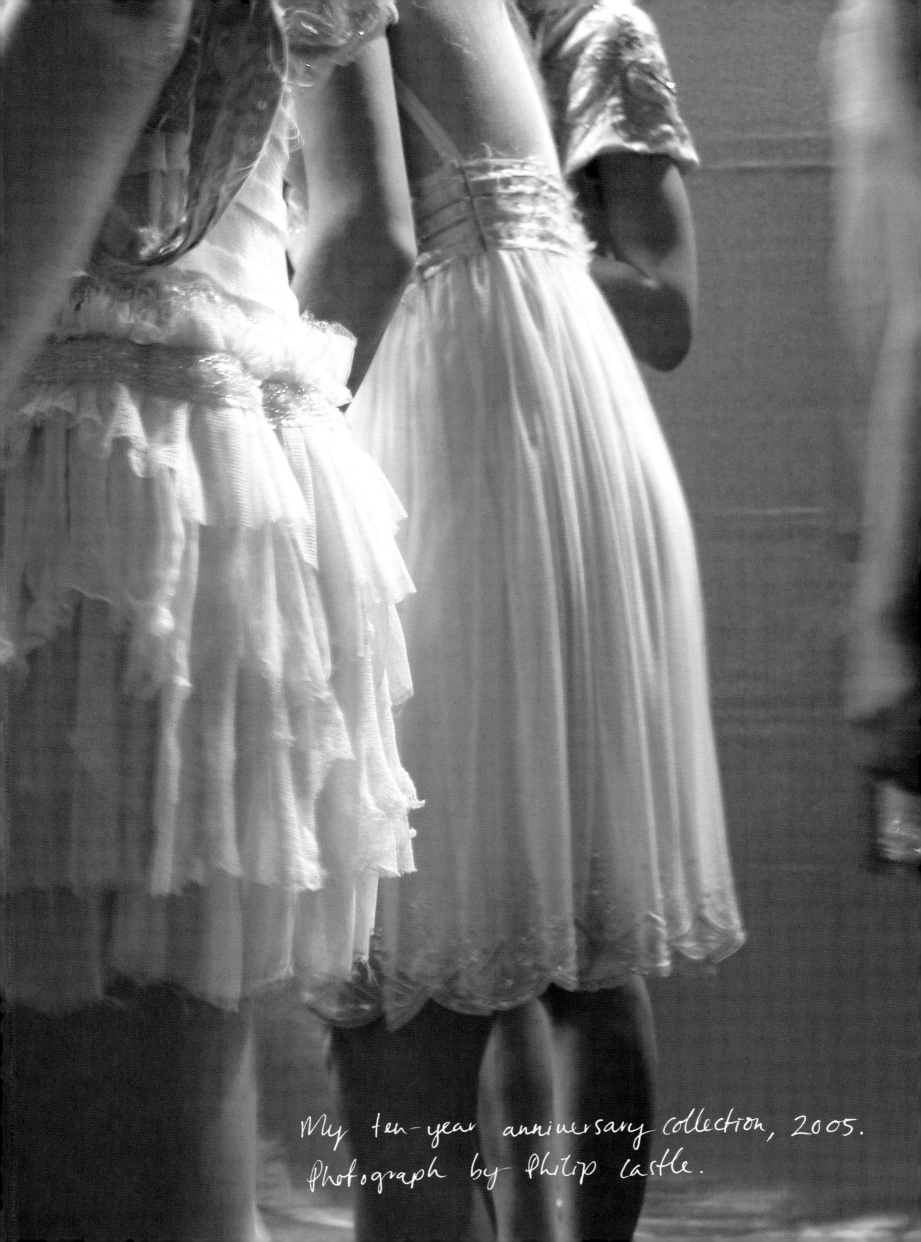

My ten-year anniversary collection, 2005.
Photograph by Philip Castle.

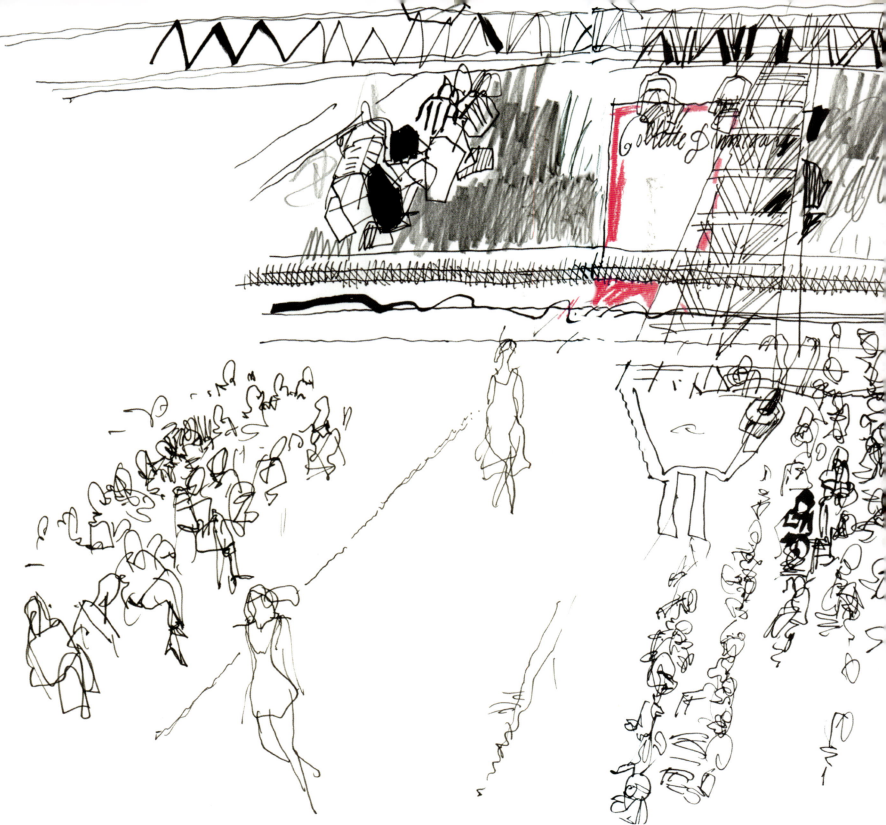

that I collapsed in the back of his car, confident that I would make it in time. Clearly my French wasn't up to scratch, as he took me straight to the American Embassy. From there I raced into the Hôtel de Crillon, where I knew the concierge, the fabulous Christian, and he took me to the nearest Métro at Place de la Concorde. I hopped on and at the station I took off my shoes and ran to the Australian Embassy.

In Paris, you never know what to expect, or who you might bump into. One night in 2004 I was hosting an after-show dinner at the legendary Prunier restaurant. As fashion columnist Maggie Alderson and I were being shown to my table in the beautiful upstairs dining room,

we walked past Yves Saint Laurent, his partner Pierre Bergé, and Catherine Deneuve, who had been Yves's muse for many years. That sort of thing happens all the time in Paris.

You never know what you might find walking the streets of Paris – and it can change the course of your life, or of your creative path anyway. New doors can open for you, you can be challenged; there is the good and the bad, the yin and the yang, the black and the white. Before I went to Paris I thought I knew everything about the world, but once I got there I realised I had a hell of a lot to learn. I hope some of it has brushed off.

Above: Illustration by Stewart Walton.

Opposite: Paris in the springtime.

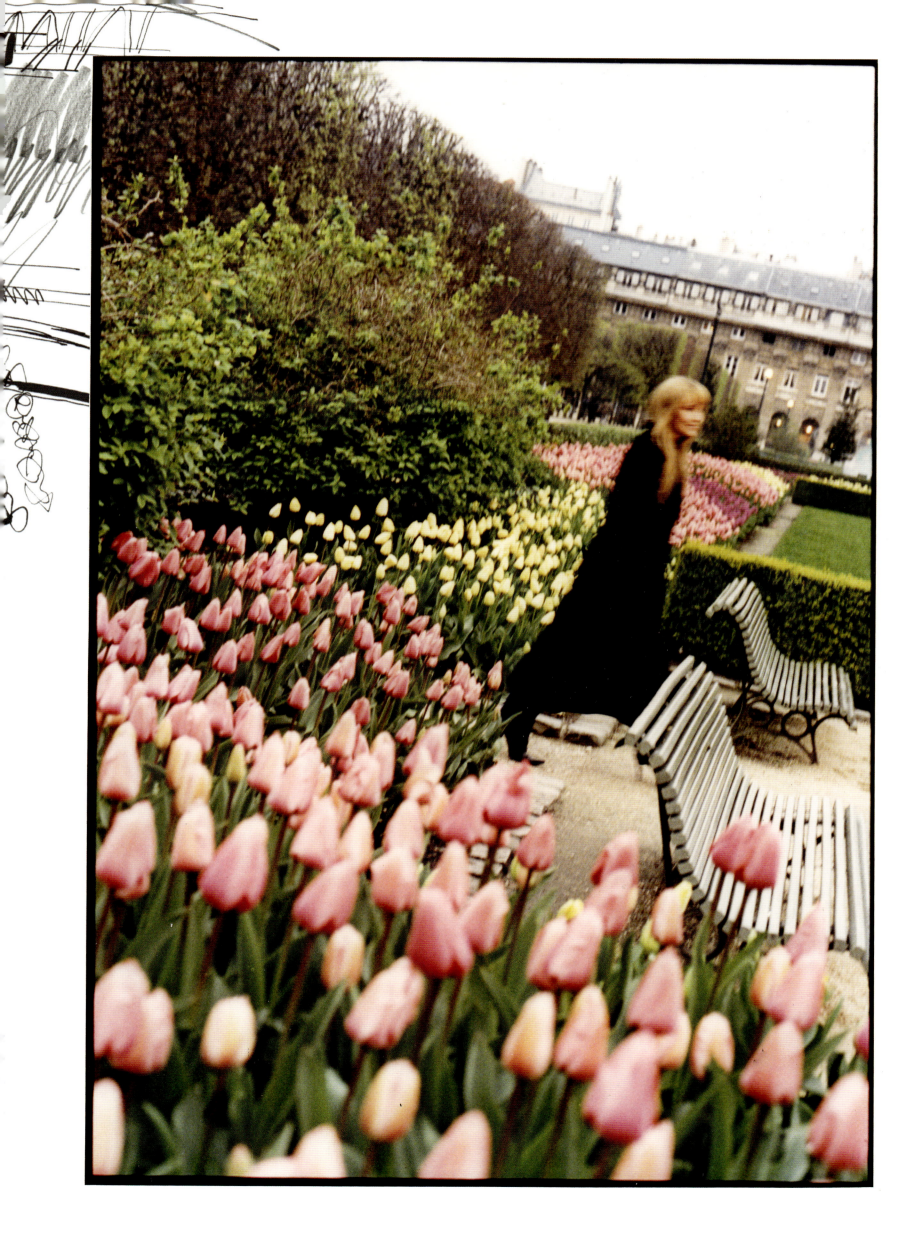

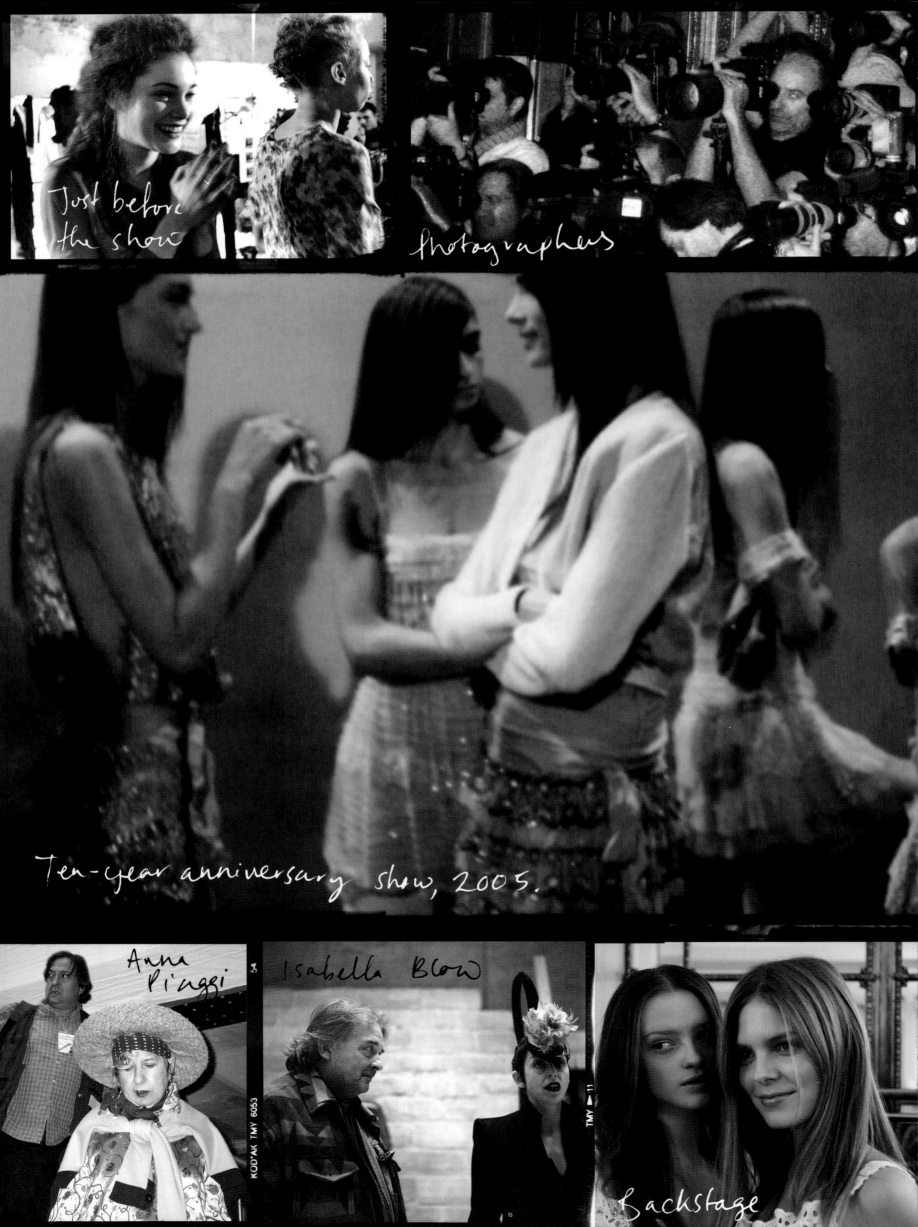

Just before
the show

Photographers

Ten-year anniversary show, 2005.

Anna Piaggi

Isabella Blow

Backstage

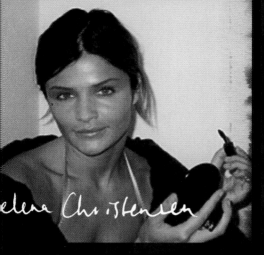

elena Christensen

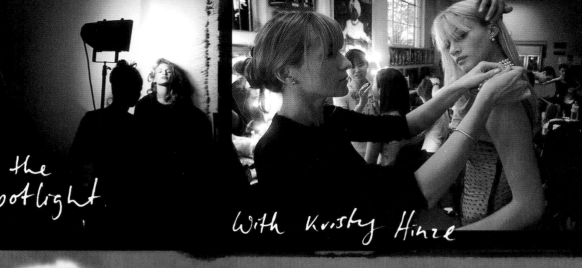

In the spotlight.

With Kristy Hinze

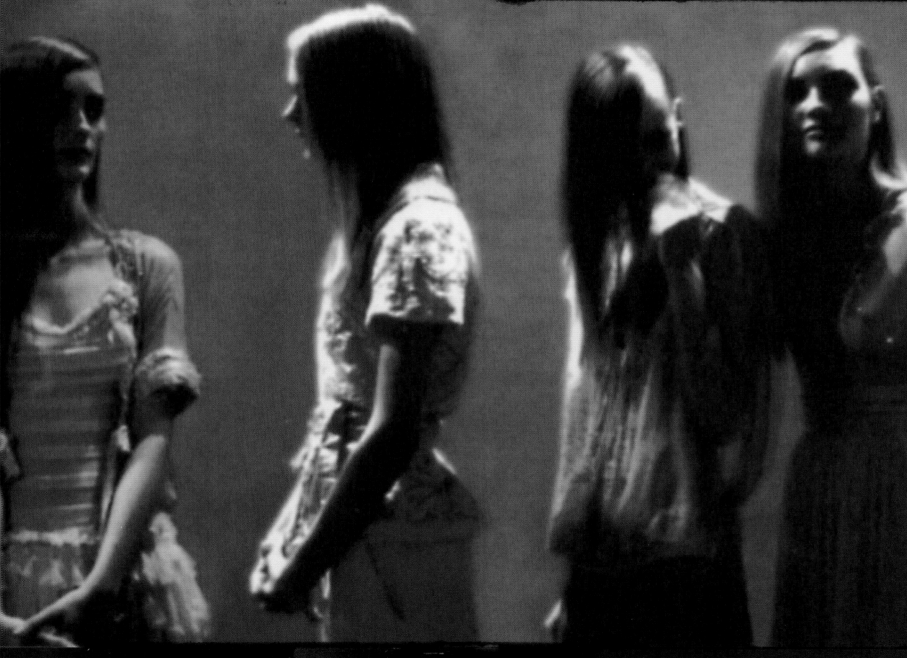

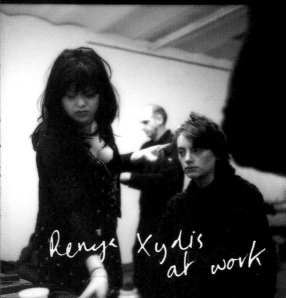

Renya Xydis at work

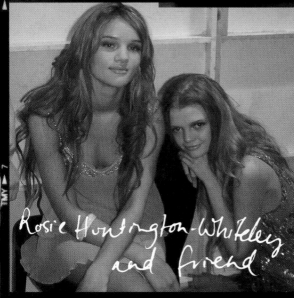

Rosie Huntington-Whiteley and friend.

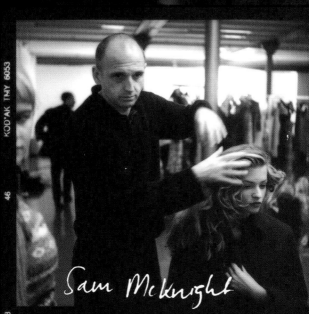

Sam McKnight

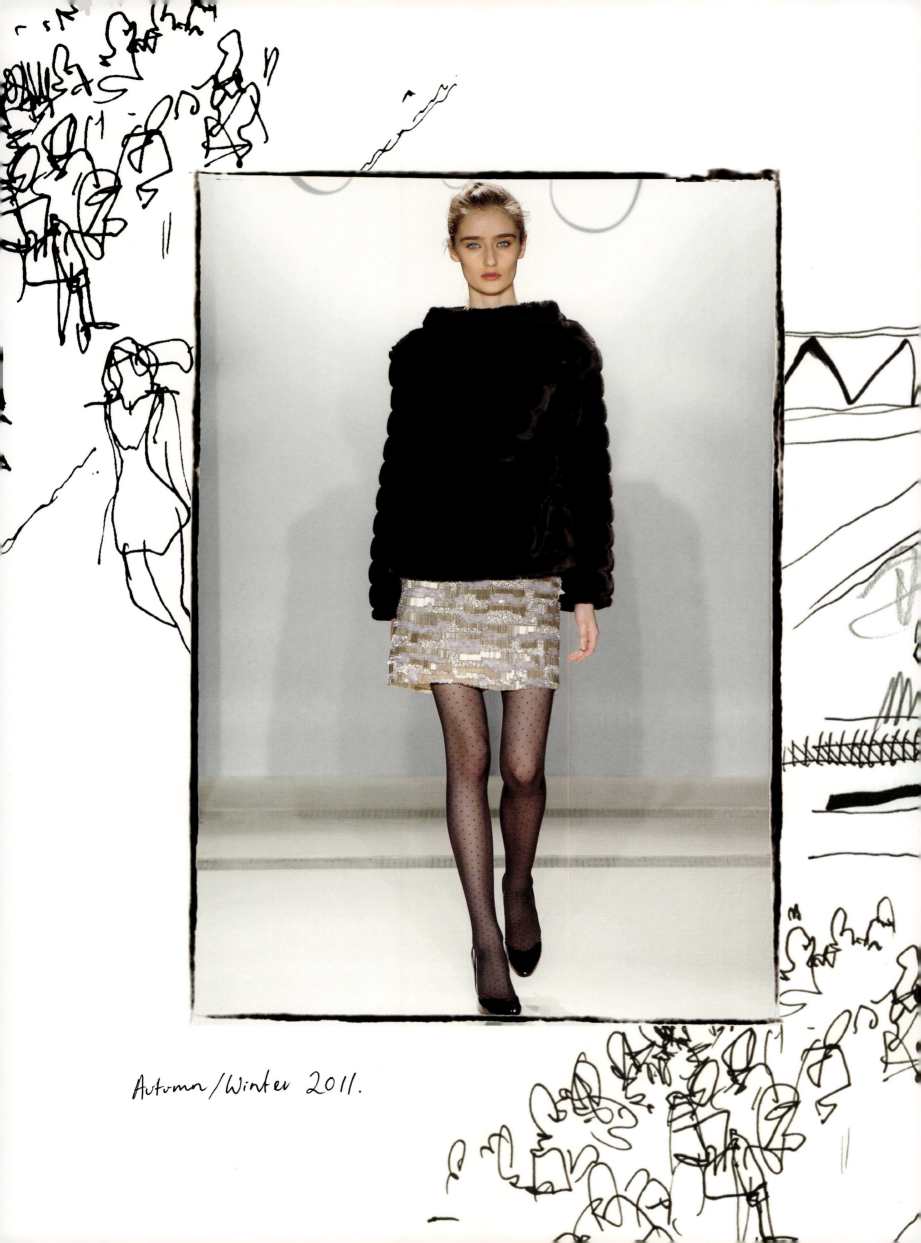

Autumn/Winter 2011.

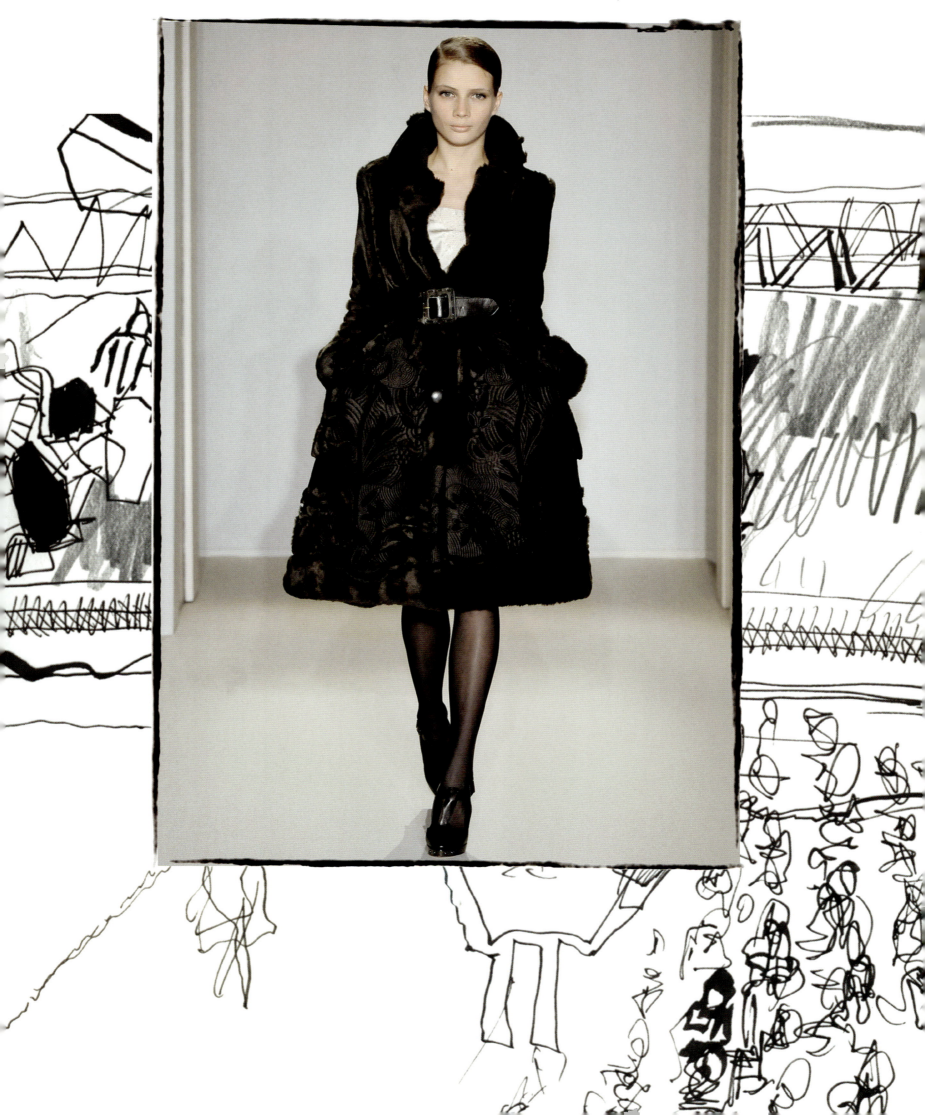

Autumn/Winter 2010.

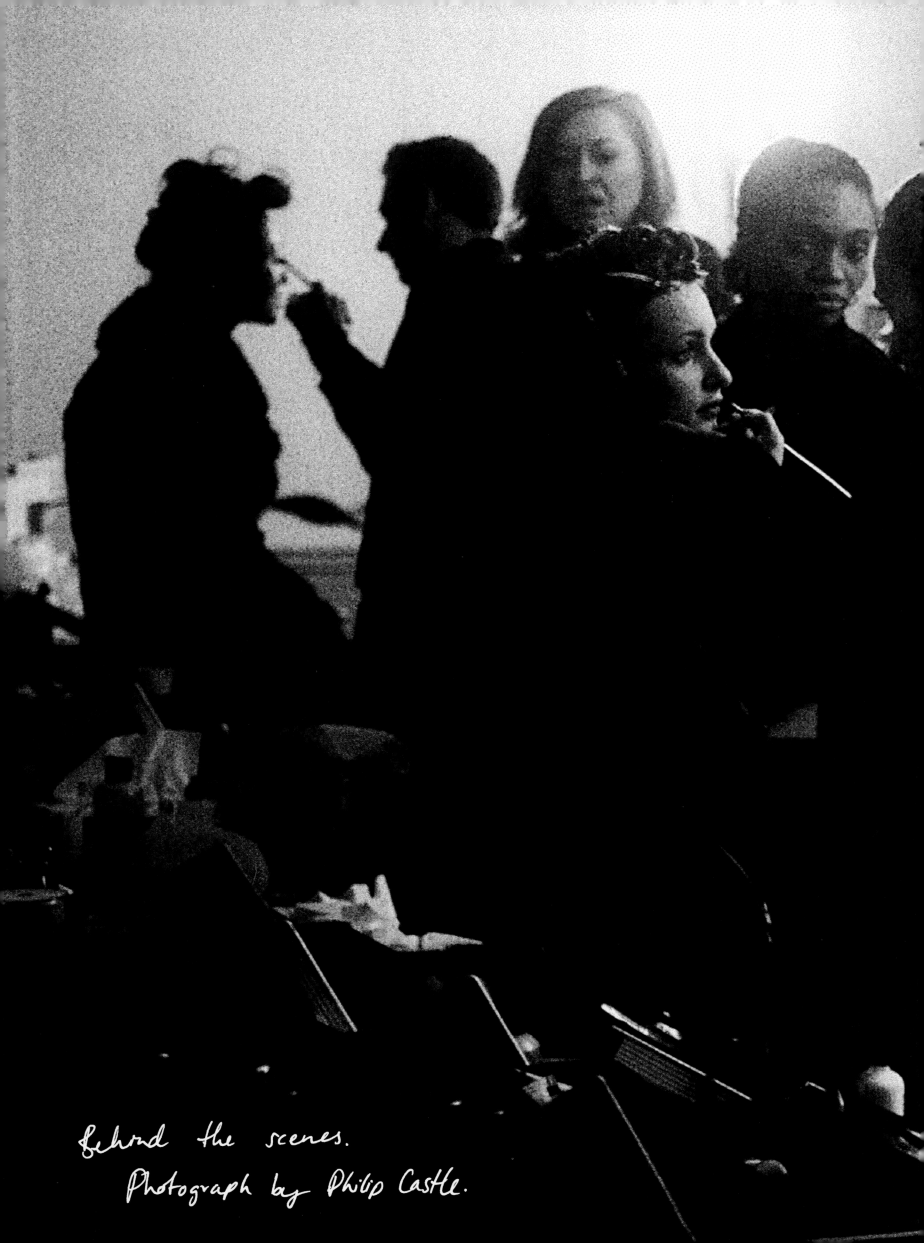

Behind the scenes.
Photograph by Philip Castle.

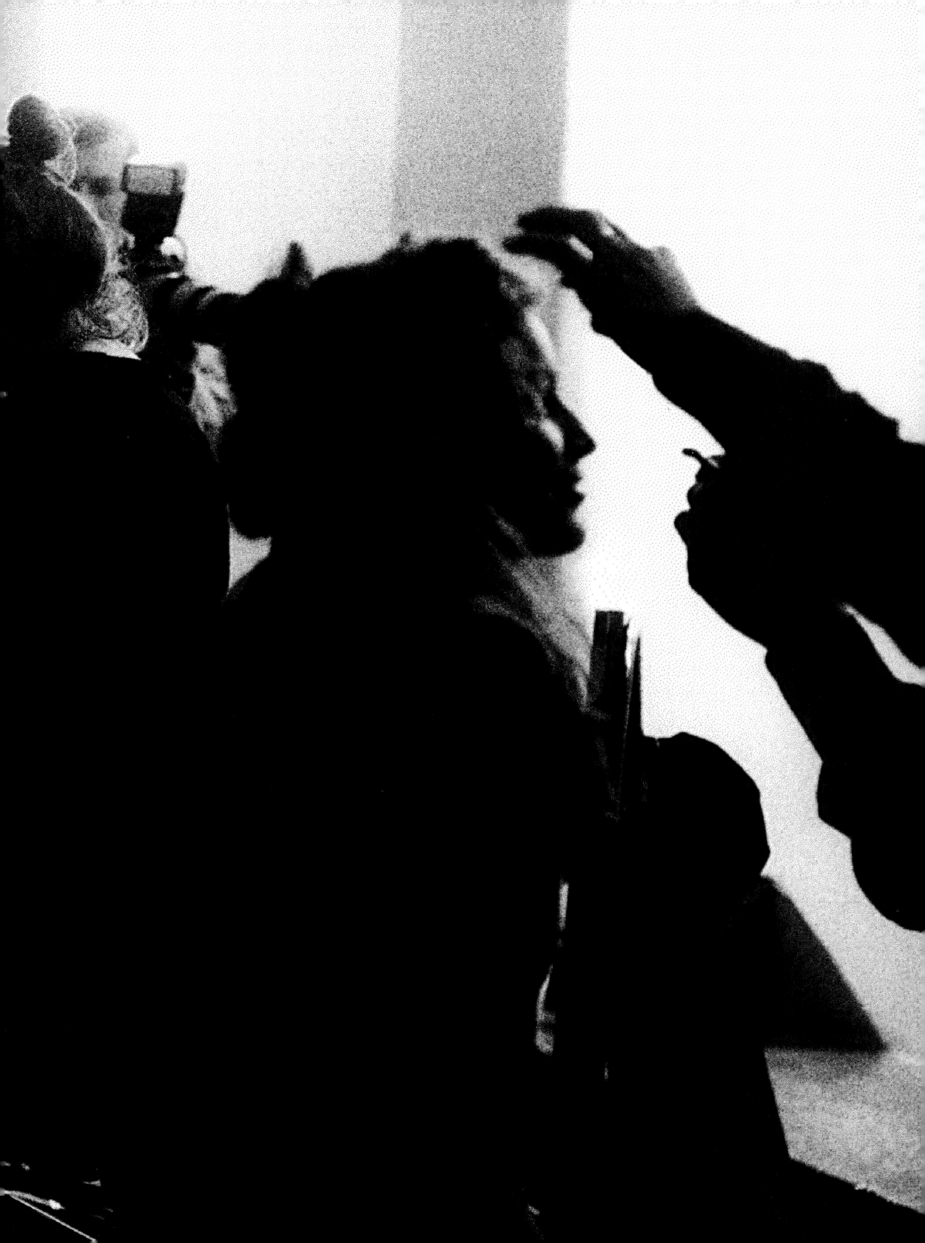

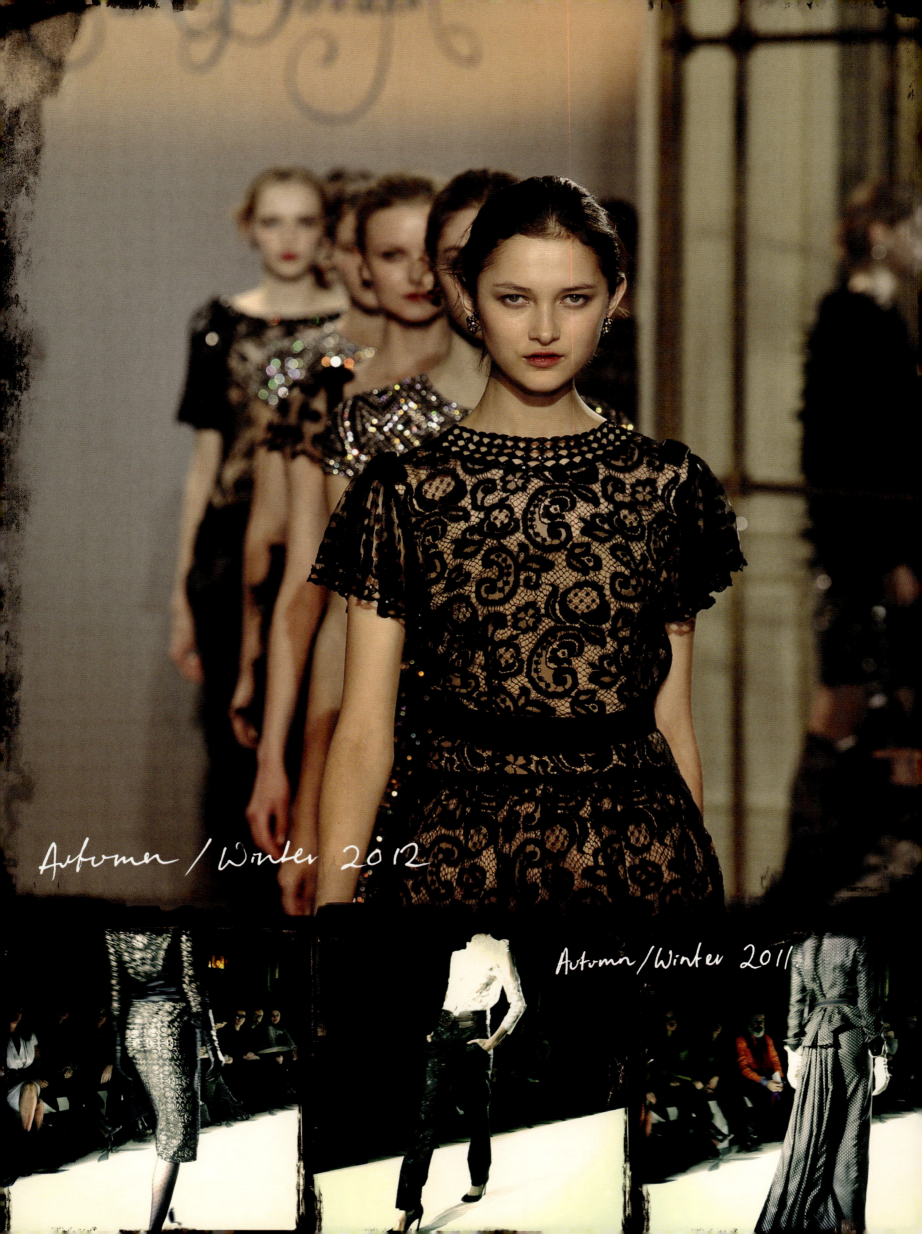

Autumn / Winter 2012

Autumn / Winter 2011

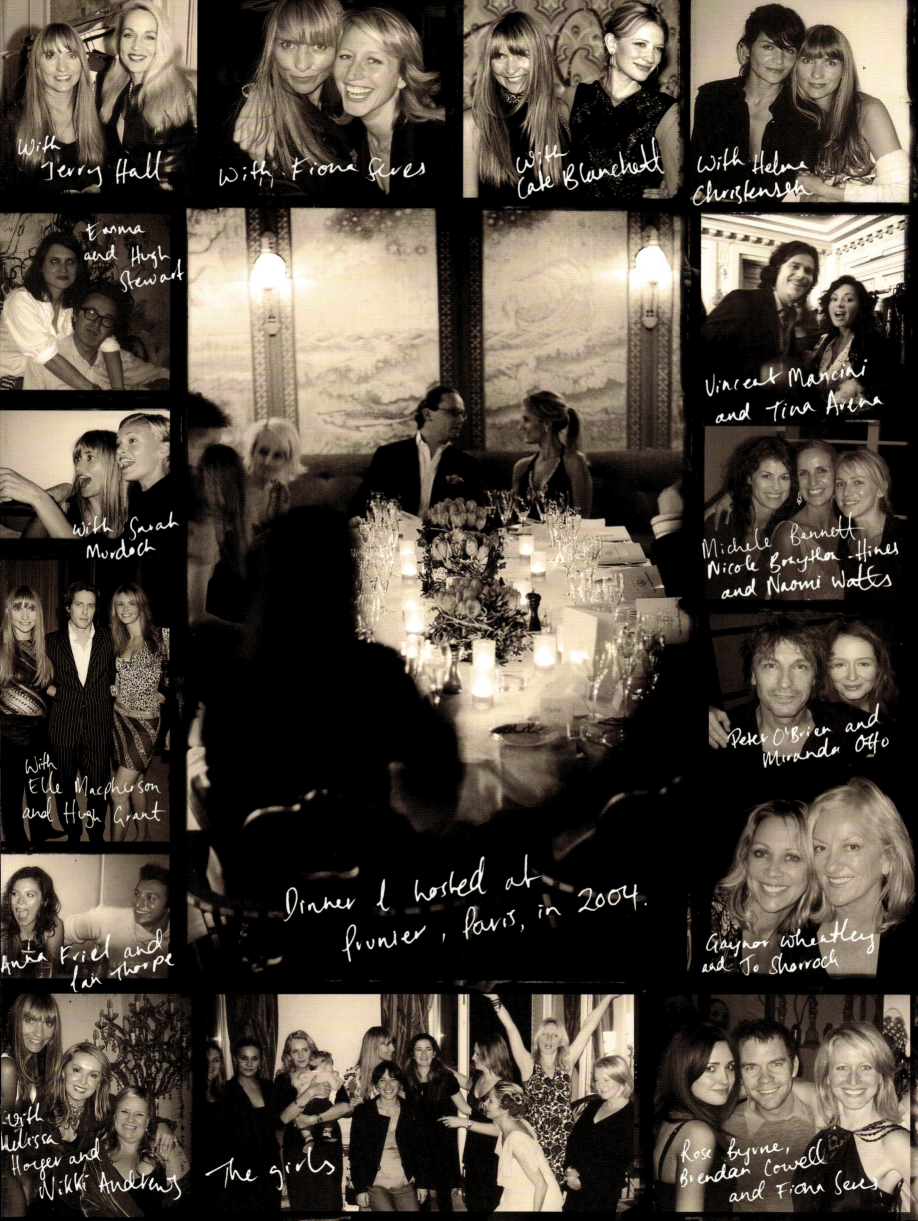

With Jerry Hall

With Fiona Scres

With Cate Blanchett

With Helena Christensen

Earma and Hugh Stewart

Vincent Mancini and Tina Arena

With Sarah Murdoch

Michele Bennett, Nicole Brayhon-Hines and Naomi Watts

With Elle Macpherson and Hugh Grant

Peter O'Brien and Miranda Otto

Anita Friel and Ian Thorpe

Dinner I hosted at Prunier, Paris, in 2004.

Gaynor Wheatley and Jo Shorrock

With Melissa Hoyer and Nikki Andrews

The girls

Rose Byrne, Brendan Cowell and Fiona Scres

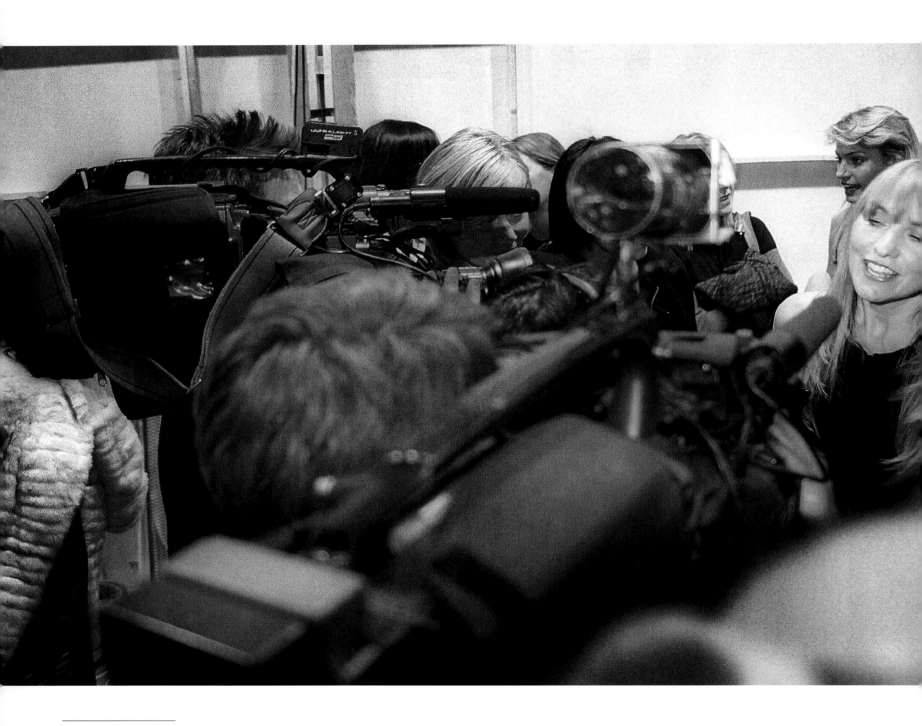

This page: Meet the press.
Photograph by Philip Castle.

Following page: With Estella, 2011.

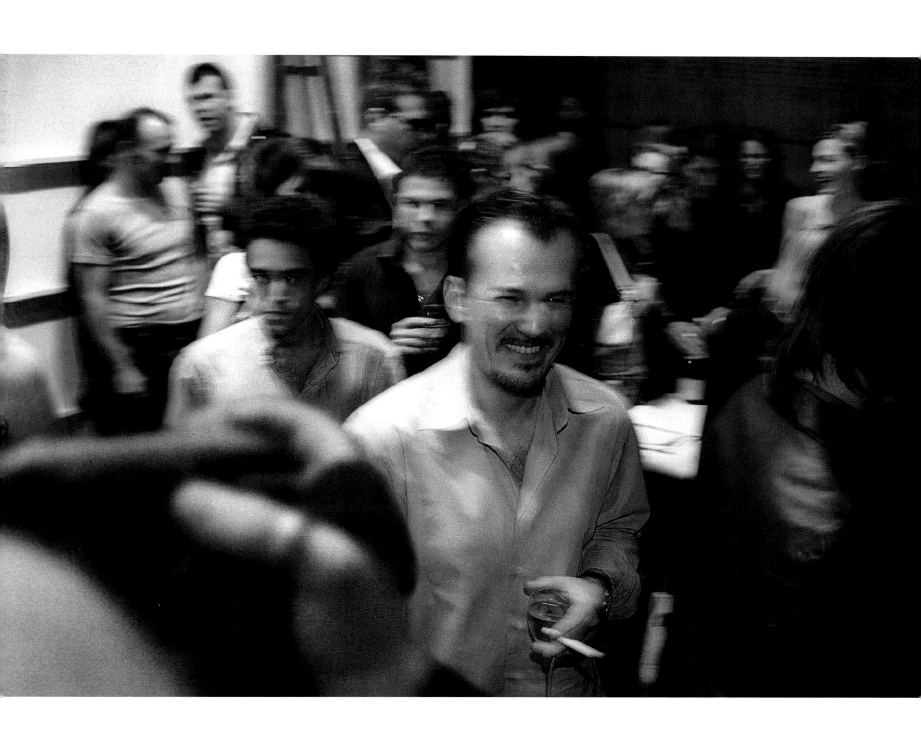

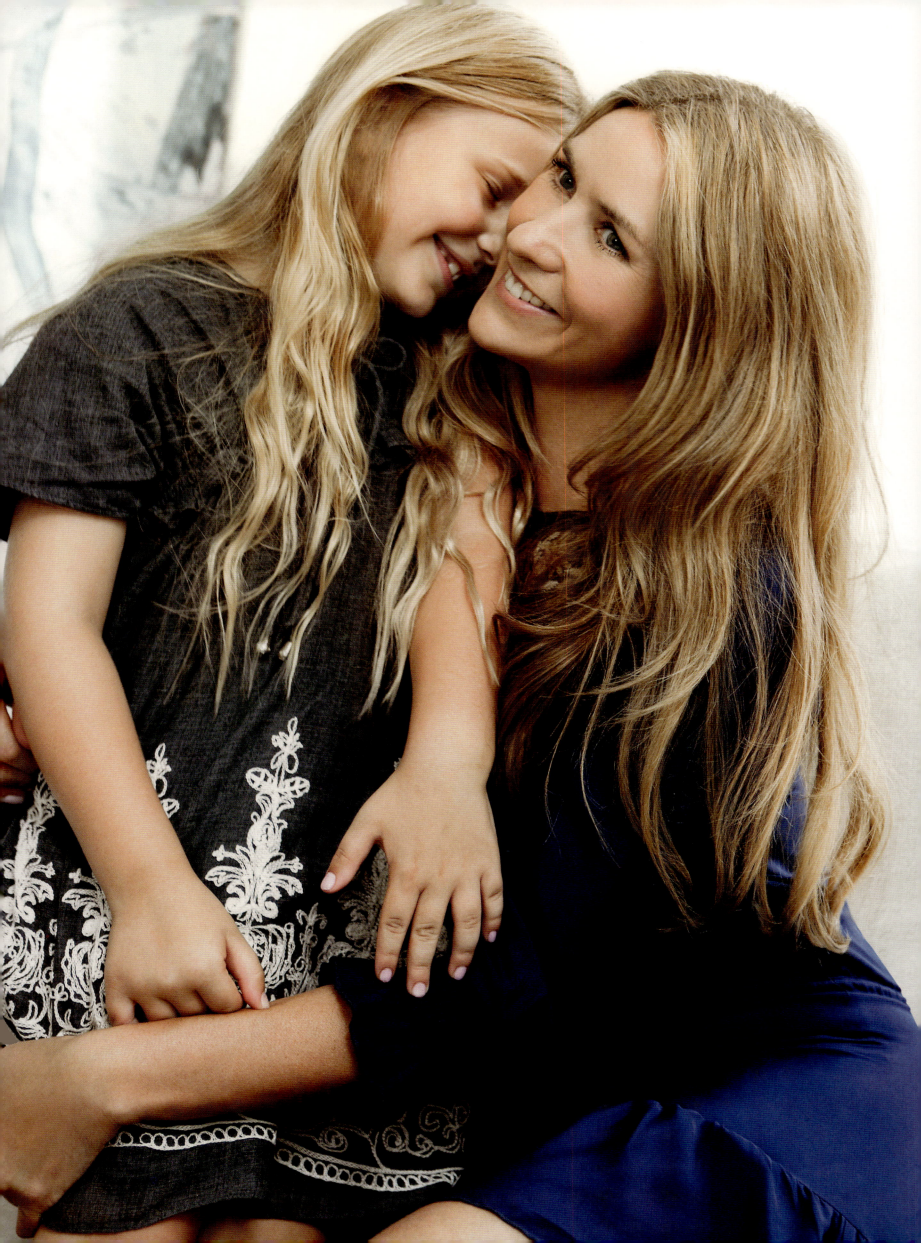

BEING A MAMA

My mother's influence;
trusting your instincts;
Estella and Hunter;
staying true to yourself.

ON INTUITION
AND INDEPENDENCE

CHAPTER 13

I LEARNT A LOT
FROM MUM; SHE WAS
SO GENEROUS AND LOVING.
She always put others first,
which is what mothers do,
AND I WAS VERY
CONSCIOUS GROWING UP
of how much she did for our family.
SHE WAS ALSO SUCH A FREE
SPIRIT, AND VERY ADVENTUROUS —
otherwise she wouldn't have married Dad,
and lived the life that she did.
I LOVE THAT ABOUT HER,
AND IT IS DEFINITELY
A PART OF MY OWN DNA.

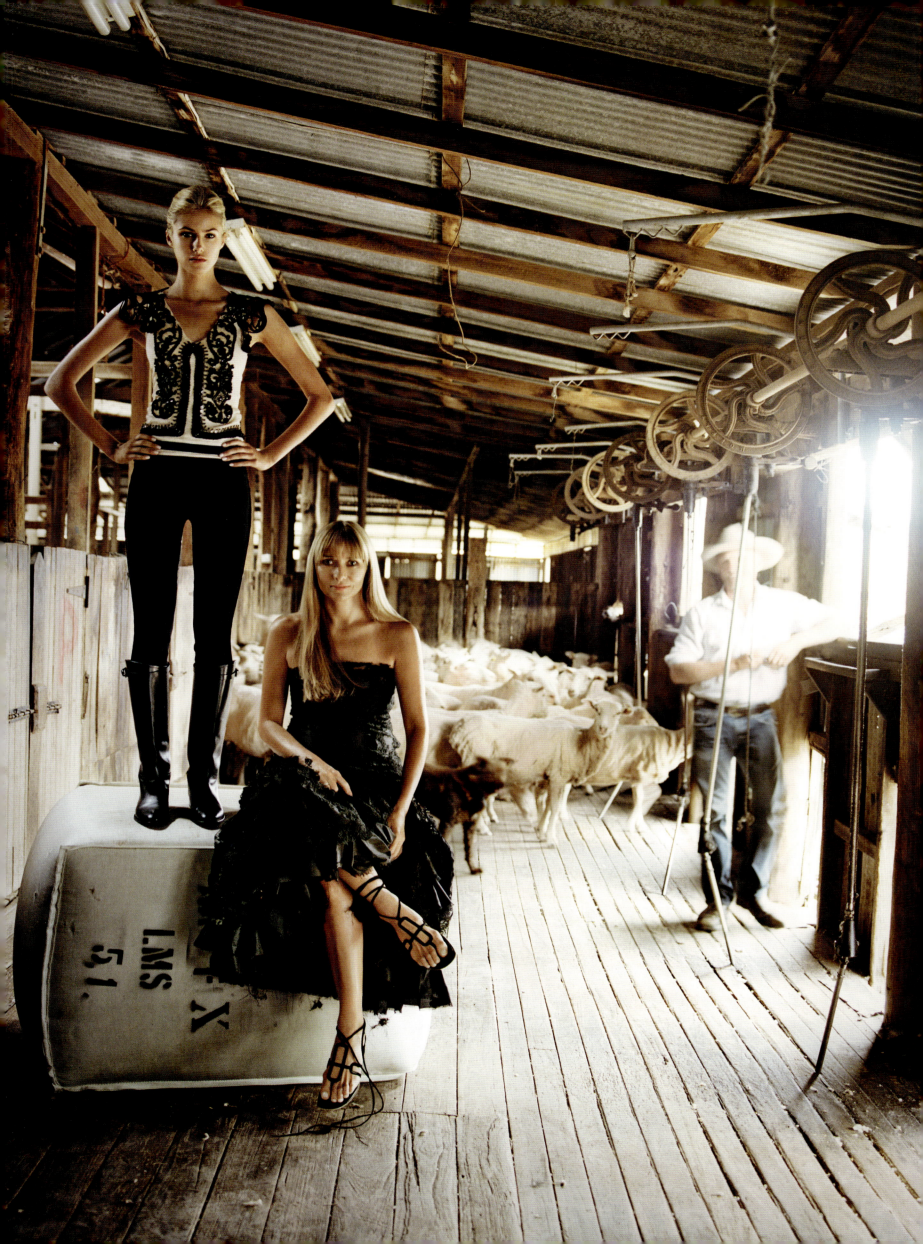

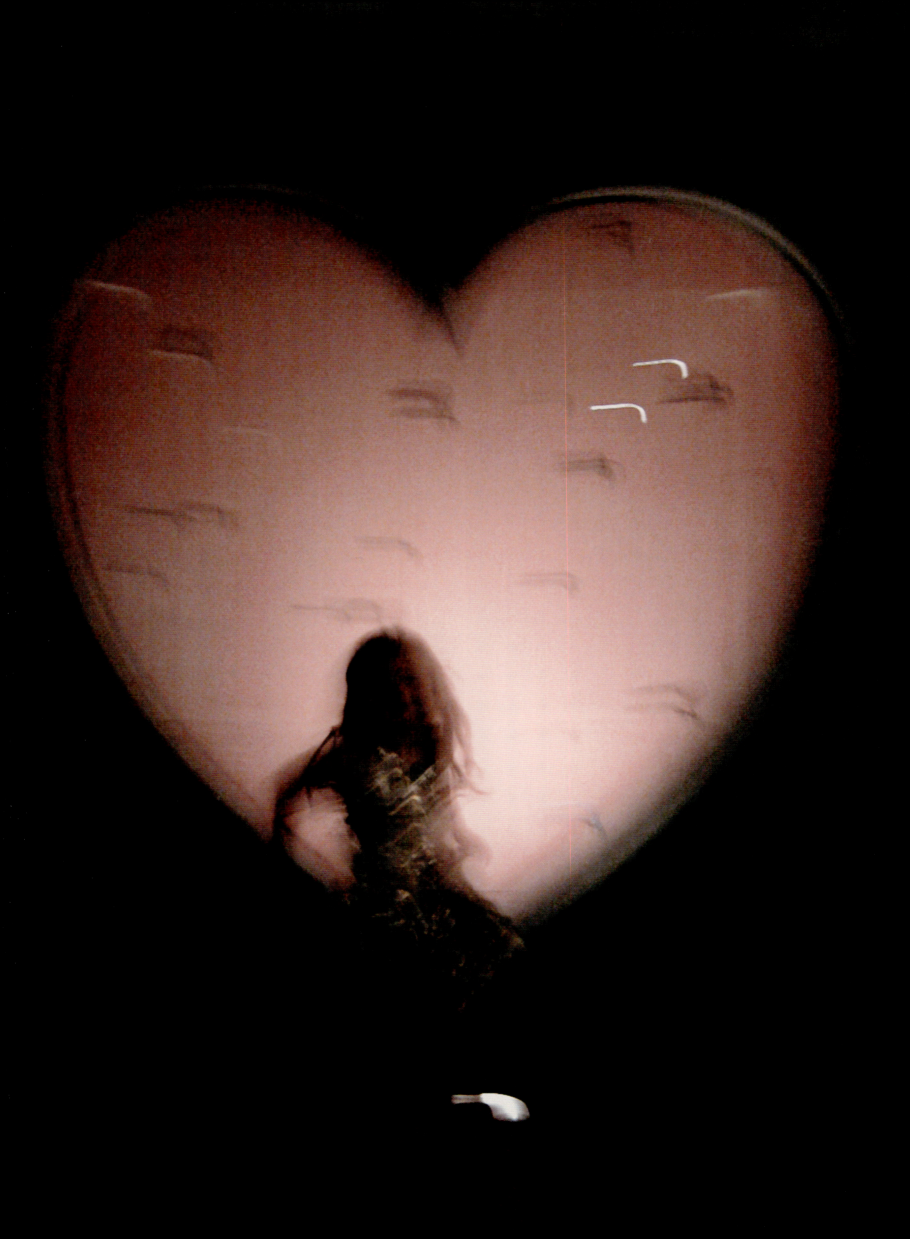

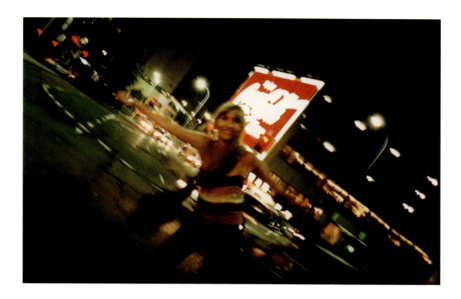

It was Mum who really encouraged me to dream, and to believe that

I could do anything I wanted to with my life. One of my oldest friends,

Andrea, says that she has never known a mother to cheer on her daughter

the way mine did. I am so grateful for that.

Mum also had a unique sense of style. She was very fig-ure-conscious, and she always looked great, whatever she wore; her favourite clothes were caftans, miu-mius and pedal pushers. I am not quite as bad as the *Ab Fab* daugh-ter, but I do care less than Mum did about how I look. I dress to be comfortable – I like to be appropriately dressed for the occasion, but that's all.

Estella is very like Mum – she has her own, highly individual sense of style. She will dress herself in lay-ers of clothes, with striped tights and knitted cardigans, and everything just mixed together – that's her thing, and I love that about her. She is big on wearing the right clothes for the right occasion. If she's riding a bike, it's shorts; if she's riding a horse, it's jodhpurs. So when it's sports day at school and everyone else wears shorts, she will wear a pretty dress, tights and something sparkly, because she thinks she needs to look her best.

I will never forget once, when she was going through her tutu stage, Bradley took her to a meeting and she wore about ten tutus, one on top of the other, with cardigans and scarves – she was so puffed-up that she barely fitted in the car. She sat through the meeting like that, lost in a sea of net and fabric, oblivious to what anyone thought. She wore the same ten-tutu outfit on a flight to Paris to meet me once – I can only imagine how uncomfortable those layers of nylon tulle must have been.

Estella is very independent, like Mum and I, but also quite shy. She will attach herself to other children, but it takes a while. She is also very creative, which comes out mainly in her storytelling and music – she sings, plays bass guitar, piano and the drums and has her own band. She is also quite stubborn, which can make her hard to handle, but I think it will help her in later life. She adores ani-mals – we have a cat, Weba, who is sixteen years old, and two dogs, Louis and Snippy. She is also mad about horses, and, to her credit, doesn't mind the hard work – she throws herself into it, cleaning out the stables, and shovel-ling manure with the best of them. When I designed my Enfant collection, she was the model for that, which was challenging at times.

Previous page: On a farm, near Goulburn in 2009. The model is wearing a Bonds singlet that I embroidered.

Opposite: Estella, dancing on stage at Petersham House, in front of a work by Damien Hirst.

Above: City lights.

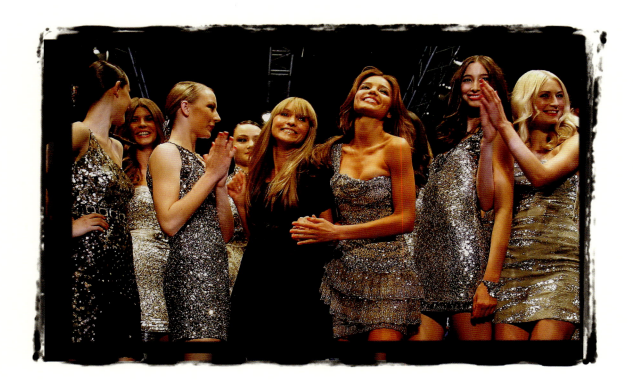

Above: Miranda Kerr and me at the finale
of the David Jones parade, 2008.

Estella spent a lot of time at the studio when she was small, and she still visits quite a bit after school. She loves playing with the fabric, and making clothes. She used to make clothes for herself – she'd cut out pieces of fabric, and drape them around herself in front of the mirrors, and everyone would help her make ball gowns. I have a funny photo of her all dressed up in a long yellow dress, wearing long gloves, and just sitting there like some matriarch. Then she went through a period of making clothes for her dolls, but now she's obsessed with making things for the dogs – saddle blankets, and mats for them to sleep on.

She has travelled with me quite a lot, from when she was a baby, but it is more difficult now that she is at school. I am a stickler for routine – children thrive on it – and I don't like to take her out of school, but on the other hand she learns so much when she travels with me. It gives her an appreciation of other cultures, and the different circumstances people live in, and exposes her to experiences she won't get at school.

I am conscious though that there are pluses and minuses to travel for her. I remember as a teenager finding it very hard to settle down after my nomadic, bohemian childhood. I needed to be stimulated all the time – I wasn't content to stay in the same surroundings. I try

to limit travel for her now to the school holidays. When I travel without my family, my trips are much shorter and more intense, and totally focussed on work, because I'm in a hurry to get home to them all.

I think the most important thing for children is that they are happy, and enjoy their childhood years. I also want Estella to be well-mannered, kind and disciplined, which she is. I don't like to see the school (or anyone else) put too much pressure on her to perform. It is just intuitive – if children are happy, they will do better. I'm like my mother in that way. She adored her children, as I do mine, and she was always more concerned about our emotional wellbeing than our scholastic performance.

A little while ago, Bradley was teasing her, saying, 'You're so good with the fabrics, Estella, you're going to have to take over the business'. She immediately said, 'No way, that's too much hard work'.

I am very intuitive – just as Mum was – and have learnt the hard way always to trust my instincts. I have made mistakes in the past, in my professional and my personal life, when I knew that someone or something wasn't right, but didn't have the courage to say so. Now I have more confidence to speak up – otherwise I just get myself into a deeper mess. In the same way, I know instinctively when

Opposite: About one month before
Estella was born, in 2004.

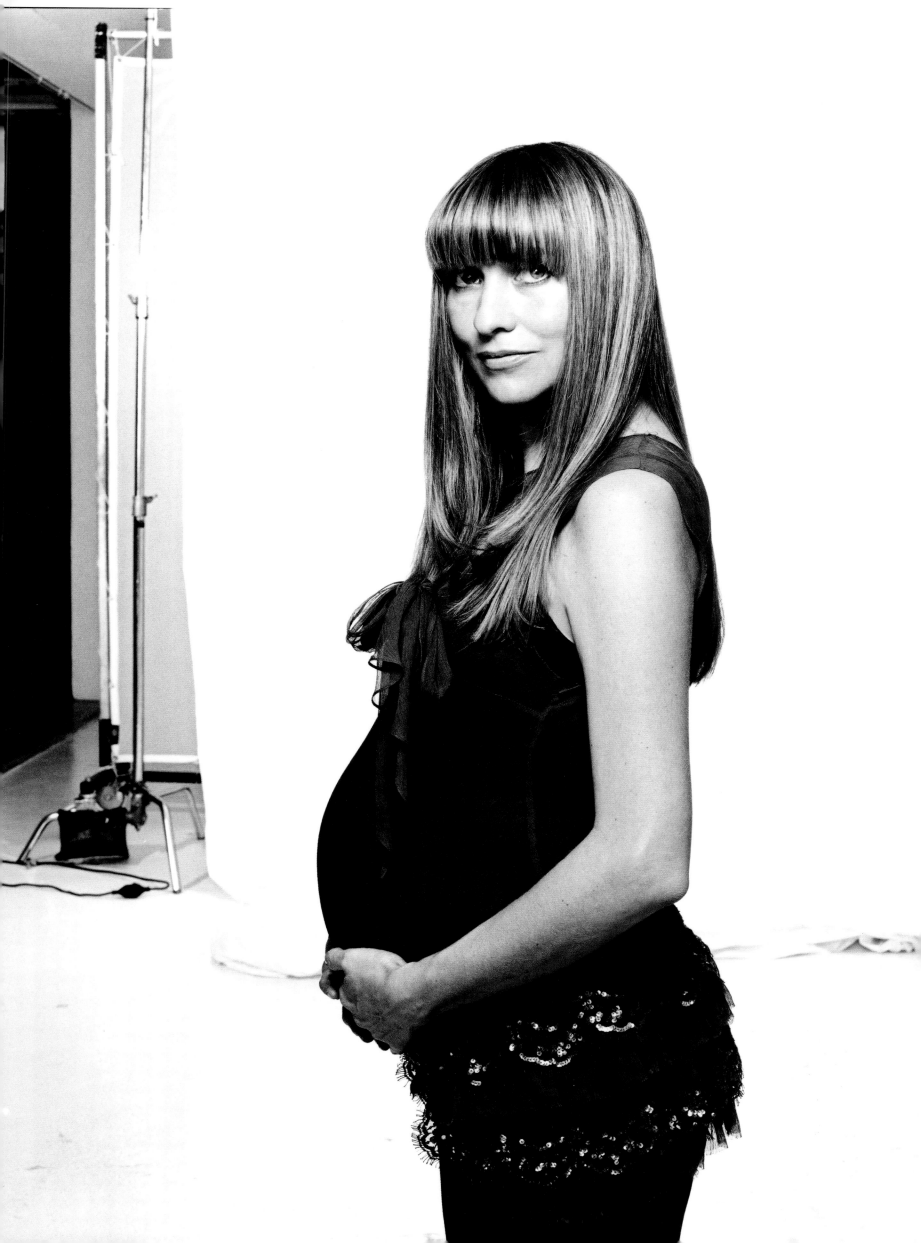

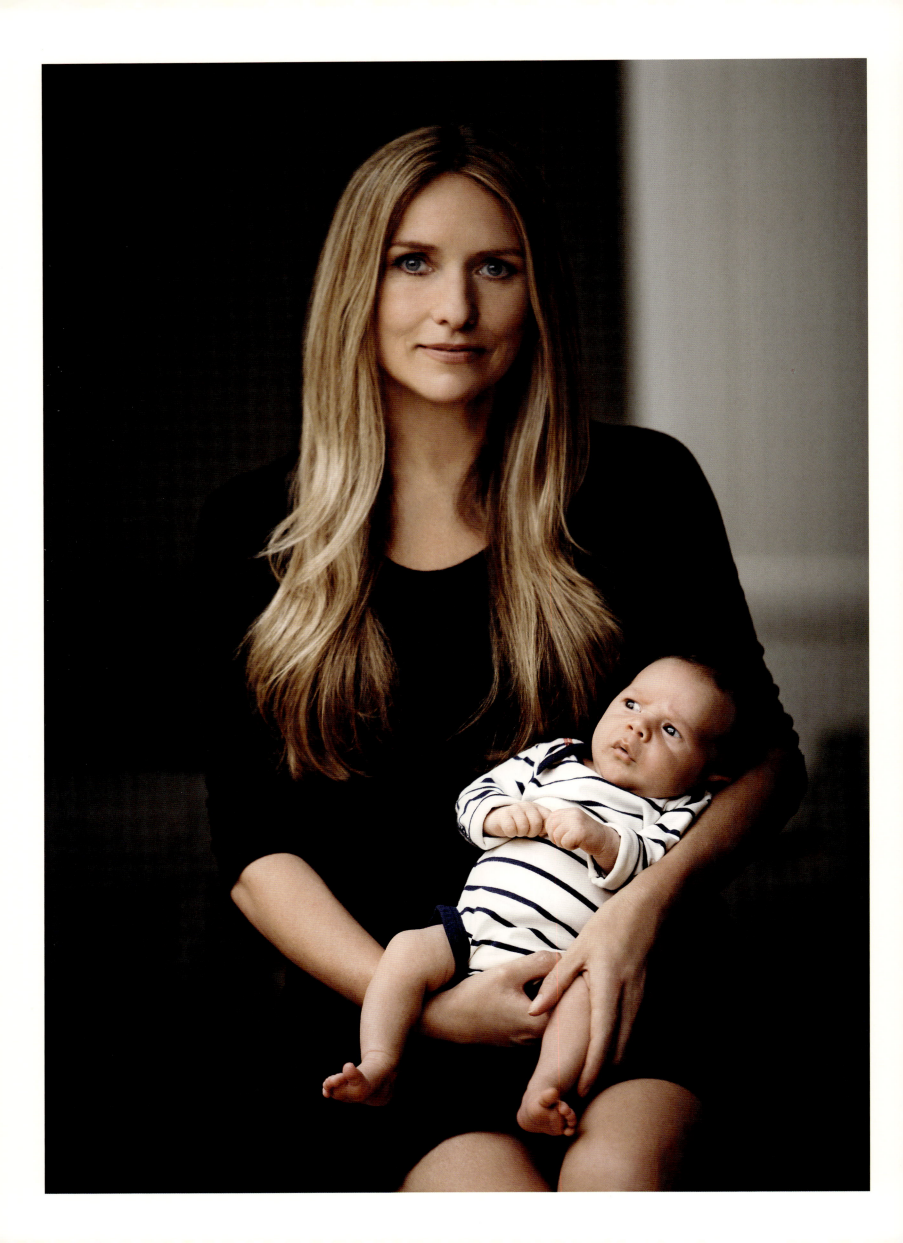

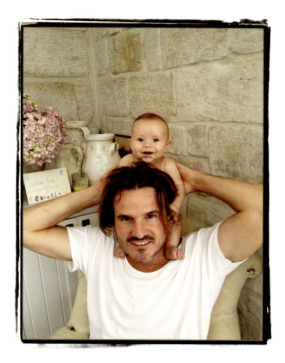

something is right. When I opened my first shop, in Paddington, I never had any doubt that I should be doing it, although I was only in my late twenties at the time. It was the same when I opened my shop in London in 2000 – people tried to talk me out of it, but I knew that it was the right location at the right time. We've now had that shop for over thirteen years, and, though it hasn't always been easy, the shop has always had great energy, and I am so glad we did it.

People sometimes ask me what is the key to my success – that's easy. You have to be passionate about what you do, and you have to be prepared to work hard. That's why there's a lot to be said for being entrepreneurial when you're young, and you think you can conquer the world – that anything's possible, that your ideas are bigger and better than anyone else's.

I was always very impatient to succeed. It used to annoy me to hear people talk about doing things, instead of just doing them. I always thought 'You don't need to tell the world. Just go out and do it. If you fail, you fail, but at least you will have learnt something.'

To succeed in the long term, you need both ability and staying power. In my business, that means working long hours a lot of the time – we often work twenty-hour days when we're doing a show. No matter how many people there are in the team, there's a lot of camaraderie, especially when you're eating pizza together at three in the morning.

Attention to detail is important, too, especially in the fashion industry. I was sometimes criticised in my early days for being too controlling, but it's not about that. People talk about 'the big picture' but that's the easy part. It's the detail, the under-the-microscope analysis, that is crucial. 'Big picture' is just an idea, and it doesn't work long-term if you don't have a quality product that provides value for money.

Creating the right work environment is important too. Working with other creative people is what keeps me going – if I am in a non-creative environment I get tired and bored. Whereas, if I am stimulated, if someone comes up with a new idea, it's like a shot of adrenaline, or a glass of champagne that keeps me going just when I think I'm about to collapse with exhaustion.

When I started out in the nineties there was a recession, and I think there are a lot of opportunities during tough times for new businesses, with good deals on leases and other benefits. I felt there was gap in the market for the kind of lingerie and dresses I was passionate about. People recognise my signature now; it comes through (I hope) in every collection. It is absolutely essential to stay true to yourself – I work hard at that. It becomes more difficult as your business grows, but as you employ new people you need to teach them what your signature is, and make sure they stay 'on brand' at all times. It's a bit of a balancing act, because in fashion you want everyone to

---

Opposite: With Hunter Desmond David
Dinnigan-Cocks, born in November 2012.

Above: Hunter and his dad.

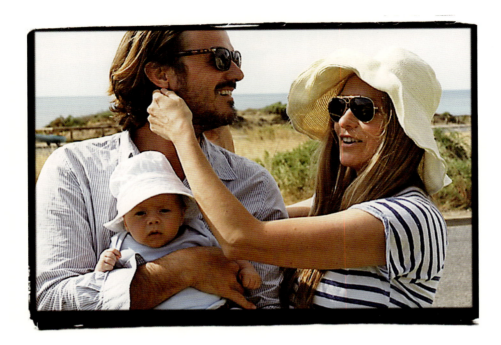

add their own personality so that you have that freshness, that new eye, but, at the same time, you must always be sure to keep the signature.

If I was to start a new business now, I would definitely team up with someone experienced in running a business, who could deal with the accounts, the staff and the human resources issues. Other than a short course I did in business organisation in New Zealand, I had no business experience to speak of – I have just learnt on the job. Over the years I have collected some trustworthy friends who have been great sounding boards for me – people like fashion luminary Peter Weiss.

Something else I am asked about is the impact on my life of having Estella (in 2004) and Hunter (in 2012). Becoming a mother changes you forever – you learn very quickly to be less selfish and impulsive, and much more organised. You also have to be on time, you can't be late, so you're always in a hurry. Balancing your work life with your home life is a bit like running a military operation, as any mother who works outside the home will tell you.

Since Estella was born, the business has grown more quickly than I anticipated – I have created my diffusion range, Collette by Collette Dinnigan, and also the bridal collection. Sometimes I forget how much work is involved in each new project. You get so much out of having children though; I wouldn't change a thing. The house is always filled with fun and laughter, and sometimes tears, and it's all about unconditional love. Being a mother, now for a second time, has certainly changed me – with everything I do now I think about how it will affect our family of four.

I suspect that being a mum this time with Hunter will be easier than it was the first time round. Shortly before Estella was born, I split up with her father, so I was a single mother. Although I did have a nanny to look after her while I was at work, when I wasn't at work I had very little support – it was just Estella and me, plus some good friends, so I was going from one full-time job to another, which was quite exhausting, physically and emotionally.

This time I have a loving partner, who is caring and nurturing with me, Hunter and Estella. From a practical point of view, it is nice just to have someone there to hold the baby, or to mind him if I need to go out for a short time. I don't know how much will change around the house. I don't think I could be any more organised with my time than I am already.

Before I had Estella, I wasn't at all maternal – my business was my baby. There was so much going on, and I was so stimulated by my travels, and the people I was meeting, that I never really stopped to consider whether I wanted a child. But once I had Estella, I wondered why I had left it so long, and I certainly hoped to have more children. I feel so incredibly blessed that Bradley and I have been able to have a child together at my age, because we tried for many years.

I guess you could say that before I had children my nurturing instinct was fully satisfied by growing my business, but now it is directed towards my family. That said, there are still business opportunities out there for me that I would like to take up, if the planets are aligned . . .

Above: At Port Willunga, South Australia, with
Bradley and baby Hunter, in January 2013.

Opposite: Our family, 2013.

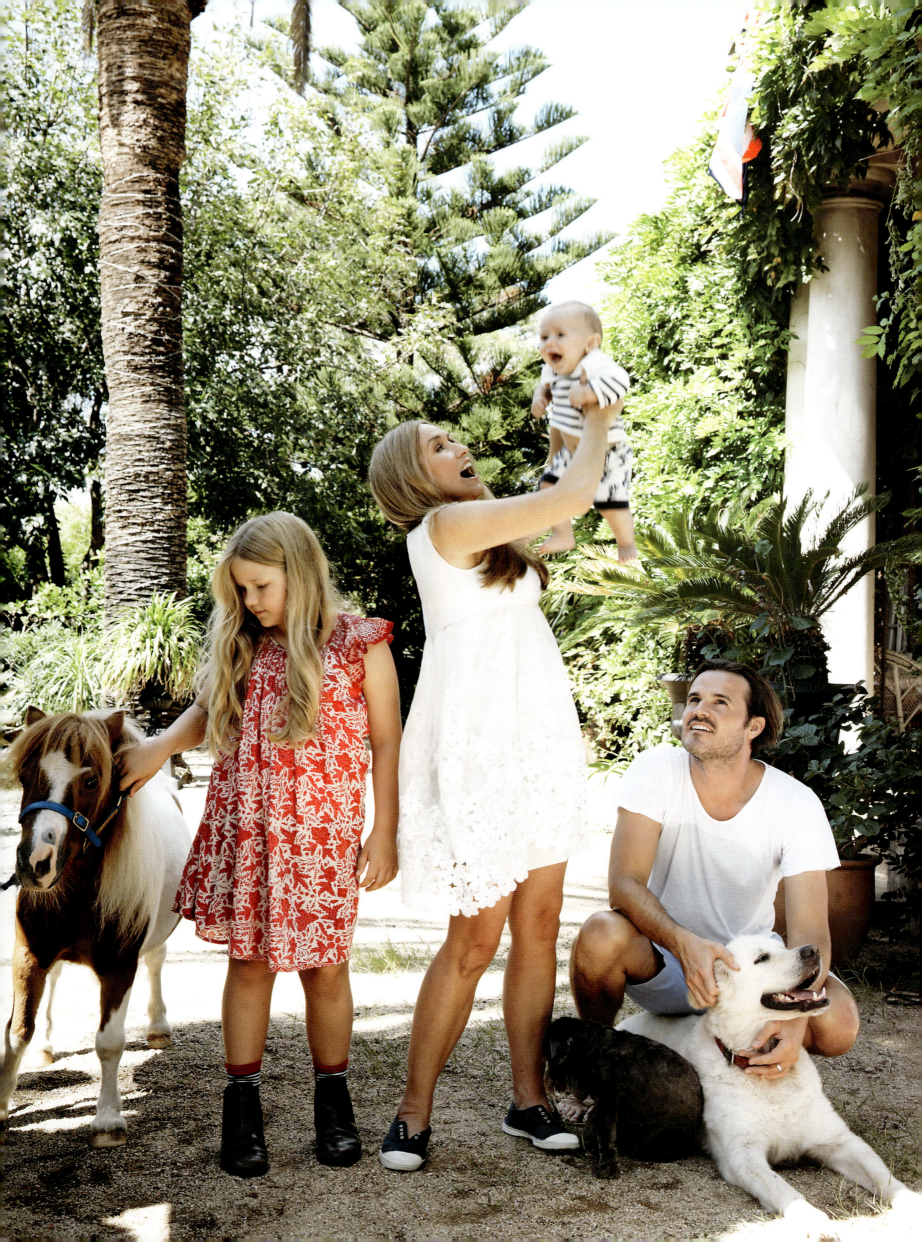

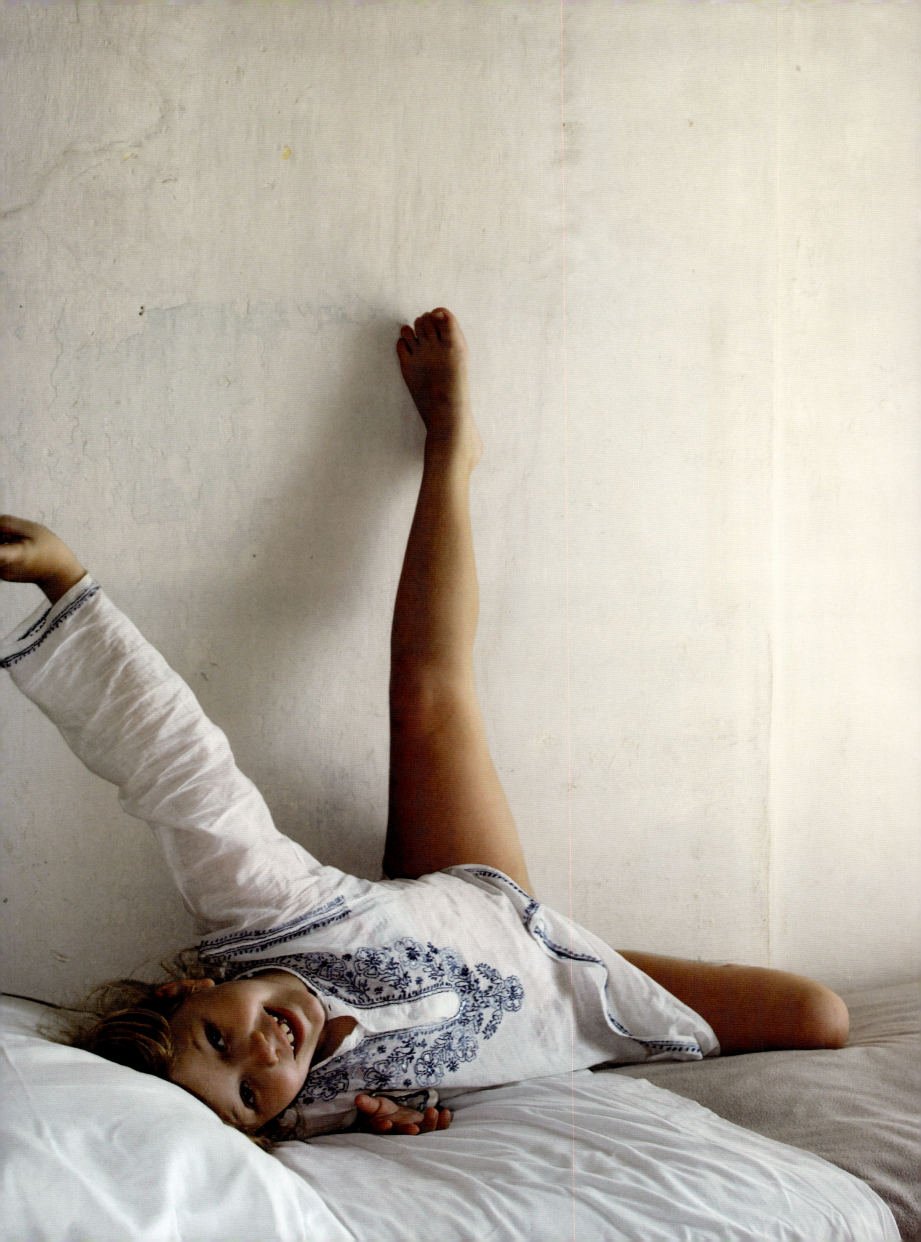

Acknowledgements

Thank you to my mother; such an inspiring woman, whom I loved so very much – I only wish she could have been here to know Estella and Hunter; to my father, whose courage and sense of adventure gave us such a unique upbringing; to my brother Seamus, whose eye for the look and feel of everything never goes unnoticed; to my husband, Bradley, for being my rock, and a great dad to both Estella and Hunter; to Estella and Hunter, you are my world; and to our dear cousin, Michele Brown, thank you for always being there.

A big thank you to Peter Weiss, whom I adore, and who still has the industry running through his veins.

Thank you to all of the Collette Dinnigan team, from the first people I employed, Sandy Parker and Paqui Cruz, to the team I have working with me now. You have all contributed significantly to the success of the brand. A special thank you to Seamus Dinnigan and Pip Dickson, who have spent many hours tracking down and obtaining approvals from all of the photographers whose work appears in this book.

Thank you also to Jamie Gordon, who helped with the opening of our London store and also worked closely with me on the creation of my logo.

Thank you to Nikki Andrews, who has been a great support, in the past as my Public Relations person, but also as a good friend and godmother to Estella.

A heartfelt thank you to the many editors, fashion directors and assistants from fashion publications all over the world for the support and encouragement you have given me from the word go. A special thank you to Alison Veness for helping me to get this project off the ground – I am so grateful.

Thank you also to the extremely talented stylists, hair stylists and makeup artists who have worked with me over the years.

Thank you to all of the photographers and artists who have made such a significant contribution to this book. Thank you also to the magazine staff, syndication departments, agents, friends and detectives who have helped with the enormous task of researching and compiling this archive of my work.

On the home front, thank you to my physiotherapist, Jo Key, and to my doctor, Bronwyn Gould, who are both amazing in helping me to deal with any health crisis, no matter how last-minute. Thank you also to the people who have given me the most wonderful help and support at home: Liz, Denise, Louisa, Sharon and Irene. Thank you to all of you for being so present and for coping with such a crazy schedule, always.

Finally, thank you to the amazing Penguin team: Publishing Director Julie Gibbs, for her wonderful energy and for believing in me, Designer Arielle Gamble for great design, Editor Nicole Abadee for her words, Publishing Manager Katrina O'Brien, Art Director Daniel New for his work on the cover, Production Controller Tracey Jarrett, Publishing Assistant Charlotte Bachali, design interns Clare O'Flynn and Jesse Chick and proofreader Carla Grossetti.

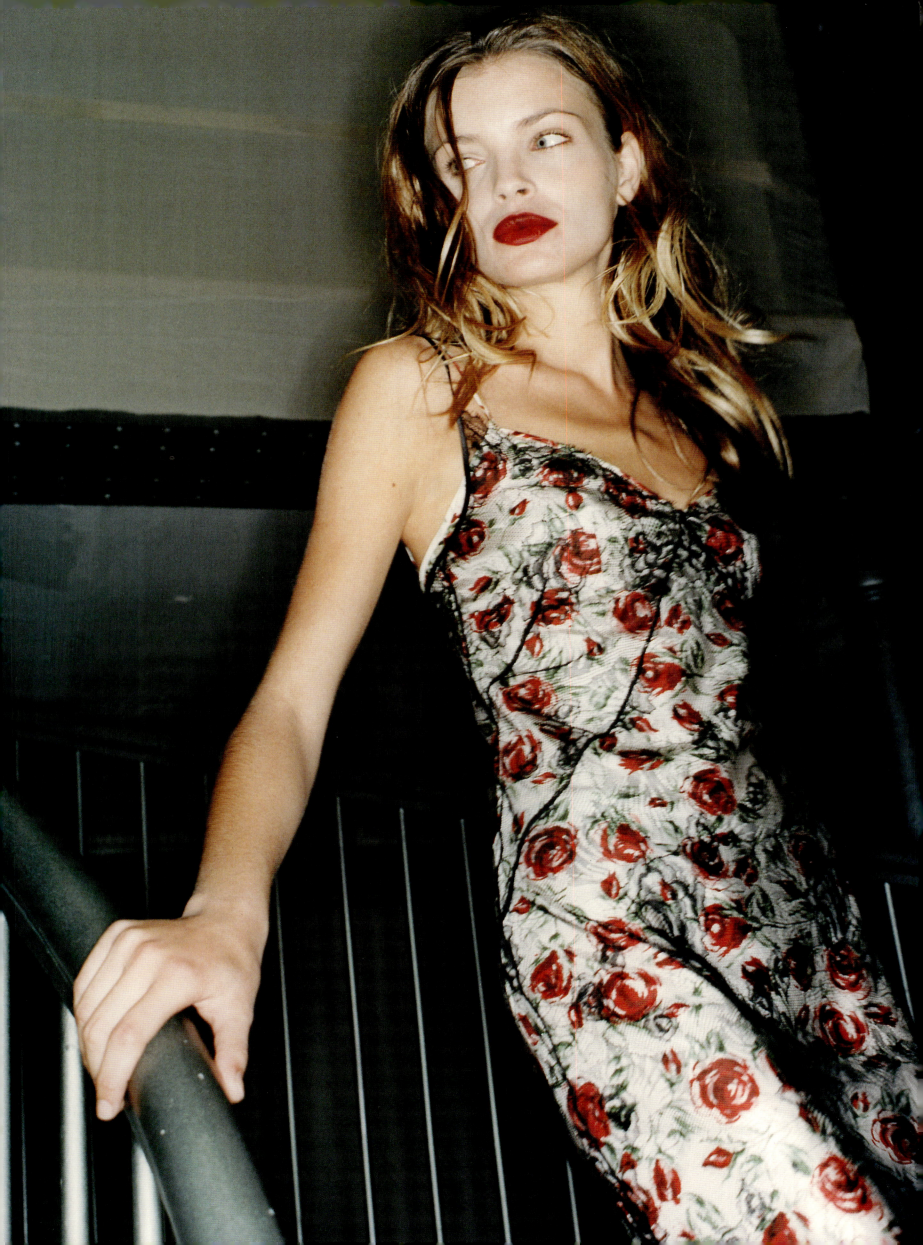

INDEX

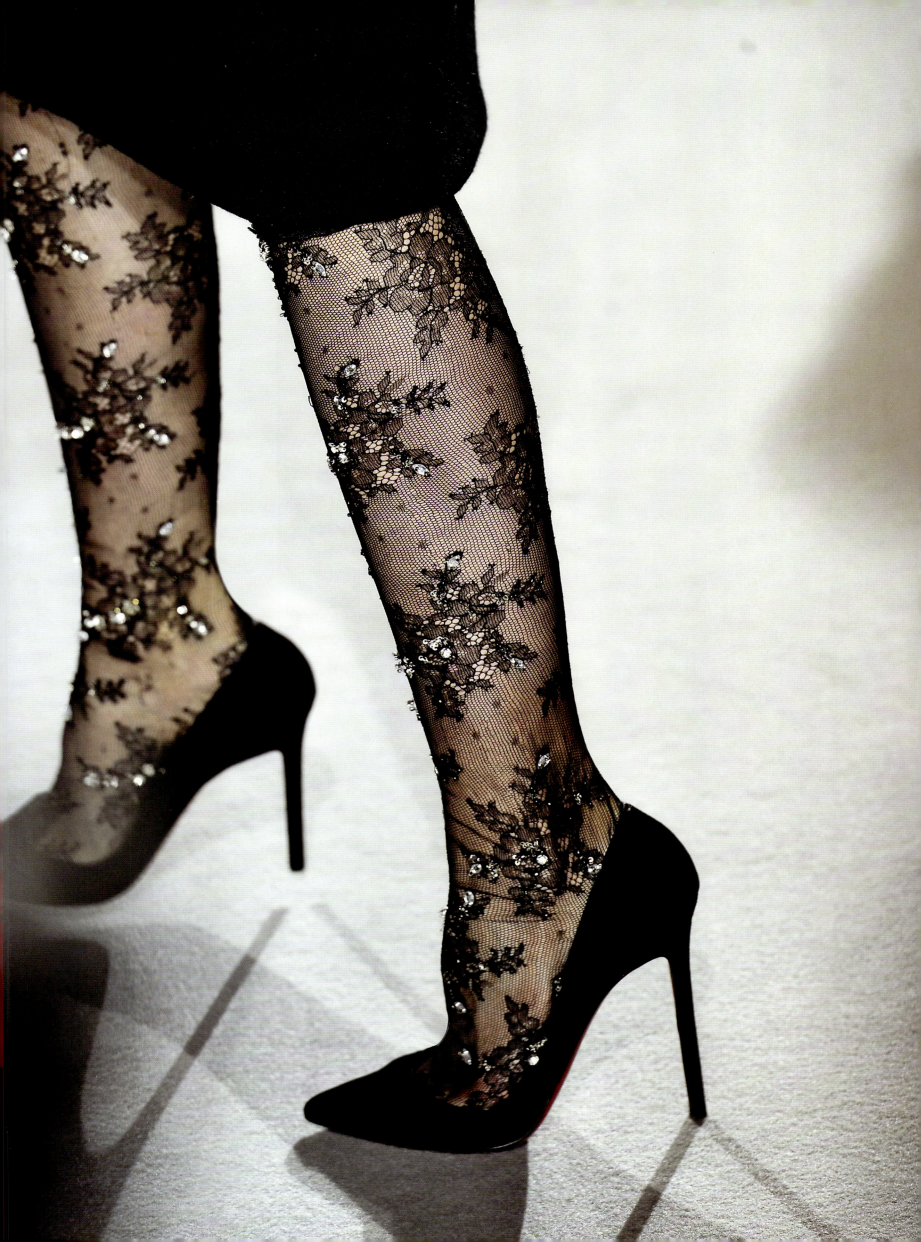

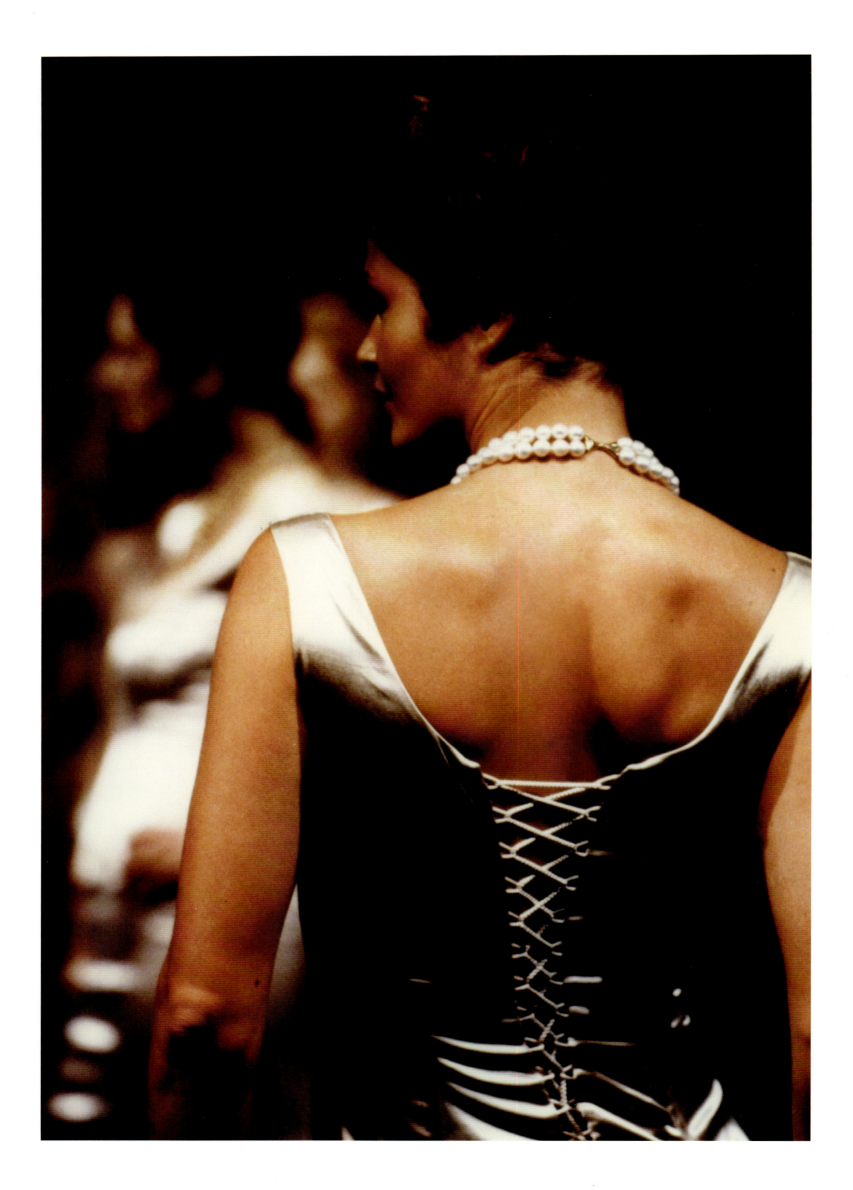

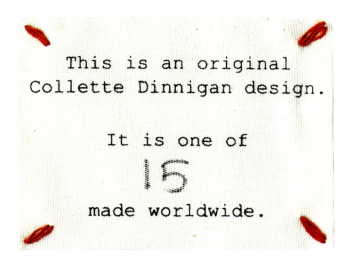

This is an original
Collette Dinnigan design.

It is one of

16

made worldwide.

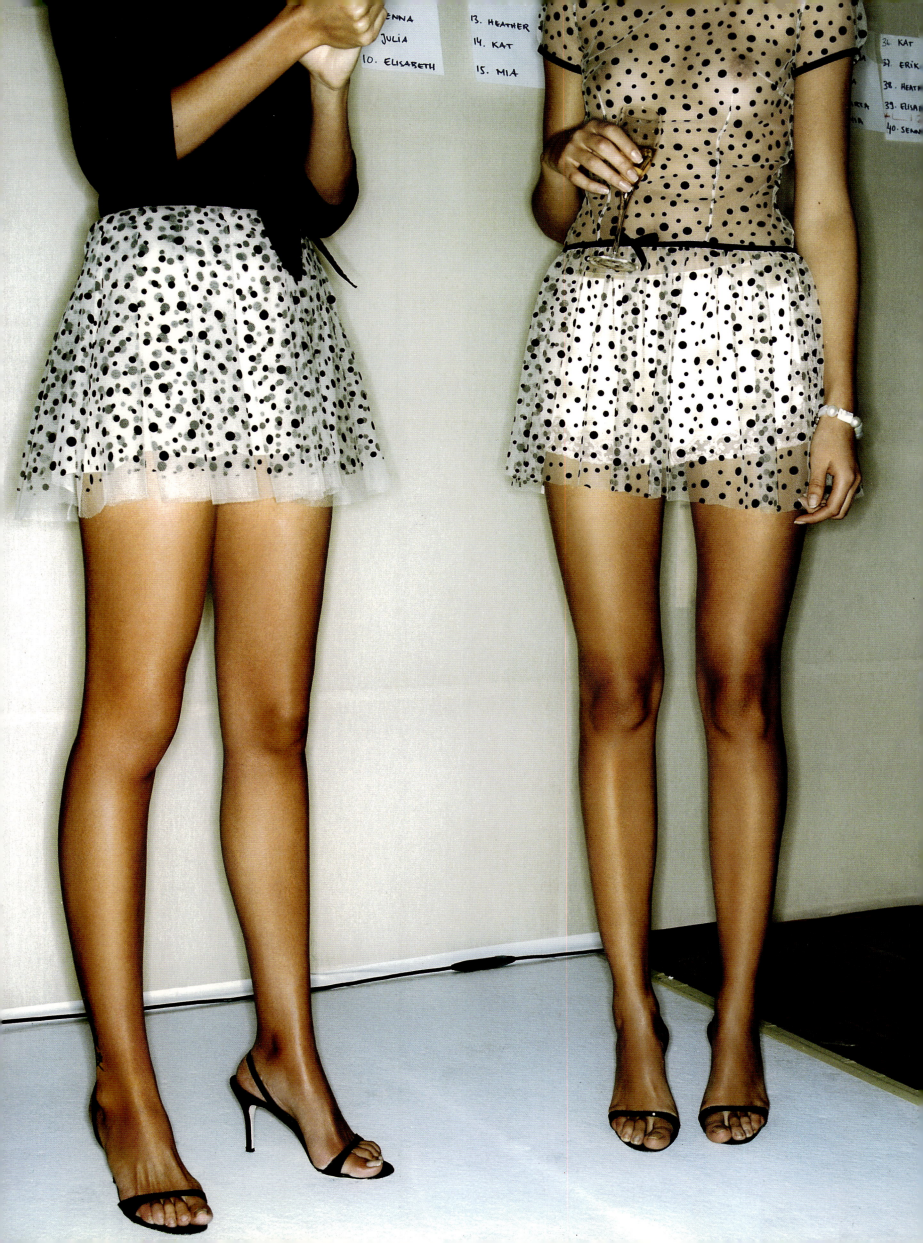

ENNA   13. HEATHER
   JULIA   14. KAT
10. ELISABETH   15. MIA

                                    34. KAT
                                    37. ERIK
                                    38. HEATH
                                    39. ELISA
                                    40. SEMON

CREDITS

Every effort has been made to contact all copyright owners prior to publication of
Obsessive Creative, to ensure that their contribution is properly acknowledged. Where we have
been unable, despite our best endeavours, to make contact we would welcome hearing from
anyone concerned, so that we may include an appropriate acknowledgement in any reprints.

Page 103: Photograph © Victor Demarchelier, published by *Harper's Bazaar*.

Pages 104–105: Photograph © David Mandelberg, published by *Harper's Bazaar*.

Page 106: All cover layouts reproduced with the kind permission of each publication: Sarah Murdoch *Condé Nast Traveller* (UK) photograph © The Condé Nast Publications Ltd; Rose Byrne *Vogue Australia* photograph © Richard Bailey; *Sydney Morning Herald Good Living Fashion* © Fairfax Syndication; Collette Dinnigan *Uno* photograph © Petrina Tinslay; *The Australian* photograph © Michelle Holden; Kylie Minogue *Cosmopolitan* photograph © Steve Shaw; Helena Christensen *Autore* photograph © Ellen von Unwerth; *Harper's Bazaar* illustration © Kerrie Hess / www.kerriehess.com; Rachel Hunter *Evening Standard Magazine* UK photograph © Sean McMenomy; Cindy Crawford *The Sunday Telegraph Sunday Magazine* photograph © Simon Upton.

Page 107: All cover layouts reproduced with the kind permission of each publication: Miranda Kerr *Harper's Bazaar* photograph © Simon Lekias; Sarah Murdoch and Collette Dinnigan *Vogue Australia* photograph © Alex Zotos; Nicole Kidman *Optimum* photograph © Albert Sanchez; Sarah Murdoch *Who Weekly* photograph © Jez Smith; Zhang Ziyi *Time Out London* photograph © Barry J Holmes; Sarah Wynter *Harper's Bazaar* photograph © Mark Liddell; *Elle Australia* photograph © Grey Zisser; *Cleo* photograph © Patric Shaw; Nicole Kidman and Robbie Williams *Hello* magazine still from video clip © Universal Music; Sarah Murdoch *Vogue Australia* photograph © Graham Shearer.

Page 108: Photograph © Patrick McMullan.

Page 111: Photograph published in *Harper's Bazaar Australia* May 2003.

Page 112: Photograph © Richard Bailey, published by *Vogue Australia*.

Page 114: Photograph on left © Jim Smeal / BEI / Rex Features; photograph in centre © Sam Levy / WireImage; photograph on right © Stewart Cook / Rex Features.

Page 115: Photograph © Chris Polk / FilmMagic.

Pages 116–117: Photograph © Marko Greitschus / Agency People Image.

Page 118: Photograph © Aller Media AS / Rex Features.

Page 119: Photograph © John Stillwell/PA Archive/Press Association Images.

Page 120: Top row from left: Charlize Theron photograph © Mark Mainz / Getty Images; Sandra Oh photograph © Frazer Harrison / Getty Images; Kate Bosworth photograph © Patrick Riviere. Second row from left: Naomi Watts photograph © AAP Image / Mick Tsikas; Emilie de Ravin photograph © Jim Smeal / BEI / Rex Features; Rachel McAdams © Jens Hartmann / Rex Features. Third row from left: Olga Kurylenko photograph © Paul Lovelace / Rex Features; Angelina Jolie © Jon Furniss / Getty Images; Emily Blunt photograph © MJ Kim / Getty Images. Bottom row from left, Taylor Swift photograph © Jason Merritt / Getty Images; Elizabeth Debicki photograph © Lisa Maree Williams / Getty Images; Ariel Winter photograph © Donato Sardella / WireImage.

Page 121: Top row from left: Elle Macpherson photograph © Richard Young / Rex Features; Pink © John Stanton / Wire Image; Jennifer Lopez photograph © Splash News. Second row from left: Julianne Hough photograph © Lester Cohen / WireImage; Kylie Minogue photograph © Dave Benett / Getty Images; Claudia Schiffer photograph © Anthony Harvey / Getty Images. Third row from left: Stacy Keibler photograph © Kevin Mazur / AMA2012 / WireImage; Kate Hudson photograph © Andrew Meares / Fairfax Syndication; Cindy Crawford photograph © Evan Agostini / Liaison. Bottom row from left: Isobel Lucas photograph © The Image Gate / Getty Images; Charlize Theron photograph © Paul McConnell / Getty Images; Rachel Bilson photograph © Jon Kopaloff / FilmMagic.

Page 122: Photograph © Jun Sato / WireImage.

Page 123: Photograph © SGranitz / WireImage.

Pages 124–125: Photograph © AAP Image / Tracey Nearmy.

Page 126: Photograph © Gerald Jenkins, published by *Australian Style*.

Page 129: Photograph © Carlotta Moye, published by *Cleo*, model Chloë Maxwell.

Page 130: Photograph © Gavin Bond, published by *Vogue*.

Page 131: Illustration © James Gordon.

Pages 132–133: Photograph © Sally Tsoutas.

Page 134: Photograph by Lucas Allen, © Australia Post.

Page 135: Photographs © Grant Matthews, published by *Vogue Australia*.

Page 136: Collette Dinnigan's private collection.

Page 137: All photographs © Sally Tsoutas, except detail of model with hands on chin and detail of model with gold face © Gerald Jenkins.

Page 138: Photograph © Simon Upton, published by *Harper's Bazaar*.

Page 139: Photograph © David Rosendale.

Page 140: Photograph courtesy of Gina Boon.

Page 141: Photograph © Earl Carter, published by *Harper's Bazaar*.

Page 142: Photograph reproduced with the kind permission of Qantas.

Page 143: Photograph © Alex Zotos.

Pages 144, 147, 148, 150–151, 152–3, 154–155, 156–7, 158–9, 160–161, 162, 163, 164–5, 166–167 (Estella at Piha beach, NZ): Photographs from Collette Dinnigan's private collection; illustrations by Clare O'Flynn and Arielle Gamble, © Penguin Group (Australia).

Page 157: Painting behind Estella in central photo by Rosie Snell – detail from 'Sea of Planes'.

Page 166: Calligraphy © Sabine Pick.

Page 168: Photograph © Hugh Stewart; painting by Tim Maguire.

Page 171: Collette Dinnigan's private collection.

Page 172: Photograph © Earl Carter, published by *Maison Magazine*.

Page 174: Photograph © Brent Young.

Page 175: Photograph © Earl Carter, published by *Maison Magazine*.

Page 176: Photograph © Geoff Lung, published by *Elle Décor*.

Page 177: Collette Dinnigan's private collection.

Page 178: Collette Dinnigan's private collection.

Page 179: Photograph © Hugh Stewart; painting by Paul Haggith.

Pages 180, 181, 182: Collette Dinnigan's private collection.

Page 183: Photograph © Petrina Tinslay.

Pages 184, 187, 188: Photographs © David Loftus.

Pages 190–191: All photographs from Collette Dinnigan's private collection except: top row from left second, third and fifth photographs; central photograph; second photograph from top in right column; and first photograph in bottom row © David Loftus.

Pages 192, 193: Photographs © David Loftus.

Page 194: Photograph © Stephen Ward, published by *Marie Claire Australia*.

Page 195: Photograph © Georges Antoni, published by *Harper's Bazaar*; model Émilie Cozette for Paris Opera Ballet.

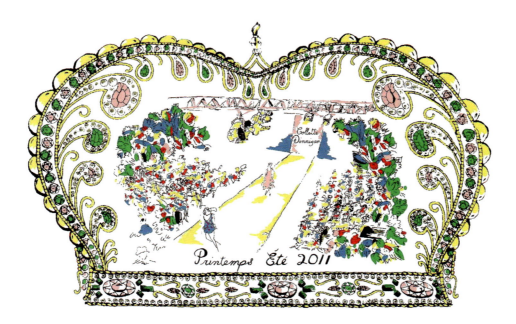

Page 196: Photograph Hugh Stewart; © Lachlan and Sarah Murdoch.

Page 197: Photograph Hugh Stewart; © Lachlan and Sarah Murdoch.

Page 198: Photograph © Lisa Tomasetti.

Page 199: Photograph Nick Haddow; © James and Erica Packer.

Pages 200–201: Mary Coustas photograph © Chris Makridis of Reid Studios; Lillian Cochrane photograph © welovepictures; Alex Gordon photograph © Janie Stevenson; Cara Jolson photograph © Tania Jovanovic; Fiona Seres photograph © Megan Seres; Nicky Oatley photographs © Liz Ham; Sarah Canet photograph © Sophie Lindsay; Tory Collison photograph © Brendan Read; Sarah Hills photograph © Tertius Pickard / New Idea; Lara Feltham photograph © Luke Feltham; Edwina McCann photograph © Hugh Stewart.

Page 202: Photograph © Sally Flegg, published by *Harper's Bazaar Brides*.

Page 203: Photograph © Cameron Bloom.

Page 204: Photograph © Gavin Bond; layout © *Vogue Australia*.

Page 207: Photograph © Seamus Dinnigan.

Pages 208–209, 210: Photographs © Gavin Bond.

Page 211: Photograph © Philip Castle.

Page 212, 213: Photographs © Frédéric Dumoulin.

Page 214: Photograph © Philip Castle.

Page 215: Photograph © Jason Lloyd-Evans.

Pages 216: All photographs © Eddy Ming, published by and layout © *Harper's Bazaar* except for bottom row, two photographs from Collette Dinnigan's private collection.

217: Top photograph © Eddy Ming; bottom row, four photographs © Frédéric Dumoulin.

Page 218: Illustration © Stewart Walton; photograph © Philip Castle.

Page 219: All photographs from Collette Dinnigan's private collection, except second row, first photograph; third row photograph; fourth row, second photograph © Philip Castle and fourth photograph © Gavin Bond.

Page 220: Photographs © Chris Moore; calligraphy © Sabine Pick.

Page 221: Photographs © David Loftus.

Pages 222–223: All photographs from Collette Dinnigan's private collection except top row, sixth photograph of Michael Hutchence and Paula Yates © Philip Castle.

Pages 224–225: Photograph © Philip Castle.

Page 226: Illustration © Stewart Walton.

Page 227: Photograph © Pascal Dolemieux.

Pages 228–229: Central photograph © David Loftus; 'In the spotlight' © Philip Castle; top left photograph © Gavin Bond; top right photograph © Brett Faulkner / Newspix; all other photographs from Collette Dinnigan's private collection.

Pages 230–231: Illustrations © Stewart Walton; left photograph © Dominique Maitre; right photograph © Shane Woodward.

Pages 232–233: Photograph © Philip Castle, model far right Laetitia Casta.

Page 234: Top photograph © Piero Biasion; bottom photographs from Collette Dinnigan's private collection.

Page 235: Central photograph © David Loftus; with Cate Blanchett © Jon Reid / AAP Image; with Elle Macpherson and Hugh Grant © Richard Young / Rex Features; all other photographs from Collette Dinnigan's private collection.

Pages 236–237: Photograph by © Philip Castle.

Pages 238: Photograph © Hugh Stewart.

Page 241: Photographs © Hugh Stewart, published by *Marie Claire*.

Page 242: Artwork Damien Hirst, Untitled, 2000, Butterflies and household gloss on canvas, 2140 x 2140 mm © Damien Hirst and Science Ltd. All rights reserved, DACS Licensed by Viscopy, 2013. Photograph from Collette Dinnigan's private collection.

Page 243: Collette Dinnigan's private collection.

Page 244: Photograph © Mike Flokis / Getty Images.

Page 245: Photograph © Justin Edward John Smith.

Page 246: Photograph © Hugh Stewart.

Pages 247, 248: Collette Dinnigan's private collection.

Page 249: Photograph © Hugh Stewart.

Page 250: Collette Dinnigan's private collection.

Page 252: Photograph © Gavin Bond.

Page 255: Photograph © Piero Biasion.

Page 256: Photograph © Sally Tsoutas.

Page 258: Photograph © Gavin Bond.

Page 261: Runway illustration inside crown border © Stewart Walton.

Page 262-5: Photograph © Philip Castle.

Endpapers: All illustrations © Nina Fuga, except for inside front endpaper illustration of girl and chandelier © Kat Macleod.

Front and back cover illustrations by Daniel New © Penguin Group (Australia).

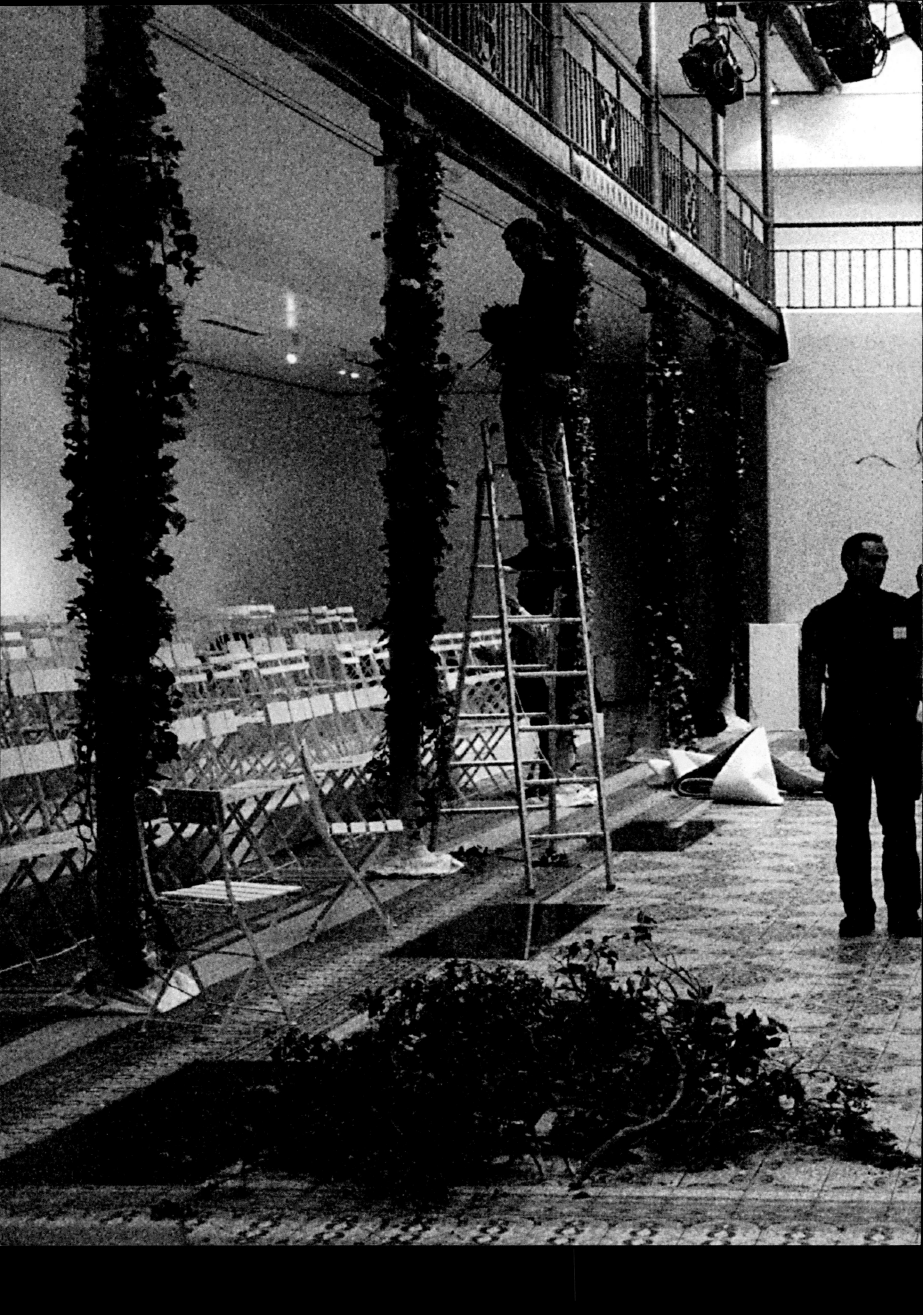

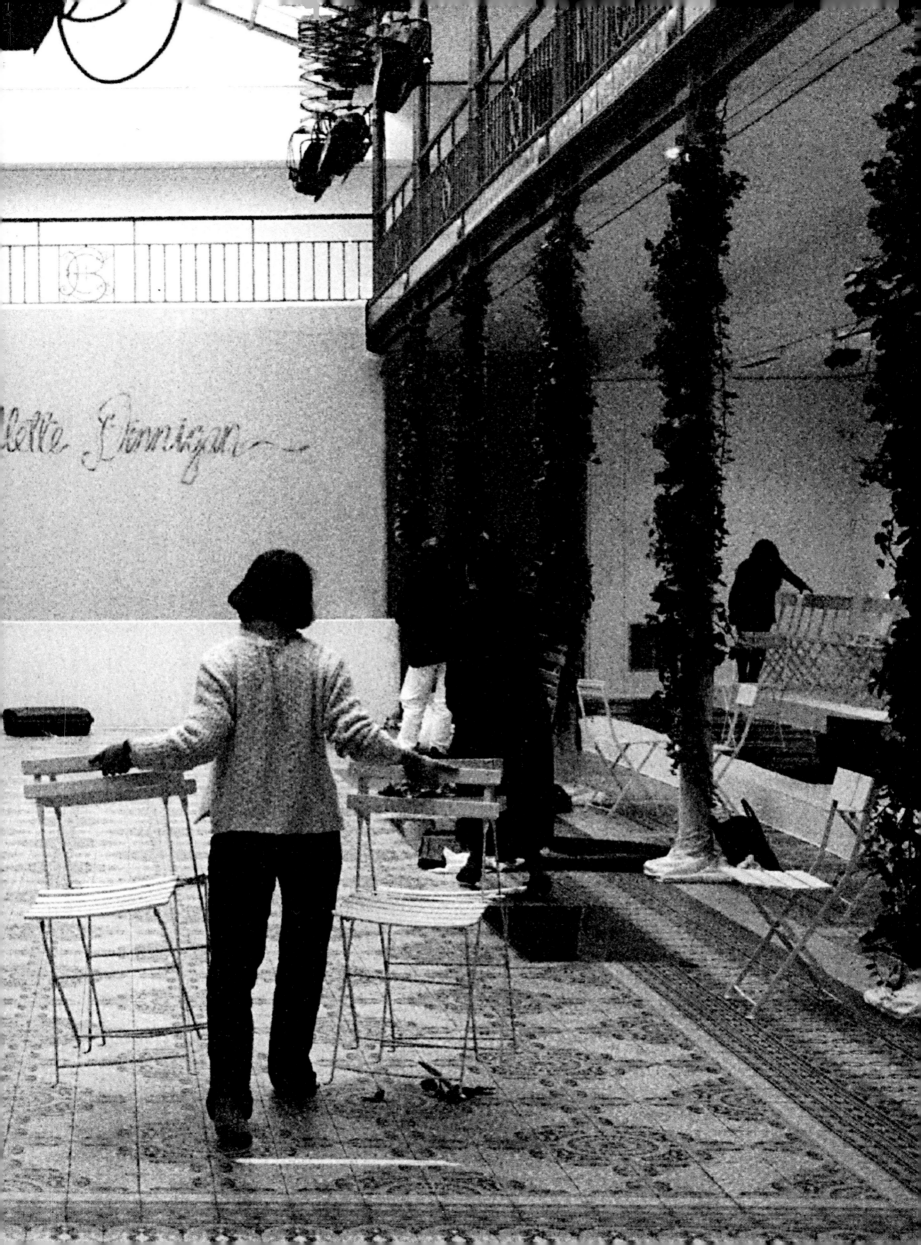

OBSESSIVE CREATIVE

HarperCollins books may be purchased for educational, business, or sales promotional use. For information please e-mail the Special Markets Department at SPsales@harpercollins.com.

First published in 2013 by Lantern, an imprint of Penguin Group (Australia).

First U.S. edition published in 2014
by Harper Design
An Imprint of HarperCollins *Publishers*
10 East 53rd Street
New York, NY 10022
Tel: (212) 207-7000
Fax: (212) 207-7654
www.harpercollinspublishers.com
harperdesign@harpercollins.com

This edition distributed by
HarperCollins *Publishers*
10 East 53rd Street
New York, NY 10022

ISBN 978-0-06-233712-2

Library of Congress Control Number: 201395341

Book design by Arielle Gamble © Penguin Group (Australia)
Cover illustrations by Daniel New © Penguin Group (Australia)
   inspired by photographs by Ellen von Unwerth of Helena Christensen
Endpaper illustrations © Nina Fuga, except for inside front endpaper
Illustration of girl and chandelier © Kat Macleod

Printed in Singapore

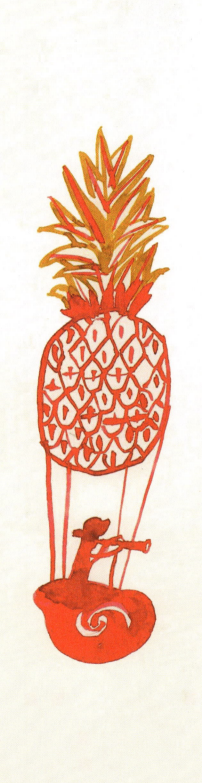

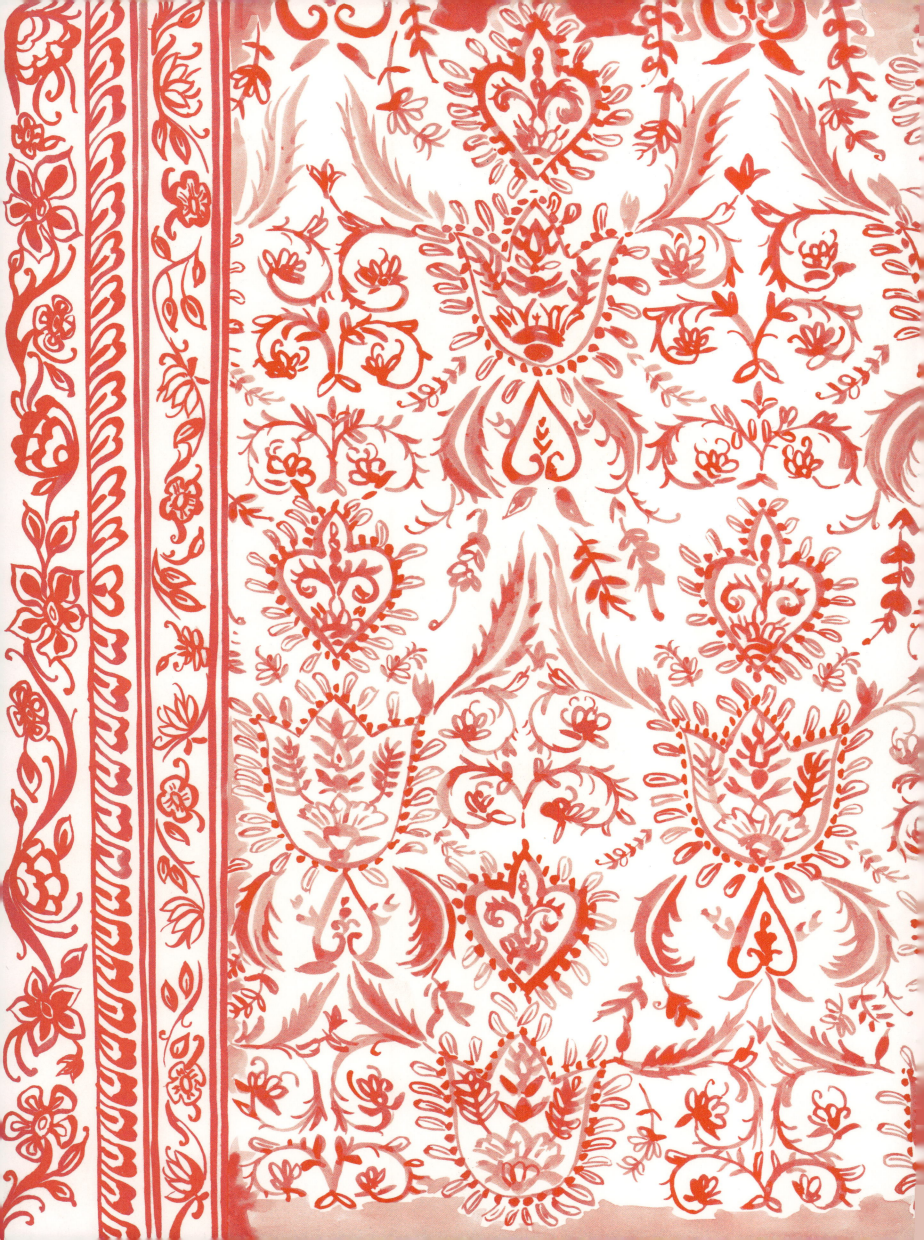